Reconstructive Foot and Ankle Surgery

Reconstructive Foot and Ankle Surgery

Mark S. Myerson, MD

Director, Institute for Foot and Ankle Reconstruction at Mercy
Mercy Medical Center
Baltimore, Maryland

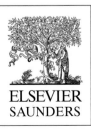

ELSEVIER
SAUNDERS

An Imprint of Elsevier

ELSEVIER
SAUNDERS

1600 John F. Kennedy Blvd.
Ste. 1800
Philadelphia, Pennsylvania 19103-2899

RECONSTRUCTIVE FOOT AND ANKLE SURGERY
Copyright © 2005, Elsevier Inc.

Notice

Surgery is an ever-changing field. Standard safety precautions must be followed, but as new research and clinical experience broaden our knowledge, changes in treatment and drug therapy may become necessary or appropriate. Neither the Publisher nor the Author assumes any responsibility for any loss or injury and/or damage to persons or property arising out of or related to any use of the material contained in this book. It is the responsibility of the treating practitioner, relying on independent expertise and knowledge of the patient, to determine the best treatment and method of application for the patient.

Library of Congress Cataloging-in-Publication Data

Myerson, Mark.
 Reconstructive foot and ankle surgery / Mark Myerson.—1st ed.
  p. ; cm.
  ISBN-13: 978–1–4160–2358–6   ISBN-10: 1–4160–2358–5
  1. Foot—Diseases—Surgery. 2. Ankle—Diseases—Surgery. 3.
 Foot—Abnormalities—Surgery. 4. Ankle—Abnormalities—Surgery. I. Title.
 RD563.M96 2005
 617.5'85059—dc22   2004065003

Acquisitions Editor: Elyse O'Grady
Developmental Editor: Janice Gaillard
Publishing Services Manager: Joan Sinclair
Project Manager: Mary Stermel
Designer: Steve Stave

ISBN-13: 978–1–4160–2358–6
ISBN-10: 1–4160–2358–5

Printed in China

Last digit is the print number: 9   8   7   6   5   4   3   2

To my beloved family, this work could not have been possible without your sacrifice. You have my enduring love, affection, and gratitude.

Contents

Video Contents

The following chapters have companion video clips on DVD-ROM.

Ch. 1–1a Chevron Osteotomy
Ch. 1–1c The Modified Lapidus Procedure
Ch. 1–1e Proximal Phalangeal Osteotomy (Akin)
Ch. 1–2 Hallux Varus
Ch. 1–3 Hallux Rigidus
Ch. 2–1 Disorders of the Sesamoids
Ch. 3–1 Correction of Lesser Toe Deformity
Ch. 3–2 Metatarsalgia
Ch. 3–3 Management of the Bunionette
Ch. 4–1 Surgery for the Diabetic Foot and Ankle
Ch. 5–1 Cavus Foot Correction
Ch. 6–1 Correction of Paralytic Deformity
Ch. 7–1 Correction of Flatfoot Deformity in the Child
Ch. 7–2 Correction of Flatfoot Deformity in the Adult
Ch. 8–1 Nerve Entrapment Syndromes
Ch. 9–1 Total Ankle Replacement

Ch. 9–3 Ankle Osteoarticular Allograft Replacement
Ch. 9–4 Reconstruction of Malunited Ankle Fractures
Ch. 10–1 Disorders of the Achilles Tendon
Ch. 10–2 Rupture of the Anterior Tibial Tendon
Ch. 10–3 Peroneal Tendon Injury and Repair
Ch. 11–1 Tarsal Coalition
Ch. 12–1 Ankle Instability and Impingement
  Syndromes
Ch. 13–1 Arthrodesis of the Hallux
  Metatarsophalangeal Joint
Ch. 13–3 Subtalar Arthrodesis
Ch. 13–4 Triple Arthrodesis
Ch. 13–5 Ankle Arthrodesis
Ch. 13–6 Tibiocalcaneal and Tibiotalocalcaneal
  Arthrodesis
Ch. 14–1 The Rheumatoid Foot and Ankle

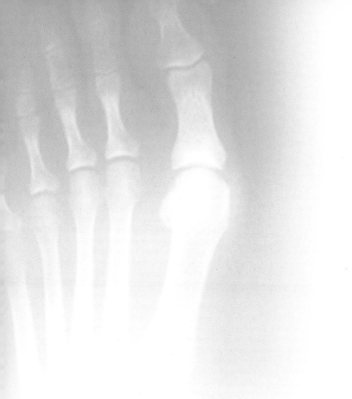

Preface

Ideas. Where do they come from? What is original thought, and what can or should be attributed to someone else? I cannot pretend to have created something novel in this textbook, and as I think about the past few decades of foot and ankle surgery, I am amazed that little of what we do has changed. Certainly, surgical approaches improve, but these are driven primarily by the technological advances that abound in our daily practice of medicine.

I have been blessed by those around me. To be an educator is a wonderful opportunity, perhaps a gift, but to be a teacher without continuing to learn is impossible. The ideas expressed in this book are therefore an amalgamation of thoughts and techniques that I have accrued from my mentors, colleagues, and fellows.

The following individuals have significantly influenced my thinking and work during the past 20 years. Melvin Jahss, with whom I completed my fellowship, taught me to question everything, to strive for intellectual honesty,

and not to accept what was written until I proved it for myself. Roger Mann, the "go-to" surgeon for many individuals, continues to set benchmarks as an educator that are worth emulating. Sigvaard Hansen taught and encouraged many to "think outside of the box" and to be innovative with surgical techniques.

To these individuals I owe my gratitude for setting the standards in foot and ankle surgery that are essential for our progress.

No work of this nature can be accomplished without assistance. I would like to thank my fellows, past and present, for their encouragement and enthusiasm for this project. In particular my sincere appreciation goes to my fellow, Dr. Naoki Haraguchi, who did a superb job with organizing and helping to edit the videos that accompany this book.

Mark S. Myerson, MD

Chevron Osteotomy

Indications

Chevron osteotomy is a procedure performed for correction of hallux valgus that is associated with a mild to moderate increase in the intermetatarsal angle. If there is any doubt as to the likelihood of this procedure "being enough," it is preferable to perform a distal soft tissue release. Some patients have a greater degree of hallux valgus than expected based upon the radiographic intermetatarsal angle. These patients usually have associated metatarsus adductus and should be treated with a chevron osteotomy (Fig. 1–1a–1).

The incidence of avascular necrosis of the metatarsal head does not increase when a soft tissue release is performed simultaneously with the osteotomy. The osteotomy can be performed in conjunction with a closing wedge osteotomy of the hallux proximal phalanx (Akin osteotomy) for patients in whom an abnormal distal metatarsal articular angle (DMAA) is present. It is preferable, however, to perform a biplanar chevron osteotomy if there is any doubt as to the congruency of the articulation with a closing wedge osteotomy (Fig. 1–1a–2). Although a lateral shift of 3 to 4 mm of the metatarsal head is usually performed, at least a 5-mm shift can be performed with careful internal fixation.

The Approach to a Standard Chevron Osteotomy

An incision is made medially at the junction of the dorsal and plantar skin, extending proximally for 3 cm from the flare just distal to the metatarsophalangeal joint. This incision is far safer and has more predictable results than a dorsally based approach, which endangers the nerve and is likely to cause an extension contracture. The incision is deepened through subcutaneous tissue. Care is taken to dissect the soft tissues carefully so that the terminal medial cutaneous branch of the superficial peroneal nerve is identified and then dorsally retracted (Fig. 1–1a–3a). It is easier to free the nerve with a hemostat, rather than with a knife or scissors.

I prefer to use an L-shaped capsular incision with the apex proximal and dorsal to the metatarsophalangeal joint. The dorsal limb is in line with the dorsal one third of the metatarsal head, and the vertical limb is level with the metatarsal neck. This incision can of course be varied, but the advantage of this capsular incision is the ability to tighten the hallux correctly after the osteotomy into both hallux varus and supination. Once the capsule is dissected off the medial eminence and medial aspect of the metatarsal head, the tibial sesamoid is visible. Inspection of the articular surface for cartilage defects or erosion is important (Fig. 1–1a–3b, c).

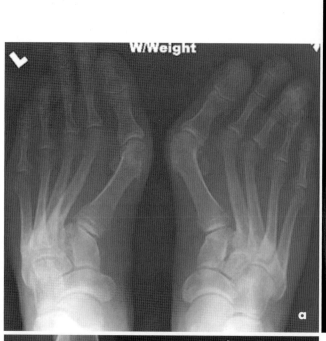

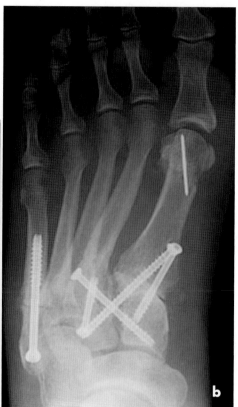

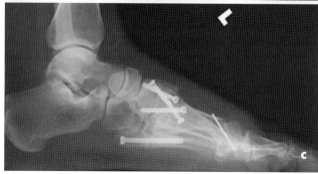

Figure 1–1a–1. *Although the deformity in this x-ray (XR) is severe, this is largely the result of metatarsus adductus, and a biplanar chevron osteotomy should be performed. There is no room to perform a proximal metatarsal osteotomy (a). The deformity has been corrected with a biplanar chevron osteotomy, and arthrodesis of the first and second tarsometatarsal (TMT) joints has been performed for correction of painful arthritis (b, c).*

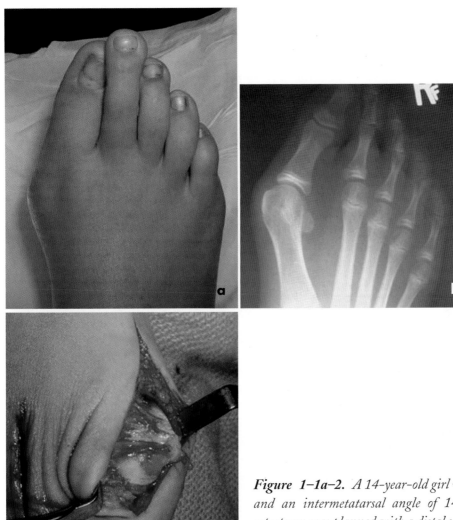

Figure 1–1a–2. *A 14-year-old girl with a hallux valgus angle of 30 degrees and an intermetatarsal angle of 14 degrees (a, b). A biplanar chevron osteotomy was planned with a distal soft tissue release. Note the severe increase in the distal metatarsal articular angle intraoperatively, which is not shown as prominently on x-ray (XR) film (b, c).*

The alignment of the first metatarsal is checked with respect to the medial eminence and the hallux, and the exostectomy is performed with a flexible chisel (Fig. 1–1a–3d). A saw blade can be used, but with a saw there is less control over the direction of the cut. The medial eminence must be cut from distal to proximal to create a smooth transition of the metatarsal head with the metaphyseal flare proximally. Avoid making the cut in the sagittal groove. Such a cut will be too lateral and will lead to the uncovering of the metatarsal head and medialization of the tibial sesamoid. This cut will lead to irritation of the sesamoid and will likely cause arthritis.

The osteotomy is planned with a cautery to mark the apex, approximately 8 mm proximal to the articular surface (Fig. 1–1a–3e). I prefer a standard cut at a 60-degree angle with the dorsal and plantar limbs of the osteotomy equidistant. Although alternative limbs of the osteotomy have been described, these offer no advantages, require more dissection, and are likely to cause more metatarsal shortening. For exposure of the dorsal surface of the metatarsal, the soft tissue is dissected dorsally with limited subperiosteal dissection. Visualizing the lateral metatarsal is unnecessary, and only the dorsal and medial aspect of the first metatarsal neck is exposed. Care should be taken not to strip any periosteum on the plantar or dorsal surface more proximal to the level of the osteotomy. A saw blade is used for the osteotomy and aligned perpendicular to the axis of the planned limbs of the osteotomy (Fig. 1–1a–3f).

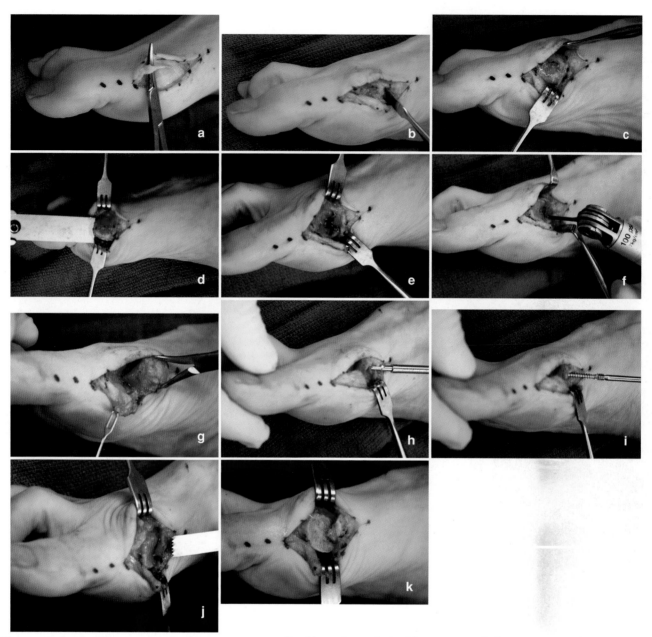

Figure 1–1a–3. *The steps in the chevron osteotomy. In this patient, the incision was marked out more distally to perform an additional phalangeal osteotomy. Following the incision, the dorsal medial cutaneous branch of the superficial peroneal nerve is identified and retracted (a). Subperiosteal dissection is performed only medially and dorsally along the metatarsal neck in the location of the plane of the osteotomy (b, c). The exostectomy is performed (d), and the osteotomy is marked with electrocautery (e). A fine, small saw blade is used to make the cut at a 60 degree angle (f). A small camp is used to grasp the metatarsal neck and the head is pushed laterally (g). A cannulated 3.0 mm headless screw (DePuy, Warsaw Ind.) is used over a guide pin and a double threaded countersink to prepare the hole and prevent splitting of the cortex (h, i). The medial overhanging ledge of bone is shaved (j) and the final appearance noted (k).*

Do *not* overperforate the soft tissues laterally, and make sure the saw blade penetrates the lateral cortex only. The metatarsal neck should be carefully held, preferably manually, because grasping with a clamp can fracture the metatarsal neck (Fig. 1–1a–3g). The metatarsal head undergoes a slight disimpaction, is retracted distally, and is then pushed over laterally. The head is now pushed laterally manually while the metatarsal shaft is held stable. This maneuver is slightly more difficult if a distal soft tissue release has been performed because the hallux and joint are effectively disarticulated. During this maneuver, the metatarsal head should not be rotated or tilted. The lateral metatarsal shift is ideally about 4 to 5 mm and should be checked radiographically. If an abnormal DMAA is present, then a biplanar chevron cut is planned with triangular jigs developed by Dr. E. Pepper Toomey (Fig. 1–1a–4). Although manually cutting a biplanar wedge is possible, it is not reliable. At

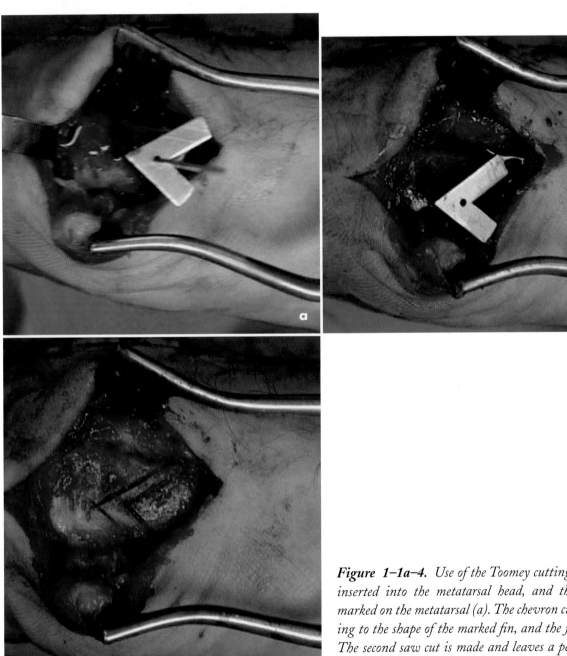

Figure 1–1a–4. *Use of the Toomey cutting jig. A K-wire is inserted into the metatarsal head, and the jig position is marked on the metatarsal (a). The chevron cut is made according to the shape of the marked fin, and the jig is inserted (b). The second saw cut is made and leaves a perfect wedge to be removed to correct the distal metatarsal articular angle (DMAA) (c).*

the completion of the first metatarsal osteotomy, the biplanar jig is inserted into the osteotomy cut, the saw is placed down on the side of jig itself, and the cut is then made against the surface of the jig. This procedure removes a perfectly formed 1-mm slice of the bone from both the dorsal and plantar limbs of the osteotomy medially.

Although the metatarsal head is often intrinsically stable, secure internal fixation is preferable, and I use a double-threaded screw (DePuy FRS screw system, Warsaw, Ind.). A guide pin is introduced at the medial border of the metatarsal just proximal to the osteotomy and checked radiographically. A drill/countersink is used to prevent fracture of the medial metatarsal neck (Fig. 1–1a–3h, i). The position of the pin is checked fluoroscopically; the length is determined; a screw, usually about 20 to 22 mm, is inserted across the guide pin; and compression is obtained. The medial overhanging bone from the osteotomy must be smoothed down with a saw by shaving or back cutting the bone (Fig. 1–1a–3j, k).

Two sutures of 2-0 Vicryl are inserted from the dorsal proximal aspect of the capsule into the plantar distal position to create an oblique suture, which pulls the hallux into slight supination and slight varus. Checking the range of motion of the hallux metatarsophalangeal joint after the capsular repair is important. If the hallux is pulled too far over medially or the range of motion is insufficient, the sutures must be removed and the repair performed again. I prefer to use absorbable sutures for skin closure, with 4-0 Vicryl for the subcutaneous tissue and interrupted 5-0 chromic sutures for skin. Radiographs are obtained following surgery at regular intervals until healing is noted (Fig. 1–1a–5).

Techniques, tips, and pitfalls

1. Even though chevron osteotomy is inherently a stable cut, internal fixation of the osteotomy is ideal, however, to prevent malunion. The technique that I have described with the double-threaded screw is reliable, stable, and allows early weight bearing and range of motion of the hallux.

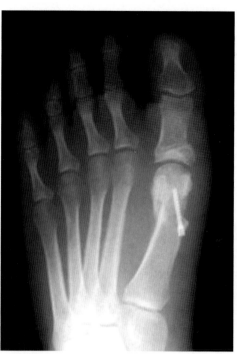

Figure 1–1a–5. Hallux correction after osteotomy. Note the addition of a closing wedge osteotomy of the proximal phalanx of the hallux (Akin osteotomy) in addition to the chevron osteotomy. Also note the slight valgus deformity of the lesser toes after correction of the hallux. I do not routinely correct these toe deformities because they are asymptomatic and over time will drift back into a more normal position.

2. Checking the position of the metatarsal head in relation to the metatarsal shaft intraoperatively is important. The metatarsal head tends to tilt either medially or laterally as impaction is performed. With either of these malpositions, the hallux tends to drift into valgus, although this is worse if any valgus impaction of the head is performed.

3. Occasionally, slight varus impaction of the metatarsal head is actually desirable to correct an abnormal DMAA. If this is deliberately performed, be careful that shortening of the metatarsal does not occur.

4. Shortening of the metatarsal may result if metaphyseal bone overlap occurs during impaction of the metatarsal head. With this shortening, transfer of weight-bearing pressure to the second metatarsal with metatarsalgia will occur.

5. Do not strip the periosteum laterally. The blood supply for the first metatarsal head enters dorsolaterally at the junction of the metatarsal neck. Avascular necrosis of the metatarsal head will not occur unless excessive periosteal stripping on the lateral aspect of the metatarsal neck is performed.

6. When exposing the dorsal surface of the metatarsal for the osteotomy, elevate the periosteum over the metatarsal where it is being cut only to insert a soft tissue retractor.

7. If intraoperative fracture of the medial edge of the distal metatarsal cortex occurs during screw insertion, either a K-wire or a suture around the fractured portion of the metatarsal can be used. A suture applied around the metatarsal is ideal, provided this does not cause any further periosteal stripping.

8. I have not found that a variation of the osteotomy cut, with a long dorsal limb, is of any advantage over the standard 60-degree cut. Although this long dorsal limb theoretically facilitates the insertion of a dorsal to plantar screw, it involves further periosteal stripping, particularly if the incision is made medially.

9. Although a dorsal incision has been described for use in a chevron osteotomy and other first metatarsal osteotomies, I would caution against its use. Frequently, this incision is associated with dorsal soft tissue contracture, which limits plantar flexion of the metatarsophalangeal joint. Furthermore, the dorsal incision places the dorsomedial cutaneous branch of the superficial peroneal nerve at risk, and scar neuroma formation is more common.

10. Correction of hallux valgus associated with any spasticity requires an arthrodesis of the MP joint. Despite healthy articular cartilage, an osteotomy for mild deformity should not be performed. Recurrence following osteotomy for hallux valgus correction in the setting of spasticity of any kind is very high.

11. Rarely, following the chevron osteotomy, instability of the first metatarsal is present, which leads to recurrent deformity. This can be corrected with a distal suture between the first and second metatarsals or with a lag type screw (Fig. 1–1a–6).

12. The addition of a distal soft tissue release to a chevron osteotomy improves the position of the hallux and the relationship of the sesamoids to the metatarsal head (Fig. 1–1a–7). This is of particular value when there is greater valgus deformity of the hallux relative to the intermetatarsal deformity. There is no increased incidence of avascular necrosis of the metatarsal head with a distal soft tissue release, which results from excessive stripping of the dorsolateral periosteum.

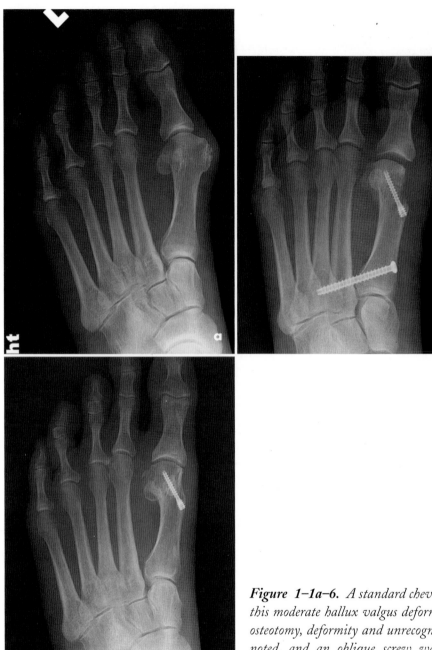

Figure 1–1a–6. *A standard chevron osteotomy was planned for correction of this moderate hallux valgus deformity (a). At surgery, following the chevron osteotomy, deformity and unrecognized instability of the first metatarsal was noted, and an oblique screw was inserted between the first and second metatarsals (b). The screw was removed at 3 months, and this is the XR appearance at two years following surgery (c).*

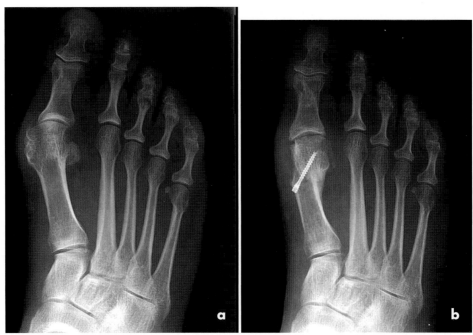

Figure 1–1a–7. *Hallux valgus deformity corrected with a chevron osteotomy combined with a distal soft tissue release performed through a separate incision in the first web space (a, b).*

The Modified Ludloff Metatarsal Osteotomy

The indication for a modified Ludloff metatarsal osteotomy is moderate to severe deformity that is not associated with instability of the metatarsocuneiform joint. The procedure is always performed in conjunction with a distal soft tissue release. No limit exists to the amount of correction that can be performed with this proximal metatarsal osteotomy. However, when there is an abnormality of the distal metatarsal articular angle, then either a double metatarsal osteotomy needs to be performed, or a closing wedge osteotomy of the hallux proximal phalanx (Akin osteotomy) is added.

Soft Tissue Release

An incision is made in the first web space; the incision extends from the cleft of the web space proximally for a length of 2.5 cm. Identify the terminal branch of the deep peroneal nerve to avoid numbness in the first web space. A small retractor is inserted into the incision. Then, a small-toothed laminar spreader is inserted between the first and second metatarsals; this insertion places the innominate-fascia on stretch to facilitate dissection. The two heads of the adductor tendon are now grasped with a small clamp and then cut sharply off the lateral edge of the fibular sesamoid. The adductor tendon is elevated into the incision; dissected free from the flexor brevis muscle and tendon, as well as the lateral edge of the sesamoid; and then cut distally. I prefer to cut the adductor tendon completely and not to reattach the tendon to the neck of the metatarsal, as some surgeons describe (Fig. 1–1b–1).

Cutting the terminal 1 cm of the adductor tendon prevents any recurrent scarring between the adductor tendon and the sesamoid complex and, therefore, recurrent deformity. The sesamoid suspensory ligament is cut with a more oblique rotation of the blade. Remember that as the hallux valgus worsens, the sesamoid rotates from a transverse plane to a more oblique or vertical position. With the sesamoid release, the blade must be inserted more obliquely as the deformity increases. The sesamoid is freed from the undersurface of the first metatarsal, the capsule is perforated sharply, and the hallux is manipulated by tearing the capsule into slight varus. It may be necessary to release the deep transverse metatarsal ligament, if the sesamoid is still tethered by the ligament and the ligament is holding the displaced sesamoid laterally. When releasing the ligament, use a Metzenbaum scissors, working from distal to proximal along the undersurface of the ligament. Be careful not to injure the common digital nerve that lies underneath the ligament.

The Capsulotomy and Osteotomy

Although the capsulotomy and exposure of the metatarsal are made initially, the exostectomy (bunionectomy) is *not* performed until the metatarsal osteotomy is complete. Subtle rotation of the metatarsal head may occur after the osteotomy, and if the exostectomy is performed first, malrotation of the metatarsal head may occur. A medial incision at the junction of the dorsal and plantar skin is preferable to one more dorsally placed (closer to

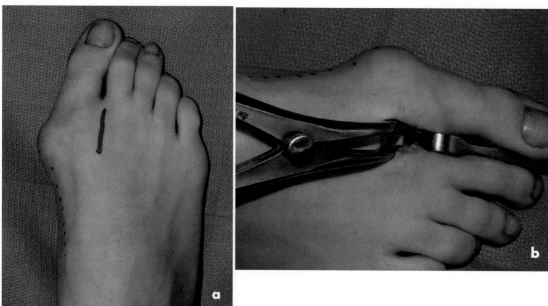

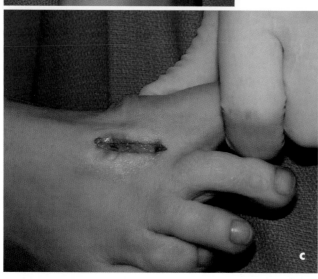

Figure 1–1b–1. *The incisions are marked as noted (a), the adductor release is performed with a laminar spreader to place stretch on the transverse metatarsal ligament (b), and the hallux is manipulated into slight hallux varus after the adductor release (c).*

the extensor hallucis longus [EHL] tendon). A more dorsal incision traumatizes the nerve and often causes dorsal scarring and contracture (Fig. 1–1b–2).

Carefully dissect the soft tissues so that the terminal medial cutaneous branch of the superficial peroneal nerve is identified. Gradually dissect the nerve free using a hemostat and retract the nerve dorsally.

Although different capsular incisions can be made, I use a straight longitudinal incision extending from the metatarsophalangeal joint proximally along the course of the first metatarsal shaft. This incision is made slightly inferiorly to leave abundant capsule dorsally for soft tissue closure. The capsule is now dissected off the medial eminence and medial aspect of the metatarsal

head; this dissection exposes the tibial sesamoid. A blunt periosteal elevator is inserted under the metatarsal head to mobilize the sesamoid.

The Osteotomy

The incision is extended proximally along the plane of the first metatarsal, and the subcutaneous dissection is performed proximally to the level of the tarsometatarsal (TMT) joint. During the dissection the more proximal terminal cutaneous branch of the superficial peroneal nerve should be retracted dorsally. Dissect off the medial and dorsal surface of the periosteum only (Fig. 1–1b–3). Turning the leg and foot so that the plane of the osteotomy can carefully be identified is helpful.

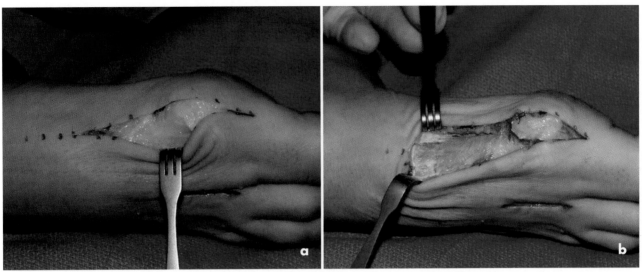

Figure 1–1b–2. *The medial incision is made at the junction of the dorsal and plantar skin, and the capsulotomy is in the plane of the metatarsal (a). Only the medial metatarsal is exposed to minimize soft tissue stripping (b).*

The osteotomy is marked out with an electrocautery and extended from the dorsal apical surface of the first metatarsal proximally at an angle of approximately 30 degrees distally. The cut is planned to exit proximal to the sesamoid complex distally over a length of approximately 3 cm. The longer the saw cut, the more likely that it will be too close to the sesamoids distally, and this cut will make screw fixation more difficult. However, as the plane of the osteotomy becomes more vertical, it is more unstable. Inserting a retractor into the proximal first web space by drawing back the EHL tendon and the soft tissues is useful. The saw blade is oriented exactly perpendicular to the axis of the first metatarsal, about 4 mm distal to the TMT joint dorsally. As the cut is made more distally, a cortical bone bridge is left on the plantar distal surface of the first metatarsal. Slight soft tissue dissection of the dorsal surface of the first metatarsal is performed, and the screw fixation is planned. I use a double-threaded cannulated screw (DePuy FRS screw, Warsaw, Ind.), with a careful countersink to prevent splitting of the dorsal surface of the first metatarsal. The more proximal the fixation, the better the axial rotation around the screw and the greater the control of correction. If the screw is inserted more distally, the metatarsal becomes banana shaped, and the likelihood of malunion and alteration of the position of the metatarsal head is increased. The screw is fully inserted, but it does not compress the osteotomy. Then, the screw is slightly "backed off" to insert the saw blade and complete the distal aspect of the first metatarsal osteotomy. A retractor is again inserted proximally between the first and second metatarsals.

When the proximal aspect of the proximal first metatarsal is pushed medially and the first metatarsal head is simultaneously directed laterally, the metatarsal direction is corrected. The value of this osteotomy is that at no time does one lose control of the plane and position of the metatarsal. Once the position of the metatarsal is corrected with good coverage of the metatarsal head distally, a second FRS screw is introduced to complete fixation. The overhanging bone is now shaved down proximally, dorsally, and medially with a saw blade. The stability of the metatarsal must be checked, and the exostectomy and capsulorrhaphy must be performed. This concept of metatarsal stability is important. Approximately 5% of the time, after an excellent correction of the metatarsal, transverse plane instability is present. This instability may not have been noted preoperatively because the ideal operation would then have been a Lapidus procedure. To some extent this instability may be controlled postoperatively with tight bandaging, but I prefer not to rely on bandaging and instead use added fixation to control the position of the metatarsal (Fig. 1–1b–3).

An exostectomy does not always have to be performed. However, even with excellent correction of the metatarsal head, gently abrading the medial head with a saw blade to facilitate stable healing of the capsule is useful. Before cutting the exostosis, check the alignment of the first metatarsal with respect to the medial eminence and the hallux. With a saw blade, the medial eminence is cut from dorsal to plantar to leave the proximal aspect of the ostectomy flush with metaphyseal flare. To prevent

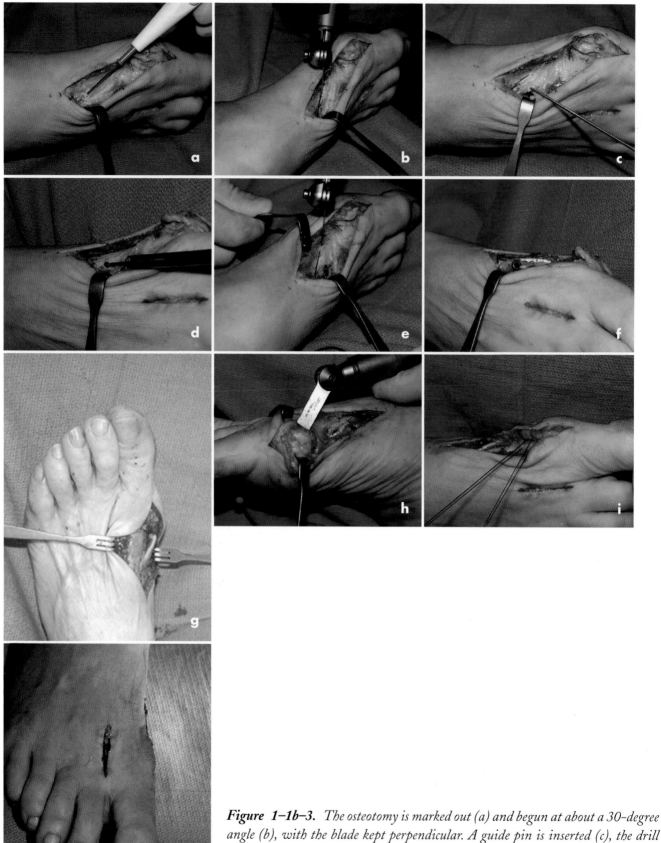

Figure 1–1b–3. *The osteotomy is marked out (a) and begun at about a 30-degree angle (b), with the blade kept perpendicular. A guide pin is inserted (c), the drill is countersunk (d), and the first screw is inserted (e). The metatarsal is then rotated around the axis of the first screw (f, g), the capsular repair is performed (h) after the overhanging bone is shaved down, and the exostectomy is performed last (i). The final appearance of the foot is noted clinically (j).*

overcorrection, hallux varus, and sesamoid arthritis, do not resect too much bone off the medial head.

The capsulorrhaphy is performed with the plantar capsular tissue with two oblique sutures of 2-0 Vicryl. These are inserted from the dorsal proximal capsule into the plantar distal position to create an oblique suture that pulls the hallux into very slight varus and supination. During the capsular repair, the hallux is maintained in a neutral position both in terms of the axial plane alignment and rotation. Before closure, make sure that the range of motion of the hallux metatarsophalangeal joint is adequate without clicking or locking, which may indicate an incongruent joint. Any clicking or locking may indicate that the distal metatarsal articular angle is not satisfactory and that an osteotomy of the hallux proximal phalanx may need to be performed.

Techniques, tips, and pitfalls

1. Malunion and nonunion are rare with the modified Ludloff metatarsal osteotomy. The major advantage of this osteotomy is that at no point during the procedure is control of the metatarsal position lost. Nonunion may occur if primary bone healing is not present, in which case periosteal bone formation is present in the early postoperative phase on x-ray (XR) film. If periosteal new bone formation occurs around the osteotomy site, it is more than likely loose, and although union of the osteotomy will occur, slight elevation and dorsal malunion may also occur simultaneously. If periosteal bone formation occurs, weight bearing should be controlled in a boot, and the foot carefully strapped.

2. The type of fixation used here is important to facilitate primary bone healing. Because of the plane of this osteotomy, bone-to-bone contact can be limited, and the plane of screw fixation is critical.

3. Rotation of the metatarsal occurs around a single axis point of the more proximal screw. Because this is an angular/rotational and not a translational osteotomy, the geometry of correction must be understood. The further proximal the osteotomy is performed or the closer the axis of rotation is to the TMT joint, the less the angular

deformity of correction is distally. For example, if the center of rotation is in the center of the metatarsal, the metatarsal is banana shaped, and the likelihood is that even with good correction, the metatarsal head will be facing more laterally. Therefore this banana-shaped metatarsal can predispose to recurrent hallux valgus.

4. The plane of the osteotomy itself is important. The saw blade must be exactly perpendicular to the axis of the metatarsal. If the saw blade is raised, the first metatarsal head will depress, and the metatarsal head will rotate into slight supination, which is desirable. The converse applies with a plane of the osteotomy where the saw blade is dropped down and the metatarsal head will tilt up. A dorsal malunion may occur with pronation of the metatarsal head and an increased likelihood of recurrent hallux valgus.

5. Occasionally, after a well-performed osteotomy, intraoperative deformity may still exist between the first and second metatarsals. Patients with this deformity have unrecognized instability of the tarsal metatarsal joint where this instability may be in the transverse and not in the sagittal plane. Unfortunately, the TMT joint cannot be stabilized with arthrodesis at this late stage. I have used two alternative techniques to do so. The first is to insert sutures between the first and second metatarsals distally. This technique has been well described for both proximal and distal metatarsal osteotomies in conjunction with the distal soft tissue release. The second technique is the insertion of a transverse screw between the first and second metatarsals proximally; this insertion does not interfere with fixation of the osteotomy. This second technique can be performed but is less reliable, and one has to watch for stress reaction of bone and possible stress fracture of the metatarsal. Strapping of the foot at weekly intervals is important to stabilize the overall alignment of the first and second metatarsals postoperatively.

6. Be aware of a contracture of the EHL tendon, which may be present even with moderate deformity as noted. The EHL tendon must be lengthened (Fig. 1–1b–4).

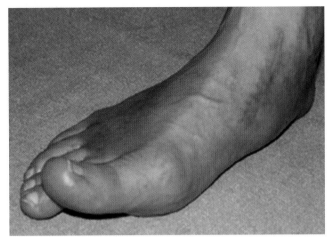

Figure 1–1b–4. *Bowstringing of the extensor hallucis longus (EHL) tendon is present, and the tendon should be lengthened at the same time as the osteotomy with a Z-step cut.*

7. Unrecognized instability of the first metatarsal may be present, which may lead to failure of the osteotomy and recurrent metatarsus varus. This instability occurs in the transverse and not in the sagittal plane. Some surgeons use firm taping of the foot postoperatively and with this strapping believe that this instability does not cause a problem. However, if the metatarsal is not corrected after the osteotomy, I do not think that taping is adequate to hold the correction. I use a lag screw (the syndesmosis screw) to lag the first to the second metatarsal (Figs. 1–1b–5 and 1–1b–6).

Figure 1–1b–5. *This patient had undergone prior simple bunionectomy with failure, hypermobility that was shown on the first XR film was not appreciated preoperatively, and a Ludloff osteotomy was performed (a). The sequence of the screw fixation (b, c) was standard, but gross transverse plane instability was noted after initial screw fixation, until a syndesmosis screw was inserted between the first and second metatarsals (d–f).*

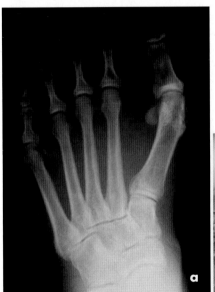

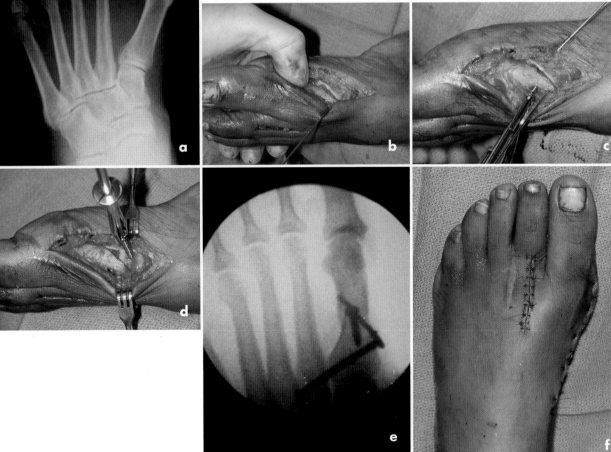

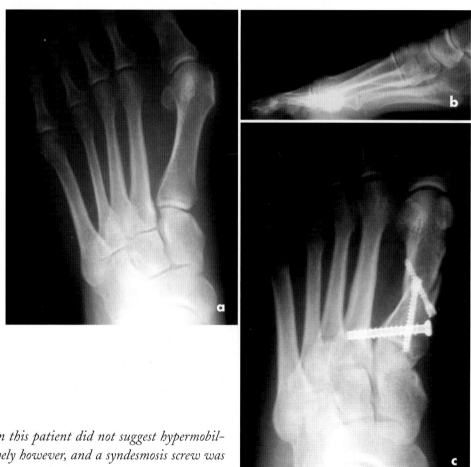

Figure 1–1b–6. *The deformity in this patient did not suggest hypermobility, which was noted intraoperatively however, and a syndesmosis screw was inserted and left in for 4 months postoperatively.*

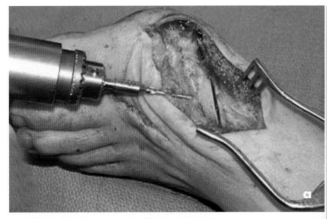

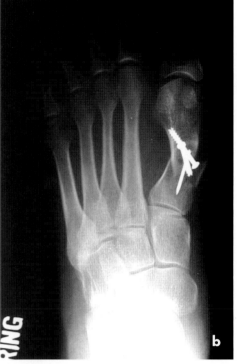

Figure 1–1b–7. *The axis of rotation in this osteotomy is too distal, and the plane of the osteotomy is too vertical (a). Note the postoperative banana shape of the first metatarsal (b).*

8. The axis of rotation of the metatarsal must be as proximal as possible to facilitate correction. If the screw is inserted too distally, the corrected metatarsal will have a banana shape, and although the alignment of the hallux with the center of the metatarsal head may be adequate, this can lead to an incongruent center of rotation and arthritis (Fig. 1–1b–7).

9. The angle of the osteotomy must be as oblique as possible without entering the sesamoid apparatus and the TMT joint. An angle that is too steep leads to an irregular correction, with an increased incidence of delayed union (Figs. 1–1b–8 and 1–1b–9).

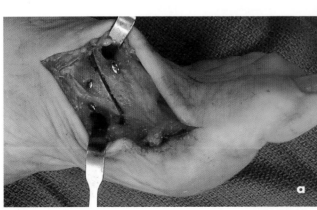

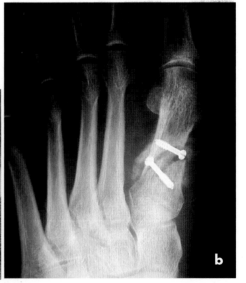

Figure 1–1b–8. *The plane of the osteotomy in this patient is too vertical (a) and increased the likelihood of a delayed union that occurred (b). Compare the XR film in b with the postoperative XR film in Figure 1–1b–6 where primary bone healing occurred.*

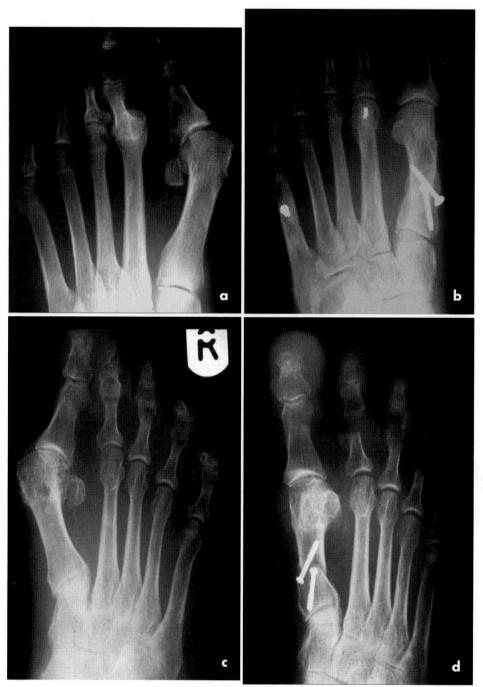

Figure 1–1b–9. *Note the primary bone healing that occurred in both of these patients (a–d) after the Ludloff osteotomy. The healing indicates stable fixation, and indirectly, the correct plane of the osteotomy is implied.*

Postoperative Course and Recovery

Patients may begin weight bearing as tolerated on the foot immediately after surgery; however, heel weight bearing is preferable. If there is any concern as to the stability and rigidity of the fixation, then a boot, rather than a postoperative shoe, is used. The foot is immobilized for approximately 4 weeks and then weight bearing in a firm accommodative shoe can be used as tolerated. Physical therapy treatments with massage, strapping, and exercise of the forefoot is useful and can begin at 6 weeks after surgery. These radiographs (Fig. 1–1b–10) demonstrate the Ludloff First metatarsal osteotomy for correction of hallus valgus and metatarsus varus. The preoperative image (*a*), is followed by the images at 6 weeks following surgery (*b, c*).

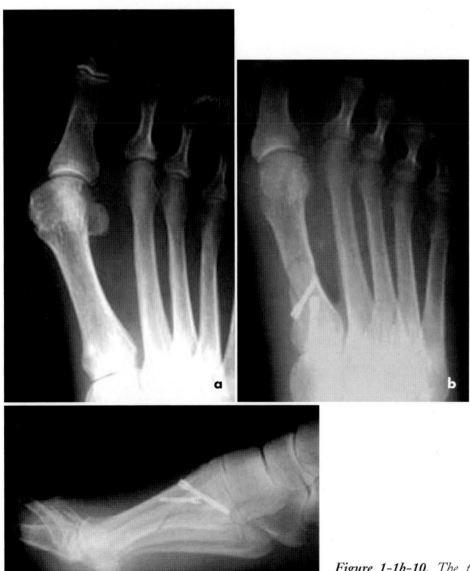

Figure 1-1b-10. *The typical correction of hallux valgus following the Ludloff First Metatarsal osteotomy is demonstrated.*

The Modified Lapidus Procedure

Overview

The indications for the Lapidus bunionectomy include hypermobility and instability of the first metatarsal on *either* the sagittal or transverse planes. Examination of the sagittal plane instability or hypermobility is best performed by stabilizing the lateral aspect of the foot and then manipulating the medial column in a dorsal or plantar direction (Fig. 1–1c–1). Radiographic parameters of instability are helpful but unreliable in planning this operation; however, instability in the transverse plane is easy to document (Fig. 1–1c–2). Patients with arthritis of the first and/or second metatarsal cuneiform joint associated with hallux valgus are best treated with an extended Lapidus procedure to include the metatarsocuneiform joints. Arthritis of the second tarsometatarsal (TMT) joint is usually the result of the instability of the first metatarsal with hypermo-

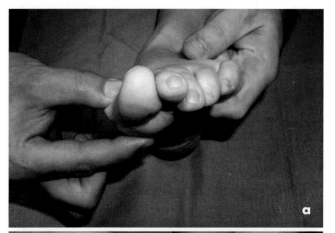

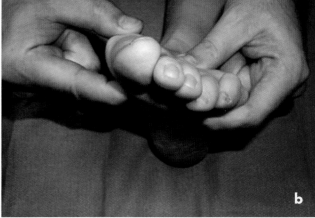

Figure 1–1c–1. Hypermobility is noted in this patient by stabilizing the lateral column of the foot firmly and then moving the first metatarsal in a plantar (a) and dorsal (b) direction. There is a "feel" to the extent of instability, and all patients with hallux valgus should have this test performed. In addition to instability in the sagittal plane, instability in the transverse plane (between the first and second metatarsals) should be examined.

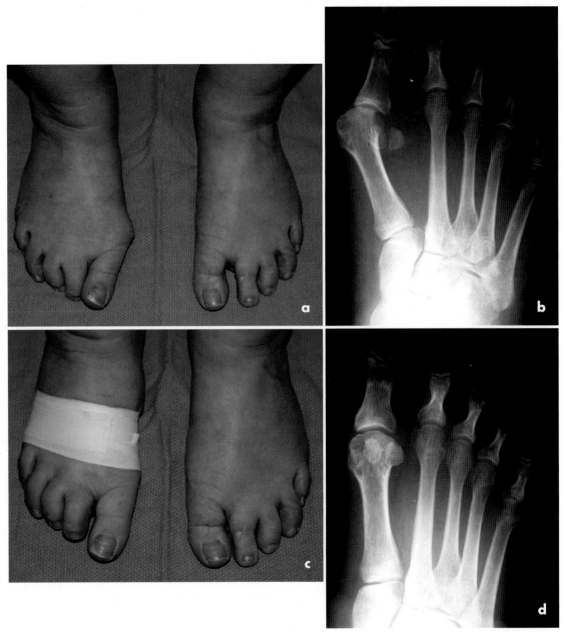

Figure 1–1c–2. *Transverse plane instability is demonstrated (a, b) and is correctable with strapping of the forefoot (c, d). A radiograph is taken with and without the strapping to confirm the presence of this excessive mobility. This is an ideal deformity to correct with the modified Lapidus procedure.*

bility leading to overload of the second metatarsal and, ultimately, arthritis. Frequently, patients with arthritis of the second metatarsal cuneiform joint have associated arthritis of the first metatarsal cuneiform joint as well, but the Lapidus procedure is indicated nonetheless in the absence of arthritis of the first metatarsal cuneiform joint. This operation should not be performed indiscriminately because the complication rate from this procedure is higher than that for other bunion operations.

Incision and Dissection

After the distal soft tissue and adductor release, the incision is extended proximally, lateral to the extensor hallucis longus tendon, without injury to the deep peroneal nerve. I find that this single midline incision is more cosmetically acceptable and facilitates exposure of the TMT joint proximally. The capsulotomy incision is not made at this time. The extensor hallucis longus tendon is retracted medially, and the incision is deepened down. With subperiosteal dissection, the dorsal surface of the articulation is identified and opened. The key to the joint debridement is *restraint*, because only the articular cartilage and minimal subchondral bone should be removed. Although the first metatarsal is moved laterally during the procedure, this movement is unnecessary through removal of any wedges of bone, which shorten the metatarsal. Instead, translation and rotation of the metatarsal base is preferable. This movement depends on the shape of the articulation, which is typically saddle shaped, and may not be conducive to this translational movement. A smooth laminar spreader is inserted into the TMT articulation, and the joint is distracted to provide visualization of the plantar of the apical surface of the first

metatarsal. The joint is much deeper than one expects, and for prevention of a dorsal malunion, the entire joint must be denuded. I prefer to use a chisel instead of a saw blade to denude the articular cartilage, and then I perforate the joint multiple times using a small drill bit down to healthy bleeding subchondral bone on both the metatarsal and cuneiform surface (Fig. 1–1c–3).

Correction of Deformity

The metatarsal is corrected with a maneuver that includes adduction and simultaneous supination. To plantarflex the metatarsal and prevent dorsal malunion, I dorsiflex the hallux to force the first metatarsal into slight plantar flexion. The first metatarsal is then squeezed to the second metatarsal, and the combination of hallux dorsiflexion and adduction of the metatarsal correct the deformity. The articular surface should be nicely impacted, and both the base of the first metatarsal

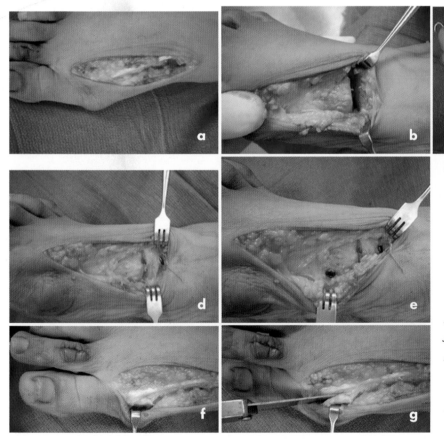

Figure 1–1c–3. A single incision can be used to perform the adductor release, the tarsometatarsal (TMT) arthrodesis, and the exostectomy (a). The entire articulation, in particular the plantar surface, is debrided (b). The hallux is dorsiflexed, and the metatarsal is pushed into alignment, while a guide pin is introduced to position the reduction of the joint (c). The first screw is inserted from the dorsal and proximal to the plantar and distal surfaces (d), and the second screw in this case was inserted obliquely from the first into the second metatarsal base (e). Once the arthrodesis was completed, an exostectomy was performed (f, g).

and the articular surface of the medial cuneiform should be well apposed. The position of the articulation is held secure with cannulated guide pins, and no instability between the first and second metatarsals should be apparent. If the alignment is corrected and no instability remains, then the fixation is planned between the first metatarsal and the medial cuneiform only. Two guide pins are inserted: the first one, which is from the dorsal proximal medial cuneiform, is aimed distal and plantar in the first metatarsal. The second guide pin is inserted from the first metatarsal dorsally and is heading slightly proximal, plantar, and lateral to the first guide pin. This articulation should now be checked fluoroscopically; note the position of the first metatarsal head in relation to the sesamoid and ensure that overcorrection is not present. I use two 4-mm fully threaded cancellous cannulated screws, with overdrilling of the proximal cortex. Countersinking the medial cuneiform is unnecessary, but it must be carefully performed in the metatarsal to prevent fracture and splitting of the proximal dorsal

apical surface of the metatarsal. If there is not only apparent instability between the first and second metatarsals, but also instability and hypermobility between the medial and middle TMT columns (i.e., between the first and second metatarsals and the medial and middle cuneiform), the pattern of fixation is different, and screws are inserted between the first metatarsal and medial cuneiform and between the first and second metatarsals. The first screw is introduced in a manner similar to that just described, with compression of the metatarsal by dorsiflexion of the hallux. The second screw is introduced from the base of the first metatarsal obliquely into the second metatarsal or middle cuneiform, depending on the plane of the metatarsal and the ability to avoid the first screw. Performing a formal arthrodesis between the first and second metatarsals, as originally described by Lapidus, is unnecessary unless there is gross instability and this is part of a more extensive arthrodesis procedure of the TMT joints (Figs. 1–1c–4 and 1–1c–5).

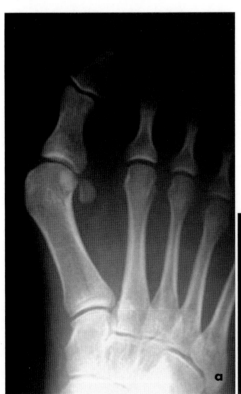
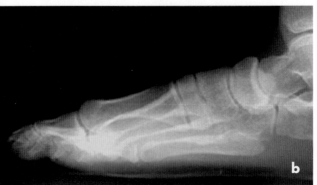

Figure 1–1c–4. *Preoperative (a, b) x-ray (XR) films of a 21-year-old woman with Down's syndrome and clinical hypermobility of the first metatarsal. Note the elevation of the first metatarsal on the lateral preoperative XR film. There was no transverse plane instability intraoperatively, and only axial screw fixation was used. Note that no exostectomy or capsulorrhaphy has been performed.*

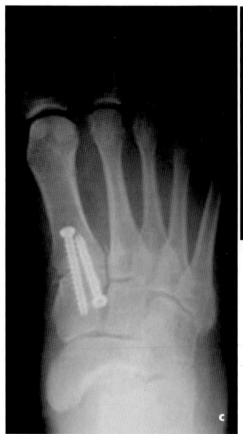

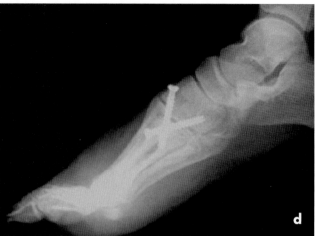

Figure 1–1c–4, cont'd. Postoperative XR film (c, d) of a 21-year-old woman with Down's syndrome and clinical hypermobility of the first metatarsal.

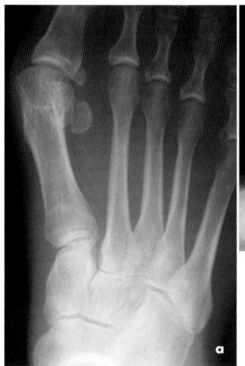

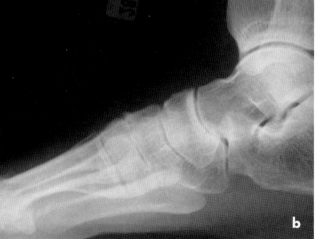

Figure 1–1c–5. This patient was treated for recurrent hallux valgus associated with painful arthritis of the tarsometatarsal (TMT) and naviculocuneiform joints (a, b).

Continued

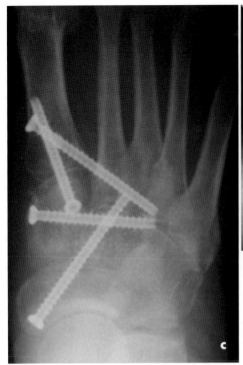
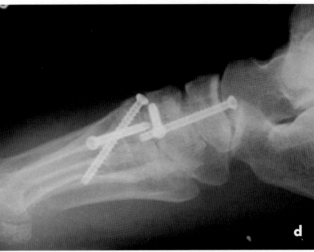

Figure 1–1c–5, cont'd. *This patient has an extended arthrodesis (c, d). Note the oblique screws that were inserted across the first and into the second metatarsal.*

Exostectomy and Capsular Repair

The alignment of the first metatarsal is checked with respect to the medial eminence and the hallux. Occasionally, an exostectomy is unnecessary (e.g., in adolescents) because the alignment is already perfect. If an exostectomy is performed, the hallux may be unstable, and hallux varus may occur. The incision is extended from the flare just distal to the metatarsophalangeal joint and extended proximally. The capsulotomy can be made in a longitudinal direction, but I prefer a more standard Λ shape with the apex proximal and dorsal, which leaves the capsule dorsal for soft tissue closure.

With a saw blade, the medial eminence is cut from dorsal to plantar to create the proximal aspect of the exostectomy flush with metaphyseal flare. Do not resect too much bone relative to the first metatarsal shaft axis because this resection will affect the position of the tibial sesamoid relative to the hallux. With the hallux in a well-aligned position relative to the first metatarsal, the capsulorrhaphy is performed, with absorbable 2-0 sutures inserted from the dorsal proximal aspect of the capsule into the plantar distal position to create an oblique suture, which pulls the hallux into slight supination.

Techniques, tips, and pitfalls

1. Be careful with the soft tissue (adductor) release with this procedure. Correction of deformity with arthrodesis is excellent, and with excessive adductor release, hallux varus will occur. Consider that a "modified or minimal" adductor release is performed for this procedure.

2. Exostectomy may not be necessary and is not performed until completion of the realignment and arthrodesis.

3. The correct positioning of the first metatarsal in the sagittal plane is imperative during this procedure. Positioning from a dorsal incision is not always easy because the base of the metatarsal cuneiform joint is not easily seen. Furthermore, when the joint surface is debrided, more cartilage may be removed dorsally than on the plantar surface, and this removal leaves the apex of the joint inferiorly intact. Leaving bone on the plantar surface of the joint automatically dorsiflexes the metatarsal and creates a dorsal malunion. This inevitably leads to a transfer of pressure and

weight on the second metatarsal with pain. To avoid this, make sure that the base of the joint is completely denuded of articular cartilage. A lamina spreader facilitates full exposure of the joint surface.

4. Rotation of the first metatarsal head must be avoided with stabilization. Ideally the metatarsal head should be slightly supinated during the stabilization and arthrodesis. Because of the plane of inclination of the first metatarsal, as it is being pushed over toward the second metatarsal, the first metatarsal tends to undergo slight pronation, rather than supination, and this must be avoided.

5. The fixation of the TMT joint can be done in one plane (from the first metatarsal into the cuneiform and vice versa), or in two planes (in order to control transverse plane instability as well). Generally speaking, the sagittal plane must be corrected primarily, and if there is additional instability in the mediolateral (transverse) plane, then an additional screw must be inserted obliquely from the metatarsal into the second metatarsal or middle cuneiform.

6. Arthrodesis of the first web space (the first to the second metatarsal and the intercuneiform space) may be unnecessary. However, if the arthrodesis is being performed as part of a procedure for correction of arthritis and deformity in which the second metatarsal cuneiform joint is included in the arthrodesis, then it is advisable to fuse between the medial and middle columns as well.

7. Rarely, despite a solid arthrodesis of the medial column (first metatarsal/medial cuneiform), the sagittal plane motion between the medial and middle columns causes instability and pain.

8. Try not to shorten the first metatarsal as part of the correction. Shortening will occur if a wedge from the metatarsocuneiform joint is resected. Depending on the shape of the articulation, the correction should be done by translation and not by resection of a bone wedge. If a bone wedge *has* to be resected,

make sure that that this shortening is compensated by plantar flexing the first metatarsal.

9. Nonunion occurs, despite contrary efforts, in approximately 8% of patients. Not all of these patients have symptoms; however, if symptoms exist, a revision with bone graft usually needs to be performed. If a revision is performed, the goal should be a solid arthrodesis, but in the *correct position*. Union may occur, but this may be at the expense of length, and a malunion does not help the patient either.

10. Revision is required for shortening of the first metatarsal, malunion, or a painful nonunion. Although revision can be accomplished with screw fixation, a small dorsally applied two-hole plate is the most useful, with bone graft inserted to realign and/or lengthen the first metatarsal.

11. The modified Lapidus procedure does not correct an abnormal distal metatarsal articular angle. The procedure is effective in correcting excessive mobility and severe deformity. If additional multiplanar deformity is present, then either a distal metatarsal or a phalangeal osteotomy must be performed (Fig. 1–1c–6).

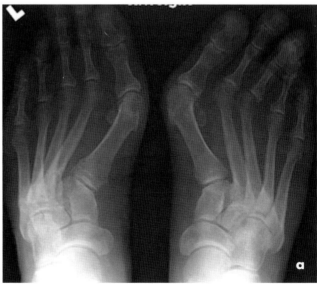

Figure 1–1c–6. *This patient had severe multiplanar deformity associated with marked metatarsus adductus and painful arthritis of the second metatarsocuneiform joint (a, b).* *Continued*

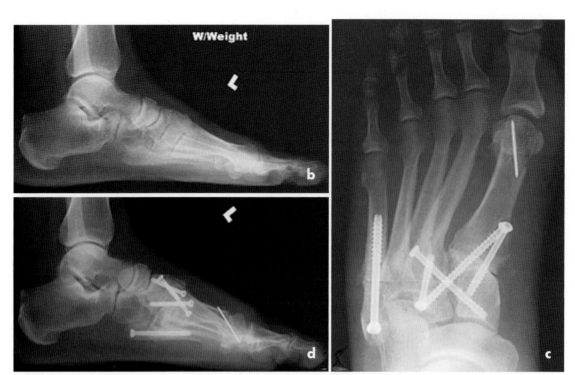

Figure 1–1c–6, cont'd. *The deformity was corrected with an extended tarsometatarsal (TMT) arthrodesis and a biplanar chevron osteotomy with the Toomey jigs. The patient had a stress fracture of the fifth metatarsal base in the interim, which was fixed simultaneously (c, d).*

Management of Complications

Whether nonunion or malunion is present, one must be able to correct residual or recurrent deformity. As previously noted, plantar flexing the first metatarsal is important during the fixation; this is best accomplished by dorsiflexion of the hallux to force the first metatarsal into plantar flexion. If dorsal malunion occurs, then this must be revised with osteotomy or interposition bone graft

(Fig. 1–1c–7). Nonunion occurs despite efforts to avoid it (Fig. 1–1c–8). The factors I have noted in development of nonunion are the following: inadequate or incorrect apposition of the bone surfaces at the TMT joint, inappropriate fixation, premature bearing of weight after surgery, and inadequate joint preparation. The surgeon may find it helpful to multiply perforate the metatarsal and cuneiform with a small drill bit to create bleeding and a slurry of bone at the joint interface.

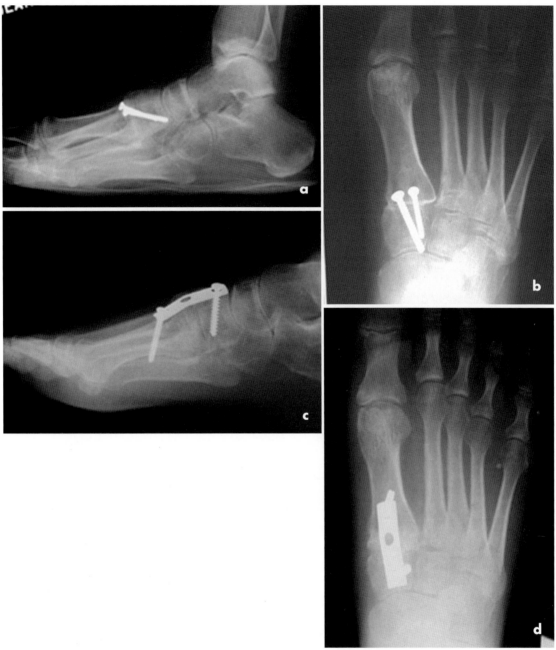

Figure 1–1c–7. *Malunion of this tarsometatarsal (TMT) arthrodesis probably occurred because of inadequate debridement of the base of the articulation (a, b). Note elevation of the first metatarsal, which caused pain under the second metatarsal refractory to padding and orthoses. This was revised with a structural triangular allograft inserted into the base of the metatarsal, with restoration of the declination angle of the first metatarsal (c, d). Note that there is not much change in the length of the first metatarsal; however, the forefoot is plantigrade. Metatarsalgia was resolved because of the plantar flexion.*

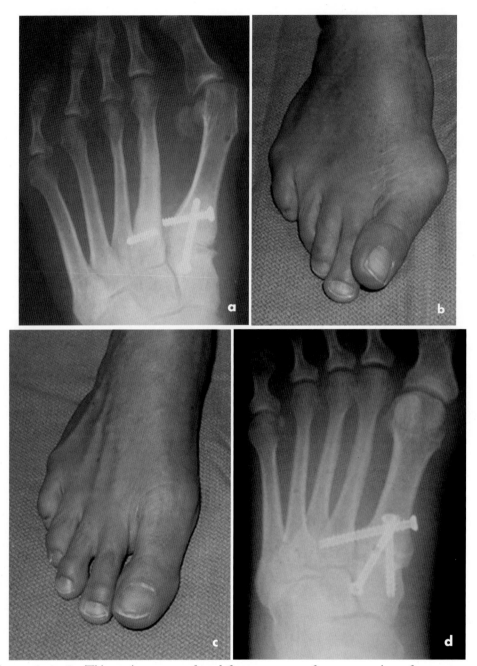

Figure 1–1c–8. *This patient was referred for treatment after a nonunion of an attempted Lapidus procedure (a, b). Note the severe deformity associated with pronation and hallux valgus. Correction was made with a revision that included bone graft and arthrodesis of the inter-metatarsal space between the first and second metatarsals (c, d).*

Suggested Readings

Faber FW, Kleinrensink GJ, Mulder PG, Verhaar JA: Mobility of the first tarsometatarsal joint in hallux valgus: A radiographic analysis. Foot Ankle Int 22: 965–969, 2001.

Myerson M, Allon S, McGarvey W: Metatarsocunei-form arthrodesis for management of hallux valgus and metatarsus primus varus. Foot Ankle 13:107–115, 1992.

Myerson MS: Metatarsocuneiform arthrodesis for treatment of hallux valgus and metatarsus primus varus. Orthopedics 13:1025–1031, 1990.

Myerson MS, Badekas A: Hypermobility of the first ray. Foot Ankle Clin 5:469–484, 2000.

Sangeorzan BJ, Hansen ST Jr: Modified Lapidus procedure for hallux valgus. Foot Ankle 9: 262–262, 1989.

Resection Arthroplasty

Overview

The indications for resection arthroplasty for hallux valgus are limited. Although this certainly has been a popular operation historically, far better procedures are available for correction of hallux valgus, even when arthritis is present. The operation is therefore limited for individuals who have arthritis associated with hallux valgus and who have good generalized forefoot function without overload of the second metatarsal. Resection arthroplasty always weakens the hallux. Inevitably, some weight bearing transfers to the second metatarsal, which will aggravate any preexisting deformity. The procedure is therefore contraindicated in patients who already have callus formation and metatarsalgia. If there is severe hallux valgus and a marked increase in the intermetatarsal angle associated with arthritis, then an arthrodesis of the metatarsophalangeal (MP) joint is the preferred procedure. Recurrent hallux valgus, as well as recurrence of the MP deformity, is likely to occur if a standard resection arthroplasty (Keller arthroplasty) is performed for correction of a greater intermetatarsal deformity. Modification of this arthroplasty is described later.

Incision and Exposure

Either a dorsal or a medial incision is used along the length of the MP joint that extends from the metatarsal neck across the metatarsal head onto the base of the proximal phalanx. The medial incision facilitates correction of the hallux valgus with the capsular repair as part of the rationale for this approach. However, a dorsal incision may also be used under some circumstances, particularly if intramedullary fixation of the hallux is used to control the position of the toe postoperatively (Fig. 1–1d–1). If a medial incision is used, then the medial cutaneous branch of the superficial peroneal nerve is identified with the dissection and retracted dorsally, and the capsule is incised longitudinally. The line of the capsular incision is slightly more toward the plantar surface to facilitate later closure with a capsular flap being well maintained dorsally. The capsule is elevated off both the medial eminence and the base of the proximal phalanx, with as much preservation of the dorsal flap as possible.

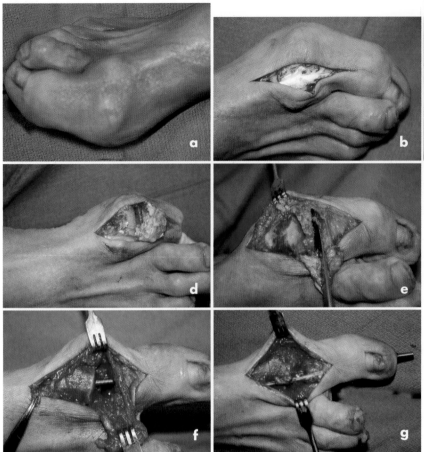

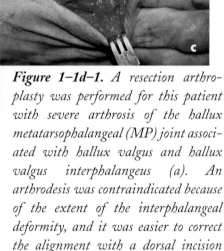

Figure 1–1d–1. A resection arthroplasty was performed for this patient with severe arthrosis of the hallux metatarsophalangeal (MP) joint associated with hallux valgus and hallux valgus interphalangeus (a). An arthrodesis was contraindicated because of the extent of the interphalangeal deformity, and it was easier to correct the alignment with a dorsal incision (b). The incision is made medial to the extensor hallucis longus (EHL) tendon, which is retracted laterally (c); the joint is exposed; and a cheilectomy is performed (d). The hallux is then plantarflexed by stripping the periosteum circumferentially around the base of the proximal phalanx, and a saw cut made, with removal of 6 mm of the proximal phalanx. An oblique cut was made on the phalanx and more medial bone was removed because of the severe hallux valgus interphanlangeus (e). After phalangeal resection, the hallux deformity persisted until the EHL tendon was lengthened. This lengthening was followed by insertion of a threaded Steinman pin, which maintained the length of the hallux (f). The soft tissue flap raised from the dorsal surface of the metatarsal head was inserted as an interposition, and the EHL tendon was repaired (g).

The medial eminence is now fully exposed with subperiosteal dissection dorsal medial and plantar to strip the undersurface of the soft tissue attachments of the flexor brevis and abductor tendons from the undersurface of the metatarsal head and neck. The base of the proximal phalanx is exposed, and although the abductor and adductor attachments have to be dissected free, the surgeon should preserve as much of the volar plate on the plantar aspect of the hallux as possible.

The problem with the saw cut is determining how much bone to resect off the proximal phalanx. If too much bone is removed, the hallux will be predict-ably weak and associated with all of the anticipated complications. However, if too little bone is removed, then the range of motion of the MP joint is limited, and pain occurs with articular impingement (Fig. 1–1d–2).

It is not possible to preserve the attachment of the volar plate, which attaches over a length of 8 mm. Try, however, to preserve this soft tissue sleeve after the bone cut is made. I remove the base of the proximal phalanx at the metaphyseal flare, which amounts to approximately one quarter of the proximal phalanx. The cut can be made slightly obliquely to facilitate slight varus posi-

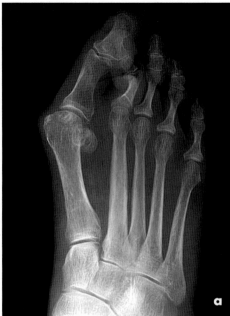

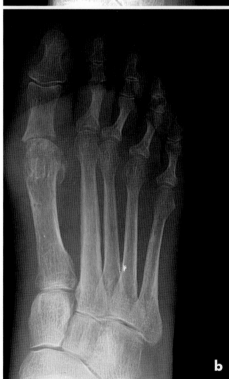

Figure 1–1d–2. A resection arthroplasty was performed for this 82-year-old patient with hallux valgus and arthritis of the MP joint (a). The alignment of the hallux was satisfactory after the arthroplasty; however, pain was present, with limited motion, perhaps because of insufficient resection of the proximal phalanx (b).

tioning of the hallux at the completion of the cut. The position of the hallux should now be checked relative to the metatarsal before the medial eminence is resected. The chisel is placed just medial to the sagittal groove, and the medial eminence is removed completely, exiting at the metaphyseal flare of the metatarsal neck. The range of motion of the hallux and the position relative to the metatarsal must now be checked. If hallux valgus persists, then lengthen the extensor hallucis longus (EHL) tendon with a standard Z-lengthening to prevent recurrent deformity of the hallux (valgus and cock-up). If the intermetatarsal angle remains wide, then the Lelièvre modification is recommended.

Lelièvre Modification of the Resection Arthroplasty

The Lelièvre modification can decrease the intermetatarsal angle and maintain the hallux in a neutral position. The premise of the Lelièvre procedure is to use the sesamoid sling to tighten up the intermetatarsal space, which then maintains the hallux in a more neutral alignment. The anatomic basis for this is the attachment of the fibular sesamoid to the second metatarsal via the deep transverse metatarsal ligament. If deformity persists at the completion of the phalangeal cut, the soft tissue around the entire undersurface of the first metatarsal neck is stripped with a periosteal elevator. The elevator is now turned to the lateral aspect of the metatarsal neck to completely liberate the sesamoid apparatus. Manual reduction of the intermetatarsal deformity is performed by squeezing the first to the second metatarsals while sutures are inserted into the inferior capsular flap and the metatarsal is held and maintained in a reduced position. When the intermetatarsal deformity is closed down, the capsule is imbricated up against the first metatarsal with a combination of sutures into the medial aspect of the metatarsal neck and into the dorsal surface of the capsular flap dorsally, which is then imbricated over the inferior layer of the capsule. Because of the extensive stripping of the lateral metatarsal neck, avascular necrosis of the metatarsal head is possible, although patients are symptom free because no articular surface is present.

Techniques, tips, and pitfalls

1. The key to resection arthroplasty is the balance of the amount of bone that is resected from the base of the proximal phalanx. Resect too much bone, and the hallux will be sloppy, unstable, and weak with transfer of weight bearing to the second metatarsal (Fig. 1–1d–3). Remove too little bone, and the hallux MP joint will be stiff and potentially painful.

2. Regardless of the amount of bone resected, it is useful to try to reattach the volar plate apparatus with the short flexor tendons attached. Reattachment can be made through holes introduced in the base of the proximal phalanx or through preservation of the periosteal sleeve between the ligamentous attachment and the base of the proximal phalanx.

3. As the severity of the hallux valgus increases, bowstringing of the EHL tendon begins. Therefore, lengthening the EHL tendon during this procedure is important to prevent recurrent hallux valgus. A simple Z-plasty lengthening of the tendon is sufficient.

4. I find it unnecessary to perform any temporary internal fixation with pin distraction of the MP joint after the arthroplasty. Provided early range of motion is started, fibrous interposition occurs regardless of any form of internal or external splinting of the hallux. Occasionally, however, temporary internal fixation is useful with correction of severe deformity (Fig. 1–1d–1).

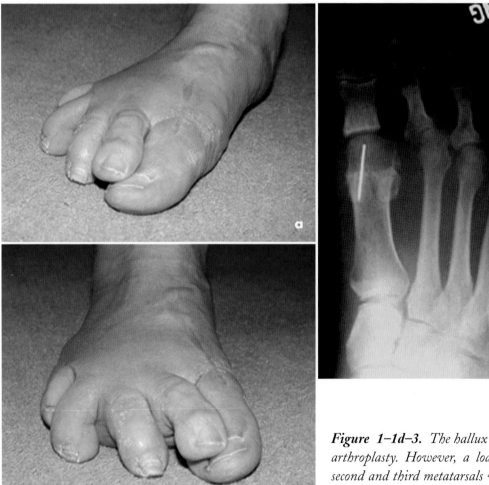

Figure 1–1d–3. *The hallux was painless after this resection arthroplasty. However, a load has been transferred to the second and third metatarsals with painful subluxation of the toes. Too much of the proximal phalanx of the hallux was resected.*

Suggested Readings

Capasso G, Testa V, Maffulli N, Barletta L: Molded arthroplasty and transfer of the extensor hallucis "brevis tendon. A modification of the Keller-Lelievre operation. Clin Orthop Nov: 43–49, 1994. Donley BG, Vaughn RA, Stephenson KA, Richardson EG: Keller resection arthroplasty for treatment of hallux valgus deformity: Increased correction with fibular sesamoidectomy. Foot Ankle Int 23:699–703, 2002.

Myerson MS. Hallux valgus. In Myerson MS (ed). Disorders of the Foot and Ankle. Philadelphia, WB Saunders, 2000.

Myerson MS, Schon LC, McGuigan FX, Oznur A: Result of arthrodesis of the hallux metatarsophalangeal joint using bone graft for restoration of length. Foot Ankle Int 21:297–306, 2000.

Vianna VF, Myerson MS: Complications of hallux valgus surgery. Management of the short first metatarsal and the failed resection arthroplasty. Foot Ankle Clin 3:33–49, 1998.

Proximal Phalangeal Osteotomy (Akin)

A commonly performed procedure for correction of hallux valgus is a closing wedge osteotomy of the proximal phalanx of the hallux that is performed in conjunction with other procedures. By itself, this procedure has few indications. When this osteotomy is performed alone, the incidence of recurrence is exceedingly high because the biomechanical deformity and imbalance around the metatarsophalangeal (MP) joint is uncorrected. However, as an adjunctive procedure with other osteotomies for correction of hallux valgus, the closing wedge phalanx osteotomy's outcome is predictable and reliable.

Although used predominantly for correction of symptomatic hallux valgus, this osteotomy is useful in conjunction with correction of a crossover second toe deformity, even when the hallux valgus is asymptomatic. The main advantage of the closing wedge phalangeal osteotomy is the preservation of the axis of the hallucal MP joint. This preservation is particularly important, for example, with the correction of an abnormal distal metatarsal articular angle. Under most circumstances, correction of the MP joint abnormality with realignment and a biplanar osteotomy of the first metatarsal is preferable. However, with the addition of the phalangeal osteotomy, the hallux shortens slightly. As a result tension on the extrinsic tendons decreases, and correction of the hallucal pronation is easier (Fig. 1–1e–1). Although the closing wedge phalanx osteotomy is of secondary importance, it does improve the cosmetic appearance of the toe.

The incision is made along the medial aspect of the proximal phalanx, extending from the capsule distally toward the interphalangeal (IP) joint, and the periosteum is split. The attachment of the capsule to the base of the proximal phalanx must be preserved to facilitate the capsulorrhaphy. After subperiosteal dissection, small retractors are inserted subcutaneously to expose the bone. Because supinating the hallux is usual, a biplanar osteotomy is generally performed, in addition to the closing wedge phalanx osteotomy. Two sets of pilot holes are now made on either side of the osteotomy with a K-wire. These are unicortical holes inserted at a 45-degree angle with respect to the plane of the phalanx. The proximal set is made in line with the medial aspect of the phalangeal shaft, and then the distal set is drilled more plantarward so that when the osteotomy is closed, the hallux is supinated and the two sets of holes line up with each other. The distal holes are approximately 2 mm inferior to the proximal holes (Fig. 1–1e–2).

The osteotomy is made in metaphyseal bone just distal to the metaphyseal flare. When the proximal cut is made, it must be exactly parallel with the base of the proximal phalanx. Because of the orientation of the phalanx, the surgeon's tendency is to aim laterally, and because of the hallux valgus, this cut has a tendency to be too close to the articular surface. The osteotomy is made in the middle of these holes, and a 2-mm wedge of bone is removed. Preserving the lateral cortex of the phalanx is important. The osteotomy should not cross

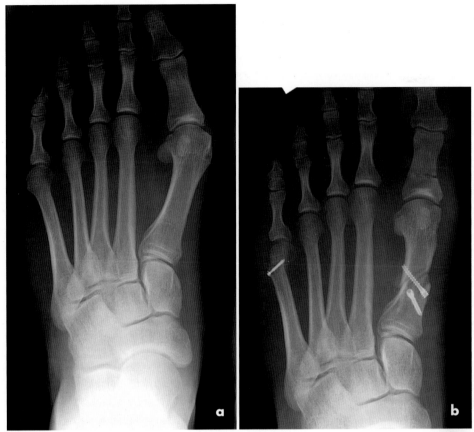

Figure 1–1e–1. *A Ludloff osteotomy was combined with a closing wedge phalangeal osteotomy for correction of this seemingly straightforward deformity that was, however, far more rigid than radiographically apparent. Despite adequate adductor release, the hallux remained in valgus, perhaps because of an incongruent metatarsophalangeal (MP) joint (a, b).*

the cortical surface but should be pried open with a small osteotome, with the lateral cortex cracked. The cortex can then be used as a hinge for closure. Once the osteotomy is complete, the hallux is supinated, and two sutures are inserted across through the predrilled holes. A tapered needle is used, and absorbable 2-0 sutures are used for closure of the osteotomy. This procedure needs neither a screw nor staples; reliable correction can be obtained simply with the suture technique. The hallux should be in the neutral position with respect to the axis of the metatarsal and in slight supination at the completion of the osteotomy (Fig. 1–1e–3).

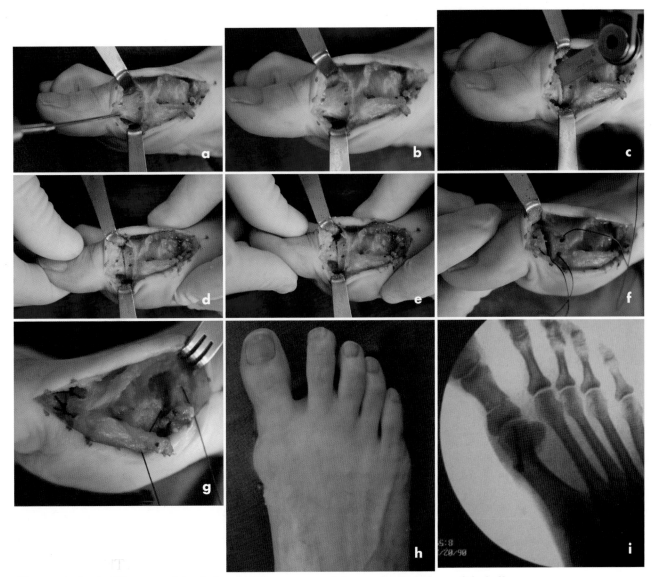

Figure 1–1e–2. *The steps of the closing wedge osteotomy of the proximal phalanx of the hallux are demonstrated. The two sets of pilot holes are balanced to facilitate rotation of the phalanx (a, b). The 1-mm wedge of bone is removed (c), and the osteotomy is closed (d). The hallux is then supinated to line up the pilot holes (e), and sutures are inserted (f). The capsule is repaired through a K-wire hole in the metatarsal cortex (g). The final intraoperative clinical and fluoroscopic appearance (h, i).*

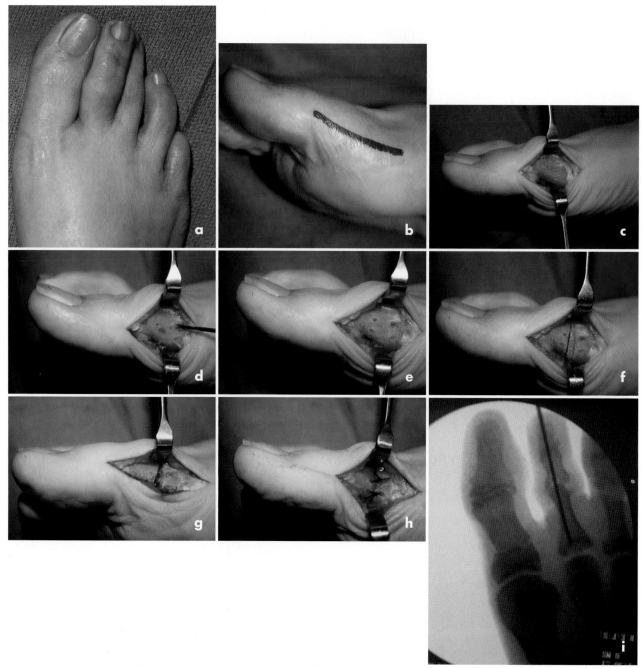

Figure 1–1e–3. *The Akin osteotomy is demonstrated in this patient with asymptomatic hallux valgus but with a deformity of the second toe that could not be corrected without realignment of the hallux (a). The incision is marked out almost to the interphalangeal (IP) joint (b), and the medial phalanx is exposed (c). Four pilot holes are introduced with a 0.062-inch K-wire at a 45-degree angle in two pairs (d, e). The wedge of bone is removed in between the pilot holes and is approximately 1 to 2 mm thick (f, g). The osteotomy is secured with two 2-0 absorbable sutures (h). The intraoperative x-ray (XR) image is presented (i).*

Management of Complications following Correction of Hallux Valgus

Nonunion

With any nonunion, an avascular segment of bone at the nonunion interface is likely, with shortening of the metatarsal, but further shortening is also likely once debridement has been performed. Debridement is required to obtain bone bleeding and healing, but this debridement inevitably leads to further shortening and the likelihood of increasing lateral metatarsalgia. Therefore the approach to correction depends on the presence of existing metatarsalgia, the amount of shortening already present in the first metatarsal, the presence of any arthritis in the metatarsophalangeal (MP) joint, and any associated soft tissue problems.

The presence of soft tissue problems, including scarring, contracture, and neuritis, must be taken into consideration with any revision of forefoot procedures. Unfortunately an increase of further scarring and stiffening at the MP joint is likely with many revision metatarsal procedures. Regardless of the bone correction and the ultimate alignment obtained, the potential for failure due to stiffness of the MP joint must be considered. Stiffness can be global and include not only the MP joint, but also the sesamoid apparatus. Although healed bones and improved alignment are worthwhile goals, potential worsening of any scarring, neuritis, and stiffness of the MP joint must be considered.

Because of this concern, arthrodesis is an appealing choice for many revision procedures. This is particularly the case when the deformity and disease involve the MP joint only. If the hallux interphalangeal (IP) joint is contracted or deformed, then MP arthrodesis may not be the preferred procedure.

With repair of a nonunion, the issues therefore are whether a structural bone graft can be used to restore length or whether primary bone healing can be obtained through supplementation of a cancellus bone graft. It is generally easier to obtain fixation of the diaphysis but easier to obtain bone healing in the metaphysis. Nonunion of a distal metatarsal osteotomy is unusual. However, repair of the nonunion and simultaneous adequate fixation of the metatarsal head in appropriate alignment are difficult.

During the operation, the surgeon must establish the correct length of the metatarsal with a laminar spreader after debridement at the osteotomy nonunion site (Fig. 1–1f–1). Once I have stretched the metatarsal back out to its appropriate length, multiple K-wires are inserted transversely among the first, second, and third metatarsals to stabilize the first metatarsal in the desired position while fixation options are explored. The same applies to repair of a malunion or nonunion of the metatarsal head after a distal metatarsal osteotomy (Figs 1–1f–2 and 1–1f–3).

41

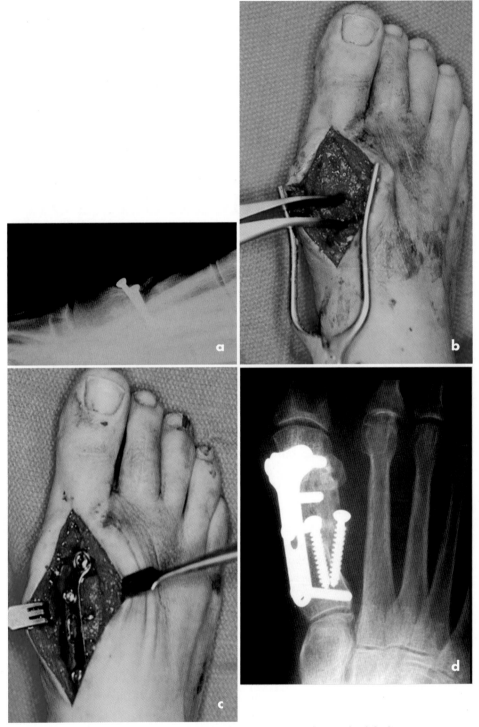

Figure 1-1f-1. *A nonunion of this metatarsal osteotomy of unknown type is noted with short-ening and elevation of the first metatarsal (a). A laminar spreader was used to establish the length of the metatarsal after debridement of the nonunion (b), followed by insertion of a tricortical bone graft and a plate to maintain the alignment (c). The final x-ray (XR) appearance (d).*

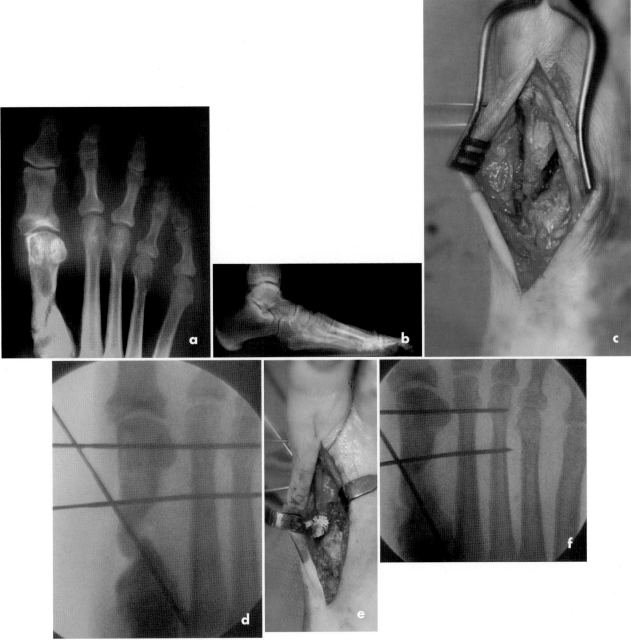

Figure 1–1f–2. *Management of this symptomatic nonunion of a proximal metatarsal osteotomy. Note the appearance of the nonunion, with elevation and shortening of the first metatarsal (a, b). The nonunion was identified and loosened, and the metatarsal was then distracted distally to restore length (c, d). Once this was done, cancellous allograft chips were inserted (e, f).*

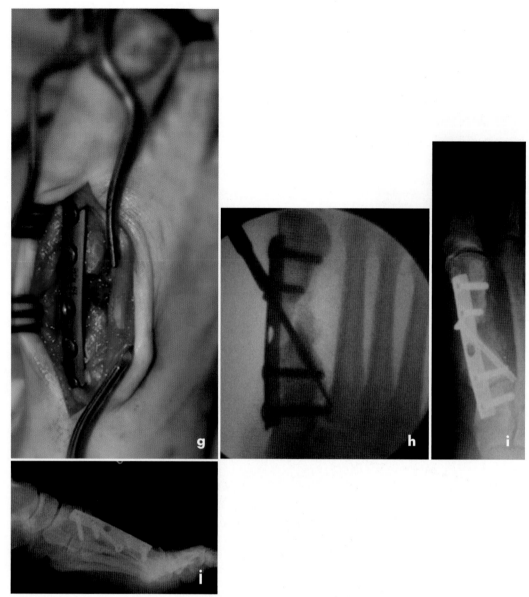

Figure 1–1f–2, cont'd. *Cannulated screw and plate fixation was performed (g, h). The final x-ray (XR) film appearance (i, j).*

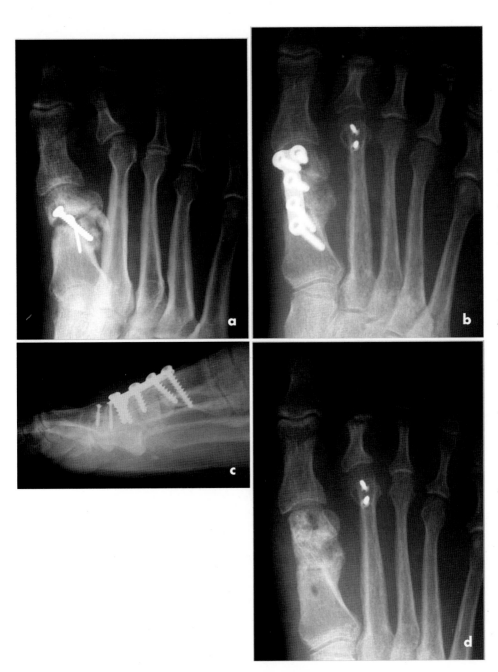

Figure 1–1f–3. *Nonunion of this distal metatarsal osteotomy was associated with marked bone loss and shortening of the metatarsal, but also preservation of the blood supply to the hallux (a). Lengthening of the first metatarsal with interposition structural allograft was performed with a small T-plate to hold the position of the reduction (b). This was combined with slight shortening of the second metatarsal (b, c). Adequate bone healing of the osteotomy occurred, and despite the radiographic appearance, no symptomatic arthritis was present, with 45 degrees of motion at the metatarsophalangeal (MP) joint after plate removal (d).*

Avascular Necrosis

Correction of avascular necrosis depends on the extent of MP joint arthritis and the shortening of the metatarsal. The decision to perform an arthrodesis depends on the extent of the avascular necrosis, but under most circumstances, this operation will be required. More important is the decision to lengthen the first metatarsal and restore the appropriate weight bearing to the hallux with an interpositional structural graft (Figs 1–1f–4 and 1–1f–5). Bear in mind that because bone often has to be resected until bleeding is obtained, the metatarsal further shortens. Wherever possible, I prefer to perform an arthrodesis without any structural graft because the rate of fusion is considerably lower with the latter approach. The decision is based on the extent of the shortening and on the metatarsalgia present. Additional procedures may need to be performed for correction of metatarsalgia, including shortening osteotomies or resection of all of the lesser metatarsal heads. The latter salvage procedure, in conjunction with an arthrodesis (a rheumatoid-type forefoot operation), should be reserved only for patients with severe forefoot deformity with involve-

Figure 1–1f–4. *Avascular necrosis occurred after this distal metatarsal osteotomy of unknown type (a, b). Severe shortening and necrosis were present, with a cock–up deformity of the hallux. This was salvaged with a bone block arthrodesis of the metatarsophalangeal (MP) joint with a structural allograft.*

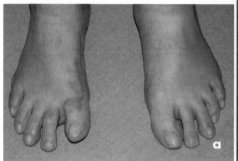
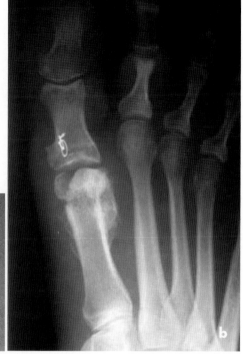

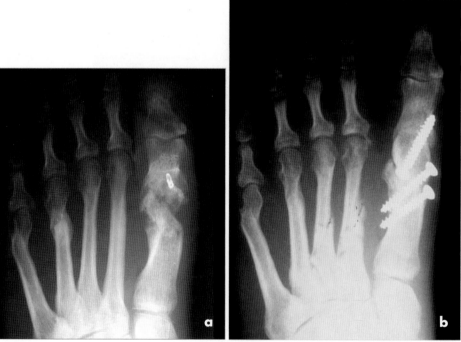

Figure 1–1f–5. *Avascular necrosis with shortening of the first metatarsal occurred in this patient after a distal metatarsal osteotomy of unknown type (a). Severe metatarsalgia of the second and third metatarsals was present (note that an osteotomy of the fourth and fifth metatarsals had been previously performed). An arthrodesis of the hallux metatarsophalangeal (MP) joint was performed with structural bone graft and screw fixation. An oblique proximal shortening osteotomy of the second and third metatarsals was performed simultaneously (b).*

ment of the lesser metatarsal heads and MP joints. This procedure does, however, give excellent relief despite the decrease in function of the lesser toes (Fig. 1–1f–6).

Infection

The approach to correction of infection depends on the extent of the bone involvement. If the infection involves the MP joint, arthroplasty or arthrodesis ultimately needs to be performed. The only problem with these single-stage procedures is the predictability of

eradication of infection before resection arthroplasty or arthrodesis is performed. For this reason, I use antibiotic-impregnated bone cement as a staged procedure and then return at 6 weeks to perform the definitive arthrodesis or arthroplasty (Figs. 1–1f–7 and 1–1f–8). If arthroplasty is to be performed, then once the cement is removed, realignment of the MP joint can be performed as an interposition arthroplasty as described elsewhere in this chapter (Figs. 1–1f–9 and 1–1f–10). One alternative with which I have recently had experience is the use of a fresh osteoarticular allograft. Once infection is under complete control, an antibiotic cement spacer is

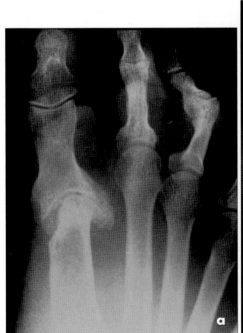
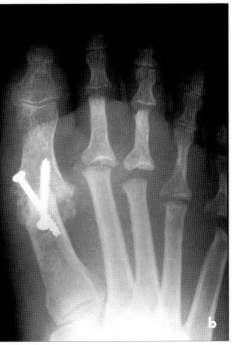

Figure 1–1f–6. Avascular necrosis was associated with severe metatarsalgia and toe deformities in this elderly patient (a). An arthrodesis was performed in situ with resection of the lesser metatarsal heads, instead of a lengthening of the first metatarsal with a graft (b).

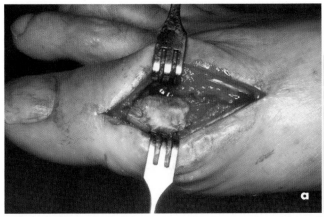
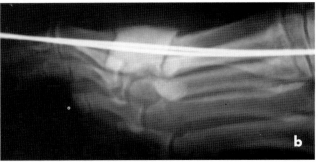

Figure 1–1f–7. Infection after an implant arthroplasty with osteomyelitis was treated with staged interposition of antibiotic cement (a). The hallux was held in alignment with K-wires (b), although these wires are not always necessary if the cement and hallux are stable.

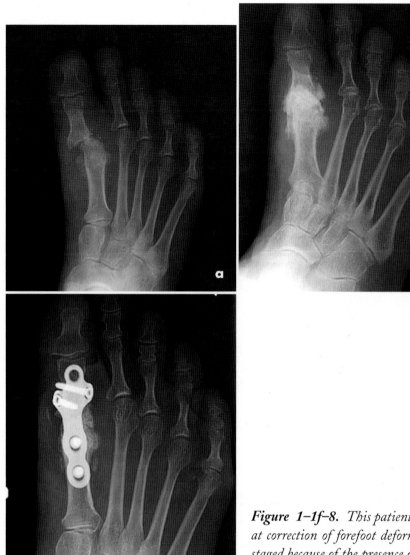

Figure 1–1f–8. *This patient had osteomyelitis after failed multiple attempts at correction of forefoot deformity (a). An arthrodesis was planned but was staged because of the presence of infection, and antibiotic–impregnated cement was used for 6 weeks as a temporary spacer (b), followed by arthrodesis with plate fixation (c).*

inserted until a suitable fresh graft is available. Bone healing at the margin of the metatarsal graft is excellent, although the range of motion of the MP joint may be somewhat limited. The long-term outcome for these grafts is unknown, but at 2 years' follow-up after these procedures, this technique remains encouraging (Fig. 1–1f–11).

Dorsal Malunion and Recurrent Deformity

The management of a dorsal malunion of the proximal metatarsal osteotomy can be difficult. Although performing a plantar flexion osteotomy of the first metatarsal may seem logical, this osteotomy is not easy to perform because of dorsal soft tissue contracture. Usually the dorsal malunion is accompanied by a shortening of the hallux extensors. With a plantar flexion osteotomy of the first metatarsal, further tightening occurs with a potential for recurrent deformity and a cock-up deformity (Fig. 1–1f–12).

The alternative procedures are an opening wedge osteotomy with bone graft, a closing wedge osteotomy through resection of a plantar-based wedge, and a dome osteotomy. A dome osteotomy can be performed from the medial aspect of the metatarsal with a crescentic saw blade inserted perpendicular to the metatarsal. This is

Text continued on p. 53

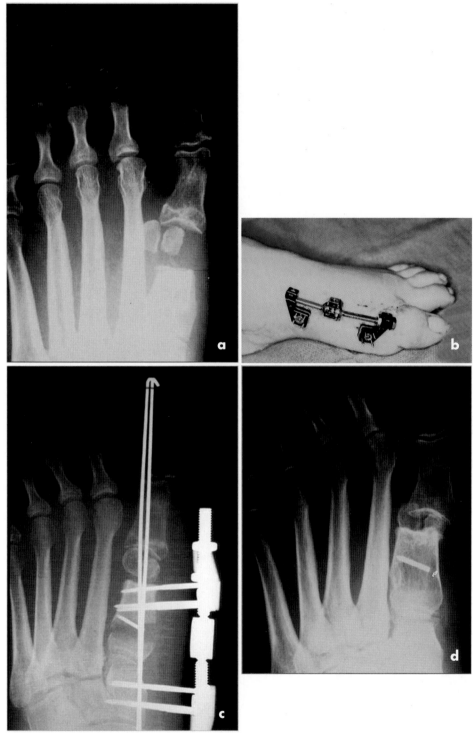

Figure 1–1f–9. *This patient had gross shortening of the metatarsal after resection of most of the metatarsal for osteomyelitis following a distal metatarsal osteotomy. The metatarsal was so short that even with an interpositional structural graft, it was considered too short for adequate function (a). For this reason, staged operations were performed, first with a lengthening with a mini-external fixator, with a length gain of 18 mm (b–d).*

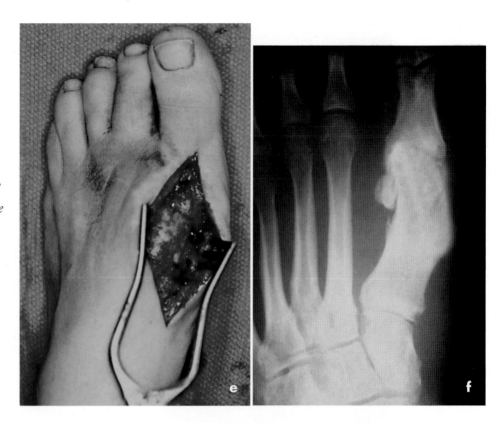

Figure 1–1f–9, cont'd.
Followed by insertion of a structural allograft (e), which was secured with large threaded pins. The final appearance of the metatarsal 2 years later, with healing of the graft and maintenance of alignment (f).

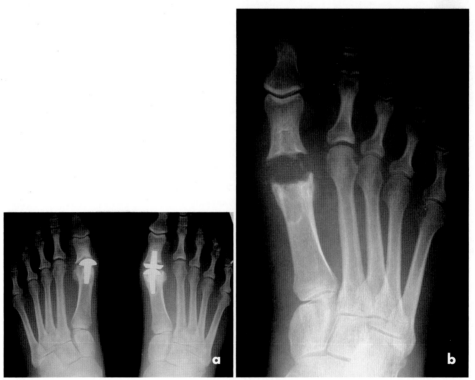

Figure 1–1f–10. *This patient received treatment for severe bilateral metatarsophalangeal (MP) joint pain with limited motion after bilateral implant arthroplasties. The right foot was infected, but the left foot was uninfected (a). The right foot was treated first with removal of the implant and a staged interposition arthroplasty with a rolled up tendon allograft (b).*

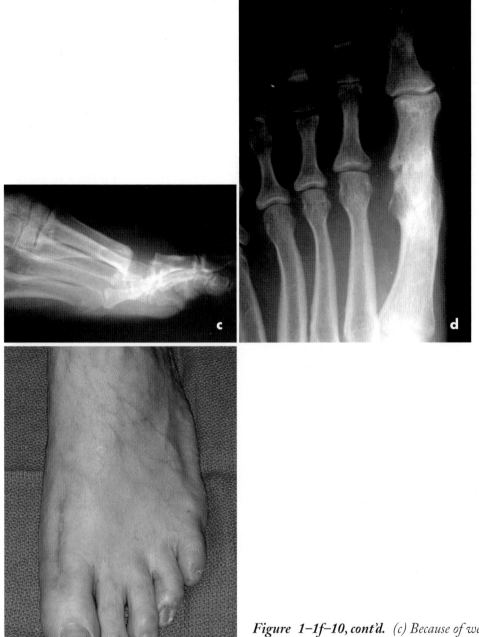

Figure 1–1f–10, cont'd. *(c) Because of weakness, the patient desired restoration of length and strength in the contralateral hallux, and an interposition arthrodesis was performed with structural graft. The images at 4 years after the latter procedure (d, e).*

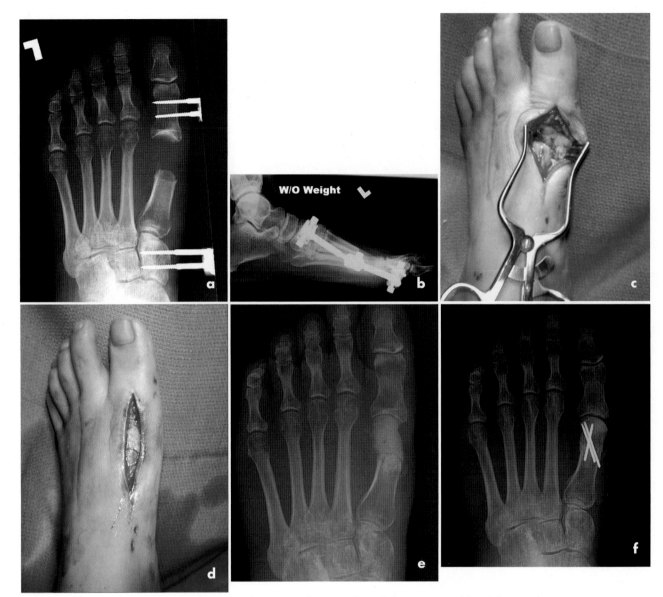

Figure 1–1f–11. *This patient underwent treatment after resection of the metatarsal head for presumed infection following a distal metatarsal osteotomy (a, b). The fixator had been applied elsewhere, and drainage from the incision persisted. The alternatives for treatment included a structural bone graft, metatarsal lengthening, and arthroplasty. After repeated bone and joint debridements (c), an antibiotic-impregnated cement spacer was inserted to maintain length (d, e), and a fresh osteoarticular allograft followed 4 months later. The radiographic appearance of the hallux 18 months later (f).*

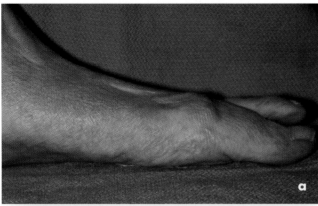

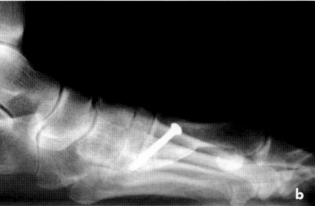

Figure 1–1f–12. Dorsal malunion after a proximal crescentic osteotomy occurred in this patient who underwent treatment of painful limitation of motion of the hallux and metatarsalgia of the second metatarsal (a, b).

an excellent technique because no further shortening of the metatarsal occurs. However, the radius of curvature of the blade is not large enough to accommodate the plain of the metatarsal. For this reason, the crescentic saw blade can be used on the plantar three quarters of the metatarsal. Then the osteotomy can be completed dorsally with a vertical step cut, through which a screw can be inserted for fixation. The other option is an opening wedge osteotomy with insertion of graft as shown for a malunion after a Lapidus procedure (Fig. 1–1f–13).

Malunion occurs for many reasons, most of which are due to incorrect use of a metatarsal osteotomy, undercorrection, inappropriate use of fixation of the osteotomy, the inherent nature or potential for instability based on the geometry of the osteotomy, or instability of the first tarsometatarsal (TMT). Figure 1–1f–14 shows an unusual case of delayed union and then malunion as a result of unrecognized neuropathy. The correction of malunion can be frustratingly difficult because of soft tissue contracture, scarring, neuritis, bone loss, and multiplanar deformity (Fig. 1–1f–15). Although I follow standard principles of correction based on the deformity, the deformity is frequently amenable to correction with a modified Lapidus procedure.

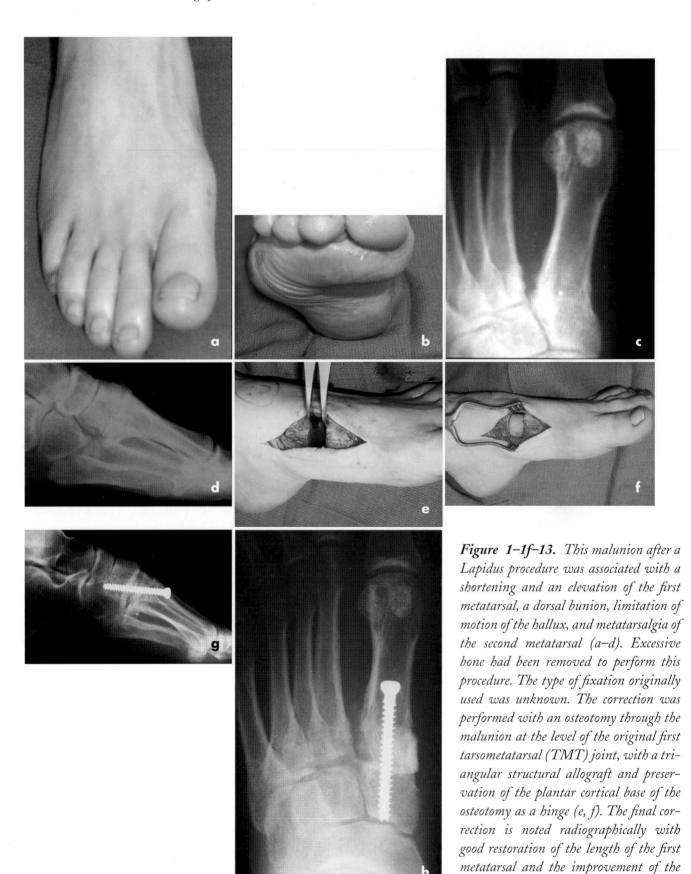

Figure 1–1f–13. *This malunion after a Lapidus procedure was associated with a shortening and an elevation of the first metatarsal, a dorsal bunion, limitation of motion of the hallux, and metatarsalgia of the second metatarsal (a–d). Excessive bone had been removed to perform this procedure. The type of fixation originally used was unknown. The correction was performed with an osteotomy through the malunion at the level of the original first tarsometatarsal (TMT) joint, with a triangular structural allograft and preservation of the plantar cortical base of the osteotomy as a hinge (e, f). The final correction is noted radiographically with good restoration of the length of the first metatarsal and the improvement of the declination and metatarsalgia (g, h).*

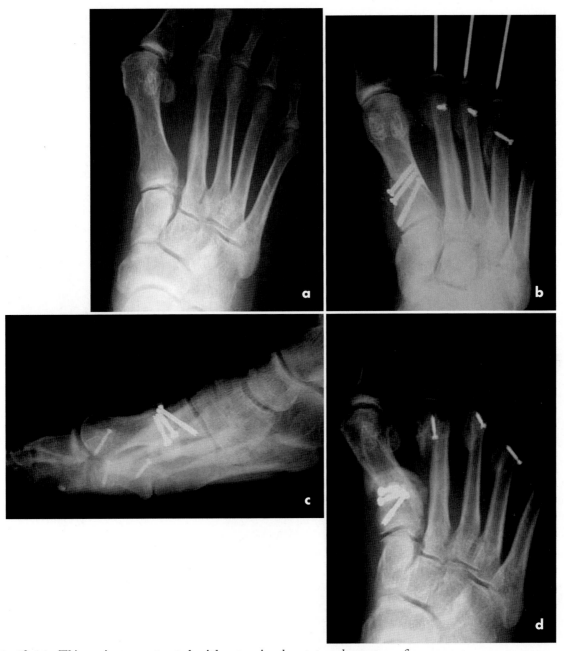

Figure 1–1f–14. *This patient was treated with a proximal metatarsal osteotomy for correction of deformity in conjunction with Weil osteotomies of the lesser metatarsals (a, b). This patient had unrecognized neuropathy, and despite adequate immobilization, delayed union and ultimately severe malunion occurred (c, d).* Continued

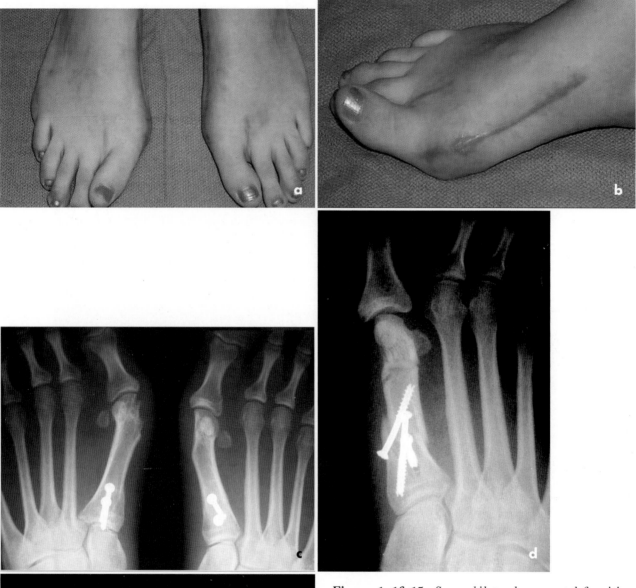

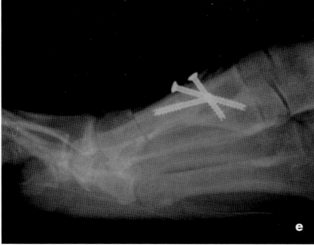

Figure 1–1f–15. *Severe bilateral recurrent deformities were present in this adolescent after what appeared to be closing wedge osteotomies of the proximal first metatarsal (a–c). Note the scarring; the hallux valgus; and, in particular, the excessive resection of the medial eminence leading to an iatrogenic increase in the distal metatarsal articular angle (DMAA) (c). The problem with this deformity is the abnormal DMAA because correction of the first metatarsal will increase the metatarsophalangeal (MP) joint abnormality. This problem was corrected with a double osteotomy, including a modified Ludloff osteotomy proximally, and a closing wedge osteotomy at the metatarsal neck to improve the DMAA. The immediate postoperative radiographs (d, e).*

Suggested Readings

Myerson MS. Hallux valgus. In Myerson MS (ed). Disorders of the Foot and Ankle. Philadelphia, WB Saunders, 2000.

Myerson MS, Miller S, Henderson MR, Saxby T. Staged arthrodesis for salvage of the septic hallux metatarsophalangeal joint. Clin Orthop 307:174–181, 1994.

Myerson MS, Schon LC, McGuigan FX, Oznur A. Result of arthrodesis of the hallux metatarsophalangeal joint using bone graft for restoration of length. Foot Ankle Int 21:297–306, 2000.

Richardson EG. Complications after hallux valgus surgery. Instr Course Lect 48:331–342, 1999.

Sammarco GJ, Idusuyi OB. Complications after surgery of the hallux. Clin Orthop 391:59–71, 2001.

Vianna VF, Myerson MS. Complications of hallux valgus surgery. Management of the short first metatarsal and the failed resection arthroplasty. Foot Ankle Clin 3:33–49, 1998.

Hallux Varus

Decision Making for Correction

The type of treatment for correction of hallux varus is determined by the flexibility of the metatarsophalangeal (MP) and interphalangeal (IP) joints. Imbalance is always present between the flexor hallucis brevis (FHB) and the extensor hallucis brevis (EHB) muscles and between the abductor hallucis and adductor hallucis muscles. With this imbalance, the deformity gradually increases, and this increase will cause a spectrum of fixed and flexible deformities of the MP and IP joints, with or without arthritis of either joint. Fortunately, the IP joint remains flexible for most hallux varus deformities. Over time, however, with increasing imbalance of the FHB and EHB muscles, a contracture of the IP joint occurs. If this contracture is rigid or if arthritis of the IP joint is present, an arthrodesis of this joint is necessary (Fig. 1–2–1). If IP contracture is present but the joint is flexible, then I would try to manipulate the joint because release of this contracture is not successful. Once an arthrodesis of the IP joint is performed, the MP joint must be corrected either dynamically with a tendon transfer or statically through restoration of ligament stability with a tenodesis.

Maintaining MP joint mobility is ideal but not always possible because of arthritis or rigid contracture. In the presence of a rigid deformity with contracture of the MP joint both in varus and extension, the likelihood of attaining soft-tissue balance with a tendon transfer is unlikely, and an arthrodesis of the MP joint is preferable for patients with this deformity. However, a resection arthroplasty of the MP joint can be considered for some patients, because arthrodesis of the MP joint should not be performed if the IP joint is deformed. This situation presents a difficult treatment decision in the occasional patient who has arthritis of the MP joint and rigid contracture of the IP joint or vice versa. The addition of an arthrodesis of the IP joint to an arthrodesis of the MP joint is not ideal because of the significant rigidity and potential problems with toe-off. For these patients, an arthrodesis of the IP joint can be combined with a resection arthroplasty of the MP joint.

Therefore, wherever possible, tendon transfer should be used to correct the deformity. However, tendon transfer is contraindicated if either arthritis or rigidity of the MP joint is present (Fig. 1–2–2).

Deformity of the first metatarsal is another contraindication to tendon transfer alone. For example, malunion of the first metatarsal, either from a distal or proximal metatarsal osteotomy, may be present but associated with a flexible MP joint. This is the result of overcorrection of the metatarsal with a negative intermetatarsal angle, leading to medial subluxation of the MP joint and hallux varus. If the malunion of the first metatarsal is left uncorrected, the tendon transfer will not correct the soft-tissue imbalance. Correction of the metatarsal alignment with osteotomy must then be performed in conjunction with a tendon transfer, which can be performed simultaneously.

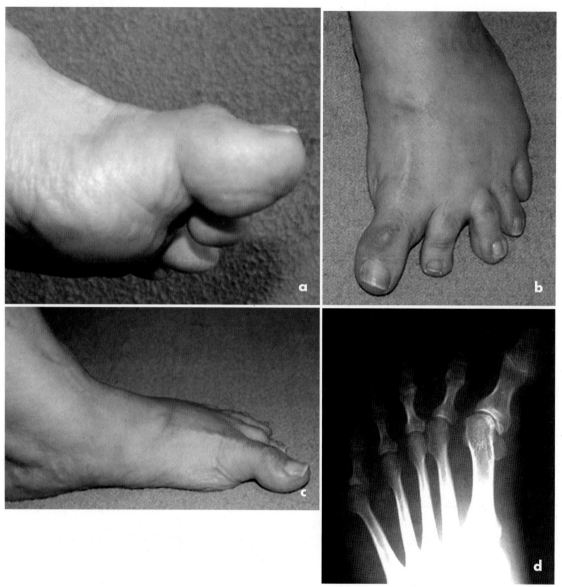

Figure 1–2–1. *The clinical and radiographic appearance of hallux varus associated with a flexible metatarsophalangeal (MP) joint but a fixed contracted interphalangeal (IP) joint. Despite the x-ray (XR) film, given the flexibility, this patient is a good candidate for an IP fusion and either a split extensor hallucis longus (EHL) or extensor hallucis brevis (EHB) tenodesis.*

Tendon Transfer and Tenodesis

I divide the surgical approach into those procedures that primarily address the soft tissues (abductor hallucis tendon release, tendon transfer, or tenodesis), the bone (first metatarsal osteotomy, hallux proximal phalangeal osteotomy), or the joint (arthrodesis of the IP joint and arthrodesis or resection arthroplasty of the MP joint). If a soft-tissue procedure is performed, the hallux MP joint must have balance around it after surgery. Therefore the abductor hallucis tendon should be lengthened or cut, and a medial capsulotomy should be performed in conjunction with the lateral stabilizing procedure. Rarely, if hallux varus occurs immediately postoperatively as a result of over-plication of the medial capsule, simple release of the abductor tendon or capsule may be sufficient. For all other situations, tendon and soft-tissue balancing needs to be performed.

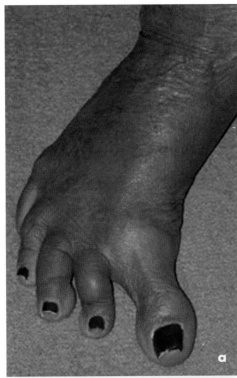

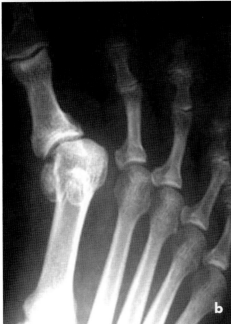

Figure 1–2–2. This deformity was flexible; however, irreversible changes have taken place in the hallux metatarsophalangeal (MP) joint, precluding correction with a tendon transfer. A fusion or arthroplasty of the MP joint is required, in addition to correction of the lesser toe deformities. Even though the hallux is flexible and will be well realigned after arthrodesis, the toes will not necessarily return to a neutral position and will require correction.

Tendon Transfers

Various tendon transfers are available for correction of dynamic deformity. The use of the entire extensor hallucis longus (EHL) tendon in conjunction with arthrodesis of the IP joint has been described in the literature. This is not my preferred procedure unless rigid deformity of the IP joint is present. In this case, arthrodesis is necessary. If the IP joint is flexible, fusing the joint is unnecessary, and in this instance, either a portion of the EHL tendon (a split transfer of the EHL tendon) or a transfer with the EHB tendon is performed (Fig. 1–2–3). Distinguishing a tendon transfer, which has the potential for dynamic correction of deformity, from a tenodesis in which the tendon is used statically is important (Fig. 1–2–4). Both procedures apply to the EHL and EHB tendon transfer. One of the problems I have experienced with the split EHL tendon transfer is that when the tendon is split from proximal to distal and the lateral half of the tendon is used for the transfer, the medial half of the EHL tendon never retains adequate tension. This imbalance and loss of tension in the

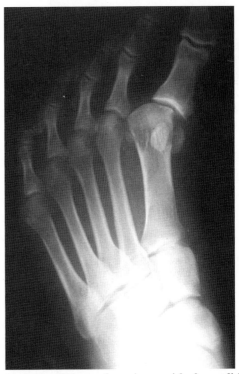

Figure 1–2–3. This patient is an ideal candidate for tendon transfer or tenodesis. However, for correction to be maintained, the lesser toes must be corrected simultaneously with relaxation of the intrinsic contracture with shortening lesser metatarsal osteotomies.

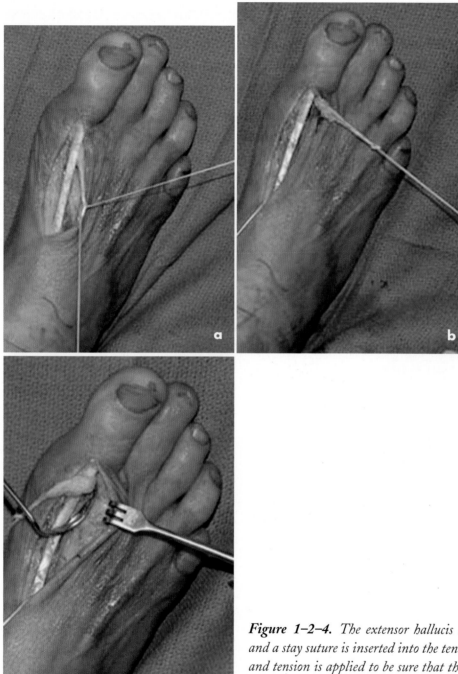

Figure 1–2–4. *The extensor hallucis brevis (EHB) is isolated proximally, and a stay suture is inserted into the tendon (a). The tendon is cut proximally, and tension is applied to be sure that this does not tear distally (b). A tapered aneurysm needle is passed from proximal to distal to grasp the suture and pull the tendon proximally (c).*

remaining half of the tendon are unavoidable. This type of transfer effectively lengthens the medial half of the tendon, leading to dorsiflexion weakness. An alternative would be to use the EHL tendon in a tenodesis procedure by splitting the tendon from distal to proximal in the same way that the EHB tenodesis is performed. Generally, keeping the EHL tendon intact is preferable, and in the presence of flexible IP and MP joints, I prefer to use the EHB tendon in a tenodesis procedure.

Through a dorsal longitudinal incision, lateral to the EHL tendon, the EHB tendon is identified and carefully dissected from the EHL tendon and extensor retinaculum. Proximally, the EHB tendon is transected just distal to the musculotendinous junction at the level of the base of the first metatarsal. The EHB tendon must be carefully dissected distal to the MP joint through the release of the extensor hood. The worst that can happen is that the EHB tendon is transected distally, and if the distal attachment of the EHB tendon is tenuous, a suture is inserted to maintain its attachment to the extensor hood. A 2-0 suture is inserted at the end of the transected EHB tendon with a fine needle, and the tendon is then passed under the deep transverse metatarsal ligament from distal to proximal. A blunt-tipped curved tapered needle (an aneurysm needle) works well here. It is not absolutely necessary to pass the tendon under the deep transverse metatarsal ligament, and any firm tether from scar tissue in the first web space is sufficient (Fig. 1–2–5).

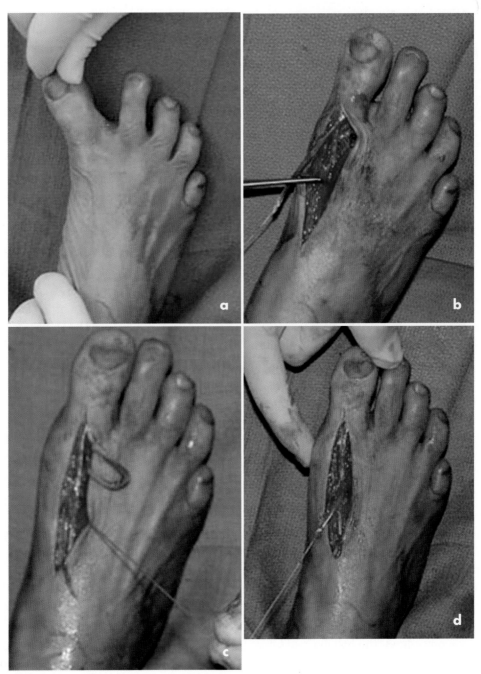

Figure 1–2–5. *This flexible deformity was corrected with a split extensor hallucis longus (EHL) procedure because the extensor hallucis brevis (EHB) tendon was absent. The hallux is flexible (a), and following the split of the tendon from proximal to distal it was passed back with an aneurysm needle (b, c). With tension applied to the tendon stump, the hallux is pulled into varus to check the stability of the tenodesis (d).*   *Continued*

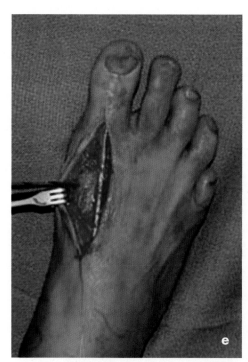

Figure 1–2–5, cont'd. *This step is completed by passing the hallux through a 3-mm drill hole in the metatarsal (e).*

A drill hole is then made from medial to lateral in the distal neck of the first metatarsal, and the tendon is passed through the drill hole and secured under tension. Before the tendon is tightened, adequate balance must be restored. I prefer to see that the hallux is lying in a neutral position after release of the medial capsule and contracted abductor tendon. The length of the EHB tendon is always sufficient to suture it back down over the dorsal periosteum with a nonresorbable suture. I use the EHL tenodesis procedure when the EHL tendon is scarred, torn, or absent. It is performed the same way as that described for the EHB tendon. More tendon from the split EHL tendon is usually available, and the tendon can be passed back onto itself over the dorsal surface of the metatarsal after passage through the drill hole.

After these tenodesis procedures, the hallux should rest in a neutral position, and it should not have to be pushed over at all. Fixing the MP joint with a Kirschner wire during surgery should not be necessary. I like to tape the hallux in a slightly overcorrected position in slight valgus for 2 months. The patients are allowed to bear weight immediately after this procedure while wearing a post-operative walking shoe. After 4 weeks patients are allowed to use a stiff soled shoe. Toe-off with bending of the MP joint should not be allowed for 8 weeks.

Arthrodesis and Resection Arthroplasty

For correction of either arthritis or rigid deformity at the MP joint, I prefer to use an arthrodesis. Occasionally, either because of a fixed, contracted IP joint or patient preference, I perform a resection arthroplasty. If either of these procedures is performed, further soft-tissue balancing is usually not required.

For the resection arthroplasty, the cut of the base of the proximal phalanx must be vertical. The surgeon should be careful with the plane of the cut to prevent any further inadvertent dorsiflexion of the MP joint, and the hallux varus deformity can be addressed with a cut perpendicular to the long axis of the proximal phalanx or with a slight valgus inclination. This arthroplasty needs to be performed in conjunction with complete release of the medial joint contracture. Arthrodesis of the MP joint is performed as described in the section on arthrodesis (see Chapter 13–1). However, because of the aberrant position of the metatarsal head, the prior medial exostectomy, and the malunion of the first metatarsal, arthrodesis needs to be carefully performed. I have found that it is difficult to accurately position the hallux as a result of various deformities around the MP joint. The normal landmarks for positioning the phalanx on the first metatarsal cannot always be followed, and using the clinical position of the hallux to guide the final position for the arthrodesis is often easier.

Note the effect of the hallux varus on the rest of the forefoot, particularly the lesser toes. If the hallux is in marked varus, over time it will pull the lesser toes into varus as well (Fig. 1–2–6). The toes will not return to a normal position even after excellent correction of the hallux deformity and must be realigned with the hallux. Standard correction of lesser toe deformity such as capsulotomy and release of the medial collateral ligament is not sufficient, even if followed by prolonged immobilization with a K-wire. I have found that the shortening of the metatarsal (which indirectly lengthens the intrinsic muscles and hence the contracture) is ideal.

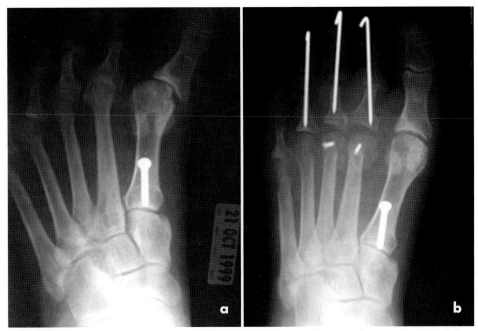

Figure 1–2–6. *This deformity was flexible. There was neither crepitus nor pain with range of motion of the hallux metatarsophalangeal (MP) joint. Dislocation of the second toe MP joint and severe subluxation of the third and fourth MP joints were present (a). These were corrected with a tenodesis procedure of the extensor hallucis brevis (EHB) tendon; arthrodesis of the second, third, and fourth proximal interphalangeal (PIP) joints; and a Weil osteotomy of the second and third metatarsals. The K-wires were removed from the toes at 4 weeks after surgery.*

Techniques, tips, and pitfalls

1. No procedure adequately corrects a hallux varus if a malunion of a metatarsal osteotomy is present, even when an arthrodesis of the MP joint is performed. The malunion must first be corrected (Fig. 1–2–7).

2. If hallux varus occurs immediately postoperatively as a result of either an excessively tight capsulorrhaphy or soft tissue release, then correction is possible with prompt taping of the hallux into valgus for 8 weeks (Fig. 1–2–8).

3. If the hallux IP joint is fixed in flexion, an arthrodesis of the IP joint must be performed. However, an array of procedures may be performed at the MP joint ranging from arthroplasty to tendon transfer. Simultaneous arthrodesis of the IP and MP joints is not desirable (Fig. 1–2–9 and Fig. 1–2–10).

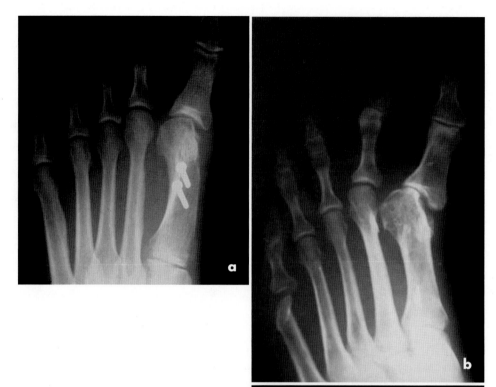

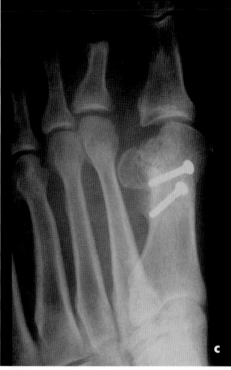

Figure 1–2–7. In each of these examples, a malunion of a metatarsal osteotomy is causing the hallux varus. In a and c, a tendon transfer was performed after correction of the malunion, and in b, an arthrodesis was performed. After the arthrodesis, which was in correct alignment, symptoms persisted because the hallux was too close to the second toe as a result of the metatarsal malunion.

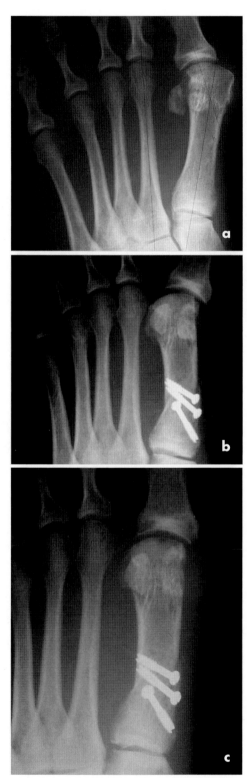

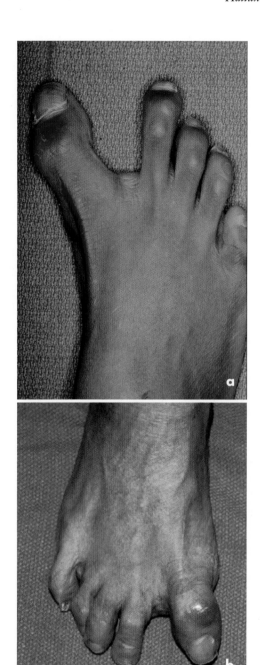

Figure 1–2–9. Fixed contracture of the interphalangeal (IP) joint was present in these patients, corrected with an arthrodesis of the IP joint in both, an extensor hallucis brevis (EHB) tendon transfer in (a), and a resection arthroplasty of the metatarsophalangeal (MP) joint in (b).

Figure 1–2–8. A Ludloff metatarsal osteotomy was performed for correction of hallux valgus, followed by hallux varus at the first postoperative evaluation (a, b). Taping of the hallux into valgus for 8 weeks resulted in excellent alignment with good scarring of the lateral joint capsule (c).

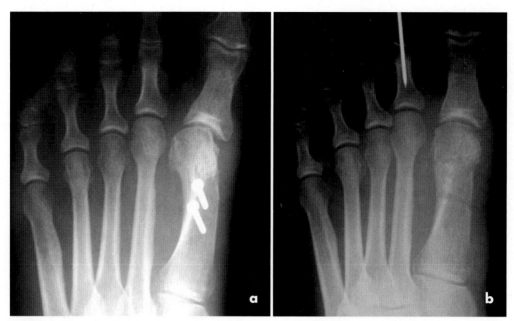

Figure 1–2-10. *Malunion of a distal metatarsal osteotomy (a) was corrected with removal of the screws, a closing wedge osteotomy of the metatarsal neck, and extensor hallucis brevis (EHB) tendon transfer (b).*

Suggested Readings

Donley BG: Acquired hallux varus. Foot Ankle Int 18:586–592, 1997.

Juliano PJ, Myerson MS, Cunningham BW: Biomechanical assessment of a new tenodesis for correction of hallux varus. Foot Ankle Int 17:17–20, 1996.

Lau JT, Myerson MS: Modified split extensor hallucis longus tendon transfer for correction of hallux varus. Foot Ankle Int 23:1138–1140, 2002.

Myerson M: Hallux varus. In Myerson MS (ed): Current Therapy in Foot and Ankle Surgery. St. Louis, Mosby-Year Book, 1993, pp 70–73.

Myerson MS: Hallux valgus. In Myerson MS (ed): Foot and Ankle Disorders. Philadelphia, WB Saunders, 2000.

Myerson MS, Komenda GA: Results of hallux varus correction using an extensor hallucis brevis tenodesis. Foot Ankle Int 17(1):21–7, 1996.

Skalley TC, Myerson MS: The operative treatment of acquired hallux varus. Clin Orthop 306:183–191, 1994.

Trnka HJ, Zettl R, Hungerford M, et al: Acquired hallux varus and clinical tolerability. Foot Ankle Int 18:593–597, 1997.

Hallux Rigidus

Overview of Surgery

Surgical correction of hallux rigidus is fairly predictable, and patient acceptance and outcome should be good. Many surgical alternatives are available, all based on the underlying anatomy, disease, and extent of arthritis. To some extent, patient needs for activities and shoe wear do play a role, but in general, these should not influence the decision making for the type of surgery. In my own practice, the cheilectomy, with or without an osteotomy at the base of the proximal phalanx (Moberg osteotomy), is the most predictable operation for correction of hallux rigidus. Although I perform arthrodesis frequently, I have experienced excellent results with interposition arthroplasty and more recently from implant hemiarthroplasty for the management of the more severe grades of arthritis. Arthrodesis continues to be a mainstay of treatment for severe arthritis, particularly if associated with deformity.

Rarely is osteotomy of the first metatarsal necessary. Elevation of the first metatarsal does not have any role in the pathogenesis of hallux rigidus (Fig. 1–3–1). However, a correlation exists between metatarsus elevatus and severe grades of hallux rigidus. In patients with both conditions, the elevation of the first metatarsal is secondary to the severe contracture of the intrinsics and retraction of the volar plate and is not a primary deformity. Although osteotomy may be required for correction of primary or congenital

metatarsus elevatus, the notion that a plantar flexion osteotomy of any sort will alleviate impingement dorsally from hallux rigidus should not be assumed. This premise is simply incorrect. The deformity is in the dorsal metatarsal head, and the arthritic segment of the metatarsal head will articulate with the base of the proximal phalanx through plantar flexion of the first metatarsal.

Cheilectomy

Incision and Dissection

An incision is made dorsomedial to the extensor hallucis longus (EHL) tendon extending over the metatarsophalangeal (MTP) joint over a length of 3 cm (Fig. 1–3–2). The dorsal medial cutaneous branch of the superficial peroneal nerve is retracted. The capsule is incised and a cuff of at least 5 mm medially is preserved for later closure. The capsule and periosteum are reflected off the metatarsal neck; this reflection exposes the hypertrophic osteophytes dorsally. Exposing the joint can be difficult because of large osteophytes, but the entire dorsal head must be exposed.

Ostectomy

I prefer to use a chisel to remove the dorsal apical surface of the metatarsal head because this gives me better control than an osteotome or saw. It is placed in the

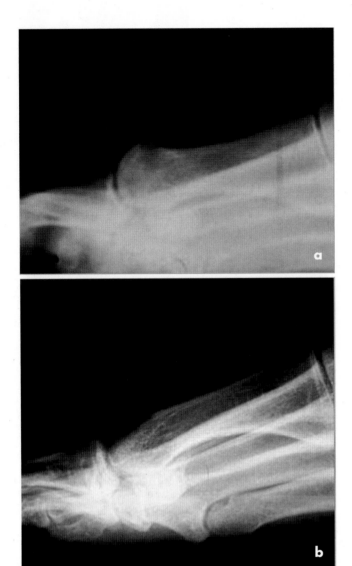

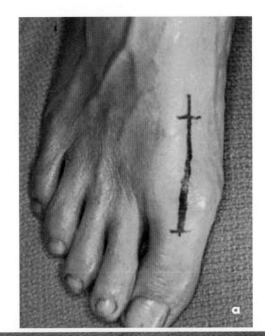

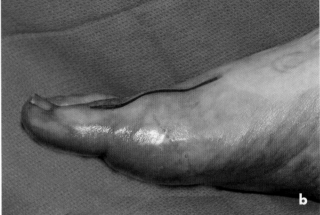

Figure 1–3–1. *Although the first metatarsal is elevated in this patient (a), a metatarsal osteotomy was not considered to be of any benefit. The metatarsophalangeal (MTP) joint was mobile, as was the first metatarsal. A standard cheilectomy was performed (b) with good results and improved motion at the MTP joint after surgery.*

Figure 1–3–2. *The dorsomedial incision is noted (a, b).*

center of the metatarsal head, and one third of the dorsal surface of the metatarsal head is removed (Fig. 1–3–3).

When the head is viewed from above, this seems like a large amount of bone to resect until an x-ray (XR) image is obtained; the image shows how little has actually been removed. The ostectomy must be performed from distal to proximal, with removal of the dorsal osteophytes, and then the medial and lateral margins of the metatarsal

head are contoured. If cysts are present in the metatarsal head, the ostectomy can be performed just dorsal to the erosion, or the head can be drilled with a K-wire, in which case the fibrocartilaginous surface may be improved (Fig. 1–3–4). Rounding off of the metatarsal head is performed with a rongeur and chisel, but the surgeon should be careful not to dissect too far proximally. If the marginal osteophytes need to be removed, they can be removed with the chisel, but going too far proximally on the lateral side of the head can cause avascular necrosis (AVN). The capsular attachment to the medial aspect to the first metatarsal head should be left intact. Dorsiflexion of the MP joint should be approximately 65 degrees after the cheilectomy.

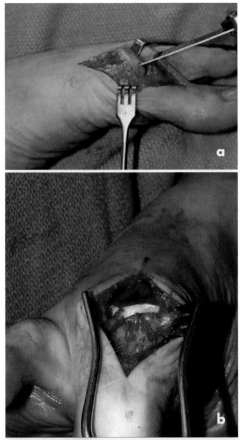

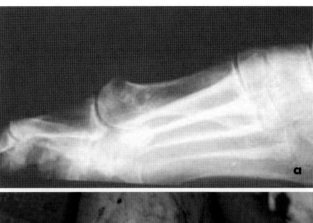

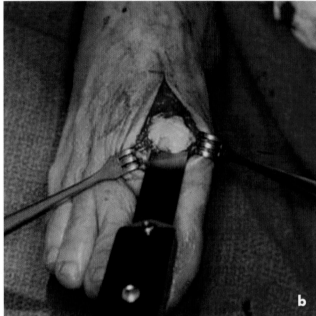

Figure 1–3–4. *A cheilectomy was performed in this patient. Cyst formation in the metatarsal head (a) indicates a more advanced form of arthritis. At surgery, a central defect in the metatarsal head was present, and a cheilectomy was performed. Note that the chisel blade is immediately under the central cartilage erosion (b).*

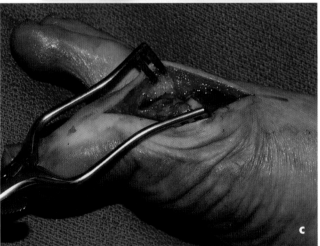

Figure 1–3–3. *The dorsal one third of the metatarsal head is removed with a chisel (a). Note the appearance of the articulation after the cheilectomy (b, c).*

Osteotomy of the Proximal Phalanx (Moberg Osteotomy)

Osteotomy of the proximal phalanx is an easy operation to perform, with a predictable outcome. The hallux is dorsiflexed approximately 10 degrees off the floor. This operation does not increase range of motion of the hallux but simply facilitates clearance of the hallux so that the starting point of the metatarsophalangeal (MTP) joint is already in slightly greater dorsiflexion. I use this operation frequently, mostly for grade II arthritis (Fig. 1–3–5). The procedure is useful when additional "movement" is desirable and, in particular, when patients need an increased dorsiflexion of the hallux because of athletic and shoe wear needs (Fig. 1–3–6). For patients with combined hallux rigidus and mild hallux valgus, a biplanar phalangeal osteotomy is performed to adduct and dorsiflex the hallux simultaneously. This osteotomy is a combination of the Akin and Moberg procedures.

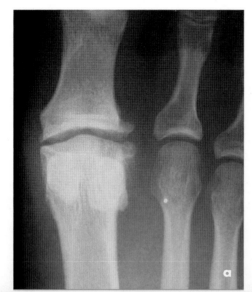

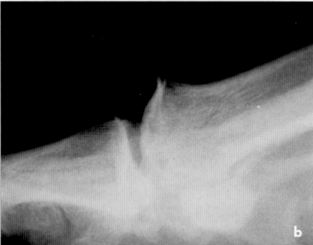

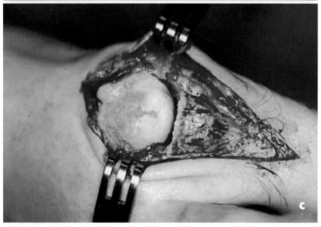

Figure 1-3-5. *Note the flattening out of the metatarsal head and proximal phalanx, a common association with hallux rigidus (a). Reasonable preservation of the joint space is present (b), and a cheilectomy is planned. This patient was a runner and desired more hallux dorsiflexion. A Moberg osteotomy was added to the cheilectomy even though a good joint space was present (c).*

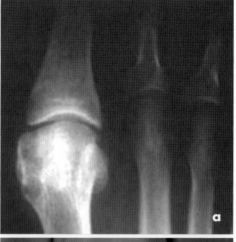

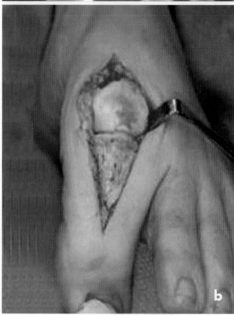

Figure 1-3-6. *The x-ray (XR) appearance of the joint in a patient with hallux rigidus, with good preservation of the joint space (a). At surgery, more erosive changes of the head were noted, and after a cheilectomy, the phalanx osteotomy was performed (b).*

The surgery is usually performed in the setting of hallux rigidus in conjunction with a cheilectomy, and the incision is simply extended more distally over the base of the proximal phalanx. The EHL tendon must be retracted laterally and protected completely during the osteotomy.

The dorsal aspect of the cortex must be well exposed, and two sets of pilot holes are inserted into the dorsal surface of the proximal phalanx. These are made obliquely at 45 degrees with respect to each other. The first set is made just distal to the articular surface, and a second set is approximately 1.5 cm distal to that. These are unicortical pilot holes to be used for later suture fixation, and the osteotomy is planned between these holes. A 1.5-mm slice of bone is removed with a saw. Once the bone wedge is removed, the base of the osteotomy is a bit more than 1.5 mm and must therefore be controlled to prevent a cock-up deformity. A 2-mm margin should be on either side of the predrilled holes after the osteotomy to prevent fracture of the hole and loss of fixation. The plantar cortex of the osteotomy is intact. A greenstick stress closure of the osteotomy is performed first through plantar flexion and then through dorsiflexion of the phalanx to completely close down the osteotomy. I open the osteotomy using an osteotome first, which loosens the plantar cortex but does not loosen the periosteal hinge. The osteotomy is secured with two 2.0-mm sutures that are introduced through the predrilled holes with a curved tapered needle that fits the contour of the holes. These sutures provide excellent stability, and screw, wire, or plate fixation is unnecessary (Fig. 1–3–7).

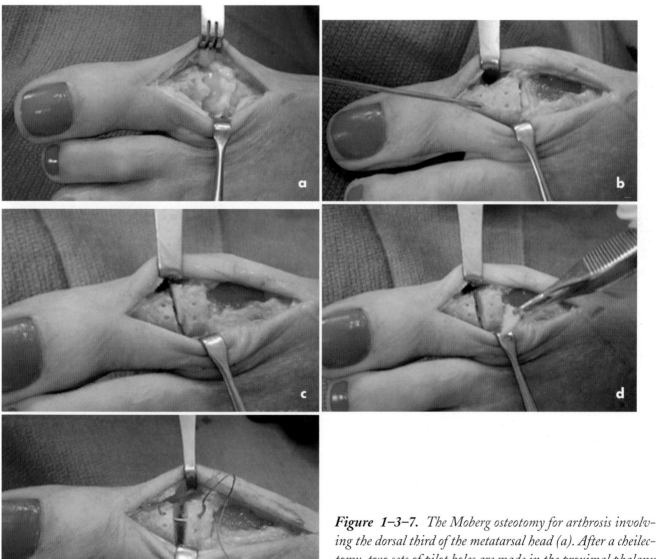

Figure 1–3–7. *The Moberg osteotomy for arthrosis involving the dorsal third of the metatarsal head (a). After a cheilectomy, two sets of pilot holes are made in the proximal phalanx with a 0.062-inch K-wire at a 45-degree angle (b). A 2-mm triangular wedge of bone is removed with a saw (c, d), and the osteotomy is secured with two 2-0 absorbable sutures (e).*

Interposition Arthroplasty

Indications

Interposition arthroplasty is a good procedure that reliably increases the range of motion of the MP joint. Regardless of the technical aspects of this procedure, the interposition of soft tissue is a good concept. This has been described with autogenous and allogeneic tissue that has been harvested locally either from the dorsal MP joint or from other adjacent autogenous tissue. This procedure is contraindicated in someone who already has a short hallux, a short metatarsal, or adjacent metatarsalgia. Clearly, some weakening and obvious shortening of the hallux occur as a result of this operation. Regardless of how the procedure is performed, plantar flexion strength is compromised.

Dissection

The incision is made dorsomedial to the EHL tendon and extends over the MP joint for about 3 cm. The dorsal medial cutaneous branch of the superficial peroneal nerve must be identified and retracted. Once the dissection through the subcutaneous tissue is complete, the extensor retinaculum is cut about 5 mm medial to the EHL tendon to maintain an adequate cuff of tissue for later closure. When the EHL is retracted, the extensor hallucis brevis (EHB) tendon, as well as the dorsal soft tissue and capsule, is exposed over the metatarsal neck. The EHB is now cut transversely as far proximally at the level of the metatarsal neck as one thick layer. The entire flap is now gradually mobilized and should include the periosteum, the EHB tendon, and the dorsomedial and dorsolateral aspect of the capsule. The flap is gradually dissected sharply off the dorsal osteophytes over toward the base of the proximal phalanx (Fig. 1–3–8).

Joint Preparation

The hallux is plantar flexed, and the osteophytes over the dorsal aspect of the metatarsal head are visualized with complete subperiosteal dissection, followed by a

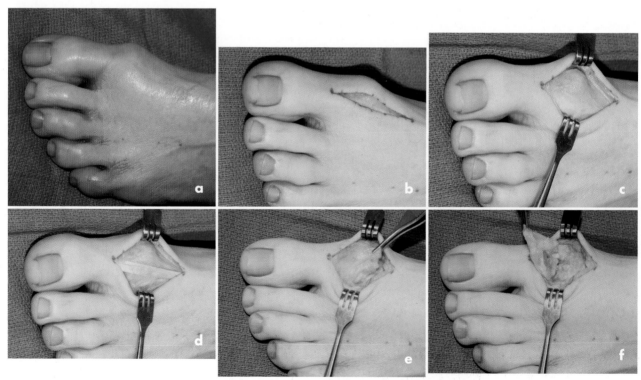

Figure 1–3–8. The incision for this patient with hallux rigidus is performed (a, b). The soft tissues are retracted (c), and the extensor hallucis longus (EHL) tendon is identified and retracted laterally (d). The flap of capsule and extensor hallucis brevis (EHB) tendon is cut and elevated distally (e, f).

cheilectomy of the metatarsal head. Resecting the dorsal one third of the metatarsal head is important, and I use a chisel, not a saw, to perform this cheilectomy. In addition to the dorsal osteophytes, the medial and lateral margins of the metatarsal head are contoured (Fig. 1–3–9). Rounding off of the metatarsal head is performed with a rongeur. Maintaining the capsular attachment to the medial aspect to the metatarsal head with this dissection is difficult if the medial eminence is removed, and if it is disrupted, a repair of the abductor tendon and capsule must be done later. Usually, however, the hallux rigidus is not associated with hallux valgus, so this repair is not an issue.

Phalangeal Bone Cut

At the completion of the cheilectomy the capsular flap is carefully elevated by holding the flap dorsally with skin hooks; a knife is used to dissect off the base of the proximal phalanx. The saw cut is made from dorsal to plantar about 8 mm distal to the articular surface, almost at the metaphyseal flare (Fig. 1–3–10). Be aware of the actual position of the joint to cut the phalanx correctly. The cut can be made slightly obliquely so that the attachment of the volar plate onto the plantar surface of the proximal phalanx is left intact. This way, the hallux may be slightly elevated off the ground at rest, but I

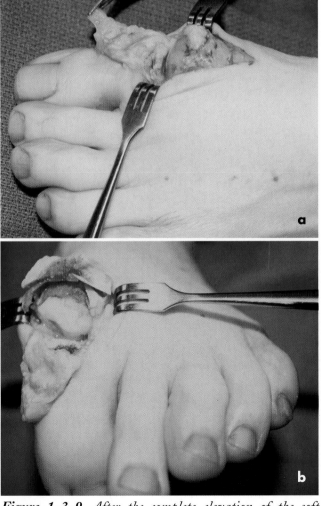

Figure 1–3–9. *After the complete elevation of the soft tissue flap (a), the cheilectomy is performed, rounding off the metatarsal head (b).*

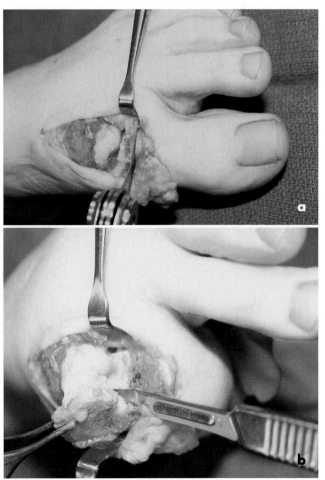

Figure 1–3–10. *The base of the proximal phalanx is cut with a saw (a) and carefully peeled off to preserve the attachment of the plantar plate (b).*

generally prefer a vertical cut to maintain contact with the ground. The base of the proximal phalanx is gradually detached from the soft tissue to prevent stripping of the attachment of the plantar plate to the remnant of the base of the proximal phalanx.

Capsule Fixation

The prepared capsular flap must now be interposed under the surface of the metatarsal head. This can be done with sutures inserted through drill holes with a K-wire (Fig. 1–3–11) or with a bone suture anchor that is inserted into the undersurface of the metatarsal head (Fig. 1–3–12). The anchor should be well impacted into the metatarsal head, and the sutures from the anchor are

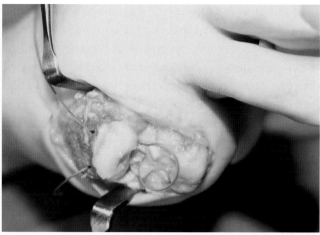

Figure 1–3–11. *Two K-wire holes are made in the metatarsal head, exiting on the plantar surface, through which a suture is inserted into the capsule.*

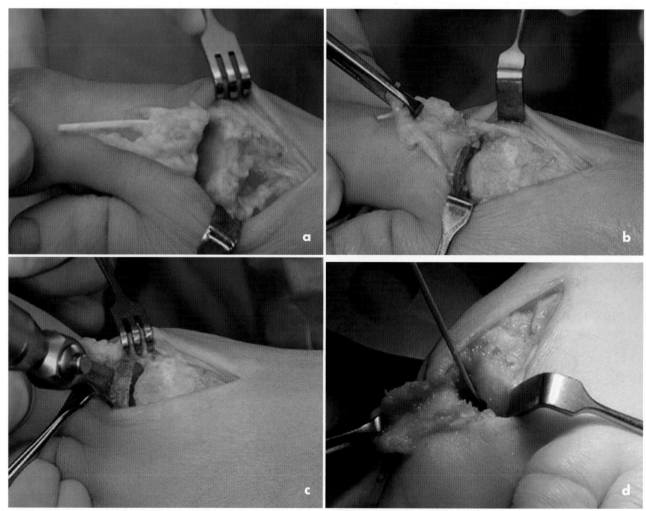

Figure 1–3–12. *The interposition arthroplasty was performed in a similar manner as in Figure 1–3–13, and after elevation of the capsule (a, b) and the saw cut of the proximal phalanx (c), a suture anchor is inserted as far under the metatarsal head as possible, which served as the anchor point for the interposition of the capsule (d).*

used to bring the dorsal soft tissue flap plantarward and line the entire MP joint. Good tension on the flap must be maintained, but the range of motion of the MP joint must be at least 60 degrees with this interposition (Fig. 1–3–13).

Implant Hemiarthroplasty

Hemiarthroplasty is a reasonable alternative for correction of end-stage hallux rigidus; an interposition arthroplasty would be the other choice. A decision as to when to perform this operation, therefore, is not really a comparison of this procedure with an arthrodesis but is interposition arthroplasty compared with implant arthroplasty. One issue to bear in mind, however, is that after implant hemiarthroplasty, the length of the hallux will be slightly longer. However, the length of the hallux must not be maintained with either procedure because of the detriment to the motion of the hallux. If the hallux's length is maintained with either type of arthroplasty, pain will continue because of impingement, arthrosis, and inflammation of the joint due to compression of the implant.

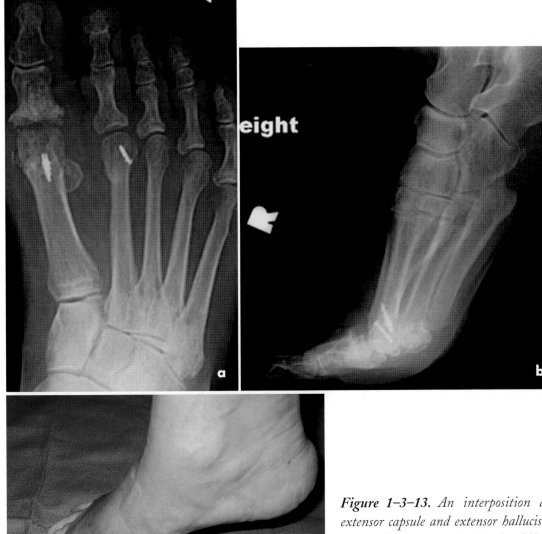

Figure 1–3–13. An interposition arthroplasty with the extensor capsule and extensor hallucis brevis (EHB) tendon was used to correct arthritis after failed Silastic joint replacement. Note the position of the bone suture anchor under the metatarsal head to which the dorsal flap is sutured (a). Dorsiflexion of the hallux is more than adequate for ambulation and shoe wear (b, c).

The history of implant arthroplasty and the hallux MP joint has certainly not been excellent, and the failure of silicone, whether with a total joint or with hemiarthroplasty, has certainly led to an awareness of potential complications of these implants. Nonetheless, a new generation of press-fit hemiarthroplasty implants is available that is thought to be excellent for operations. The clear advantage of implant over interposition arthroplasty is the maintenance of some of the lengths of the hallux. Although this may not appear to be significant, the extra 3 mm of length does change the overall appearance and possibly the function of the hallux. From a technical standpoint, exposure is identical to that of an interposition arthroplasty with the exception of the elevation of the dorsal soft tissue flap (Figs. 1–3–14 and 1–3–15). A 5-mm cut of extensor capsule is maintained on the medial aspect of the EHL tendon, and the soft tissues are elevated off the joint in a routine manner followed by cheilectomy. Removing the dorsal osteophytes from the base of the proximal phalanx is helpful to maintain the correct orientation of the saw cut. The saw must be perpendicular to the axis of the proximal phalanx. Inclining the cut off the perpendicular to facilitate dorsiflexion and keep some of the plantar capsule intact is not advantageous because this incline will only create a cock-up toe deformity if the incline is excessive. The key seems to be in the amount of bone that is resected. When I first started performing this procedure, I attempted to preserve as much length of the hallux and attachment of the volar plate as possible. Although the hallux was indeed longer, this led to more substantial soft tissue impingement, contracture, limited dorsiflexion, pain, and ultimately failure of the joint.

Today I remove approximately 6 to 7 mm of the base of the proximal phalanx. This would be about 1 cm of a space in the joint on distraction of the hallux once the proximal phalanx is cut, and after the insertion of the appropriate reaming tool, the broach, a trial implant is inserted. The implant comes in three sizes and is oriented to the shape of the base of the proximal phalanx. Before the prosthesis is inserted, the joint should be assessed for any disruption of the medial capsule and abductor tendon. To avoid postoperative hallux valgus, I predrill the medial base of the proximal phalanx with two K-wire holes through which a suture is inserted. Once the prosthesis has been inserted and impacted to obtain a good press-fit, I use the sutures that are already in the phalanx to repair the medial capsule. After surgery, the hallux is maintained in a neutral, well-padded position, and ambulation is begun as tolerated. Range of motion is initiated to tolerance after 2 weeks, and then vigorous dorsiflexion exercises with physical therapy are recommended in patients able to make the transition into a comfort shoe by 3 to 4 weeks after surgery.

Metatarsal Osteotomy

As previously noted, the indications for metatarsal osteotomy in the setting of hallux rigidus are rare. However, if a patient has metatarsus primus elevatus and gross elevation of the first metatarsal, limited dorsiflexion, and no arthritis, then a plantar flexion osteotomy can be performed (Figs. 1–3–16 and 1–3–17). The key to understanding this is that arthritis on the dorsal aspect of the metatarsal head is going to further limit and compromise the ability of this type of osteotomy to work.

Clearly some osteotomies, which have been described, can be performed in the distal portion of the metatarsal, but these can accentuate the problem by virtue of the change in the center of motion of the metatarsal head and the increase in pressure not only on the sesamoids but also on the dorsal aspect of the MTP joint. If an osteotomy must be performed, I perform this proximally through a proximal closing wedge. The base of the wedge is approximately 5 mm. A medial incision is used to perform this osteotomy, and after elevation of the periosteum, the entire base of the metatarsal is visible, including the metatarsal cuneiform joints. The plantar base wedge is now removed, and the dorsal cortex is intact. Only about 4 mm should be removed during the initial part of this wedge. With the wedge resected, the hallux is dorsiflexed, and as it dorsiflexes, pressure is exerted on the metatarsal head and the distal metatarsal is pushed down into plantar flexion. With increasing dorsiflexion of the hallux, greater plantar flexion force is exerted on the metatarsal and vice versa. From here, the fine adjustments can be made to the amount of bone removed through the wedge. If limitation and dorsiflexion are still present, then the saw blade can be inserted again into the partially closed osteotomy so that it will just access the saw blade. Then, with the saw blade

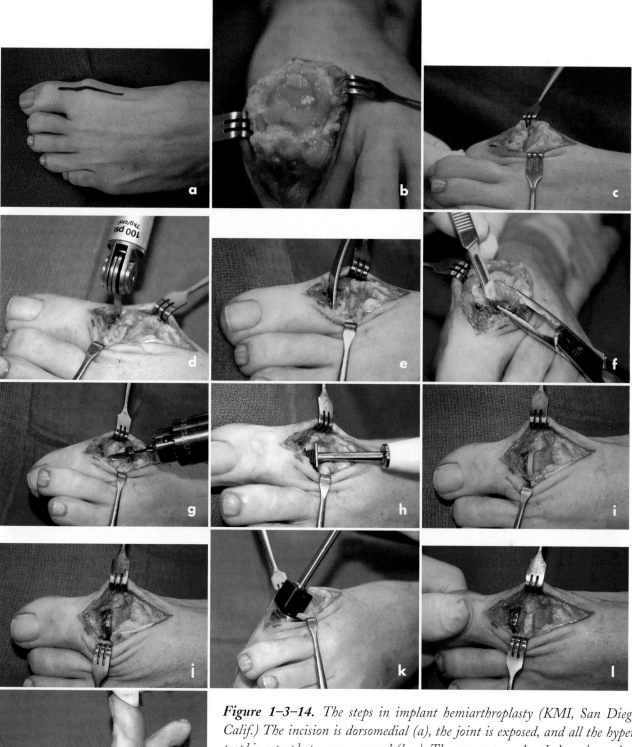

Figure 1-3-14. *The steps in implant hemiarthroplasty (KMI, San Diego, Calif.) The incision is dorsomedial (a), the joint is exposed, and all the hypertrophic osteophytes are removed (b, c). The saw cut on the phalanx is made at the metaphyseal flare (d); then the base of the phalanx is lifted off the soft tissues with a periosteal elevator (e); and then finally a knife is used to sharply divide the remaining attachment of the volar plate (f). A reamer is used to perforate the phalanx (g), followed by a broach to prepare the canal for the prosthesis (h). A trial implant (i) is followed by an insertion of the regular implant (j), which is tamped into place to secure a press-fit of the prosthesis (k). On distraction of the hallux, a sizeable gap is noted, which is the result of release of the soft tissues around the joint and is to be expected (l), and the range of motion is checked, which should be at least 60 degrees of dorsiflexion (m).*

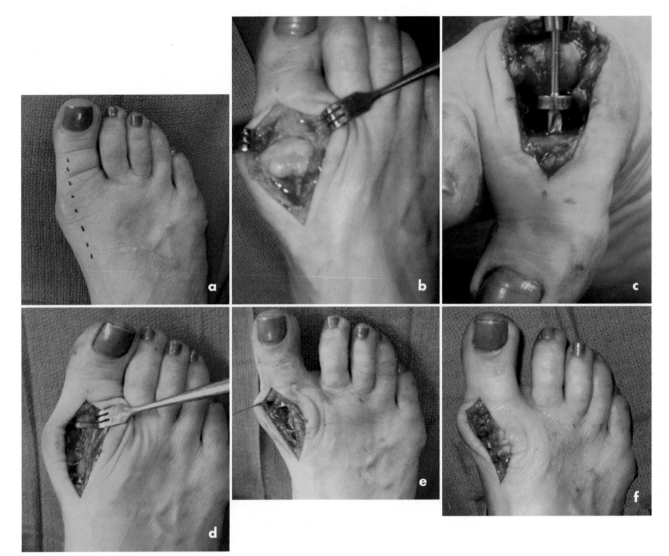

Figure 1–3–15. *The implant arthroplasty for a patient with slight hallux valgus and hallux rigidus. The incision (a) is similar for other approaches to the hallux, and after exposure of the metatarsal head (b), a cheilectomy is performed. The proximal phalanx is cut at the metaphysis, with removal of 6 mm of bone, and the phalanx is drilled with a broach to facilitate insertion of a trial prosthesis (c). Note that with insertion of the implant, the hallux lies in valgus, which occurs from release of the capsule and abductor (d). The implant was removed, sutures were placed through the phalanx into the capsule to tighten the medial joint (e), and the final position of the hallux is noted (f).*

Figure 1–3–16. *A cheilectomy was performed for this patient without success, and although arthrosis of the metaphalangeal (MP) joint was not present, limited dorsiflexion was present.*

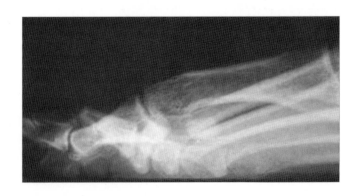

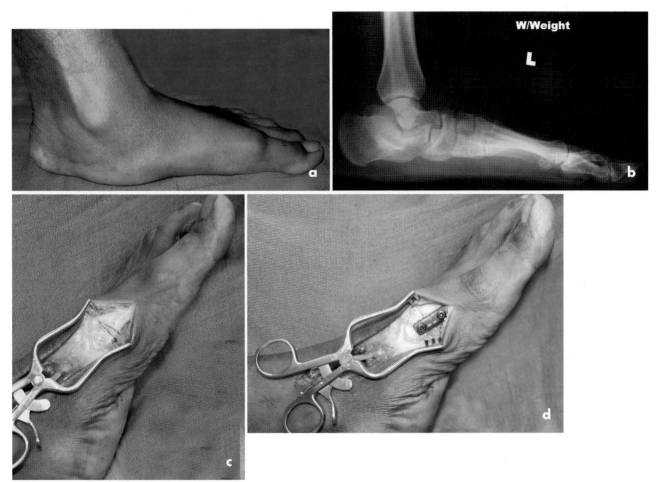

Figure 1–3–17. *In addition to significant symptoms from the flatfoot, limited dorsiflexion of the hallux was present, with a functional hallux rigidus present. The hallux is fixed in plantar flexion because of elevation of the first ray and contracture of the short hallux flexors (a, b). Note the plantar closing wedge osteotomy of the base of the first metatarsal (c), fixed with a two-hole, one-third tubular plate (d).*

repeatedly passing through the closed osteotomy, an increase in the plantar flexion of the distal metatarsal occurs with a reciprocal increase in the dorsiflexion of the hallux. Rarely does a cheilectomy need to be performed in conjunction with this procedure. The premise for this operation is to decrease the intrinsic contracture that is present as a result of the elevation of the first metatarsal. With this metatarsus elevatus, the short flexor contracts, and contracture occurs in the volar plate apparatus. Through resection of the wedge, the relaxation that occurs in the plantar musculature and ligaments facilitates motion. Fixation is performed under tension. I have tried to use dorsally inserted K-wires and screws in the past, but these seem insufficient to maintain the metatarsal in the plantarflexed position and keep the osteotomy closed. A small key plate works well, as does a plate applied to the plantar surface of the first

metatarsal. Patients need to be kept non–weight bearing for approximately 6 weeks after surgery until the osteotomy is healed to prevent any gaps in the osteotomy and any malunion with recurrent dorsal impingement.

Techniques, tips, and pitfalls

1. The goal of cheilectomy is to decrease pain. Although an increase in the range of motion is desirable, it should not be the goal for surgery.

2. The range of motion obtained during cheilectomy does not persist after surgery and decreases about 30%.

3. Removing too much bone during the cheilectomy is difficult. Obtaining a lateral

intraoperative XR image to confirm adequate bone removal is helpful.

4. The use of a nonsteroidal medication postoperatively decreases the inflammation and postoperative fibrosis.

5. A cheilectomy is a reversible procedure, and because other surgical alternatives are available if arthritis worsens, this is the procedure of choice for grade II and sometimes even early grade III arthritis. The patients' improvement over the years after this surgery is surprising, despite the appearance of arthritis on XR film.

6. In the presence of a central osteochondral defect, I try to remove enough of the metatarsal head and then, if necessary, drill the defect or perform a microfracture.

7. A patient with little range of motion preoperatively will appreciate the increase in motion postoperatively. Conversely, treating a patient with good motion preoperatively with an arthrodesis is not desirable.

8. Management of hallux valgus and associated hallux rigidus is difficult. If the valgus deformity is mild and the medial eminence needs to be removed, then the removal can be part of the cheilectomy. If the deformity is more severe, then an arthrodesis may have to be performed.

Suggested Readings

Brage ME, Ball ST: Surgical options for salvage of end-stage hallux rigidus. Foot Ankle Clin 7:49–65, 2002.

Coughlin MJ, Shurnas PS. Hallux rigidus: Demographics, etiology, and radiographic assessment. Foot Ankle Int 24:731–743, 2003.

Coughlin MJ, Shurnas PS: Hallux rigidus. Grading and long-term results of operative treatment. J Bone Joint Surg Am 85-A:2072–2088, 2003.

Coughlin MJ, Shurnas PJ: Soft-tissue arthroplasty for hallux rigidus. Foot Ankle Int 24:661–672, 2003.

Haddad SL: The use of osteotomies in the treatment of hallux limitus and hallux rigidus. Foot Ankle Clin 5:629–661, 2000.

Hamilton WG, Hubbard CE: Hallux rigidus. Excisional arthroplasty. Foot Ankle Clin 5:663–671, 2000.

Horton G: Hallux rigidus. In Myerson MS (ed): Foot and Ankle Disorders. Philadelphia, WB Saunders, 2000.

Horton GA, Park YW, Myerson MS: Role of metatarsus primus elevatus in the pathogenesis of hallux rigidus. Foot Ankle Int 20:777–780, 1999.

Lau JT, Daniels TR: Outcomes following cheilectomy and interpositional arthroplasty in hallux rigidus. Foot Ankle Int 22:462–470, 2001.

Mann RA: Intermediate to long term follow-up of medial approach dorsal cheilectomy for hallux rigidus. Foot Ankle Int 21:156, 2000.

Claw Hallux Deformity

The various degrees of a claw hallux deformity range from an interphalangeal (IP) and metaphalangeal (MP) joint that is flexible to one that is fixed with severe subluxation of the MP joint. In other variants of claw hallux deformity the MP joint is in neutral position, but a fixed flexion contracture is present as a result of tethering of the flexor hallucis longus (FHL) tendon, the intrinsics, or both. This tethering arises as a result of a scar in the distal third of the leg associated with a tibia fracture, or it is the consequence of a compartmental syndrome of the foot. The approach to correction is based entirely on the flexibility of the hallux at either joint, whether dynamic function of the hallux is present. For example, in the setting of severe fibrosis of the intrinsics after a compartmental syndrome, the approach would be different from one for an intrinsic minus deformity that is present simply as a result of intrinsic weakness (e.g., associated with Charcot-Marie Tooth disorder).

If the IP joint is fixed in flexion, an arthrodesis of that joint needs to be performed. Flexion of the hallux then occurs through the long flexor tendon (if functioning) and does not rely on the flexor hallucis brevis tendon, which is usually compromised in these claw hallux deformities. If a severe cock-up deformity is present with the IP joint fixed in flexion, I will transfer the FHL tendon around or through the base of the proximal phalanx to improve MP flexion strength, in addition to performing an IP arthrodesis. This transfer moves the axis point for flexion of the hallux more

proximally. This procedure must be combined with a dorsal soft tissue release with a lengthening of the extensor hallucis longus (EHL) tendon and a capsulotomy of the MP joint (Fig. 1–4–1). In some deformities the MP joint is severely hyperextended, and a decision must be made about whether a fusion would be preferable to a soft tissue release. The latter may be reasonable, but function of the hallux is never good. The dilemma, however, arises when both the MP and IP joints are fixed because arthrodesis at both the MP and IP joints is not ideal. If I perform a soft tissue release for correction of severe claw hallux deformity, then, in addition to an EHL lengthening or transfer (to the metatarsal neck as a Jones procedure), the dorsal capsule and the collateral ligaments are completely released. A curved periosteal elevator is inserted into the joint to forcibly plantarflex it and release the sesamoids. Motion after this procedure is never good, but the operation still may be preferable for the patient who needs an IP fusion for correction of a severe fixed claw hallux deformity.

Correction of a claw hallux deformity after a compartmental syndrome can be extremely difficult. A fixed flexion contracture is usually at both the MP and IP joints. The EHL tendon is usually functioning, but again, the fixed flexion contracture has little power to dorsiflex the hallux. I have attempted various soft tissue releases and have ultimately concluded that the only way the hallux can be repaired is by completely releasing the sesamoid complex. The approach is through a medial

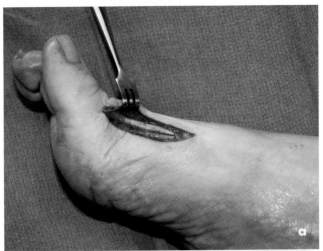

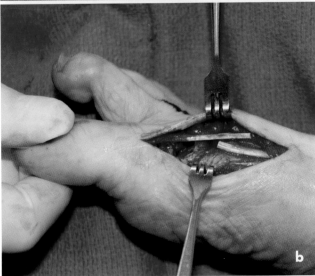

Figure 1–4–1. A cock-up extension deformity of the hallux was associated with a fixed extension contracture at the metaphalangeal (MP) joint, and the deformity was corrected with a lengthening of the extensor hallucis longus (EHL) tendon (a, b), followed by a transfer of the flexor hallucis longus (FHL) tendon to the base of the proximal phalanx.

incision similar to that for a sesamoidectomy, and the branch of the medial plantar nerve is identified and retracted. The abductor tendon and the volar plate are cut, and this cut reveals the FHL tendon. Once the FHL tendon is retracted, the volar plate ligament is cut completely, and the sesamoids are allowed to retract proximally. The hallux is then passively dorsiflexed. At this time, at least 45 degrees of passive dorsiflexion should be present with the ankle in neutral position. If this dorsiflexion is not present, then the FHL tendon needs to be lengthened. A proximal lengthening is preferable. It should be proximal to the medial malleolus either

through a fractional lengthening at the musculotendinous junction or by a standard Z-lengthening of the tendon. If a Z-step cut lengthening is performed, then at least 60 degrees of passive dorsiflexion of the hallux must be present or deformity will occur postoperatively. Once the volar plate has been completely released, the effect of the contracture on the IP joint must be observed. Is this is a fixed contracture, or is there a passive tenodesis effect of the FHL that is eliminated with plantar flexion of the ankle? To determine this, plantarflex the foot and assess the amount of dorsiflexion that occurs through the IP joint. If the IP joint can be completely straightened with the foot plantarflexed but the hallux flexes at the IP joint with the foot in neutral position or in dorsiflexion, then a tenodesis effect is present. If a fixed flexion deformity is present, then an arthrodesis of the IP joint must be performed.

Interphalangeal Arthrodesis Technique

Arthrodesis of the IP joint is performed through a longitudinal incision over the dorsal aspect of the hallux medial to the EHL tendon. Distally, the attachment of the EHL is important and one must not injure the germinal matrix at the base of the nail. The incision can either be cut in an L or a T shape to facilitate exposure, and then the EHL tendon can be retracted. I pull the EHL tendon over to one side with a skin hook after incising the extensor hood. The EHL tendon always remains partly tethered to the extensor retinaculum and will not retract far proximally even if cut at the level of the IP joint (Fig. 1–4–2).

Correction of a claw hallux deformity invariably includes arthrodesis of the IP joint of the hallux. Rarely, this deformity is flexible, and arthrodesis may not need to be performed. The correction of the deformity depends more on the extent of the contracture at the metatarsophalangeal joint than at the IP joint. Because the IP joint is invariably fixed and an arthrodesis is performed, the issue of the remaining treatment algorithm then depends on the flexibility at the MP joint.

A longitudinal incision is made medial to the EHL tendon dorsally and to the subcutaneous tissue that retracts the tendon laterally. If a fixed deformity of the hallux is present with a severe hyperextension deformity, then the EHL tendon does not need to be preserved and

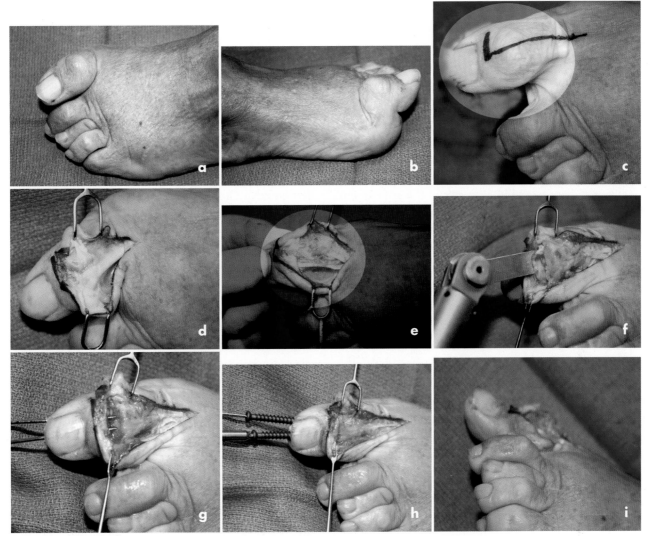

Figure 1–4–2. *The approach for correction of a claw hallux deformity with interphalangeal (IP) arthrodesis and extensor hallucis longus (EHL) tendon lengthening (a, b). The incision is marked out as a long L shape (c), and the EHL is exposed and retracted laterally (d). Because of the extension contracture of the metaphalangeal (MP) joint, a Z-step cut lengthening of the EHL tendon is performed (e). After the saw cut of the proximal phalanx, the distal phalanx is cut slightly obliquely to dorsiflex the IP joint (f). Two guide pins are inserted out the tip of the hallux and then passed back proximally (g), and then a 4-mm, fully threaded screw is inserted (h). Note the corrected position of the hallux at both the MP and IP joints after IP arthrodesis, and MP capsulotomy and EHL lengthening (i).*

is transferred proximally into the first metatarsal. Generally, however, the EHL tendon will be retracted laterally and an attempt made to preserve the tendon. Even with slight extension at the MP joint, once the IP joint is fused, an increased force develops across the MP joint in plantar flexion through the IP arthrodesis and the FHL tendon. The incision is turned laterally to create an L or T shape for facilitation of the arthrodesis exposure of the IP joint. The distal corner of the

attachment of the EHL tendon and extensor hood to the base of the proximal phalanx is incised, and then the soft tissue flap is elevated to raise the EHL tendon and move it laterally. This procedure is best made with a small skin hook. Then with subperiosteal dissection, the medial to lateral ligament is cut, and the joint is finally exposed. The EHL tendon can be lifted up off the proximal phalanx and then retracted laterally while the head of the proximal phalanx is completely delivered into the incision. The proximal phalanx is then cut with only the articular surface removed. This cut can be made slightly obliquely to create some dorsiflexion in the arthrodesis, but I usually do this once a second cut on the base of the distal phalanx has been made when I know how much bone to resect.

The cut on the distal phalanx is not as easy because the lateral attachment of the EHL tendon is now at risk. The tendon is detached, and it can be repaired because it does not slide proximally as a result of the attachment of the EHL tendon to the extensor hood. The base of the distal phalanx curves slightly proximally under the proximal phalanx, and this cut always includes slightly more bone on the plantar than dorsal surface even if made perpendicular to the axis of the hallux. Once the bone surfaces are cut, the apposition of the distal to the proximal phalanx is checked, and fixation is performed with a single cannulated, 4 mm, partially threaded screw. A fully threaded screw can also be used provided the hallux is compressed manually during insertion of the screw. A guide pin is inserted antegrade distally out the distal phalanx and then back across into the proximal phalanx; this insertion ensures that the hallux is well centered over the middle of the phalanx. A skin incision is now made over the guide pin but must be made transversely in line with the skin creases. If the incision is made vertically, this creates more of a scar, which can be potentially painful. When the screw is introduced, the screw may push the distal phalanx away from the proximal phalanx; the proximal phalanx should be held in position manually. If there is a slight gap, I take the screw out, oppose it manually, and then reinsert the screw under manual compression.

If the hallux tends to cock-up at the MP joint after the arthrodesis, then an EHL tendon lengthening or transfer must be performed. Be careful about performing a transfer of the entire EHL tendon if the extensor hallucis brevis (EHB) tendon is not functioning well. This is common in severe claw hallux deformity, and the best that could be hoped for is a hallux that functions passively but lies in a more neutral position with respect to the metatarsal on the weight-bearing surface of the floor. With severe claw hallux deformities, dysplastic changes usually take place in the MP joint because the head is compressed slightly dorsally and adequate range of motion may never be regained. Nonetheless, performing a complete transverse dorsal capsulotomy and then an EHL lengthening or tendon transfer as necessary is important. Flipping the undersurface of the volar plate and the sesamoid apparatus to loosen the attachment to the metatarsal neck may be necessary. Then, the sesamoid will slide more proximally under the head with plantar flexion of the hallux, which was previously blocked as a result of the extension contracture. To look at the type of motion at the MP joint in plantar flexion is useful. A gliding motion is ideal; the joint "booking" open as the hallux is plantarflexed is unwanted. This latter motion occurs because of dysplastic changes in the metatarsophalangeal joint from the chronic extension contracture.

Disorders of the Sesamoids

Tibial Sesamoidectomy

When sesamoid disease is present, I am more inclined to perform a sesamoidectomy than to attempt other procedures, including sesamoid shaving, bone grafting of the sesamoid, or removal of one pole of the sesamoid. Regardless of whether a tibial or fibular sesamoidectomy is performed, one has to be aware of the mechanical changes that take place around the hallux. After tibial sesamoidectomy, the hallux tends to drift into slight hallux valgus with a weakness in push-off strength; possibly even dorsiflexion contracture occurs. After fibular sesamoidectomy, hallux varus, as well as a weakness in push-off strength, may occur. However, bone grafting of the sesamoid (e.g., in the setting of a chronic nonunion of the sesamoid) can work. However, because of the morbidity that follows this particular procedure with requirements for non–weight bearing and the potential for persistent nonunion after prolonged rehabilitation, sesamoidectomy is a more appealing procedure. The only time that I will not perform a sesamoidectomy for sesamoid disease is after acute fracture with diastasis of the end of the sesamoid (e.g., in the setting of a severe turf toe injury where the volar plate has retracted proximally and a cerclage suture technique is used around the sesamoid to facilitate healing), assuming that comminution is not present. If sesamoid comminution exists, then I would perform a sesamoidectomy.

Skin Incision and Dissection

An incision is made over the medial aspect of the metatarsophalangeal (MTP) joint just dorsal to the plantar skin. Following this landmark is essential to avoid injury to the cutaneous nerve. This incision must be carefully deepened, and skin hooks are then inserted into the plantar skin flap and retracted inferiorly. With a hemostat, the subcutaneous tissue is gradually divided down to the fascial layer, which is perforated and spread until the common digital nerve to the hallux is identified and retracted. A longitudinal incision is made directly just above the abductor tendon and through the medial joint capsule to enter the articulation of the MTP joint. Identifying the abductor tendon is important because this may be used later for repair and reconstruction of the plantar medial ligament deficit (Fig. 2–1–1).

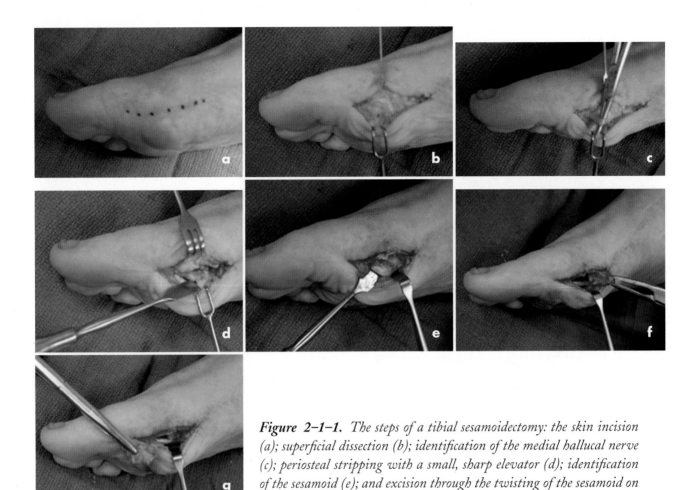

Figure 2–1–1. *The steps of a tibial sesamoidectomy: the skin incision (a); superficial dissection (b); identification of the medial hallucal nerve (c); periosteal stripping with a small, sharp elevator (d); identification of the sesamoid (e); and excision through the twisting of the sesamoid on its pedicle (f, g).*

Sesamoid Excision

The sesamoid is not easy to excise because the periosteal fibers (Sharpey fibers) are adherent and no simple plane for dissection exists. The sesamoid is grasped with a small skin hook, and with a distal to proximal approach, the sesamoid is gradually dissected free. Grasping the sesamoid with a clamp and twisting it in one direction or another to mobilize it are helpful. Usually, I detach the distal portion of the sesamoid first and then peel it away, trying to preserve the layer of the fibers of the flexor hallucis brevis tendon (Fig. 2–1–2). Inspecting the flexor hallucis longus tendon and making sure that it is completely intact are important.

Reconstruction of the Medial Joint and Capsule

The remaining attachment of the medial head of the flexor hallucis brevis tendon must be imbricated. At times, there is sufficient tissue for imbrication with a simple suture and for attachment to the base of the proximal phalanx, while the integrity of the volar plate is maintained. If there is a more substantial defect, then this must be repaired to prevent hallux valgus. I use the abductor hallucis tendon to strengthen the plantar-deficient flexor hallucis brevis ligament. The tendon can be detached from the medial phalanx and then advanced into the plantar aspect of the base of the proximal phalanx with a suture anchor. The medial joint capsule must then be reinforced with 2-0 nonabsorbable sutures to maintain the joint in neutral. If the flexor hallucis brevis complex is reparable, then the abductor/capsular tissue is carefully tightened with interrupted, overlapping, figure-eight, 2-0 nonabsorbable sutures. Tension is applied while repairing the abductor and capsule flaps to preserve the hallux in slight plantar flexion and in a neutral position in the transverse plane.

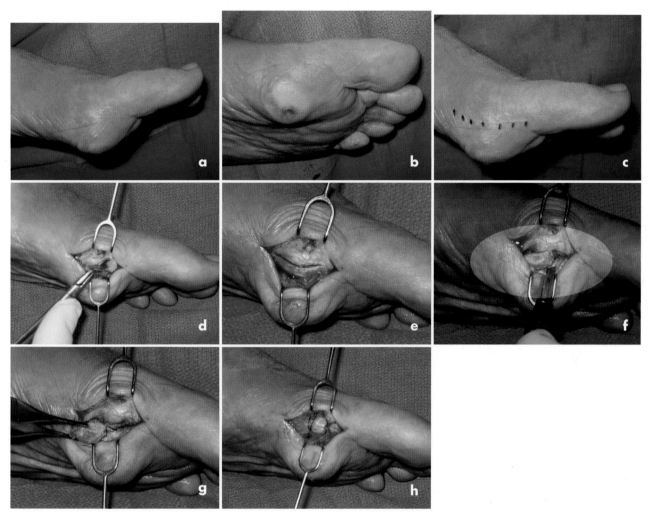

Figure 2–1–2. *The tibial sesamoid was excised in this patient with diabetes for intractable bursitis associated with recurrent ulceration. The slight hyperextension of the hallux is noted with the enlarged bursa (a, b), and the incision is marked out (c). The terminal hallucal nerve is isolated (d), and the abductor tendon is incised longitudinally (e). The abductor and flexor hallucis brevis tendons are sharply divided from the sesamoid (f), the sesamoid is removed (g), and the abductor tendon is repaired (h).*

Postoperative Course and Treatment

The hallux is taped into slight varus for the first 3 weeks and then taped with a figure-eight strap for an additional 6 weeks into a neutral position. Weight bearing may begin immediately after surgery in a surgical shoe and in a thick-soled running shoe worn at 3 weeks. Exercise may start at 4 weeks without any push-off strength because passive dorsiflexion of the hallux must not take place for 8 weeks. Cycling and other static exercise machines may be used as tolerated, but again, no dorsiflexion of the hallux must occur.

Techniques, tips, and pitfalls

1. Protecting the terminal branch of the medial plantar nerve to the hallux is essential. Injury to this nerve will cause a debilitating neuroma. Once the nerve has been identified, it must be retracted and protected.

2. Strapping of the hallux is essential postoperatively. This should be done into slight hallux varus and into slight plantar flexion, and limitation of dorsiflexion for the first 2 months is important. A stiff-soled shoe, with an orthosis including a Morton's extension, is also helpful.

3. Be careful about a sesamoidectomy performed for a patient with a forefoot cavus or fixed plantar flexion of the first metatarsal. Although the pain from the symptomatic sesamoid may abate, pressure under the first metatarsal may occur, with transfer of pain to the fibular sesamoid.

Fibular Sesamoidectomy

The main issue with respect to fibular sesamoidectomy is the surgical approach (i.e., dorsal or plantar). Usually, the diseased sesamoid sits directly underneath the metatarsal head, and a dorsal approach is difficult. On the other hand, one has to recognize the potential morbidity from a plantar incision, and therefore a dorsal incision can at times be used. From this dorsal incision, however, it is far more difficult to repair the sesamoid complex. Provided that the nerve on the plantar aspect of the foot is protected, the plantar incision is the preferred approach.

Plantar Incision and Dissection

The sesamoid is approached through a vertical incision made lateral to the weight-bearing surface of the first metatarsal head. The incision is therefore made almost under the first web space, and with dissection, the plantar aspect of the fatty tissue is gradually retracted until the plantar terminal hallucal nerve is identified. The nerve is larger than one imagines and can be found by sweeping a curved hemostat under the tissue until it delivers the nerve into the incision. The nerve is generally retracted laterally with a retractor and should be protected through the rest of the dissection.

The sesamoid is encased in periosteum and surrounded by the adductor complex and the attachments of the lateral head of the flexor hallucis brevis tendon. I incise the periosteum, and then, with as much protection as possible of the lateral head of the flexor hallucis brevis tendon and the adductor tendon, the sesamoid is gradually removed. The attachment of the sesamoid to the intersesamoid ligament has to be cut before removing the sesamoid. The size of the defect is unpredictable, but a repair should be attempted. For some patients with mild hallux valgus, the hallux is less likely to drift into hallux varus, and a repair is unnecessary. However, if a defect is present, the adductor tendon should be sutured into the short flexor tendon, and a cerclage suture should be made between the flexor hallucis brevis tendon and the volar plate and the distal aspect of the intersesamoid ligament. In this way, the slight plantar flexion and valgus positioning of the hallux was maintained.

Dorsal Incision

The dorsal incision should be used sparingly and only when the sesamoid is accessible in the web space; otherwise, a repair of the sesamoid sling as previously described is difficult. A dorsal incision is made in the first web space, over a length of 2.5 cm. The terminal branch of the deep peroneal nerve is identified and retracted laterally, and the soft tissues gradually dissected. A small retractor facilitates exposure, and the innominate fascia is cut to expose the adductor complex in the deeper soft tissues. The plane of the sesamoid depends on the presence of hallux valgus and associated disease. A knife is inserted between the sesamoid and the undersurface to the metatarsal head, and the sesamoid suspensory ligament is cut. The sesamoid is grasped with a clamp and is then gradually dissected free of the attachment to the intersesamoid ligament. Once the sesamoid is detached from its soft tissue attachments, the adductor complex is repaired. The distal stump of the adductor tendon is grasped and reattached to the distal head of the flexor hallucis brevis tendon with a tapered needle and 2-0 braided Dacron suture. Checking the stability of the hallux and noting any absence of deformity (in varus) with stress applied to the hallux are important (Fig. 2–1–3). The repair of a volus plate rupture is shown in Fig. 2–1–4.

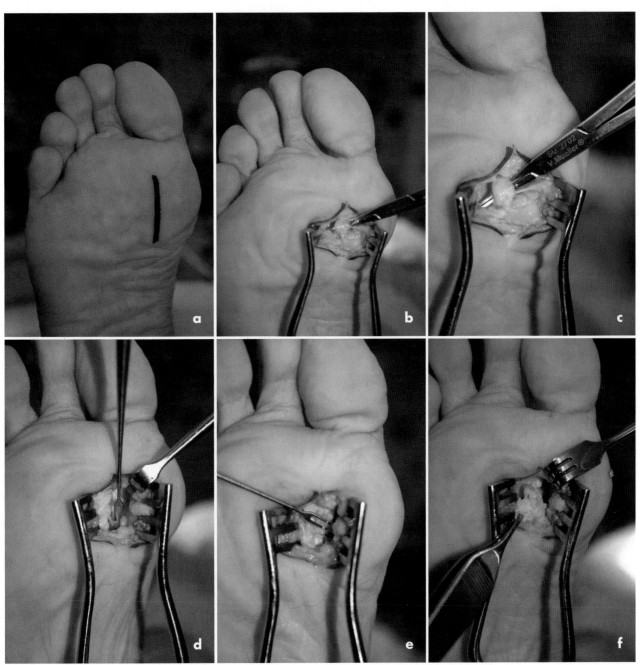

Figure 2–1–3. *Steps in a fibular sesamoidectomy. Note the incision slightly lateral to the weight-bearing surface of the first metatarsal (a). The superficial dissection must initially identify the terminal branch of the medial plantar nerve, which is large and easy to retract (b, c). A small skin hook is used to retract the corner of the sesamoid because the plane for subperiosteal dissection is not easy to identify because of a lack of Sharpey fibers (d, e).* Continued

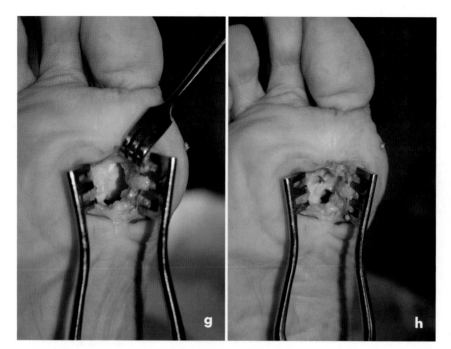

Figure 2–1–3, cont'd. The sesamoid is then removed sharply, the flexor hallucis longus tendon is identified (f, g), and the retinaculum and adductor tendon are repaired (h).

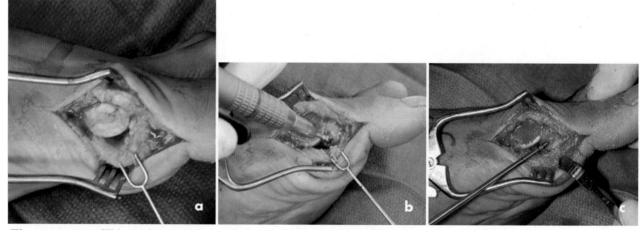

Figure 2–1–4. This patient was a professional football player who sustained a traumatic rupture of the medial collateral ligament and the medial aspect of the volar plate off the hallux, followed by weakness, pain, and hallux valgus. Note the defect in the volar plate and the attachment of the abductor hallucis tendon (a). The base of the proximal phalanx was burred to create a bleeding bed for the ligament (b), and a suture anchor was inserted (c).

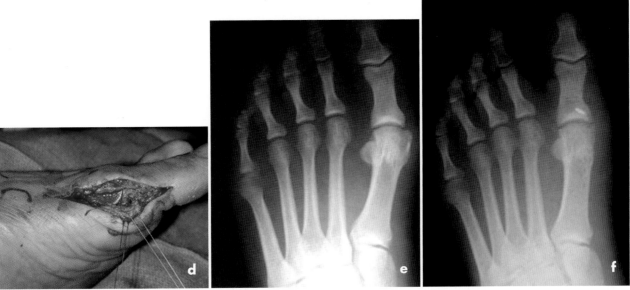

Figure 2–1–4, cont'd. *The repair was performed and was followed by an osteotomy of the base of the proximal phalanx to improve the rotation of the hallux (d, f). The preoperative x-ray (XR) film is shown for comparative purposes (e).*

Suggested Readings

Jahss MH: The sesamoids of the hallux. Clin Orthop 157:88–97, 1981.

Leventen E: Sesamoid disorders and their treatment. Clin Orthop Aug: 236–240, 1991.

Richardson EG, Brotzman SB, Graves SD: The plantar incision for procedures involving the forefoot. An evaluation of one hundred and fifty incisions in one hundred and fifteen patients. J Bone Joint Surg 75:726–731, 1993.

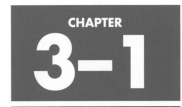

Correction of Lesser Toe Deformity

Claw Toe and Hammertoe Correction

I follow a simple algorithm for correction of claw toe and hammertoe: Is the deformity fixed or flexible, and is the deformity at the interphalangeal (IP) joint, the metatarsophalangeal (MP) joint, or both? For most patients, I perform a resection arthroplasty of the IP joint. Arthrodesis is performed under the following circumstances:

1. For recurrent deformity
2. For deformity of the IP joint in the transverse plane
3. For correction of neuromuscular deformity
4. In the absence of adequate flexion strength at the MP joint where stiffness of the IP joint will be acceptable to the patient

Functionally, there does not appear to be much difference between arthroplasty and arthrodesis of the IP joint. Strength is certainly improved with an arthrodesis because the force of the long flexor tendon is then transmitted to the MP joint to improve plantar flexion of the MP joint. The grip strength of the toe at the level of the IP joint is better with an arthroplasty provided the toe remains flexible. However, the toe is rarely flexible. The potential for complications of both arthroplasty and arthrodesis also has to be considered. Although arthrodesis leaves the toe rigid, it is indeed straight, and depending on how the operation is performed, arthrodesis can avoid the toe shortening that is inherent with some arthroplasty procedures. Bear in mind the potential for complications of an IP arthrodesis includes a fixed flexion deformity of the distal interphalangeal (DIP) joint. A mallet toe occurs in approximately 10% of patients as a result of overpull or contracture of the flexor digitorum longus (FDL) tendon on the DIP joint.

Correction of the Metatarsophalangeal Joint Contracture

I approach the MP joint release sequentially. This begins with a release of the long and short extensor tendons, followed by a transverse dorsal capsulotomy. If a contracture still persists, then I release the collateral ligaments dorsally and then, finally, release the volar plate contracture, if present. If the joint is unstable or dislocated, soft tissue releases as described for a contracture are not sufficient, and a shortening osteotomy of the metatarsal needs to be performed (Fig. 3–1–1). If the MP release is performed as an isolated procedure, in the absence of correction of the IP joint, then a decision has to be made whether to secure the MP joint with a K-wire. I use a K-wire if any instability persists. Do not use the K-wire to reduce an unstable joint because the subluxation will recur promptly once the wire is removed. In other words, the K-wire can facilitate scarring of the MP joint, but it should not be relied on to correct deformity.

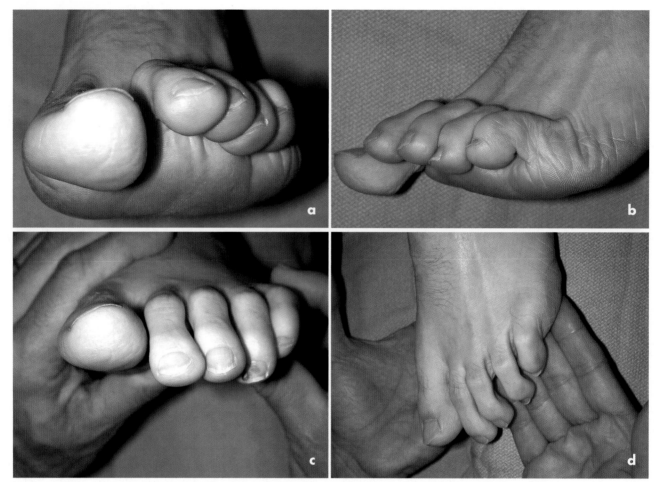

Figure 3–1–1. *I use this "push up test" to help with decision making in the surgical procedure. The toe deformities are presented in a non–weight-bearing position (a, b). Pushing up under the metatarsal heads (c, d) simulates weight bearing. Minimal deformity of the metatarsophalangeal (MP) joints, which are flexible, can be seen, and fixed deformity is present in the proximal interphalangeal (PIP) joints. A resection arthroplasty or arthrodesis of the PIP joints will be sufficient here, followed by intrinsic strengthening exercises.*

Posterior Interphalangeal Resection Arthroplasty and Arthrodesis

Either a longitudinal or transverse elliptical incision is made over the posterior interphalangeal (PIP) joint, over a length of about 1 cm. I use small hooks to retract the skin and then incise the extensor hood either longitudinally or transversely. This incision depends on whether an arthroplasty or arthrodesis is performed and whether K-wire fixation of the joint is used. In elderly patients, I prefer to use strapping instead of a K-wire to stabilize the toe, and in these patients, I use a transverse ellipse over the PIP joint and can close the ellipse to help with the alignment of the toe. This transverse incision does, however, cause some thickening of the PIP joint, which

is permanent. Once the distal portion of the PIP joint is identified, the collateral ligaments on either side are cut. Cut in toward the joint to prevent accidental laceration of the neurovascular bundle. A curved periosteal elevator (named a *shmogler* by Dr. Melvin Jahss) is inserted into the IP joint to strip the soft tissue from the medial lateral surface and undersurface of the phalangeal neck.

Bone Cuts

I prefer to use a small bone cutter instead of a saw to remove no more than the distal one quarter of the proximal phalanx. A bone cutter will, however, cause minor crushing of the edges of the condyle, and this crushing leads to painful ridges on the margins of the point unless these are trimmed. A smooth contour of the distal remnant of the proximal phalanx should be created. The PIP joint must be stabilized, and this stability can be performed with a suture in the extensor hood or a K-wire. If the MP joint has been opened, the K-wire is best introduced antegrade from the MP joint distally through the PIP joint arthroplasty, out through the toe, and then driven back retrograde into the metatarsal. Depending on the need for MP stability, the K-wire can be left in the phalanx or driven across the MP joint. If a K-wire is used, palpate the condyles over the PIP joint through the skin to make sure that no minor mediolat-

eral deviation of the joint, which will always be painful, is present. If this deviation is present, then the K-wire must be redirected, or the spur must be trimmed with a burr (Fig. 3–1–2). The alignment of the toe is, however, more important, and if there is any transverse plane deviation, then the K-wire must be repositioned. If a K-wire is not used, then the toe must be stabilized with a suture through the extensor hood and capsule. I use two figure-of-eight sutures with 4-0 absorbable material. I prefer to use absorbable 5-0 chromic sutures for the skin closure. If a K-wire is not used, then the toe must be held stable with a bandage or splint for 3 weeks postoperatively.

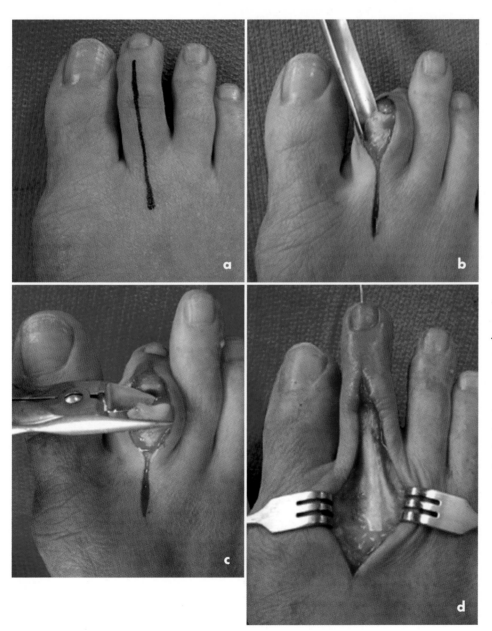

Figure 3–1–2. *The proximal interphalangeal (PIP) arthroplasty incision is marked out to be performed with release of the metatarsophalangeal (MP) joint (a). A curved periosteal elevator (shmogler) is inserted into the edge of the joint to release the collateral ligament (b), and 4 mm of bone is removed with a bone cutter (c). A K-wire is inserted into the PIP joint but not across the MP joint because a crossover toe deformity is present and it must still be corrected (d).*

Posterior Interphalangeal Arthrodesis

I use an arthrodesis of the PIP joint to correct fixed contracted deformity following, for example, a compartment syndrome (Fig. 3–1–3), a neuromuscular deformity, instability associated with good IP joint flexion, and some recurrent deformities. The goal of the procedure is to realign the toe and make use of the long flexor tendon to improve plantar flexion of the MP joint. This arthrodesis is particularly valuable for severe failure of resection arthroplasty of the PIP joint, when too much bone has been removed and an interposition arthrodesis of the PIP joint with graft is performed (Fig. 3–1–4). If an arthrodesis of the PIP joint is performed, then I prefer to use a 3-mm burr and not a saw to cut and fashion the joint into a cup and cone shape. Use of

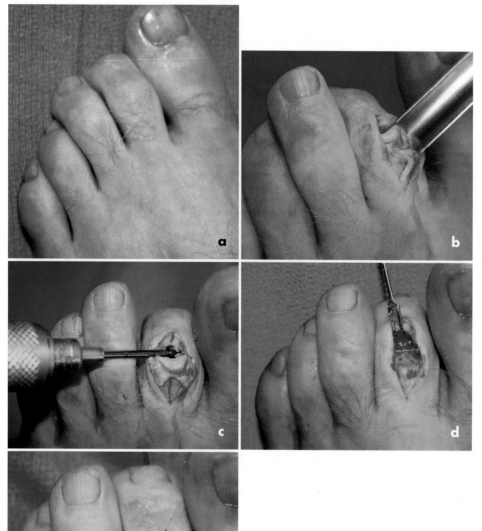

Figure 3–1–3. Arthrodesis of the proximal interphalangeal (PIP) joint of the second toe for a fixed claw deformity after a compartment syndrome (a). After exposure through a dorsal longitudinal incision, a curved shmogler is inserted into the edge of the joint to free up the collateral ligament (b). A 4-mm burr is then used to contour the edges of the proximal phalanx, followed by creation of a reciprocal defect in the middle phalanx (c). A pilot hole is now made in the center of the proximal phalanx with a K-wire (d), and the wire is inserted out the tip of the toe and then moved retrograde into the predrilled hole in the proximal phalanx (e).

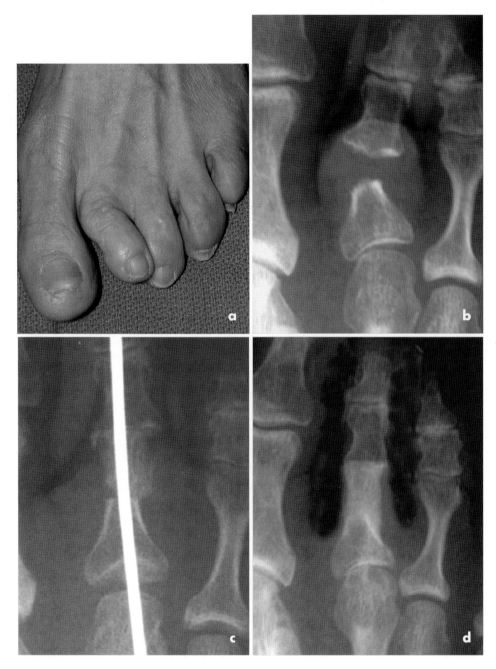

Figure 3–1–4. Recurrent deformity of the second toe occurred in this patient after attempted resection arthroplasty. The toe is short, curved, and painful (a). Note the excessive bone resection, the medial deviation of the metatarsophalangeal (MP) joint, and the slight MP subluxation (b). An interposition bone graft harvested from the ipsilateral calcaneus was performed to lengthen the toe fixed with a single K-wire (c). The final appearance is noted with good alignment of the toe and improved length (d).

a burr minimizes bone loss and does not widen the toe at the PIP joint. The condyles and the articular cartilage are removed, but the medial and lateral cortical margins are preserved. The burr is then compressed into the middle phalanx to create a reciprocal cup shape for the phalanx. A number of alternatives are available for fixation of the PIP joint. If the MP joint is unstable, then a K-wire is used. It is introduced from the MP joint distally and then is moved retrograde across both the PIP and MP joints. Alternatively, if only the toe is be fixed,

a guide hole is first prepared with a K-wire in the proximal phalanx and is then introduced antegrade across the IP joint and then retrograde across the previously drilled K-wire hole. The reason for the predrilled hole in the proximal phalanx is to facilitate the correct passage of the wire across the IP joint. If it is not perfectly in the center of the toe, then a malunion of the fusion occurs, and the malunion creates a painful medial or lateral deviation. Other types of fixation that bury the fixation in the phalanges are appealing but must be used carefully. These alternatives include a buried bioresorbable pin, a buried intra-articular screw, and a snap-off threaded pin. All of these avoid fixation, which exits the toe, and therefore avoid the potential for infection.

Arthrodesis of the PIP joint creates a toe that is straight, and for some patients, this may not be physically or cosmetically acceptable. Slight flexion is preferable but not easy to accomplish with standard methods of fixation. If small threaded snap-off pins are introduced and cross the IP joint obliquely, the toe can be positioned in slight flexion, and the pins can be left out percutaneously.

Managing Arthritis of the Lesser Toe Metatarsophalangeal Joint

Management of arthritis of the lesser toe MP joint, in particular the second toe, has to be approached as a salvage operation because little can be done to maintain a healthy, flexible joint. The goals should therefore be to relieve pain, to maximize range of motion and, most important, not to compromise the stability of the joint. The arthritis occurs in the setting of chronic subluxation, Freiberg's osteochondrosis, or both and frequently occurs after a prior operation of the toe or joint. Options for treating this include a complete metatarsal head resection, a partial metatarsal head resection, and shortening of the metatarsal head or shaft. Wherever possible, I try to preserve the MP joint, and, if possible, a shaft shortening osteotomy or a Weil osteotomy works well, depending on the extent of joint arthritis. Why a Weil osteotomy would work in the setting of arthritis is puzzling, but clearly, the shortening of the metatarsal through release of the pressure on the intrinsic tendons decompresses the pressure on the joint. The Weil osteotomy has a role in the treatment of joint arthritis for the described conditions and in the setting of rheumatologic deformity. The management of the lesser toe MP joints in rheumatoid arthritis is discussed in a separate chapter. Metatarsal head resection is never a good alternative to manage arthritis of a single joint. It can, however, be combined with resection of *all* of the lesser metatarsal heads. This resection is a salvage operation and is usually performed as such for more diffuse metatarsalgia and arthritis and not for correction of a single isolated arthritic joint.

Interposition Arthroplasty

I use an interposition arthroplasty combined with partial shaving of the anterior aspect of the metatarsal head when the joint cannot be preserved. This is an operation that works well and accomplishes the goals previously described through maintenance of motion and stability. This operation must be used cautiously in the setting of a dislocation of the MP joint associated with arthritis because subluxation may persist. The key to the interposition arthroplasty is to resect the appropriate amount of the metatarsal head and to leave the undersurface of the condyles of the head intact to maintain a plantigrade weight-bearing surface. Clearly, if too much of the head is removed, adjacent metatarsalgia will occur. Dissect off and retract the long extensor tendon. Then, transversely cut the periosteum, the capsule, and the extensor brevis tendon as far proximally on the metatarsal neck as possible. This entire soft tissue flap is then lifted up and raised in a Y-shape with a distal base that remains attached to the base of the proximal phalanx. Once the flap has been elevated off the metatarsal head, the joint must be completely reduced with a shmogler (Fig. 3–1–5).

The joint is then exposed, and the metatarsal head is cut with a saw contouring the cuts to maintain a circular shape of the head. I remove approximately 4 mm of the metatarsal head. This amount must, however, be enough to ensure motion without compression on the head with range of motion. Provided the condyles are left intact, more of the metatarsal head can, in fact, be removed. The soft tissue flap that has been raised is now used for an interposition and is anchored underneath the metatarsal head in one of two ways: Either a small suture anchor is inserted into the undersurface of the metatarsal head, or two K-wire holes are made in the head. A U-shaped suture is inserted through the K-wire holes to capture the flap. The flap is then pulled underneath the metatarsal head at the appropriate tension. The remaining tissue of the flap must sit underneath the metatarsal head so that the flap can then function as a tenodesis maintaining the reduction of the MP joint (Fig. 3–1–6).

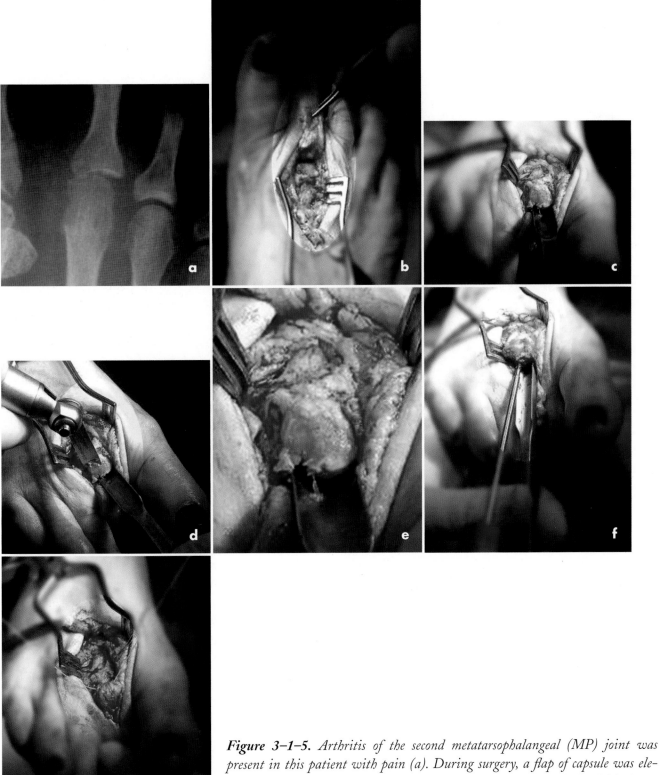

Figure 3–1–5. *Arthritis of the second metatarsophalangeal (MP) joint was present in this patient with pain (a). During surgery, a flap of capsule was elevated (b), and a curved periosteal elevator was inserted under the head (c). A saw was used to contour the head (d), and with the elevator under the head, a small suture anchor was inserted into the undersurface of the head (e, f). The capsule was finally inserted under the head with the anchor (g).*

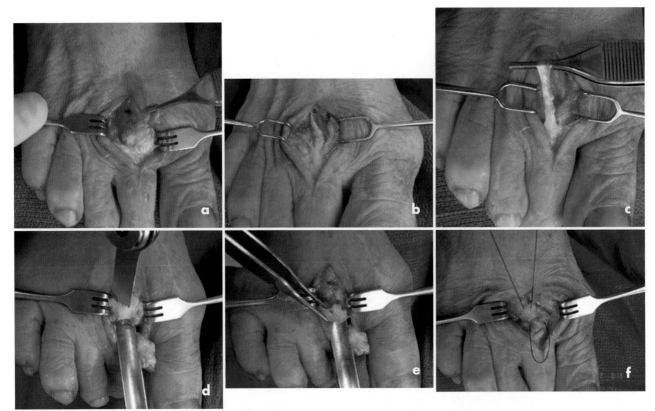

Figure 3–1–6. *Arthritis of the second metatarsophalangeal (MP) joint was treated here with an interposition arthroplasty. Note the arthritis and the hypertrophic capsule and scar around the joint (a, b). Preserving the long extensor tendon, which is first dissected off the scar and retracted, is important (c). A curved periosteal elevator (shmogler) is inserted, and the contour of the head is resected with a saw (d). The head is resected with the contour maintained (e), and a Y-shaped suture is inserted through K-wire holes in the head (f).*

Osteochondrosis of the Metatarsal Head

Management of arthritis of the lesser metatarsal head associated with osteochondrosis does not mandate resection arthroplasty or metatarsal head resection. Even for severe arthritis, an osteotomy of the metatarsal head itself can invariably be performed. With this triangular osteotomy, a wedge is removed from the metatarsal head, the avascular sclerotic bone is resected, and the intact cartilage is rotated from the undersurface of the head. The plantar cartilage is almost always healthy, and this is shifted up into an anterior facing position so that the plantar surface of the metatarsal head now articulates anteriorly with the proximal phalanx (Fig. 3–1–7). The size of the osteotomy is based on the extent and location of the avascular necrosis. Generally, the arthrosis and avascular bone are in the dorsal anterior aspect

of the metatarsal head. I start the osteotomy just inferior to this and aim the saw blade back plantar and posterior, preserving at least 5 mm of the articular surface of the metatarsal head. The wedge is then resected from the more dorsal aspect of the head and a triangular piece is removed with a base that measures approximately 4 to 6 mm. Fixation of the head is performed with a suture. I drill the dorsal distal metatarsal with a single small K-wire hole and then insert an absorbable suture first through the articular cartilage and then out the predrilled hole to secure the metatarsal head. The head does not require any more fixation than this, and I would not suggest using a K-wire, which can spin the small segment of the head right off. The operation is interesting, and the blood supply always seems to be sufficient either through the articular surface itself or through the distal metatarsal head to nourish the small osteochondral piece.

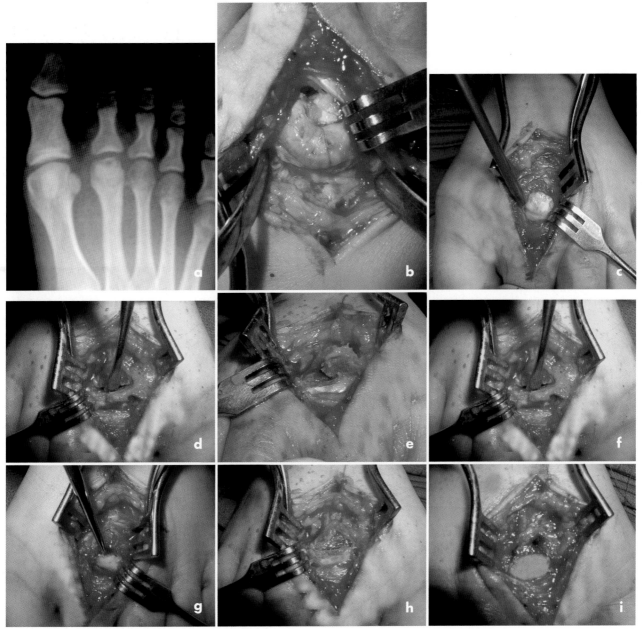

Figure 3–1–7. *Osteochondrosis of the metatarsal was treated in this 24-year-old patient with an osteotomy of the metatarsal head. Extensive necrosis of the metatarsal head was noted on x-ray (XR) film (a) and on gross examination of the head (b, c). The metatarsal head was cut with a knife blade instead of a saw because of the necrosis (d). The wedge of bone was removed (e), and it was pried open with a smooth elevator (f). The head was gently debrided with a small curette, but the plantar cortex was maintained intact (g). The osteotomy was then closed (h, i) and repaired with two 4-0 absorbable sutures.*

Techniques, tips, and pitfalls

1. Bone loss after excessive resection arthroplasty of the IP joint can be corrected with arthrodesis. This arthrodesis will shorten the toe even further, and an arthrodesis with interposition structural bone graft is necessary. I have harvested this graft from a small piece of the posterior calcaneus, which is shaped with a saw into the size required to fit the defect. This small bone block arthrodesis must be performed with threaded K-wire fixation, and the pin should be left in for at least 8 weeks.

2. A longitudinal incision over the PIP joint leaves the toe narrower, and the toe can be further tapered through excision of a longitudinal ellipse from the PIP joint. However, if a longitudinal skin incision is used, then some sort of fixation of the IP joint must be used. The fixation can be with a K-wire or through placement of a suture in the extensor hood. Alternatively, a transverse ellipse can be made through the skin, subcutaneous tissue, and extensor hood, and when closed, this type of ellipse facilitates the position of the toe. However, this type of approach will lead to a slight widening of the toe, which may be undesirable.

3. Arthrodesis of the PIP joint leads to a straight toe. This is not always well tolerated and, if possible, slight flexion should be incorporated into the arthrodesis. With the antegrade-retrograde technique with the K-wire, this flexion is not possible, and an alternative form of fixation must be used. Small threaded K-wires can be introduced obliquely across the crossing of the PIP joint and either buried flush with the bone or left out percutaneously.

4. If infection of the PIP joint occurs postoperatively, this may lead to a swollen inflamed toe, which always remains slightly thickened and uncomfortable. Interstitial fibrosis occurs, so even with resolution of the infection, permanent widening of the toe is present. This may necessitate revision surgery with scar resection and realignment.

5. Some patients benefit from correction of hammertoe, but for them, the correction cannot be accomplished without realignment of the hallux. The decision of realignment is difficult, for example, in elderly patients who have an asymptomatic bunion but a painful fixed deformity of the second toe. For these patients, I advocate an amputation of the second toe. It is quick, recovery is easy, and the procedure is remarkably well accepted by patients, particularly elderly patients. Usually, the hallux has already drifted as far as it can go, it is abutting the third toe, and the second toe is no longer functional. Amputation improves shoe wear and decreases pain without compromising forefoot function.

6. Be careful in the patient who has rigid deformities of all of the lesser toes with or without MP joint dislocation. These occur not only in some elderly individuals, but also in patients after crush injuries. In the patient with severe contracture without dislocation, the tendency is to perform a soft tissue release with realignment of the PIP joint. This seems reasonable; however, the incidence of wound complications is high in these patients because of stretching of the skin. The other option is to shorten the metatarsal, with either a metatarsal head resection or Weil osteotomy. However, even these operations are associated with an increased incidence of skin healing problems.

7. Scarring of the MP joint can be difficult to treat with revision surgery. Despite bone shortening, recurrent contracture may be present, and a skin Z-plasty may be helpful to aid in the soft tissue release and realignment (Fig. 3–1–8).

8. Amputation of the second toe is an excellent procedure for management of fixed deformity, particularly in elderly patients, when the toe is dislocated and the hallux deformity is asymptomatic (Fig. 3–1–9).

9. Some toe deformities are severe although they are asymptomatic. These often require

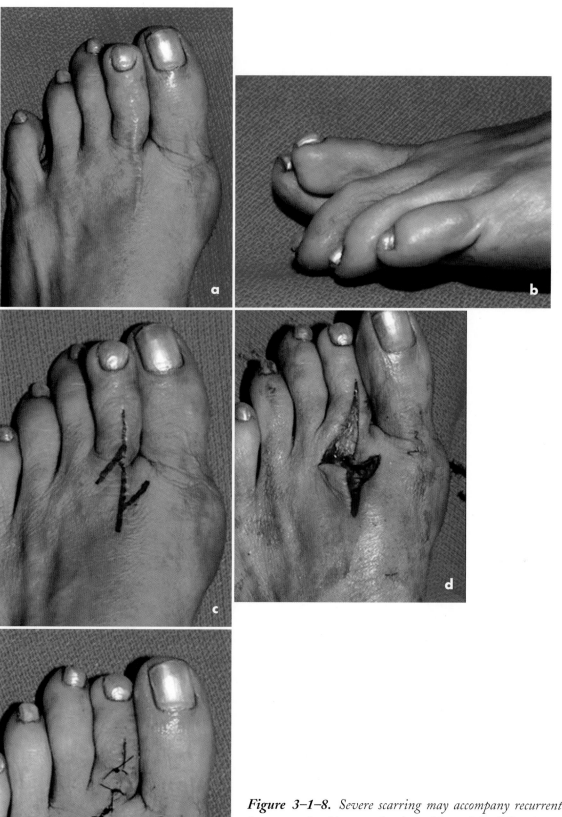

Figure 3–1–8. *Severe scarring may accompany recurrent deformity of the lesser toes. In this case, simple revision of the deformity may not be possible (a, b). For realignment of the toe, in addition to whatever tendon lengthening, capsulotomy, and bone procedure must be performed, a Z-plasty of the skin may be necessary. The skin is marked out first for the longitudinal incision, and then the Z-plasty incisions are marked at a 45-degree angle with the center located over the metatarsophalangeal (MP) joint (c). The flaps are cut (d) and sutured (e). The apex of the flaps should be sutured first to prevent retraction of the skin.*

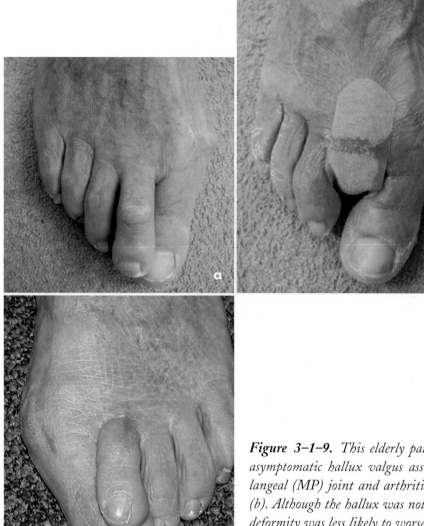

Figure 3–1–9. *This elderly patient had severe pain in the second toe and asymptomatic hallux valgus associated with a rigid hallux metatarsophalangeal (MP) joint and arthritis (a). A second toe amputation was selected (b). Although the hallux was not as deformed as in some patients, the hallux deformity was less likely to worsen because of the rigidity of the MP joint. In contrast, this patient had undergone prior operations to both the hallux and second toe with recurrence of deformity (c). Although the hallux is in severe valgus, it was asymptomatic, and a second toe amputation was performed.*

correction, not necessarily for cosmetic purposes, but for prevention of recurrent deformity of the hallux (Fig. 3–1–10).

10. Fixed toe deformity at both the MP and IP joints should be corrected with shortening of the toe or metatarsal. Frequently, the deformity is of such a magnitude that even metatarsal shortening osteotomy is not realistic, and metatarsal head resection is preferable (Fig. 3–1–11).

Correction of Crossover Toe Deformity

Crossover toe deformity cannot be corrected in the same way as a claw toe or hammertoe. If this correction is done with a standard MP joint release and arthroplasty of the IP joint, the deformity recurs because the deformity (contracture) is in the transverse plane (Fig. 3–1–12).

Ideally, stability in the transverse plane should be enhanced, but at the same time, flexibility of the MP joint and control of any sagittal plane instability should be maintained. To some extent, the success of the

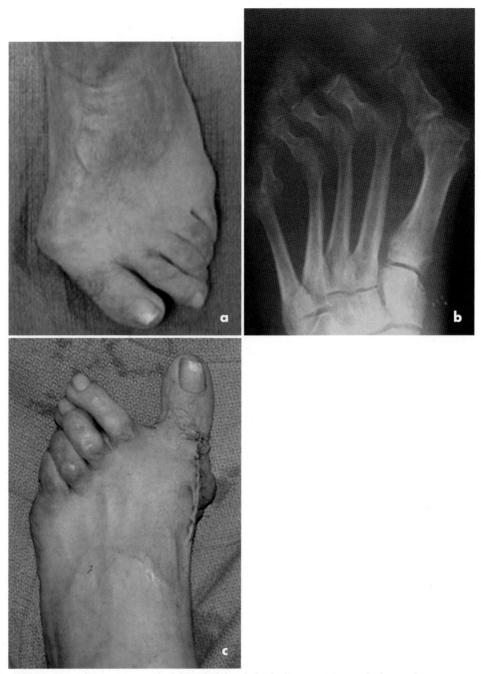

Figure 3–1–10. *This patient had severe painful arthritis of the hallux metatarsophalangeal (MP) joint associated with asymptomatic lesser toe deformities (a, b). Once the hallux had been realigned with arthrodesis, the magnitude of the lesser toe deformity was more apparent (c). The toes must be corrected, and this can be accomplished with either resection of the lesser metatarsal heads or with shortening osteotomy of the lesser metatarsals, followed by proximal interphalangeal (PIP) arthroplasty.*

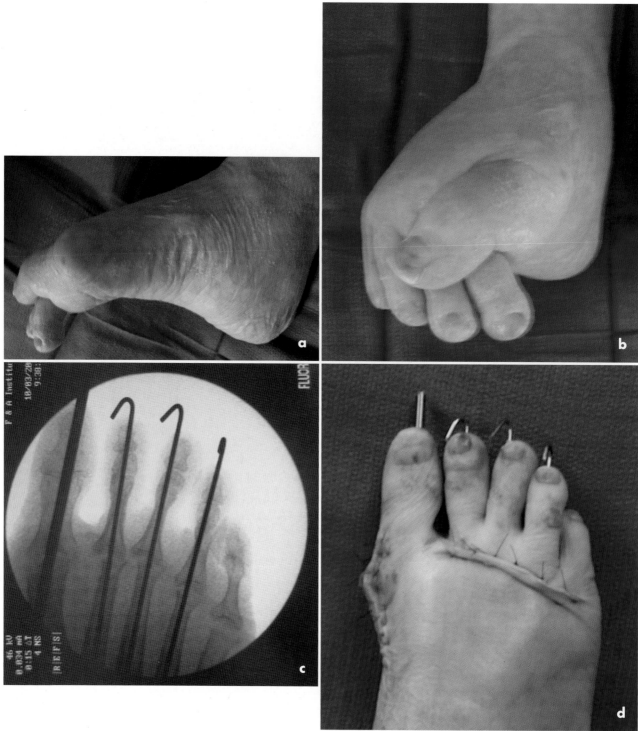

Figure 3–1–11. *This 76-year-old patient had severe rigid contracture associated with a neurological disorder (a). The toes were fixed, and a rigid flexion contracture was present at the metatarsophalangeal (MP) joints. Correction included resection of all of the metatarsal heads, including the first head, without an MP fusion to facilitate immediate ambulation (b–d). In addition to resection of the metatarsal heads, all of the flexor tendons had to be cut.*

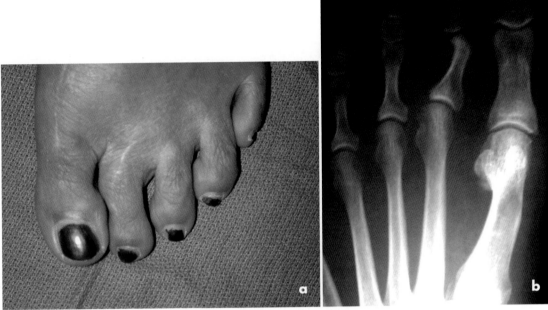

Figure 3–1–12. *This patient underwent a bunionectomy and distal metatarsal osteotomy for correction of hallux valgus and a second proximal interphalangeal (PIP) resection arthroplasty for correction of a presumed claw toe, with recurrent deformity. This is a crossover toe deformity and cannot be treated in the same way as a claw toe (a, b).*

operation will depend on the cause of the deformity. The pathogenesis of this condition is assumed to be a result of a rupture of the lateral collateral ligament, followed by varying degrees of rupture of the plantar lateral volar plate, followed by dorsomedial deviation. If this is associated with a long second metatarsal, then the second metatarsal should be shortened. Shortening the metatarsal relieves the medial joint contracture because pressure is taken off the intrinsic tendons (Figs. 3–1–13 and 3–1–14).

Repair of the ruptured lateral collateral ligament and volar plate is technically difficult and probably unrealistic. For the repair to be performed, the suture must be inserted into the lateral collateral ligament without restraint of the joint and creation of a dorsiflexion contracture.

Incision and Dissection

The incision begins at the MP joint, with an adequate soft tissue release of the dorsal and medial contracture. The extensor hood is identified and is incised longitudinally medial to the extensor digitorum longus tendon,

which is retracted laterally. The attachment of the extensor hood to the base of the proximal phalanx must be maintained, and a transverse dorsal capsulotomy is performed. On the dorsal medial aspect of the MP joint the collateral ligament is now released. This can be cut at its attachment to the proximal phalanx or the metatarsal head, but the volar plate ligament should be maintained (Fig. 3–1–15).

Extensor Digitorum Brevis Tendon Transfer

If the instability of the toe is predominantly in the transverse and not the sagittal plane, then the extensor digitorum brevis (EDB) tendon and not a flexor to extensor tendon transfer is preferred. The EDB tendon and the extensor digitorum longus tendon are identified proximally and dissected free of each other by a longitudinal split of the extensor hood with Metzenbaum scissors. A 6-cm length of the EDB tendon is selected, and before division of the tendon, two nonabsorbable 4-0 sutures are inserted on either side of the tenotomy to stabilize the tendon after the division for transfer. A tenotomy is now performed in between these two sutures, and the distal portion of the EDB tendon is now gradually

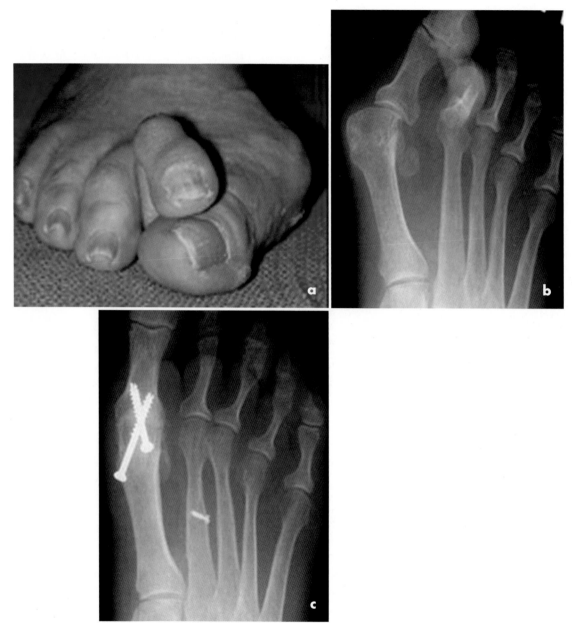

Figure 3–1–13. *A severe grade of crossover toe deformity was present associated with dislocation of the second metatarsophalangeal (MP) joint and arthritis of the hallux MP joint (a, b). Correction of the second toe can only be accomplished with shortening of the metatarsal to reduce the intrinsic contracture. A midshaft osteotomy was performed, in conjunction with a flexor to extensor tendon transfer and arthrodesis of the hallux MP joint (c).*

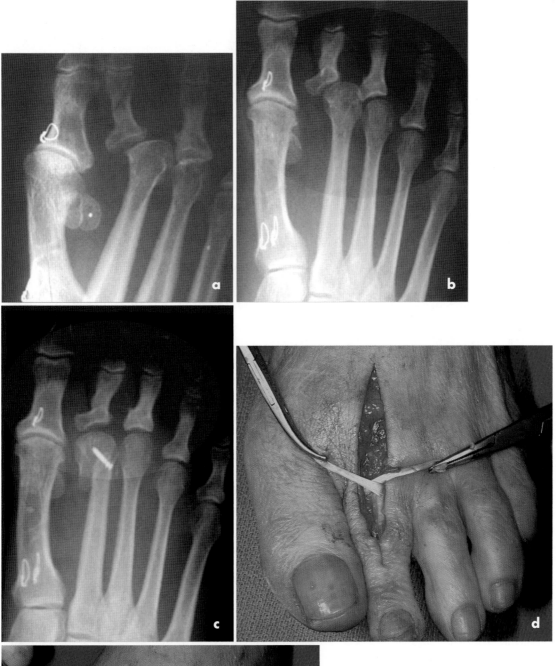

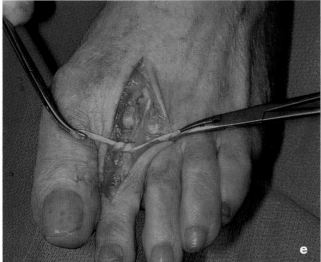

Figure 3–1–14. *In conjunction with various procedures for correction of hallux valgus, a crossover toe deformity was treated with some type of lateral closing wedge osteotomy of the base of the proximal phalanx of the second toe (a, b). This procedure did not realign the toe, and the patient was referred for subsequent correction, which was performed with a shortening osteotomy of the second metatarsal (c). At the time, an unstable second toe metatarsophalangeal (MP) joint was addressed with a flexor to extensor tendon transfer. Note the use of a knot in the tendon; this knot allows the toe to be pulled laterally to correct the transverse plane deviation (d, e).*

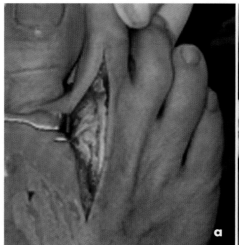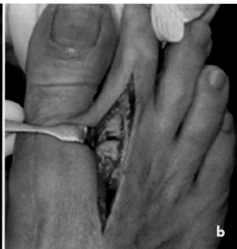

Figure 3–1–15. *The dissection of the metatarsophalangeal (MP) joint is performed initially with a dorsal capsulotomy and release of the contracted medial collateral ligament (a, b).*

mobilized. It is dissected free more distally from the extensor hood. Its attachment to the extensor hood overlying the base of the proximal phalanx must be maintained (Fig. 3–1–16).

If this tears or looks as if it will separate, then a stay suture can be inserted between the distal tendon and the extensor hood. With the work now being done in the lateral web space, a curved, blunt-tipped (aneurysm) needle is passed from proximal to distal and below the deep transverse metatarsal ligament. The needle is then curved up into the soft tissue, and the suture attached to the EDB tendon is passed through the needle, which is then delivered proximally. The EDB tendon is now pulled deep to the soft tissue tether and passed proximally. As the tendon is pulled, the toe should assume a normal alignment, with good correction in both the transverse and sagittal planes. Because of the axis of the tendon transfer, the toe may supinate slightly, and this supination must be noted (Fig. 3–1–17).

Now, two options are available for stabilization: either a dynamic transfer of the EDB tendon or the use of the transferred tendon as a tenodesis. Generally, I prefer a more dynamic use of the EDB tendon, and the proximal stay suture is now used to tie the tendon transfer back down onto itself for this tendon transfer. If the tendon suture does not hold, then the EDB tendon can be inserted either into the dorsolateral periosteum or through a drill hole in the metatarsal neck. Once the toe is aligned, consider using a K-wire across the MP joint to further temporarily stabilize the toe.

The Flexor to Extensor Tendon Transfer

At the completion of the soft tissue release as previously described, the stability of the MP joint is examined. If it is unstable in both the sagittal and the horizontal planes, then a flexor to extensor tendon transfer can be performed. A flexor to extensor tendon transfer can be used for other indications, but instability, subluxation, or dislocation of the MP joint should be present.

INCISION AND DISSECTION.   A transverse incision is made on the plantar surface of the proximal flexion crease, and the small vein in the center in the incision is cauterized. Small soft tissue retractors are inserted on either side of the incision, medially and laterally. The flexor tendon sheath is identified when the fatty tissue is pulled out of the way. The sheath is cut longitudinally from proximal to distal, with the tendons exposed. A curved hemostat is inserted through and under both flexor tendons, and when they are placed on stretch, the distal phalanx is flexed. A percutaneous tenotomy of the longus flexor tendon is performed at the level of the DIP joint.

TENDON PREPARATION.   A second hemostat is now passed under the long flexor tendon proximally, and the tendon is pulled into the incision. The distal tendon stump is grasped on both sides with two hemostats, and the tendon is split in half along the median raphe. This split can be made with a knife or with the pulling of the clamps separating the tendon. The split tendon is now passed from plantar to dorsal with a small clamp that is

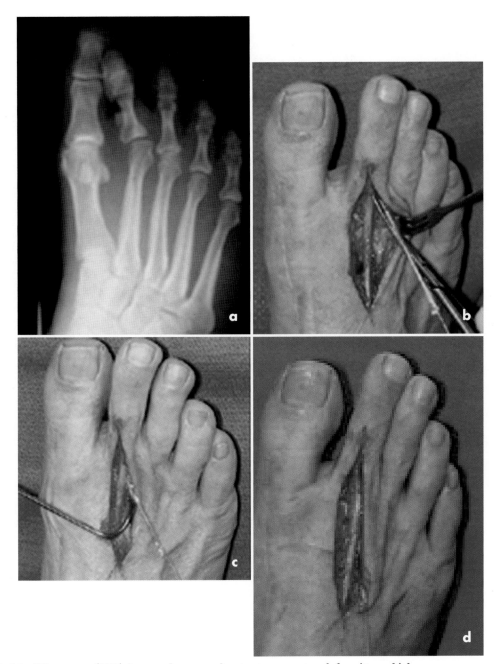

Figure 3–1–16. *The x-ray (XR) image shows moderate crossover toe deformity, which was corrected with an extensor digitorum brevis (EDB) tenodesis (as opposed to a tendon transfer) (a). The EDB tendon is cut proximally, and a 4-0 stay suture is inserted into the tendon (b). A curved needle (aneurysm needle) is passed under the deep metatarsal ligament, grasping the suture (c), and the tendon is pulled under the ligament proximally (d).*

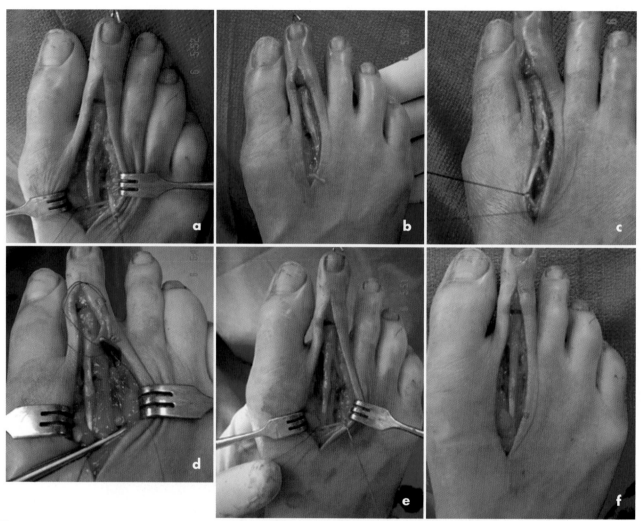

Figure 3–1–17. The extensor digitorum brevis (EDB) tendon transfer was performed in this patient for a grade II crossover toe deformity. A posterior interphalangeal (PIP) arthrodesis had been performed, and the K-wire was inserted across the PIP, but not the metatarsophalangeal (MP) joint (a). With pressure under the metatarsal head, the dynamic instability of the second MP joint is visible (b). The EDB tendon is exposed with more proximal dissection, two 4-0 stay sutures are inserted, and the tendon cut in between the sutures (c). A curved tapered needle is passed under the deeper soft tissue in the second web space (d). Note that when the EDB tendon is pulled, the toe now assumes a more normal position under tension (e) and the final appearance of the repair (f).

passed from dorsal to plantar along the base of the proximal phalanx and out the plantar incision. The clamp must hug the edge of the phalanx to prevent vascular injury. Each end of the flexor tendon is inserted into the tip of the clamp and then passed from plantar to dorsal on each side of the phalanx. The tendon ends are then looped superficially to the extensor hood, and a knot is tied in the tendon. By tensioning the knot (pulling on the medial slip of the tendon pulls the phalanx more lat-

erally), the surgeon can correct the frontal plane alignment into a neutral position. Immediately before the suture is tensed, a K-wire is introduced antegrade across the MP joint and out the tip of the toe. Once the suture has been tied and the tension on the flexor tendon transfer is corrected, the K-wire is then inserted retrograde back across the MP joint to stabilize the toe further. For tension of the transfer and prevention of tightness of the MP joint, the tendon is sutured with the toe in approximately 30 degrees of dorsiflexion while the ankle is held in neutral dorsiflexion. The tendon is now secured with two interrupted nonabsorbable 4-0 sutures both to itself and to the extensor hood (Fig. 3–1–18).

Oblique Metatarsal Head Osteotomy (Weil Osteotomy)

The indication for this procedure is instability of the MP joint in either the sagittal or transverse plane. The goal of the operation is to slightly shorten the metatarsal head. The intrinsic contracture on either side of the MP joint is therefore relaxed, and alignment is facilitated.

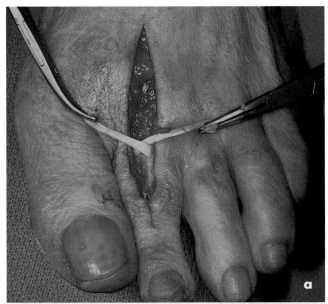

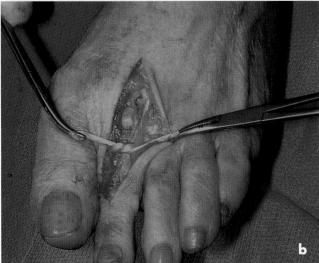

Figure 3–1–18. The flexor to extensor tendon transfer.

This procedure is also performed in conjunction with subluxation or dislocation of the MP joint, occasionally in the setting of metatarsalgia, when instability is present simultaneously.

Despite its popularity and indeed my own extensive experience, the problem with this osteotomy is the unpredictability with respect to the axial alignment of the toe after surgery. This type of osteotomy has been shown both in the clinical and in the laboratory setting to cause slight elevation of the axis of the intrinsic tendons dorsal to the center of the metatarsal head. The extensor tendons are then augmented by the slight dorsal shift in the intrinsic tendons, which do not as effectively plantarflex the MP joint. The toe is therefore slightly shortened and also slightly elevated off the ground.

To some extent this elevation can be obviated with vigorous plantar flexion exercises of the MP joint that begin soon after surgery. The flexor to extensor transfer is not a panacea for correction of instability because this, too, may be associated with complications, including stiffness and dissatisfaction with the use of the toe. Nonetheless, in the presence of a dislocated MP joint, a shortening osteotomy of the metatarsal of some type is necessary, and the Weil osteotomy is an effective procedure to reduce this dislocation. I do not think that this is an ideal procedure for correction if isolated metatarsalgia is present because alternative osteotomies are available that do not elevate the toe. Surprisingly, given the plane of the osteotomy, avascular necrosis of the metatarsal head is extremely rare, and although arthritis of the MP joint may occur, it is uncommon.

The incision is made and located according to the number of metatarsals corrected. If a single metatarsal is addressed, an incision is made directly over the MP joint. If two adjacent metatarsals are corrected, then the incision is made between them (e.g., in the second interspace). Although performance of the central three metatarsal osteotomies through a single incision located over the third MP joint is possible, this creates too much stretching of the skin with the potential for wound breakdown, and I prefer to use two incisions, one medial to the second MP joint and then one slightly lateral to the fourth. The incision is deepened through the subcutaneous tissue, and the extensor tendons are lengthened, particularly in the setting of any subluxation, dorsiflexion contracture, or dislocation. A dorsal capsulectomy is performed to expose the metatarsal head, and a curved periosteal shmogler is inserted into the MP joint if it is dislocated. As it is levered down, the metatarsal head becomes visible. Take care not to injure the articular surface with the periosteal elevator as the shmogler is inserted. If the joint is dislocated the volar plate must be stripped off the underside of the metatarsal head to facilitate scarring under the neck. With the metatarsal head visible, the cut is planned at the apex of the metatarsal head 1 to 2 mm inferior to the articular edge. The cut is made at a 30-degree angle, but this varies according to the declination of the metatarsal. It is typically made over a length of about 2 cm, which corresponds to the length of the saw blade used. The cut is not completed, and a second cut is made just inferior to this so that a slice of bone of approximately 2 mm is removed. Depression of the metatarsal head with the plane of this osteotomy is inevitable. The extent of this depression correlates with the plane of the osteotomy. The resection of a small wedge of bone is therefore an important part of this procedure unless significant shortening of more than 8 mm is performed, in which case depression of the metatarsal head and metatarsalgia does not occur. After removal of the small slice of bone, the saw is reintroduced and the cut completed. This cut is tactile because the plantar surface of the metatarsal is perforated, and the metatarsal head is then grasped with a small-toothed clamp and pushed proximally by the desired amount. This amount is usually 5 mm, but it will be determined according to the length of each metatarsal, prior trauma, and the need for shortening. The metatarsal is held firmly with the clamp, and a screw is inserted with a small threaded twist-off screw from the dorsal aspect of the distal metatarsal, which does not require predrilling. Rarely, two screws are used. The screw should be aimed into the metatarsal head and not directly plantarward so that the screw threads are buried and not protruding. This protrusion can cause metatarsalgia or irritation of the volar plate with limitation and dorsiflexion. The overhanging bone is then trimmed off either with a saw or small bone cutter, and the motion of the MP joint is assessed for stability and impingement at the osteotomy interface (Fig. 3–1–19).

On the basis of the remaining stability, further procedures can be performed, including a flexor to extensor tendon transfer or an EDB tendon transfer. Although a K-wire can be used, the plane of the osteotomy is such that the K-wire can displace the metatarsal head during insertion. Positioning the toe in the axis of the metatarsal is difficult, because the toe protrudes into the shoe. If stability is essential and the use of a K-wire is thought to be important, then the toe has to be plantarflexed in line with the metatarsal, and then a cutout of the shoe is made to support the pulp of the toe and prevent it from getting irritated on the shoe itself. The K-wire is left in for approximately 3 weeks to stabilize the volar plate and prevent recurrent instability. Leaving the K-wire in also facilitates scarring down the volar plate and the intrinsic tendons so that dorsal subluxation is less likely to occur (Figs. 3–1–20 and 3–1–21).

Techniques, tips, and pitfalls

1. As an alternative to passing the split tendon along the sides of the proximal phalanx, it can be passed through a drill hole in the base of the proximal phalanx. The hole is made at a 30-degree angle with respect to the phalanx and begins dorsally at the base of the proximal phalanx just distal to the articular surface and then exits slightly more distally in the region of the incision on the plantar surface of the proximal flexion crease. A suture passer is inserted through the drill hole dorsally into the plantar aspect of the soft tissue, and the flexor tendon is then grasped and pulled dorsally. The tendon is now split along the median raphe and then tied dorsally over the extensor hood.

2. In correction of crossover toe deformity, establishing the correct tension is difficult. Overcorrection can occur if the tendon transfer is too tight, with limitation of dorsiflexion. There is a fine balance between establishing adequate tension and stability, and then a tension that limits passive dorsiflexion of the MP joint. This problem with the tension applies to any procedure for which the flexor to extensor tendon transfer is performed, whether associated with vertical (sagittal plane) instability, subluxation, or dislocation. Ideally, 45 degrees of passive

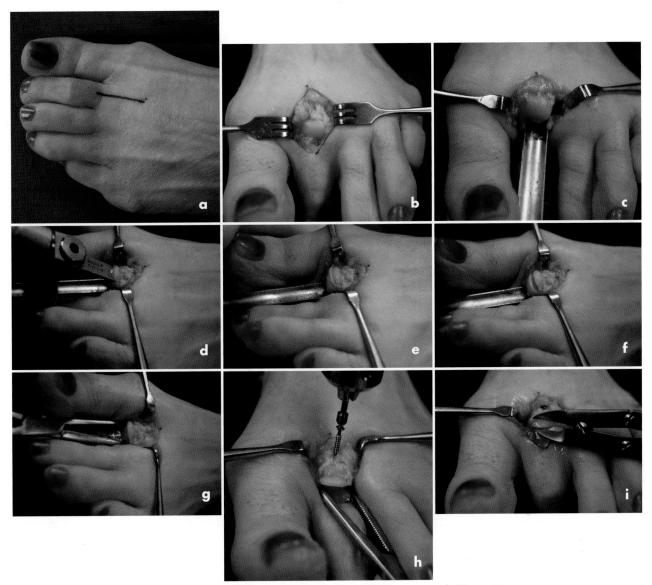

Figure 3–1–19. *The steps of the oblique metatarsal head osteotomy (Weil osteotomy). The incision is centered over the metatarsophalangeal (MP) joint (a), and the metatarsal head is exposed (b). A curved periosteal elevator (shmogler) is inserted under the head (c), and the first cut is made 1 mm inferior to the dorsal surface of the metatarsal head (d). A 2-mm wedge of bone is removed (e, f), the osteotomy is completed, and the head is shifted proximally by the desired amount (g). The osteotomy is secured with a twist-off screw (DePuy, Warsaw, Ind.) (h), and the dorsal bone lip is removed with a bone cutter (i).*

dorsiflexion of the toe is wanted, with the ankle in a neutral position, mimicking toe-off.

3. Stability is also important postoperatively and a K-wire should be used, but it should not be left in more than 2 to 3 weeks.

4. The axis of the transfer of the flexor tendon must be as proximal to the MP joint as possible so that the force vector is at the correct location. If the tendon transfer is done in the middle of the proximal phalanx, the force on the MP joint is minimized and, in fact, will lead to further dorsal subluxation of that joint. An alternative technique is to pass the flexor tendon through a drill hole at the base of the proximal phalanx.

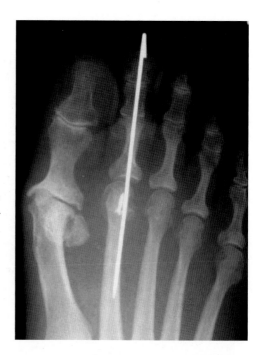

Figure 3-1-20. *This patient was treated for asymptomatic arthritis of the metatarsophalangeal (MP) joint caused by avascular necrosis and symptomatic dislocation of the second MP joint with a Weil osteotomy. Despite the use of a flexor to extensor tendon transfer, the second MP joint remained unstable, and a K-wire was used. Note, however, that the wire hit the screw for fixation of the osteotomy and then caused lateral subluxation of the MP joint.*

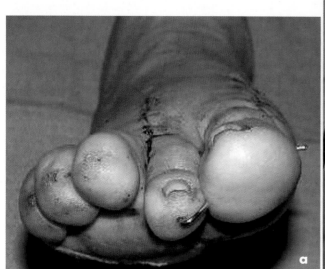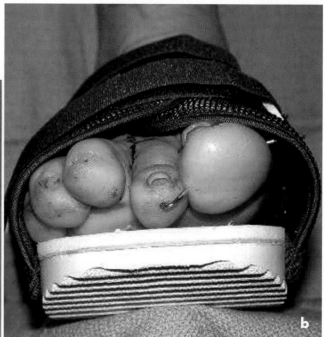

Figure 3-1-21. *A K-wire was used to stabilize the metatarsophalangeal (MP) joint after a Weil osteotomy. For the wire to be positioned in the metatarsal shaft, the toe was plantarflexed (a). Plantar flexion causes impingement of the toe against the postoperative shoe, which may be cut to provide room for the toe (b).*

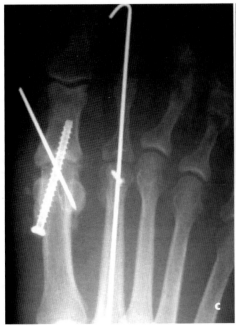

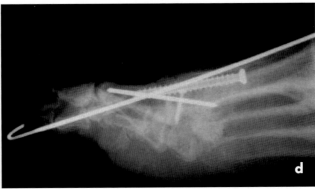

Figure 3–1–21, cont'd. Note the radiographs, with the position of the second toe, and the MP fusion where a screw and a pin were used for fixation. A single screw was not sufficient, and no room was available for a second screw because of the bone loss after a prior bunion procedure (c, d).

Suggested Reading

Cohen I, Myerson MS, Weil LS Sr. Flexor to extensor tendon transfer: A new method of tensioning and securing the tendon. Foot Ankle Int 22:62–63, 2001.

Myerson MS, Shereff MJ. The pathological anatomy of claw and hammer toes. J Bone Joint Surg Am 71:45–49, 1989.

Trnka HJ, Nyska M, Parks BG, Myerson MS. Dorsiflexion contracture after the Weil osteotomy: Results of cadaver study and three-dimensional analysis. Foot Ankle Int 22:47–50, 2001.

Metatarsalgia

Metatarsal Condylectomy

Condylectomy of the metatarsal is performed rarely and only for isolated metatarsalgia resulting from a prominent condyle. Because other procedures are more effective to correct a more global metatarsalgia, the condylectomy should be limited to the more focal painful callosity under the metatarsal head. This type of callosity is linear, as opposed to oval or more diffuse, which is under one or more metatarsals. The disadvantage of a plantar condylectomy is the destabilization of the volar plate, with potential instability followed by arthritis.

An incision is made over the dorsocentral aspect of the metatarsophalangeal (MP) joint, the extensor retinaculum is incised longitudinally adjacent to the extensor tendon, and the plantarflexed toe exposes the metatarsal head. A curved periosteal elevator (shmogler) is inserted into the MP joint, and the head is fully exposed while the elevator is maintained underneath the metatarsal head. A 1-cm chisel is inserted into the plantar condyle, and approximately 3 mm is removed with a clean cut of the underside of the metatarsal head. Working with a chisel and not an osteotomy and initiating the cut with the beveled edge, with the aim up into the metatarsal shaft, are useful. If an osteotome is used, the bevel will direct the cut out of the condyle prematurely, and insufficient bone will be removed. Once the cut is initiated, the chisel is then turned around with the bevel aiming

plantarward, and in this way, a fracture of the metatarsal is prevented. The trick is to remove the condyle and not lose it in the plantar soft tissues. The chisel is now worked against the periosteal elevator with the condyle in between. With a gradual twist of the chisel blade, the condyle is then "delivered" anteriorly and removed.

The joint must now be tested for stability. If it is grossly unstable, then a K-wire should be used for 3 weeks to help maintain stability and facilitate scarring down of the volar plate onto the metatarsal neck. The problem occurs if the volar plate is detached and then slight dorsal subluxation of the phalanx occurs on the metatarsal head through mobility of the MP joint. Scarring will occur dorsally, leading to a fixed extension contracture of the MP joint. If a K-wire is not used, plantar flexion exercises need to begin soon after surgery.

Dorsal Wedge Osteotomy of the Lesser Metatarsals

A dorsal wedge osteotomy of the lesser metatarsals is performed for specific conditions of isolated metatarsalgia. Although alternatives for correction of metatarsalgia are available, such as the Weil osteotomy, a shortening diaphyseal osteotomy, and a shortening proximal metatarsal osteotomy, each procedure is associated with potential problems. I have found that the Weil osteotomy can be used for correction of isolated metatarsalgia, but it is not predictable because of the varied position of the toe in the sagittal plane. For specific relief of metatarsalgia, either a condylectomy or a dorsal wedge osteotomy is more predictable. However, the potential for transfer metatarsalgia must be considered. Although no osteotomy is so precise that it can avoid transfer of weight, the dorsal wedge osteotomy remains a reasonable procedure for correction after a prior fracture, stress fracture, or prior osteotomy of an adjacent metatarsal.

An incision is made over the neck of the metatarsal, and the dorsal aspect of the metatarsal head is visualized. The soft tissues, including the periosteum and extensor tendons, are retracted, and two pilot holes are inserted. These are unicortical holes, made with a 1-mm Kirschner wire at a 45-degree angle to each other and placed approximately 1 cm apart. The osteotomy is performed in between these pilot holes. Not more than 1 mm of bone must be removed. This means that, including the thickness of the saw blade, the actual base of the osteotomy is about .5 mm thick. A greenstick cut is performed, and the plantar cortex *must* be left intact. I prefer to complete the osteotomy with a fracture maneuver that actually opens up the osteotomy using manual dorsal pressure on the head of the metatarsal. This preserves a nice periosteal bridge on the plantar surface and prevents excessive dorsal shift of the metatarsal head. Fixation of the osteotomy is performed with a stout suture of 2-0 absorbable material on a tapered needle, which is easily passed through the predrilled holes. More extensive fixation is not necessary (Fig. 3–2–1). Although I have performed this for more than one metatarsal at a time, multiple dorsal wedge osteotomies need to be carefully planned because the presence of transfer metatarsalgia increases as the number of these osteotomies is performed, and multiple Weil osteotomies is preferable.

Oblique Metatarsal Head Osteotomy (Weil Osteotomy)

This osteotomy is indicated for many conditions, ranging from subluxation and dislocation of the MP joint, to crossover toe deformity, correction of rheumatologic deformity of the MP joint, and metatarsalgia. Be aware of the anatomy of the osteotomy, because the pressure under the metatarsal head can actually increase as the head is translated proximally. To avoid this, I

routinely remove a 1- to 2-mm slice of bone from the metatarsal head. Numerous anatomic cadaveric studies have been performed in which the pressures under the metatarsal heads were checked. The osteotomy can cause a change in pressure under either the operated or the adjacent metatarsal. Clinically, however, transfer metatarsalgia does not seem to occur, provided the principle of the osteotomy is understood.

The issue then arises as to whether an isolated second metatarsal osteotomy should be done or whether the third and possibly the fourth should be included. The decision depends, of course, on the preexisting disease. Generally, I will perform the osteotomy for most cases only on the second metatarsal. Other decision factors include if the third and/or the fourth toe appears to be too long, callosity is under the metatarsal head, or subluxation of the third MP joint is present. The same considerations apply to correction of transverse plane deformities of the second, third, and fourth toes that are accompanied by either severe hallux valgus or hallux varus, for which osteotomies of all three middle metatarsals should be performed (Figs. 3–2–2 and 3–2–3).

If only the second metatarsal is to be cut, then the incision is centered over this joint. If the second and third metatarsals are to be cut, then the incision is based in the second web space. The difficulty with the incision planning occurs if the second, third, and fourth metatarsals are cut. A central incision can be made over the third metatarsal, but be careful with the skin retraction. The alternative is to have the first incision slightly medial to the second metatarsal and the second incision slightly lateral to the fourth metatarsal to include as wide a skin bridge as possible; however, this method makes it difficult to address the middle and third metatarsal osteotomy.

The Incision, Bone Cut, and Fixation

Before the osteotomy, the metatarsal head must be fully exposed and the collateral ligaments cut. They do not need to be completely transected, but released dorsally, and then stretched as the joint is subluxated inferiorly. If the joint is dislocated, then it must be reduced with a curved periosteal elevator (a shmogler); the proximal

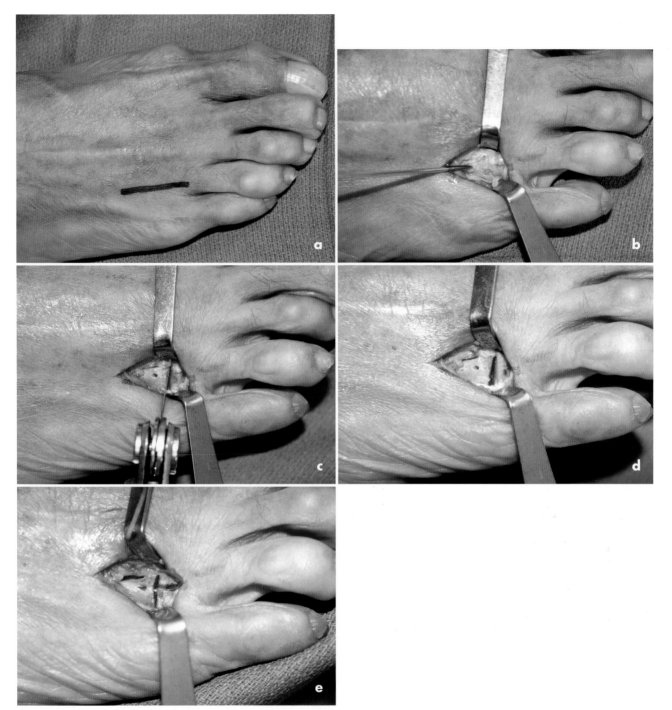

Figure 3–2–1. *A dorsal wedge osteotomy of the fourth metatarsal is shown for this patient with isolated fourth metatarsalgia after a stress fracture to the third metatarsal. The incision is marked along the distal metatarsal (a), and two unicortical pilot holes are made in the neck of the metatarsal at an angle of 45 degrees to the metatarsal (b). A saw is used to resect a 1-mm wedge of bone (c, d). The metatarsal neck is then pushed up across an intact plantar cortex, and a suture is inserted through the predrilled holes for fixation (e).*

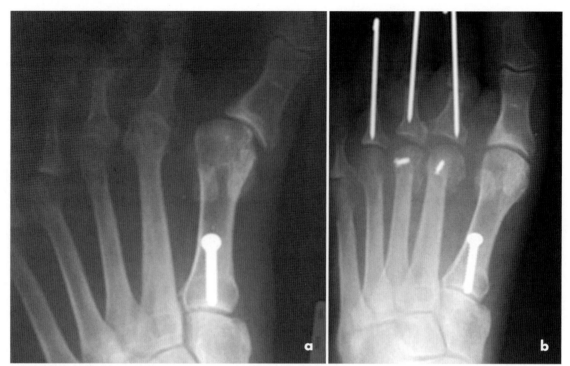

Figure 3–2–2. *Severe hallux varus occurred after a proximal crescentic osteotomy in this patient, accompanied by adductus of the lesser toes (a). The toe deformities must be corrected simultaneously, and the best way to decrease the tension on the intrinsic contracture is with a Weil osteotomy, performed on the second and third metatarsal (b).*

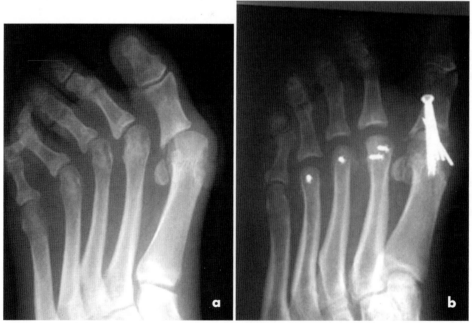

Figure 3–2–3. *Preoperative (a) and postoperative (b) x-ray (XR) images of a patient with severe valgus deformity of the lesser toes associated with subluxation of the lesser toe metatarsophalangeal (MP) joints and arthritis of the hallux MP joint after a failed resection arthroplasty. This was corrected with an arthrodesis of the MP joint and Weil osteotomies of the lesser metatarsals.*

phalanx should be pushed under the head to expose the head for the osteotomy. If no subluxation is present, then the phalanx can be bent downward to expose the dorsal surface for the osteotomy. The cut in the metatarsal head is made at the dorsal apical surface of the head just inferior to the dorsal joint cartilage. The cut is made with a saw at an angle approximately 25 degrees with respect to the metatarsal shaft. This angle may vary, however, according to the declination angle of the metatarsal so that if a 25-degree cut is used and the second metatarsal is in equinus, then metatarsalgia will occur. The angle of the osteotomy has to increase toward the more lateral metatarsals, which are always "flatter" than the declination of the second metatarsal.

The cut is not completed, and a second saw cut is made just inferior to the first cut so that a wedge or slice of bone is now resected measuring approximately 1 to 2 mm. The slice of bone is then removed, and the first cut is completed on the more dorsal surface of the metatarsal. Sensing that the osteotomy is completed is easy because when the metatarsal is perforated on its plantar surface, the head suddenly shifts and retracts to a more proximal position.

The metatarsal head must be held securely in the desired position; either use a clamp or push up under the head with the phalanx to compress the osteotomy. The head should be shortened approximately 5 mm, although this amount depends entirely on the underlying disease. While the metatarsal head is held in the corrected position, a twist-off screw (DePuy, Warsaw, Ind.) is inserted through the metatarsal neck. Usually a 12-mm screw is sufficient. It can be introduced slightly eccentrically to insert a K-wire through the head and avoid the screw in the metatarsal. The dorsal overhanging bone shelf of the metatarsal head osteotomy is now trimmed with either a small bone cutter or a saw until the shelf is smooth.

The stability of the MP joint must always be evaluated, and if instability is excessive, then a flexor to extensor tendon transfer could be considered. The toe should resume a more normal position, and the articulation should be well centered over the MP joint. As an alternative to the flexor to extensor tendon transfer, a K-wire can be used and inserted as far proximally as possible.

Techniques, tips, and pitfalls

1. For correction of a crossover toe deformity with the Weil osteotomy, the metatarsal head can be rotated slightly laterally to change the center of motion of the MP joint and direct the toe slightly laterally. This technique does not, however, apply to the osteotomy when it is performed for correction of sagittal plane instability or dislocation.

2. If a K-wire is used to stabilize the MP joint, the dilemma is how to position the toe for maximum stability. For the K-wire to be run all the way into the metatarsal, the toe has to be in the same plane as the metatarsal, and the toe is plantarflexed in relation to the forefoot. As such, the toe is jammed into the postoperative shoe. The forefoot will have to be elevated to prevent any pressure under the tip of the toe. This elevation can be done with a pad proximal to the metatarsal or with the removal of the end of the postoperative shoe.

3. A frequent complication of this osteotomy is elevation of the toe off the ground with slight dorsal contracture (Fig. 3–2–4). The reason for this complication has been demonstrated in the clinical setting and in the laboratory. As a result of the shortening of the metatarsal, the axis of the intrinsic muscles shift dorsal to the center of the metatarsal head, and these begin to function as an extensor instead of a flexor of the MP joint. This complication can be prevented to some extent with a K-wire across the MP joint, the application of tape to the toe, or vigorous massage. This massage in plantar flexion should begin as soon as tolerated and continue for 2 months after surgery. Therapy modalities are also helpful to strengthen the plantar flexion of the toes.

4. Despite the severity of dissection around the MP joint, avascular necrosis of the metatarsal head is extremely rare. The blood supply in the surrounding tissues seems to be sufficient to heal the osteotomy without vascular compromise.

5. The head should be fully visualized before the osteotomy is made. The use of the curved

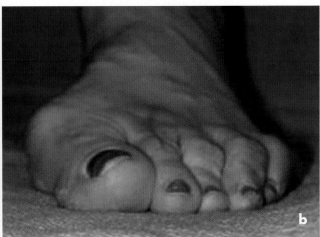

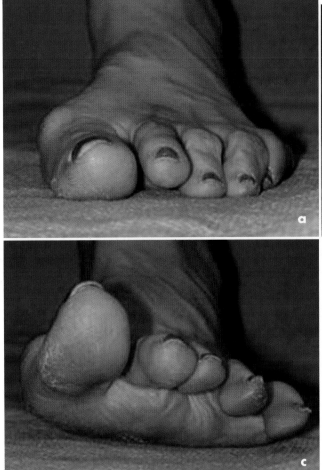

Figure 3–2–4. This patient was treated with a Weil osteotomy and a flexor to extensor tendon transfer for a dislocated second metatarsophalangeal (MP) joint. Note the attitude of the toe (a), which is slightly extended at rest but has very good flexion strength with good ground contact (b) and good extension (c).

periosteal elevator (shmogler) under the metatarsal head also strips the synovial attachment of the volar plate, and this allows it to shift more proximally with the osteotomy. Some surgeons believe that this step is important to loosen the volar plate and facilitate realignment of the metatarsal head.

6. The angle of the osteotomy must differ according to the angle of declination of the metatarsal so that the plane of the cut will be flatter for the third and fourth metatarsals.

7. The shift of the head is approximately 5 mm, and although it is not precise, there is a "feel" to the amount of shortening that is ideal. If an osteotomy of the third and fourth metatarsal heads is also performed, then each of the more lateral metatarsals should have about 1 mm less shortened.

Correction of Brachymetatarsia

I correct brachymetatarsia according to the age of the patient and the number of metatarsals involved. Although gradual distraction of the metatarsal can be performed successfully, I prefer, wherever possible, to perform a single (nonstaged) lengthening using interpositional graft. This is certainly preferable when more than one metatarsal is involved because the application of distraction to two adjacent lesser metatarsals is impractical. Nonetheless, gradual distraction is a reliable technique, provided it is tolerated by the patient.

If isolated brachymetatarsia is present, correction of the dorsiflexed and extended lesser toe must be performed simultaneously. This operation is usually done with an extensor tendon lengthening and MP joint release with percutaneous stabilization of the toe across the MP joint with a K-wire. If the toe is not stabilized at the MP joint, gradual hyperextension of the MP joint will occur with worsening deformity of the toe during lengthening.

Correction with an external fixation device begins with assembly of the fixator before the bone cut. Performing the osteotomy once the fixator is attached is far easier than working on a loose, unstable metatarsal during insertion of the pins. With minimal periosteal stripping, an osteotomy is performed with a sharp osteotome or a saw after a 1-cm incision. The distractor is then aligned, and the plane of distraction is checked. The correction of any toe deformity must be performed at this time with internal fixation across the MP joint.

Lengthening as a single-stage procedure with insertion of structural bone graft has an advantage in that the exact length of the toe can be attained in one setting. The only limiting factor is the actual length that can be obtained without the potential for ischemia of the toe, but I am usually able to obtain about 18 mm of length of a single metatarsal without jeopardizing perfusion to

the toe. A lamina spreader is inserted while the circulation to the toe is watched as the spreader is gradually distracted. Once the desired length has been attained, then temporary K-wires are inserted in multiple planes across the metatarsals for temporary fixation to keep it out to length with insertion of the graft. The graft can be held secure with a small dorsal plate or with K-wires inserted exteriorly. Because the K-wire has to be inserted across the MP joint anyway for stabilization of any toe deformity, using a long K-wire is advantageous; the wire should be inserted across into the cuboid or cuneiform joint and maintained for at least 8 weeks. Allograft bone seems to be sufficient, and I supplement this by soaking the graft in the Symphony platelet system (DePuy, Warsaw, Ind.) (Fig. 3–2–5).

With either a single-stage lengthening or with the use of an external fixator, the MP joint is stiff at the completion of the lengthening, and physical therapy will be required. Function of the toes, however, is good on resolution, and rarely is a flexion contracture of the toe present.

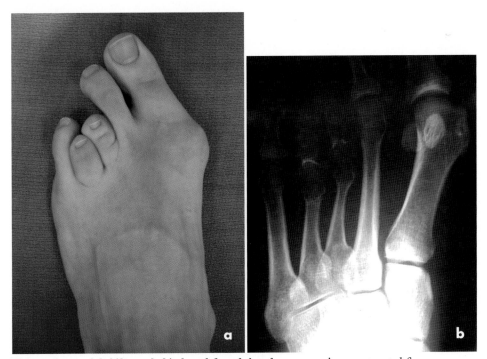

Figure 3–2–5. This patient with bilateral third and fourth brachymetatarsia was treated for correction of hallux valgus and second metatarsalgia, in addition to the short third and fourth metatarsals (a, b).

Continued

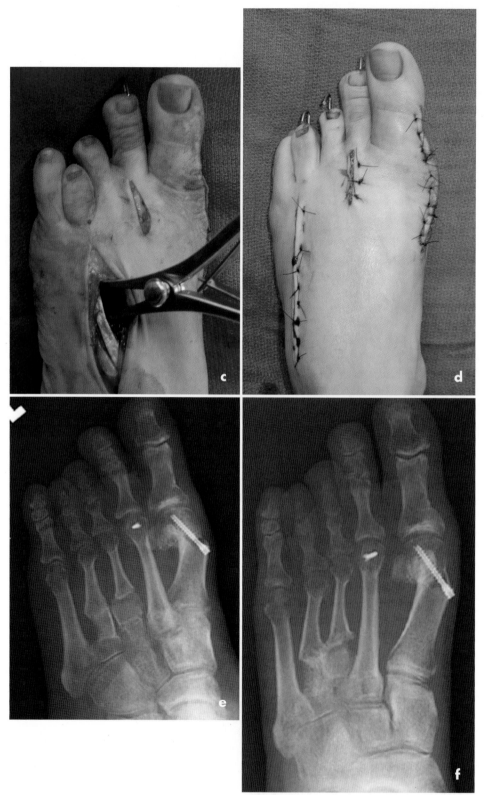

Figure 3–2–5, cont'd. *A shortening Weil osteotomy of the second metatarsal and a biplanar chevron osteotomy of the hallux were performed, followed by a one-stage lengthening osteotomy of the third and fourth metatarsals with interposition allograft and application of Symphony platelet system (DePuy, Warsaw, Ind.) (c, d). The final oblique and anteroposterior (AP) x-ray (XR) images are noted 3 months after surgery (e, f).*

Suggested Reading

Davies M, Saxby TS. Metatarsal neck osteotomy with rigid internal fixation for the treatment of lesser toe metatarsophalangeal joint pathology. Foot Ankle Int 20:630–636, 1999.

Feibel JB, Tisdel CL, Donley BG. Lesser metatarsal osteotomies. A biomechanical approach to metatarsalgia. Foot Ankle Clin 6:473–489, 2001.

Magnan B, Bragantini A, Regis D, Bartolozzi P. Metatarsal lengthening by callotasis during the growth phase. J Bone Joint Surg Br 77:602–607, 1995.

Melamed EA, Schon LC, Myerson MS, Parks BG. Two modifications of the Weil osteotomy. Analysis on sawbone models. Foot Ankle Int 23:400–405, 2002.

O'Kane C, Kilmartin TE. The surgical management of central metatarsalgia. Foot Ankle Int 23:415–419, 2002.

Trnka HJ, Nyska M, Parks BG, Myerson MS. Dorsiflexion contracture after the Weil osteotomy: Results of cadaver study and three-dimensional analysis. Foot Ankle Int 22:47–50, 2001.

Management of the Bunionette

Surgical Approach

Correction of the bunionette depends entirely on the magnitude and type of deformity. Clearly, ostectomy is a reasonable alternative, but caution is needed with a simple ostectomy because of recurrent deformity and the removal of too much of the metatarsal head, which causes instability and further deviation of the first toe with or without arthritis. Although I rarely perform an ostectomy on its own, the operation can be considered when the fifth metatarsal head, including the plantar condyle, is painful. For patients with this condition, an ostectomy can be performed. A condylectomy that countours the first metatarsal head can be included. The removal of an excessive amount of bone, however, will lead to the development of instability of the joint with or without avascular necrosis.

Chevron Osteotomy

For any deformity that involves a curvature of the metatarsal with widened intermetatarsal angle, an oblique metatarsal osteotomy is preferred. For all other deformities, a distal metatarsal osteotomy, either simple translation at the neck of the metatarsal or a chevron osteotomy, can be performed.

For either procedure, fixation of the metatarsal is preferable. Only temporary fixation is required. Despite the initial radiographic appearance, the bone healing that

invariably occurs in nonunion of the distal metatarsal osteotomy is rare. The fixation can be performed with a small twist-off screw, a buried or percutaneously introduced K-wire, or a bioresorbable pin. The Chevron cut that is performed in the fifth metatarsal head is technically no different than that made in the first metatarsal head for correction of a hallux valgus and bunion.

I try to have maximum bone-to-bone position and try to ensure that the angle of the cut is no less than 60 degrees. With a smaller angle cut, more cortical and less metaphyseal bone contact is made, and this contact leads to the possibility of instability (Fig. 3–3–1).

Oblique Fifth Metatarsal Osteotomy

An oblique shaft metatarsal osteotomy is performed for a wider fourth to fifth intermetatarsal angle or a deformity that involves bowing with a lateral curvature to the metatarsal. The osteotomy is made in the same plane as that for correction of a modified Ludloff first metatarsal osteotomy. (In fact, I got the idea for the oblique first metatarsal osteotomy while performing this fifth metatarsal osteotomy as described by Coughlin.) The cut is made from proximal dorsal to distal and plantar at an angle of approximately 30 degrees with respect to the metatarsal shaft. The cut should be made according to the location of deformity, and ideally it should be as far proximal as possible to gain the maximum correction. This proximal cut is not always necessary if only a

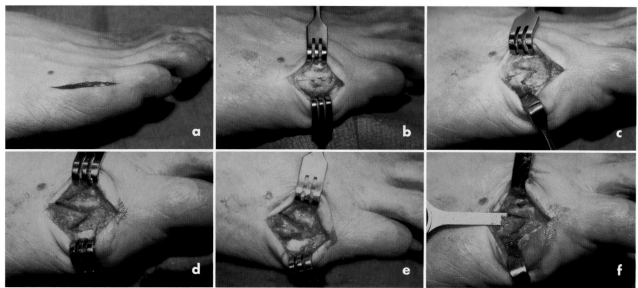

Figure 3–3–1. *The chevron osteotomy for correction of a bunionette. The incision is longitudinal as is the capsulotomy (a), and the metatarsal head is exposed (b). The cut is marked out with electrocautery (c) and completed with a small saw blade (d). The metatarsal head is shifted medially by 4 to 5 mm (e) and secured with an 11-mm twist-off screw. The lateral edge of the bone is trimmed with a saw (f).*

more moderate deformity is present, in which case the osteotomy can be in the midshaft of the metatarsal. As with the first metatarsal (Ludloff) osteotomy, the key to this procedure is to swivel the metatarsal around the hinge point of a K-wire, pin, or screw. Once two thirds of the osteotomy has been cut, the screw is inserted, and this screw maintains control of the osteotomy. Once the screw has been inserted and the osteotomy is stabilized, the cut on the metatarsal is then completed, and correction is performed through rotation of the metatarsal around the axis of the screw, which is then tightened. The overhanging bone on the lateral and dorsal aspect of the metatarsal is then shaved down with a saw blade. This osteotomy can simultaneously correct fifth metatarsalgia and a prominent bunionette when the plane of the osteotomy is changed. Normally, the saw blade cut is made exactly perpendicular to the axis of the fifth metatarsal. However, in the presence of metatarsalgia, the saw blade can be dropped slightly. For the aim to be medial and dorsal so that the metatarsal is rotated medially, the blade is also inclined dorsally. This technique is an effective means of correcting metatarsalgia. Fixation of the fifth metatarsal osteotomy can be more difficult than the first, and it requires many fragment screws or K-wires. Countersinking any screw is impor-

tant because these screws can be prominent, and unless the hardware is protected, this is always painful subcutaneously and will need to be removed postoperatively (Fig. 3–3–2).

Techniques, tips, and pitfalls

1. A simple exostectomy is not ideal for correcting a bunionette. Recurrence is common, and with this, subluxation of the fifth metatarsophalangeal (MP) joint will occur.

2. The healing of a distal metatarsal osteotomy that is shown on an x-ray (XR) image lags behind the clinical healing, and although the XR image may not show consolidation, the latter is usually clinically stable.

3. The oblique diaphyseal osteotomy is easy to perform, provided the fixation is stable. As with the first metatarsal modified Ludloff osteotomy, the correction is obtained through rotation of the axis of the metatarsal around the

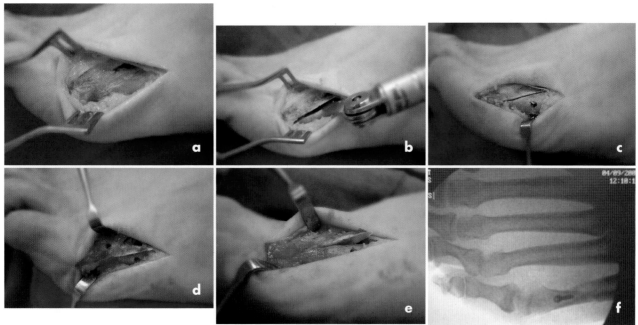

Figure 3–3–2. *The oblique metatarsal osteotomy for correction of a bunionette associated with an abnormal metatarsal shaft angle. An incision is made along the length of the metatarsal through the capsule to expose the shaft (a). The saw cut was made in this case with a saw blade that was slightly inclined dorsally to simultaneously correct the fifth metatarsalgia (b). The cut was not completed, a screw was inserted, and the distal metatarsal was rotated around the axis of the screw (c–e). The screw was then tightened, and the lateral overhanging bone was resected (f).*

screw. Here the use of a small bone reduction clamp is helpful to hold the metatarsal during fixation.

4. For failure of exostectomy, an osteotomy can still be performed, unless a considerable amount of the fifth metatarsal head is uncovered, in which case a resection of the fifth head is preferable.

Suggested Reading

Coughlin MJ. Treatment of bunionette deformity with longitudinal diaphyseal osteotomy with distal soft tissue repair. Foot Ankle 11:195–203, 1991.

Diebold P. Basal osteotomy of the fifth metatarsal for the bunionette. Foot Ankle 12:74–79, 1991.

Kitaoka HB, Holiday AD Jr, Campbell DC II. Distal chevron metatarsal osteotomy for bunionette. Foot Ankle 12:80–85, 1991.

Koti M, Maffulli N. Bunionette. J Bone Joint Surg Am 83:1076–1082, 2001.

Surgery for the Diabetic Foot and Ankle

Decision Making with Midfoot Neuroarthropathy

Although classifying the Charcot process as acute, sub-acute, and chronic is helpful from a practical standpoint, the definitions of these stages have no practical value because I treat the foot according to the magnitude of the deformity and the presence of periosteal new bone formation. The latter is important because the presence of periosteal new bone formation, which occurs after a month or so following injury, is often associated with marked osteopenia and bone fragmentation. Surgery in this setting may be extremely complicated and perhaps unrealistic if considerable osteopenia is present, even if the deformity is amenable to open reduction and internal fixation. If the foot is warm, surgery should be deferred because the warmth is an indicator of bone activity and periosteal new bone formation (Fig. 4–1–1).

If the deformity becomes chronic and stable, the midfoot is unlikely to deform; however, bone prominence is often present on the plantar aspect of the midfoot, which may lead to ulceration or infection. By *chronic*, I mean stable, with an absence of swelling and inflammation. In these chronic arthropathies, the apex of the deformity is some-where on the plantar foot. Occasionally, if the first metatarsal, cuneiform, or navicular joint dislocates medi-ally, the forefoot abducts and the bone prominence is directly medial. This type of deformity is easier to treat with an ostectomy than those where bone prominences are on the lateral or plantar midfoot. The more lateral

rocker bottom deformity occurs when the navicular joint and cuneiforms are crushed or dislocate dorsally. These changes lead to a shortening of the medial column and a laterally based prominent rocker deformity with the apex at the plantar cuboid.

The rationale of operative treatment is to decrease the deformity and thereby minimize the likelihood of com-plications of deformity such as infection and amputa-tion, which otherwise may be imminent. Certainly, the reduction of acute dislocation makes sense, and, for example, this would include patients with acute frank dislocation of the midfoot who clearly benefit from this more urgent operative treatment. For patients with chronic but stable neuropathic deformity of the midfoot, the indication for surgery is more specific, and surgery is performed when deformity cannot be controlled and ulceration and infection is recurrent because many of these patients can be treated with appropriate shoes, orthoses, and braces. Occasionally, patients experience pain from the deformity, and although a misnomer in the setting of neuropathy, some patients do at times experience a sense of deep discomfort and aching asso-ciated with the deformity. Justifying surgery in patients with chronic deformity who have recurrent problems is always easier, but this too seems to be related to the effi-ciency with which an orthotic and prosthetic treatment program is able to decrease the morbidity of deformity.

As a generalization, I have modified my approach to surgery over the past two decades. During the 1980s, I

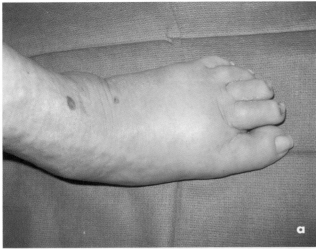

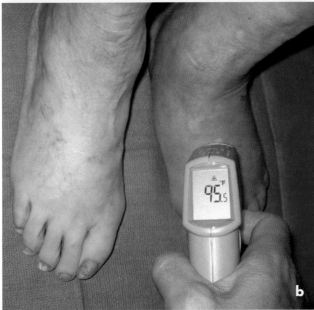

Figure 4–1–1. *The appearance of an inflamed and swollen foot as a result of acute neuropathic arthropathy. Note the swelling and erythema (a) and the temperature reading 95° F of the midfoot, indicative of severe inflammation (b).*

operated on many neuropathic deformities, believing that without surgery, infection, ulceration, and eventual amputation would be imminent. Over the past decade, I have gradually come full circle in my approach to the treatment of both acute and chronic deformities, and fewer operations now seem to be justified. Patients who had undergone surgery for acute fracture or dislocation seemed to need the same vigilant monitoring for complications of deformity. With an increased patient acceptance of modified shoe wear and braces, those who were not treated operatively for the acute dislocation may have fared as reasonably as those treated operatively.

My approach to surgery seems to have a better delineation for those cases that are clearly operative and nonoperative, but a "gray-zone" remains where the decision between these two is controversial.

Realistically, a "feel" to the foot develops that helps guide the type of treatment needed. Patient compliance, weight, extent of neuropathy, perfusion, skin condition, family support, opposite limb function, mobility of the ankle, and the distance a patient has to travel for foot care are all factors that should be used when planning surgery for either the acute or chronic stages of neuroarthropathy. Decision making regarding the chronic stage is a bit more straightforward. If shoes or braces can be worn on the foot, conservative management should be pursued if the patient does not undergo an operation. The degree of deformity determines the ability to wear a shoe or brace. During the acute phase, some absolute indications for surgery exist, including medial dislocation of the cuneiform or navicular, which causes skin necrosis. Initially, the associated swelling masks the bone prominence, but with resolution of swelling, a pressure sore or full-thickness skin loss occurs (Fig. 4–1–2).

Complete bone extrusions must be operatively reduced and stabilized. For one type of acute neuropathic injury of the midfoot with dislocation, the indication for surgery is not as clear-cut, and the reduction is performed to prevent the later deformity and neuropathic process. In patients with these injuries, the issue is whether the potential morbidity of surgery outweighs the likelihood of complications that will occur later.

The key to operative treatment, however, is to take careful note of the quality of the bone. From a practical standpoint, knowing the onset of the injury is difficult because many patients are unaware of the initial event anyway. It is preferable to use the appearance of the bone as an indication of both the onset of the neuropathic injury, but also the possibility for surgery. Performing surgery on the midfoot where the bones are crumbling as a result of osteopenia can be difficult, if not frustrating and complicated. Therefore I am more inclined to correct a subluxation or dislocation than multiple fractures around the midfoot. The traditional methods of reduction and fixation of these injuries do not work well here because recurrent deformity seems to occur, unless combined with arthrodesis.

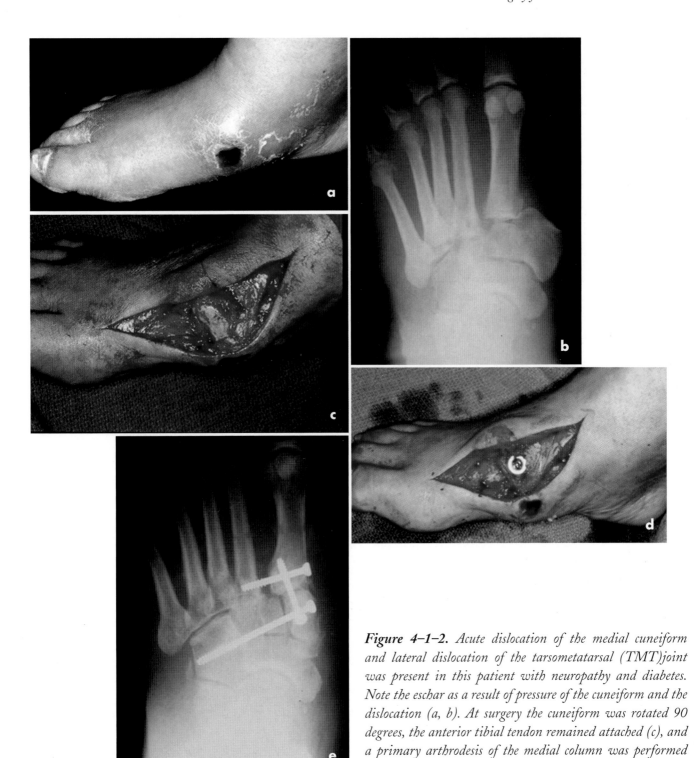

Figure 4–1–2. *Acute dislocation of the medial cuneiform and lateral dislocation of the tarsometatarsal (TMT) joint was present in this patient with neuropathy and diabetes. Note the eschar as a result of pressure of the cuneiform and the dislocation (a, b). At surgery the cuneiform was rotated 90 degrees, the anterior tibial tendon remained attached (c), and a primary arthrodesis of the medial column was performed (d, e).*

Surgical Approach

I prefer to leave large segments of the subchondral bone of the midfoot bones intact and use a burr to remove selected portions of the articular surface. I do not advise using either a chisel or an osteotome because the ligamentous support is friable and tenuous, and bone may literally fall out. More often than not, neuropathic fracture, dislocation, or fracture-dislocation of the midfoot results in loss of medial column length as a result of a comminuted intercalary segment (Fig. 4–1–3).

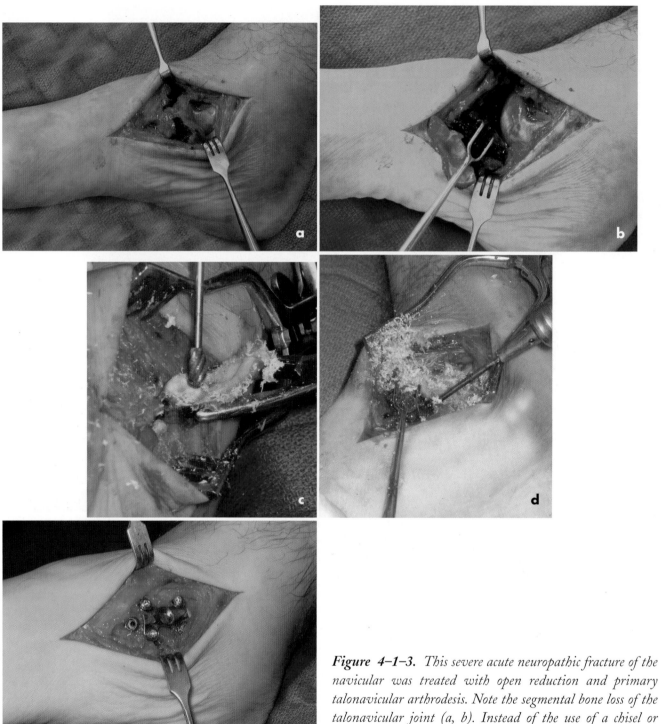

Figure 4–1–3. *This severe acute neuropathic fracture of the navicular was treated with open reduction and primary talonavicular arthrodesis. Note the segmental bone loss of the talonavicular joint (a, b). Instead of the use of a chisel or osteotome to denude cartilage, a burr was used to prevent further bone fragmentation (c, d). Fixation is accomplished with a combination of cannulated screws and a medially applied plate (e).*

If bone quality is sufficient, the medial column length can be maintained. Traditional bridge plating from the talus to the cuneiforms or first metatarsal may be inadequate to maintain length because the inherent lack of rigidity risks loss of fixation and hardware failure. However, with primary fusion denuding to the subchondral bone is a must, often on both sides of these midfoot bones, leaving bone structure behind with a likelihood of medial column shortening and a lateral rocker bottom deformity.

When the deformity involves the midfoot, an extended talonavicular-cuneiform arthrodesis has to be performed. Be careful, however, with the arthrodesis because shortening of the medial column occurs and it may be preferable to include the calcaneocuboid joint in the arthrodesis to avoid deformity. If the subtalar joint is involved with accompanying hindfoot valgus and forefoot abduction, a triple arthrodesis should be performed. I try to apply compression across the arthrodesis sites using lag screw fixation, but this is frequently not possible because of bone loss, and plates are necessary (Fig. 4–1–4).

A complete transverse tarsal joint dislocation with dorsal dislocation of the cuneiform commonly leads to a floppy, unstable forefoot. This deformity results because the forefoot is placed into dorsiflexion by the pull of the tibialis anterior tendon, whereas the Achilles tendon forces the hindfoot into equinus. The combination of these deformities results in a foot that is ineffective at both heel strike and toe-off, and the midfoot is at risk for ulceration. A second deformity that frequently requires surgery in the chronic phase is the midfoot rocker bottom deformity that is associated with supination of the forefoot. This deformity results from the heel cord pulling the foot into equinus and subsequent weight bearing on the lateral aspect of the foot. To minimize the effect of the equinus contracture, I routinely perform a lengthening of the Achilles tendon.

If the navicular is substantially fragmented and unable to be maintained as a part of the fusion mass, a naviculectomy with subsequent talocuneiform arthrodesis with similar surgical principles should be performed.

Ostectomy

Ulcers develop as the result of bony prominence or unstable joints that produce a prominence during weight bearing, and if ulcers are intractable, ostectomy should be considered to treat the bone prominence. This ostectomy works well, provided there is no associated instability. If the bone prominence is resected and is followed by an unstable midfoot, then the problem with recurrent ulceration will invariably recur. Ostectomy can only be performed if stability of the midfoot is present. Because this is a much easier and quicker procedure to recover from with less morbidity, I prefer to perform an ostectomy as opposed to an arthrodesis wherever possible. If I am unable to get the ulcer to heal before the ostectomy (even with a total contact cast), then the ostectomy is not contraindicated. However, the incision has to be made carefully to avoid extension of the ulcer and the possibility of infection. Technically, the ostectomy is not difficult, and the only issue is to try to minimize postoperative soft tissue problems. Rarely I approach the ostectomy through the open ulcer. Usually, the skin has healed over the ulcer from a total contact cast program, and the incision is made off the weight-bearing surface of the foot, whether medial or lateral. Large skin flaps are preserved, and full-thickness dissection should be used to reach the prominence with a broad periosteal elevator. I use a combination of an oscillating saw, osteotomes, and a rongeur to create a contoured surface amenable to ambulation (Fig. 4–1–5). Be careful not to resect too much bone or the result will be instability, which is particularly prone to occur on the inferior aspect of the midfoot joints. A large solid neuropathic bone mass may be present but is unlikely; resection of the undersurface of unfused midfoot joints may have the effect of worsening the deformity and secondarily exacerbating the deformity.

Fixation Options for the Midfoot

External fixation is only used to provide reduction and fixation when an ulcer cannot be healed before arthrodesis, and I do not use an external fixation construct when the soft tissue is healed without ulceration. Occasionally, the internal fixation obtained is poor and is understandably worrisome in a noncompliant patient. For these patients, I occasionally add an external fixator using half rings

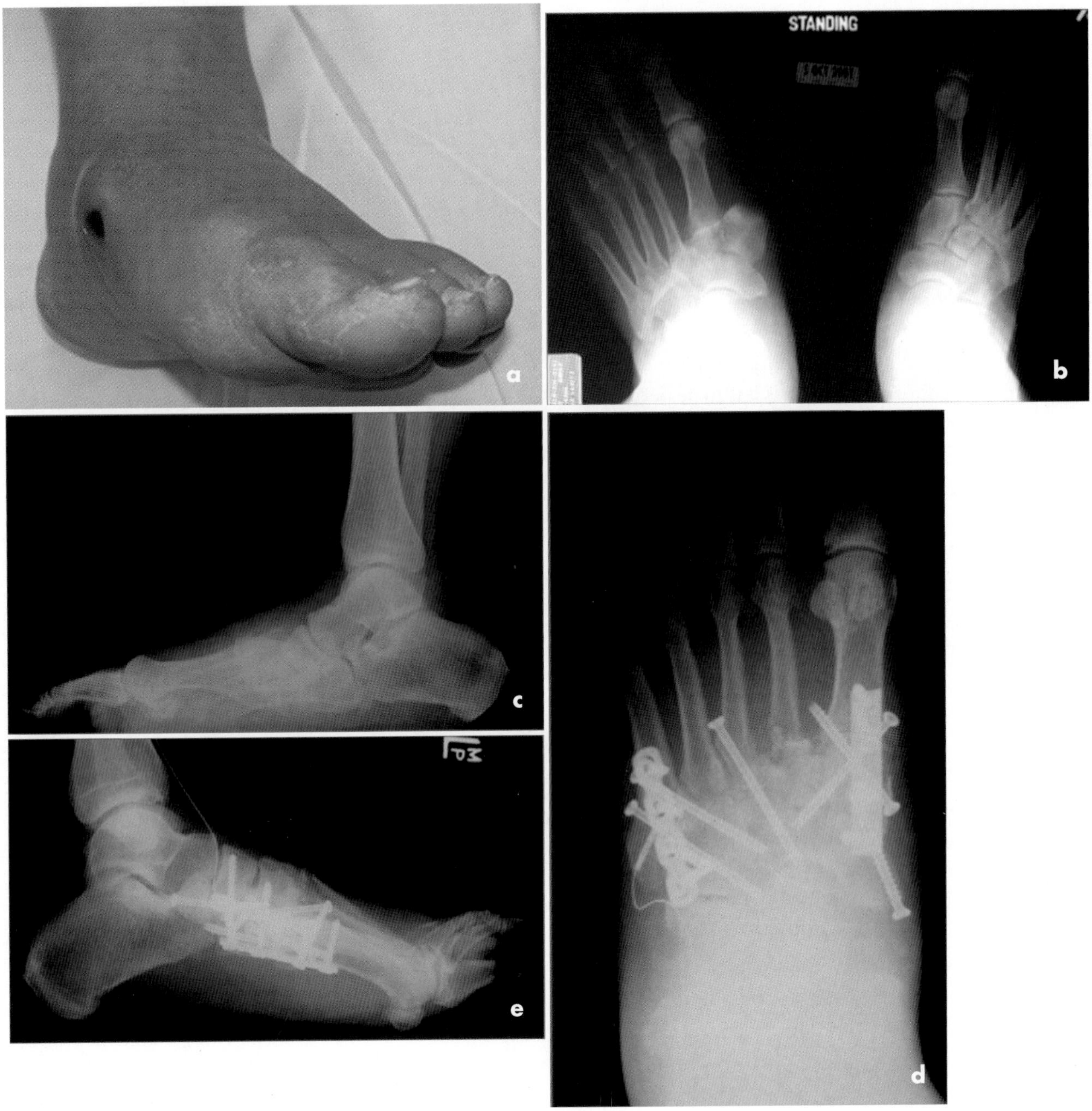

Figure 4–1–4. *A chronic midfoot dislocation was present in this patient, and despite adequate protection in a protective boot, skin breakdown was present. Note the dislocation of the entire midfoot (a–c). This dislocation was fixed with two plantar plates applied to the undersurface of the medial and lateral columns, combined with internal fixation and an implantable bone stimulator (d, e). This figure has been provided courtesy of Dr. Lew Schon, who was instrumental in developing the concept of application of a plate on the plantar surface for this type of correction.*

applied to the midfoot (DePuy Ace, Warsaw, Ind.). I use the same half ring external fixator to treat open infection or ulceration with associated osteomyelitis. In the case of indolent osteomyelitis, resection of the infected bone is usually the first step in establishing a clean wound bed that is essential for healing the associated ulcer. The dilemma comes in removing enough necrotic bone without causing destabilization of the medial column of the foot, and usually extensive ostectomy is required, followed by arthrodesis with the external fixator.

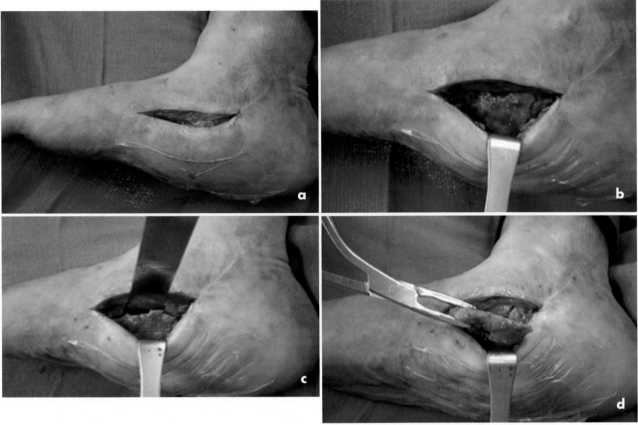

Figure 4–1–5. *Ostectomy of the nonspecific plantar bone mass was performed for this patient via a medial incision off the weight-bearing surface of the foot (a). The flap is kept as thick as possible, and with subperiosteal dissection, the mass of bone is exposed (b). A curved 2-cm osteotome is used to remove the bone mass as one piece (c, d).*

Wherever possible, I use a tension-banding effect of a plate applied on the plantar surface. This does require more stripping of the medial soft tissues and abductor hallucis muscle, but it is a stable construct (Fig. 4–1–6). An alternative is to use large cannulated screws as described by Sammarco, which are inserted from distal to proximal. Once the reduction is complete and the midfoot alignment is obtained, the guide pins are inserted antegrade through the metatarsal at the level of the tarsometatarsal (TMT) joint from proximal to distal. The midfoot is reduced, the guide pins are then redirected proximally across the midfoot, and the screws are introduced through the metatarsal heads and buried in the metatarsal shaft. I expect that in the future, locking plates will provide a logical way to obtain rigid fixation through the use of their "internal fixator" function in the midfoot.

Dressings and sutures are removed 2 to 4 weeks after the operation. After appropriate healing of incisions has been confirmed, a non–weight-bearing, below-the-knee plaster or fiberglass cast is applied. This is maintained with frequent cast changes for at least 2, but often 4, months. Thereafter a weight-bearing cast is applied and maintained until bridging trabeculation is observed at the surgical site. Patients need, on average, 6 to 12 months for union of arthrodesis of the midfoot. Once healing is evident, it is advisable to use a polypropylene ankle-foot orthosis for up to 1 year, which will lessen the effects of direct pressure and shear stresses encountered in normal weight bearing on the abnormal midfoot.

Correction of Neuropathic Deformity of the Hindfoot and Ankle

Unlike the Charcot midfoot deformity, once collapse of the hindfoot and ankle occurs, deformity is often inevitable, necessitating surgery. The decision then is not as much whether surgery has to be performed, but rather

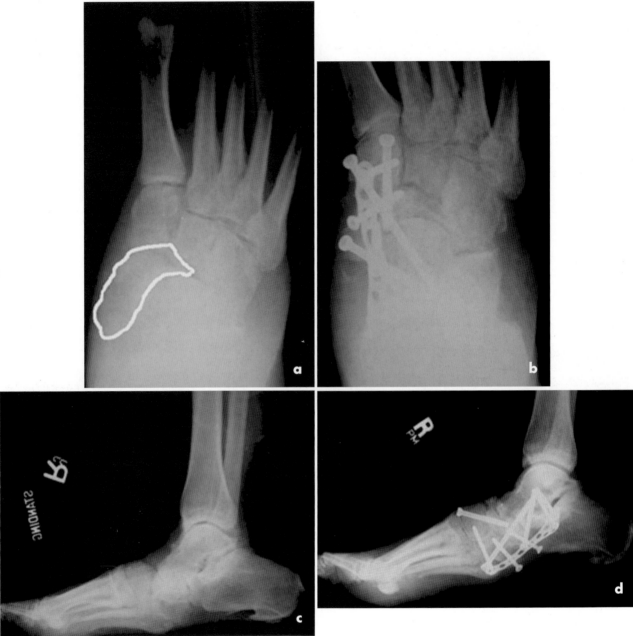

Figure 4–1–6. *Chronic dislocation of the midfoot with plantar and medial subluxation of the navicular joint led to ulceration of the medial foot, which was refractory to all methods of non-surgical care. Note the dislocation of the navicular joint associated with a flatfoot and a rocker bottom deformity (a, c), which was corrected with open reduction, and arthrodesis of the medial column of the foot with a plantar plate (b, d).*

how it has to be performed. A number of fixation options are available, and decision making here depends to some extent on the magnitude and type of deformity and the individual surgeon's preference. Clearly, in the presence of sepsis, external fixation is ideal. However, we have demonstrated that even in the presence of ulceration of the fibula, for example with a severe varus deformity of the ankle, that the arthrodesis can be performed with internal fixation. For example, in the presence of the severe varus ankle, if the fibula is exposed, infected, or both, it is totally excised as part of the procedure followed by internal fixation. For these patients I routinely mix antibiotic powder with the cancellous bone graft. Perhaps it is a matter of degree of the infection and a concern for the presence of osteomyelitis that would then prompt the use of an external fixator for management of the infection and the use of alignment for correction of deformity. The Ace ring fixator (DePuy Ace, Warsaw, Ind.) is versatile, easy to apply, and utilitarian in the setting of neuropathic deformity.

Application of the DePuy Ace–Fischer Ring Fixator

The DePuy Ace-Fischer Ring Fixator is a useful device for management of the diabetic patient with infection, avascular necrosis of the talus, hindfoot and ankle deformity, and wound problems associated with osteopenia where internal fixation might not be sufficient. The external fixator may be considered for use in a patient who has neuropathy or osteopenia where, for example, internal fixation may be indicated. However, a concern about this external fixation is the ability of the patient to remain non–weight bearing.

Numerous configurations of the external fixation ring are used. The standard foot and ankle frame is the most versatile, but other techniques for application of this external fixator, including a small foot ring and a tibio-calcaneal ring, are also available, depending on the magnitude and location of infection or deformity.

Regardless of the type of deformity and the type of ring being used, I prefer to close all the wounds before application of the external fixator. It is easier to close the incision before application of the fixator, and closing gives a better sense of where the cross pins are going to be because I prefer not to have pins going through the incision. Clearly, in the presence of infection, this part of the incision will not be closed. For example, in the presence of a severe varus deformity with exposed fibula, an incision would be made over the distal fibula to perform the cheilectomy for the tibiocalcaneal arthrodesis. The incision that is extended proximally and distally

would be closed, but the original open wound would be left open.

Assembly of the Fixator

The frame is constructed by first assembling the foot ring. The pins are placed in the plane of the plantar surface of the foot, beginning in the tuberosity of the calcaneus. Try to watch the axis of the insertion of the pins if there is, for example, a valgus deformity because with correction, the frame will be shorter on the medial than on the lateral side of the foot; planning the connecting rods will be difficult. It does not matter whether one begins medially or laterally, but the first pin should be at an angle of approximately 45 degrees with respect to the calcaneus. While the second pin is inserted, the anchor-distractor is placed on the ring, which then connects the pin to the foot ring frame. Take at look at the bolts and become familiar with the anchors and the distractors. When an anchor is used to attach the pin to the frame, the square bolt is farthest away from the foot, and the opposite is the case when a distractor attached to the pin and frame is used.

Sufficient space is needed posteriorly behind the ring in the back of the heel. Whether the pins are on the plantar or dorsal side of the ring is unimportant, although for convenience, the pins are usually on the undersurface of the ring. The next set of pins is inserted. The second pin should be perpendicular to the axis of the first pin, and the third perhaps somewhere in between, although this depends on the soft tissues, the location of incisions, and the ability to actually insert the pins depending on deformity. All three pins are inserted into the calcaneus. When the second and third pins are attached to the frame, applying either a 2.5- or 5-mm washer between the anchor distractor and the ring is useful, but not necessary, to provide clearance so that the pins do not hit each other as they cross through the calcaneus. For this reason, it is helpful to attach the anchor distractor onto the ring first and then insert the pins through this with the washer attached as an offset. The bolts that attach to the external fixator come in different lengths, and when an offset washer is used, a longer bolt is used. For convenience, the anchors are all on one side of the frame, and the distractors are on the other (Fig. 4–1–7).

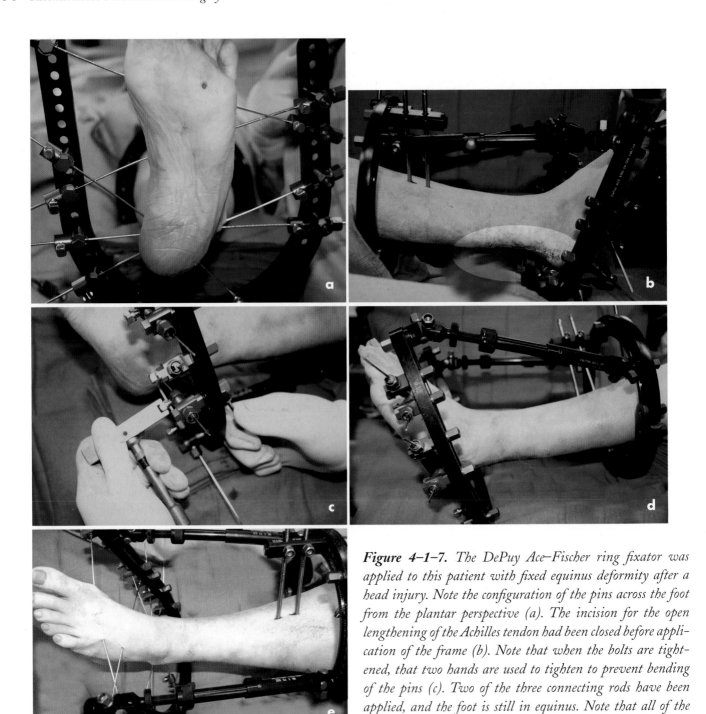

Figure 4–1–7. *The DePuy Ace–Fischer ring fixator was applied to this patient with fixed equinus deformity after a head injury. Note the configuration of the pins across the foot from the plantar perspective (a). The incision for the open lengthening of the Achilles tendon had been closed before application of the frame (b). Note that when the bolts are tightened, that two hands are used to tighten to prevent bending of the pins (c). Two of the three connecting rods have been applied, and the foot is still in equinus. Note that all of the tensioning nuts are on one side of the frame (d, e).*

Once the three pins are inserted into the back to the calcaneus, the ring is usually stable enough that one can assess the need for the remaining two or three pins in the midfoot. Again, these are inserted on the basis of the availability of bone and the presence of foot deformity. Generally, I start with the pin going obliquely from the first metatarsal into the fifth metatarsal from distal to proximal. While inserting the metatarsal pins, try to visualize the convex arc of the metatarsals in the midfoot. Typically, if a pin is inserted perpendicular to the axis of the metatarsals, it will enter the first metatarsal, miss the central three metatarsals, and then exit from the fifth metatarsal. Nothing is wrong with this, provided good fixation is obtained in these two metatarsals. Generally, I do use a fifth pin also, in the forefoot. Inserting a pin exactly transversely across the metatarsus is not important because if the frame slides across the metatarsal, the result is loosening of the pin.

Tensioning of the Pins

Once all the pins are inserted, make sure that the space is sufficient on either side of the foot and that no potential for abutment exists once the wires are tensioned. The wires must not be bent over at all, and if a bend is present, the wire needs to be straightened or replaced. When the wires are tensioned, care must be taken to avoid any bending of the wires (see Fig. 4–1–7c). I do this with open-ended wrenches on both the anchor distractor and the bolt. The same thing is done with an open-ended wrench on the square bolt on the wire itself, making sure that you have counterpressure under the bolt with another open wrench to prevent bending of the wire. It is preferable to have all of the anchors on one side and the distractors on the other. When beginning the tensioning for the distractor device, make sure that the threaded part of the distractor is open as far as possible so that there is as much thread length exposed with the square neck adjacent to the foot. This ensures maximum potential for compression for full tightening of the wire using the T handle with counterpressure on the bolt itself.

The Connecting Rods

The connecting rods are applied in a manner to facilitate wound care, application of a free flap, or a vacuum-assisted wound closure device. Once the wires and the foot ring are tensioned, three or four connecting rods are connected to the foot ring. Small, medium, or large connecting rods can be used depending on the amount of tibia to be spanned. Usually I use the medium connecting rods. Opening up the connecting rod as far as possible ensures the ability for maximum compression. Unlock the hexagonal nut on the connecting rod and then unscrew the compression distraction wheel maximally. Position the connecting rods anywhere around the circumference, but try to anticipate the position for compression so that the rods are almost equal, circumferentially around the frame.

Ideally, the connecting rods should be spaced circumferentially around the limb as far away from each other as possible. Sometimes this is not possible because of the configuration of the frame and the desire to maintain wound access. As a rule, these fixators are applied to maintain the hindfoot and limb in some means of compression, generally for arthrodesis-type procedures. If a compression-type frame is applied, then the telescoping portion of the connecting rod is opened completely to facilitate maximum compression. Alternatively, if this is a neutralization frame, it does not matter as much to what extent the distraction telescoping tubes are opened.

The Tibial Half Pins and Compression of the Frame

Before the proximal tibial half pins are inserted, the circular ring is loosely connected to the connecting rods to determine the location for insertion of the tibial half pins. Although single, double, or triple pin holders can be used to attach the ring to the half pins, I prefer to use a three-pin holder below the ring and use only two of these holes, leaving the little hole open just in case an infection occurs in one of the pins, in which case the pin location can be changed. The half pins are inserted in the standard manner, as perpendicular to the surface of the medial tibia as possible. Whenever possible, try to avoid inserting the pins as unicortical pins; this kind of insertion may lead to a stress riser of the tibia and possible fracture. Once the two half pins are inserted in the tibia, a decision can be made about whether a third half pin is to be inserted through a separate pin holder. This insertion can be proximal to the ring, preferably, again, at right angles to the plane of the tibia. Once all of the pins are attached, then the connecting rods are assembled to the leg ring, the limb and foot are placed in alignment, and the bolts are tightened. If compression is desirable, the foot is positioned and then manually compressed while the connecting rod bolts are tightened. These pin insertions apply particularly to the telescoping rod, which will then be clamped. Final added compression can be obtained with the wheel with a tommy bar. At the completion of the assembly of the ring, all the pins are bent over to prevent any sharp protruding points and extensive dressing applied in a standard manner (Figs. 4–1–8 and 4–1–9).

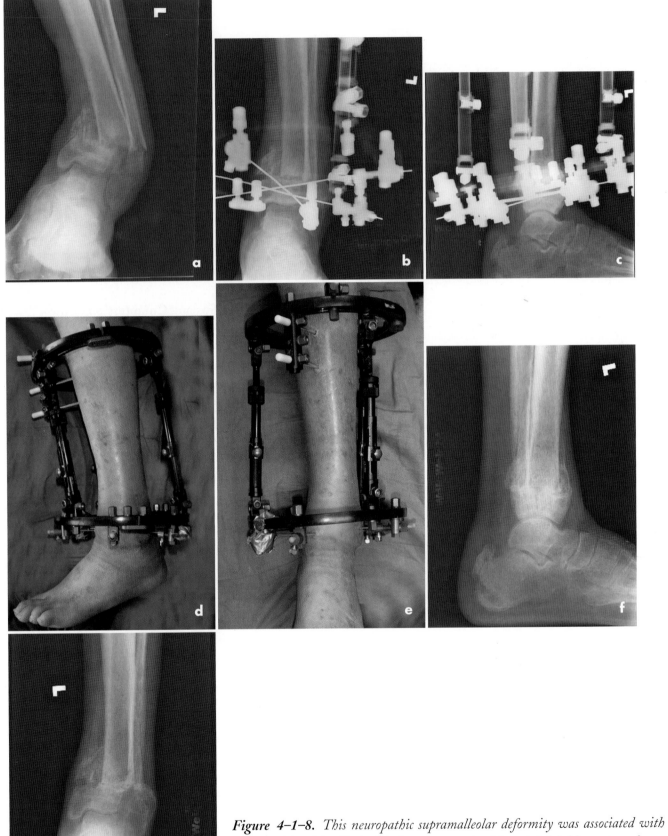

Figure 4–1–8. *This neuropathic supramalleolar deformity was associated with osteomyelitis of the fibula (a). It was treated with serial debridements and corrected with a ring fixator (DePuy Ace, Warsaw, Ind.) (b–e). The final radiographic appearance is noted at 4 months after initiation of treatment and at 1 month after removal of the fixator (f, g). The limb was immobilized in a removable boot for an additional 6 months.*

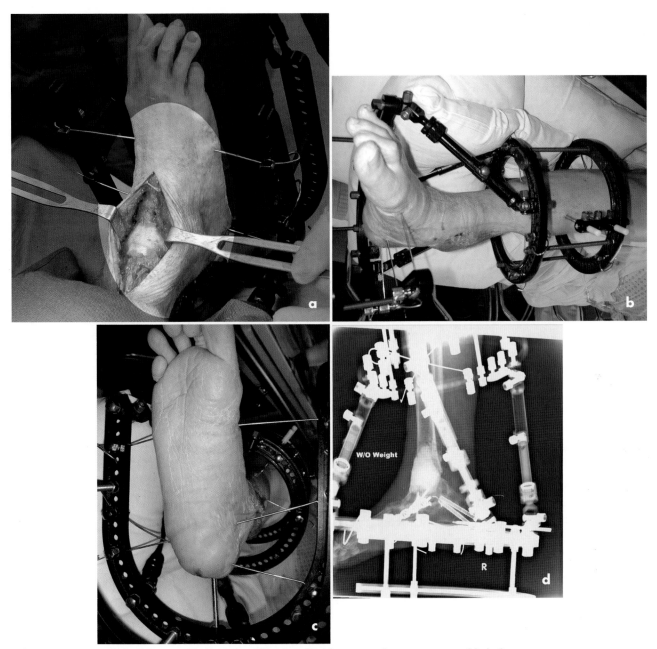

Figure 4–1–9. *A ring fixator (DePuy Ace, Warsaw, Ind.) was used to reconstruct this infection of the distal tibia. The patient had undergone successful prior hindfoot arthrodesis, and osteomyelitis of distal tibia was present 2 years later. Antibiotic-impregnated bone cement was used to fill the void after serial debridements and application of the ring fixator (a–d).*

Fixation Options for the Hindfoot

The issue arises as to the ideal means of fixation for stabilization of the hindfoot. Clearly the external fixator is useful if not necessary in the presence of sepsis, and at the opposite end and in the absence of severe deformity, cannulated screw fixation is most versatile. When there is gross instability that involves the ankle and/or subta-

lar joint, a blade plate or intramedullary rod is preferable. Originally, I had used the blade plate for most of these procedures because control of rotation was not possible with an intramedullary rod. The older intramedullary fixation systems permitted only transverse screws through the calcaneus. If severe erosion was present in the calcaneus, as is frequently the case with neuropathic deformity, then it is difficult, if not impossible, to maintain control of rotation. With the advent of improved intramedullary fixation, the problem does not exist because the Versa nail (DePuy Ace, Warsaw, Ind.) has the capacity for lateral or posteroanterior insertion of the locking screws in the calcaneus and talus. Therefore the decision to use intramedullary fixation depends on other factors such as the type and location of the deformity, ability of the patient to comply with non–weight bearing, and factors that include the bone quality. Remember that the primary goal for correction of neuropathic deformity is stability. This applies whether or not surgery is performed. Therefore although arthrodesis is desirable, the absence of arthrodesis does not in any way defeat the purpose of surgery nor lead to failure. Under these circumstances, intramedullary fixation may be preferable in the setting of a patient who has significant deformity and a total inability to comply with restricted mobility postoperatively.

The indication for surgery in this patient group is far easier to define. Almost all patients are treated initially with a brace of some sort to maintain the alignment of the foot under the tibia. Even gross deformities may be immobilized indefinitely in this manner, and despite the inconvenience, the brace is well tolerated. When ulceration occurs despite adequate brace use, then surgery is indicated. Surgery is deferred until there is no evidence of clinically active infection and until swelling had decreased. If the limb is swollen, diuretic agents, bed rest with limb elevation, and a Unna bandage (Carapace, Inc, Toledo, Ohio) are used for 48 hours before surgery. In patients with documented osteomyelitis, the treatment should be initiated with culture-specific intravenous antibiotics and local wound care. Although the infection cannot always be eradicated in these patients, drainage or surrounding erythema at the time of reconstructive surgery should be minimal.

Surgical Exposure

For most severe dislocations of the hindfoot and ankle, I use a blade plate for fixation (Fig. 4–1–10). Although an intramedullary rod can be used (Fig. 4–1–11), the blade plate has been shown clinically and biomechanically to be more stable, and this remains my fixation of choice for most neuropathic deformities. A curvilinear incision is made over the distal 10 cm of the fibula and is extended distally toward the sinus tarsi. Whenever possible, existing incisions should be used. A full-thickness skin flap is developed without regard for the sural and superficial peroneal nerves in the patient with neuropathy. These nerves and even the peroneal tendons are therefore cut to prevent excessive skin retraction and dissection. The distal 10 cm of the fibula are resected after an oblique osteotomy with an oscillating saw. If not associated with ulcer or infection, the fibula is harvested for bone graft using an acetabular reamer. The remnants and fragments of the talus are excised. Specifically, the fragmented body of the talus is always removed, although the head of the talus may be protected and preserved provided it is vascularized and not involved with a medial dislocation of the talonavicular joint or infection. The articular surface of the distal tibia is prepared by making a flat cut with an oscillating saw, and a flexible chisel is used to debride the articular cartilage on the dorsal surface of the calcaneus. Great care is then taken to establish precise alignment of the foot under the leg. After the deformity is reduced, it is stabilized initially with two 1.6-mm guide pins. One guidewire is inserted through the heel posteriorly into the distal tibial metaphysis anteriorly. The second guidewire is inserted posteriorly through the distal tibial metaphysis into the talar head (if present) or the navicular joint. I try not to incorporate the talonavicular joint into the arthrodesis. Wherever possible in the setting of neuroarthropathy, limited motion is preferable, and this applies to the talonavicular joint and to a tibiocalcaneal arthrodesis.

The blade plate is then placed on the lateral calcaneal subchondral bone in the region of the thalamus. Care is taken to position the hindfoot in neutral because the calcaneus tends to displace into slight valgus as compression is applied to the plate proximally. I typically apply compression to the plate through the two most proximal screw holes. If added stability is required, a fully threaded 6.5-mm cannulated cancellous screw is placed over a guide pin from the calcaneus posteriorly to the anterior distal tibia proximally.

Allograft or autograft bone, or a combination thereof, is used; the choice is determined by the amount of bone harvested from the fibula and the size of the defect to be filled. The bone graft is then mixed with 400 mg of tobramycin and 500 mg of vancomycin powder. The antibiotic bone graft mixture is firmly packed between the bone surfaces anteriorly, in addition to the posterior

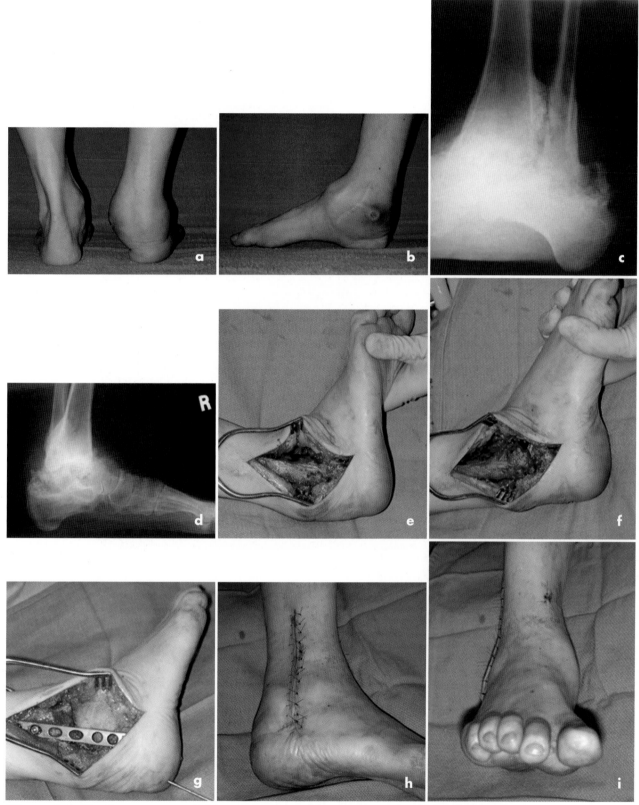

Figure 4–1–10. *Severe uncontrollable neuroarthropathy was present in this patient with ulceration and hindfoot collapse (a, b). Note the profound hindfoot valgus and necrosis of the talus (c, d). When the tibiotalocalcaneal (TTC) arthrodesis is planned with the blade plate, correct positioning of the foot is essential because the foot tends to move into dorsiflexion and valgus, putting the hindfoot in calcaneus (e, f). The easiest way to correct and maintain position is with a structural allograft. A femoral head graft was used to correct the deformity, and arthrodesis was performed with a blade plate (g–i).*

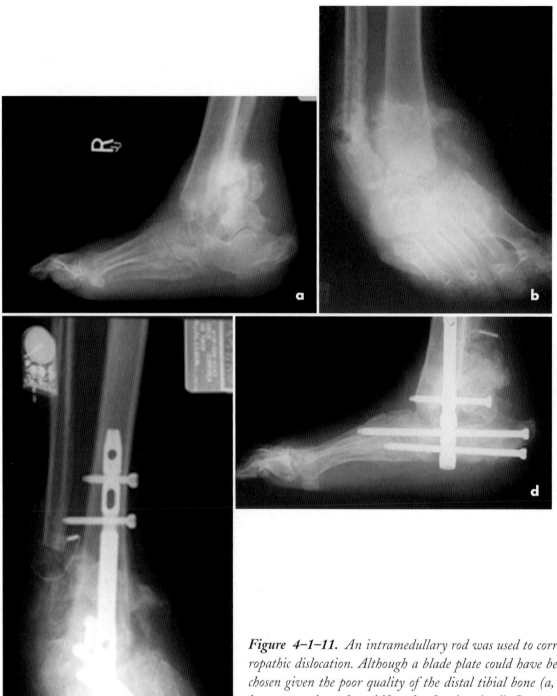

Figure 4–1–11. *An intramedullary rod was used to correct this severe neuropathic dislocation. Although a blade plate could have been used, a rod was chosen given the poor quality of the distal tibial bone (a, b). Note the use of long screws into the midfoot for fixation (c, d). Long screws are not ideal because the foot becomes rigid. However, after insertion of the rod, there was little rotational stability until these long screws were inserted.*

aspect of the tibia and calcaneus, to facilitate an extra-articular and an intra-articular arthrodesis. The back of the tibia is debrided by raising a thick osteoperiosteal flap that extends down onto the dorsal surface of the calcaneus posteriorly. Graft is packed here as well. The wound is closed in layers with 2-0 absorbable sutures, and 3-0 nylon sutures are used for the skin. If tension is present on the skin edges during closure, it may be due to the change in shape of the hindfoot or the added subcutaneous bulk of the plate, and the peroneal tendons may need to be removed.

Suggested Readings

Bibbo C, Lee S, Anderson RB, Davis WH: Limb salvage: The infected retrograde tibiotalocalcaneal intramedullary nail. Foot Ankle Int 24: 420–425, 2003.

Cooper PS: Application of external fixators for management of Charcot deformities of the foot and ankle. Foot Ankle Clin 7:207–254, 2002.

Farber DC, Juliano PJ, Cavanagh PR, et al: Single stage correction with external fixation of the ulcerated foot in individuals with Charcot neuroarthropathy. Foot Ankle Int 23:130–134, 2002.

Jani MM, Ricci WM, Borrelli J Jr, Barrett SE, et al: A protocol for treatment of unstable ankle fractures using transarticular fixation in patients with diabetes mellitus and loss of protective sensibility. Foot Ankle Int 24:838–844, 2003.

Myerson M: Arthrodesis for diabetic neuroarthropathy. In Myerson M (ed): Current Therapy in Foot and Ankle Surgery. St Louis, Mosby-Year Book, 1993, pp 116–122.

Myerson MS: Diabetic neuroarthropathy. In Myerson M (ed): Foot and Ankle Disorders. Philadelphia, WB Saunders, 2000.

Myerson MS: Salvage of diabetic neuropathic arthropathy with arthrodesis. In Helal B, Rowley DI, Cracchiolo A III, Myerson MS (eds): Surgery of Disorders of the Foot and Ankle. London, Martin Dunitz, Ltd, 1996, pp 513–522.

Myerson MS, Alvarez RG, Lam PW: Tibiocalcaneal arthrodesis for the management of severe ankle and hindfoot deformities. Foot Ankle Int 21:643–650, 2000.

Myerson MS, Henderson MR, Saxby T, Short KW: Management of midfoot diabetic neuroarthropathy. Foot Ankle Int 15:233–241, 1994.

Myerson MS, Levine S: Management of infection and ulceration in the diabetic foot. In Myerson M (ed): Foot and Ankle Disorders. Philadelphia, WB Saunders, 2000.

Papa J, Myerson M, Girard P: Salvage, with arthrodesis, in intractable diabetic neuropathic arthropathy of the foot and ankle. J Bone Joint Surg 75:1056–1066, 1993.

Schon LC, Easley ME, Weinfeld SB: Charcot neuroarthropathy of the foot and ankle. Clin Orthop Apr:116–131, 1998.

Cavus Foot Correction

Overview

Correction of the cavus foot can be daunting. However, as long as basic principles are adhered to, the foot can usually be well corrected and dynamically balanced, with as much motion as possible maintained. Where is the apex of the deformity? Is this a midfoot or a forefoot cavus? Is the forefoot in equinus; is this a global equinus; or does this involve only the first, or perhaps the middle, metatarsals? How mobile is the first metatarsal? Is the foot rigid, or can the foot be passively correctible? Surgeons rely on a type of a block test to determine flexibility of the hindfoot and forefoot. This test is certainly acceptable, but I also prefer to manipulate the heel and to see the effects of the hindfoot on the forefoot. If I can reduce the heel into heel valgus, then perhaps less correction will need to be done in the hindfoot and more in the forefoot. Most important, what are the additional deforming forces on the foot? Invariably, the peroneus longus muscle is stronger than the anterior tibial muscle, and the posterior tibial muscle is stronger than the peroneus brevis muscle with varying degrees of contracture of the gastrocnemius and soleus muscles present.

Decision Making

Generally, I perform a combination of a calcaneal osteotomy, a first metatarsal osteotomy, and a plantar fascia release. I then add whatever else is necessary to complete the correction, including a resection of the base of the fifth metatarsal, an ankle ligament reconstruction, or a midfoot osteotomy. It is rare that a triple arthrodesis needs to be performed. In fact, this arthrodesis, while not contraindicated, is associated with numerous long-term complications, particularly ankle arthritis. The mobility of the hindfoot must be preserved.

Although it is possible to perform an anatomic correction of the foot initially, these procedures are insufficient in the long term if muscular imbalance remains. Integral to the success of any of these procedures is a corrected foot, a plantigrade hindfoot relative to the forefoot, and muscle balance. Even with perfectly executed surgery, if the posterior tibial muscle is overactive relative to the evertors of the hindfoot, the foot will ultimately "fail," and further adductovarus deformity will occur. The posterior tibial muscle must therefore be transferred in many of these procedures. Frequently, a cavus deformity is associated with slight weakness of the anterior tibial muscle, and the posterior tibial tendon can be transferred as part of this corrective procedure. Usually, the transfer is performed to the dorsal aspect of the foot through the interosseous membrane. Occasionally, however, if the anterior tibial muscle is strong and the predominant deformity is adductovarus, then a split posterior tibial transfer can be performed with the lateral limb being transferred into the peroneus brevis tendon. Not much of the split tendon is needed for the transfer; enough is needed so it can pass behind the tibia and fibula and hook into the peroneus brevis tendon with an effective suture tenodesis. The separate components of the reconstruction of the cavus foot are discussed later.

Plantar Fascia Release

The plantar fascia release is an integral part of correction of the cavus foot deformity, and this is usually the first procedure that I perform as part of the correction. Correcting the position of the calcaneus is difficult without first releasing the plantar fascia. From a technical standpoint, although I used to make an incision directly under the arch of the foot medial to the fascia, I found this counterproductive. Although this incision was easy to perform, it always left a large hypertrophic nodular scar, almost like fibromatosis, which would then develop and which was difficult to soften, even with aggressive rehabilitation. Subsequent to this, I attempted the entire plantar fascia release from the lateral incision inferior to the calcaneal osteotomy. This worked fairly well, but getting the medial bundle is difficult. If there is severe cavus deformity, the medial band over the abductor fascia cannot be released. The incision does, however, remain a reasonable way to perform the fascia release. This modification of the original Steindler procedure is performed by extending the incision for the calcaneal osteotomy slightly more distally and cutting across the fascia transversely with Metzenbaum scissors.

The easiest procedure for me is a complete fascia release through a medial longitudinal incision adjacent to the heel, which is made slightly more distally at the junction of the dorsal and plantar skin. Unfortunately, some patients may experience a small patch of numbness on the medial aspect of the heel pad from this incision, and the potential for this must be explained to patients preoperatively. The incision is made over a 2-cm length. With the incision kept longitudinally in the axis of the foot, no problems occur with wound healing during the lengthening and flattening of the medial column; problems would occur if a vertical incision were made along the axis of the tarsal canal.

The branch of the lateral plantar nerve is not usually visible and does not need to be looked for. A copious fatty tissue under the incision needs to be reflected with a large soft tissue retractor until the fascia is visualized. I then split the fascia directly off the calcaneus using scissors from a medial to lateral direction. The scissors are advanced without a cutting motion until both the medial and lateral bands are completely released (Fig. 5–1–1).

For severe deformity, where cavo-adducto-varus is present, the fascia of the abductor hallucis tendon must also be completely released. For some of these severe deformities, the intrinsics must be stripped off the calcaneus completely, in addition to the fascia release. The stripping can be done with scissors or a broad periosteal elevator from the same medial incision where the intrinsics are completely released and elevated off the calcaneus.

Calcaneus Osteotomy

The incision for the calcaneal osteotomy varies according to the type of procedure performed. If an osteotomy alone is performed, then a shorter incision is made directly inferior to the peroneal tendons (Fig. 5–1–2). Usually, however, the calcaneal osteotomy needs to be performed with additional procedures, including repair of the peroneal tendon, reconstruction of lateral ankle instability, and a peroneus longus to brevis tendon transfer. For these cases, the incision is simply extended posteriorly along the axis of the peroneal tendons behind the fibula.

The incision is deepened through subcutaneous tissue in the plane between the peroneal tendon and the sural nerve. The nerve can be retracted either superiorly or inferiorly depending on its position. The periosteum needs to be elevated over a broad area because a wedge is going to be removed. I insert a retractor to separate the soft tissues and then place two small, curved retractors on either side of the calcaneus to expose the entire lateral tuberosity. A saw, not an osteotome, should be used to make the cut; a wide, fan-shaped saw blade should be used. The cut is first initiated perpendicular to the axis of the calcaneus at a 45-degree plane to the tuberosity. I use a punching action with the saw blade so that I can feel the medial cortex as it is perforated. Once the first cut has been made, the second cut is made at an angle to this of approximately 20 degrees, but this angle depends on the size of the wedge.

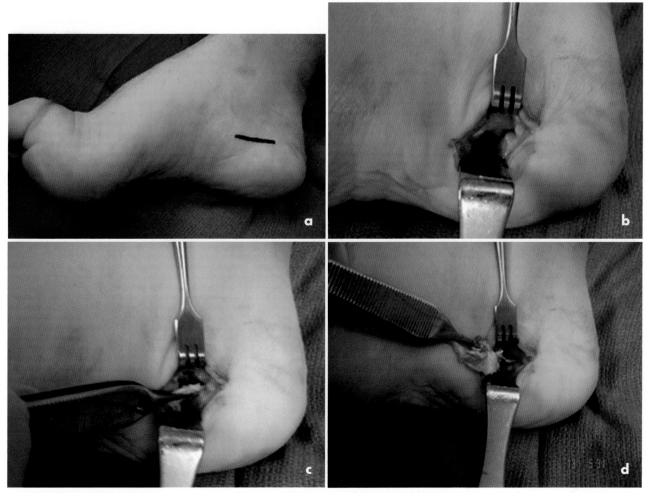

Figure 5–1–1. *The plantar fascia release is shown with the incision marked (a), the reflection of the fatty tissue (b), the grasp of the partially cut fascia (c), and the removal of a segment of the fascia after the fasciotomy (d).*

It is far easier to start out with a smaller wedge and remove more bone, if the correction is not sufficient (Fig. 5–1–3).

Once the wedge or bone has been removed, I then pull the heel into valgus. The osteotomy rarely closes down perfectly at this time, and additional perforation of the calcaneus needs to be made so that it is closed down smoothly. This perforation can be made by reinserting the saw blade while the osteotomy is partially closed. The cuts are then completed with multiple minor perforations (curfing). Depending on the deformity, the calcaneus is moved in two or three planes. The valgus closing wedge osteotomy is the first plane. The tuberosity is then always shifted lateral to its axis under the subtalar joint, which improves the weight-bearing axis of the hindfoot. The third plane is a cephalad shift and is

added according to the pitch angle of the calcaneus. I try to flatten out the talocalcaneal angle, and the calcaneus-first metatarsal angle in particular flattens as the calcaneal tuberosity is moved cephalad.

I use two guide pins to hold the calcaneus in the corrected position. The first guide pin is inserted centrally into the body of the posterior tuberosity, which is then manipulated into the corrected position (Fig. 5–1–3e). While the guide pin is being held and the heel is forced into the desired position, a second guide pin is introduced for screw fixation. It is best to insert the screw from slightly posterior lateral to slightly anterior and medial to gain maximal compression. Tamping the overhanging inferior ledge of bone is unnecessary, but this can be done with a small bone tamp to prevent any irritation on the peroneal tendons.

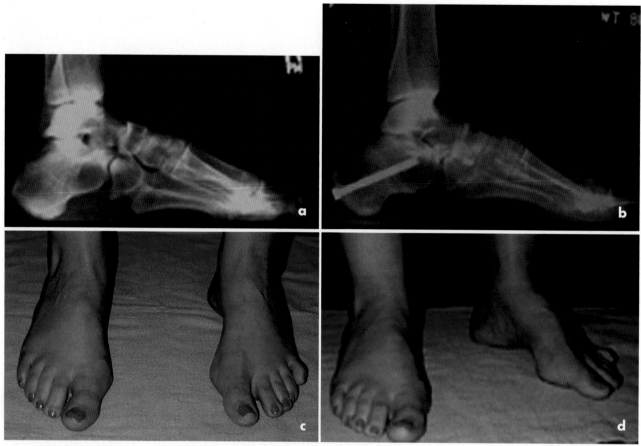

Figure 5–1–2. For some patients all that is required is a calcaneus osteotomy combined with a plantar fascia release for correction of a symptomatic heel varus (a–d). Note the correction of the varus and calcaneal pitch of the right foot after a biplanar calcaneus osteotomy.

Peroneus Longus to Brevis Tendon Transfer

The peroneus longus to brevis tendon transfer is a useful procedure when the peroneus longus muscle is working and is flexible. Regardless of the strength of the peroneus brevis tendon, this transfer augments the weakness of the peroneus brevis muscle. Ideally, this procedure is done in younger patients and even in children to achieve maximal advantage. If the brevis tendon is scarred, torn, or absent, the longus tendon can still be transferred to the stump of the base of the brevis tendon. The peroneus longus tendon is cut under direct vision as it passes underneath the cuboid. A stay suture is then inserted into the tendon, and it is pulled distally to obtain the correct tension. I pull on it maximally, and then when I have maximal tension, I release it slightly and perform the tenodesis at this tension (Fig. 5–1–4).

The sutures are inserted by burying the notch either as interrupted sutures or as a continuous locking whip suture. Four or five sutures seem to be sufficient. When I have drawn back on one of these tenodesis procedures, a modest fibrous scar appears between the two tendons, but the union of the tendons is never complete. A strong nonabsorbable zero suture should be used (Fig. 5–1–5).

First Metatarsal Osteotomy

As the heel is brought into valgus, increased pronation of the forefoot occurs with an increased plantar flexion of the first metatarsal. Occasionally I will perform a valgus calcaneal osteotomy without a first metatarsal osteotomy, but a decision has to be made on the basis of the deformity of the foot. More important is the balance that one is attaining with the combination of the calcaneal osteotomy, the peroneus longus to brevis tendon transfer, and the first metatarsal osteotomy. With the

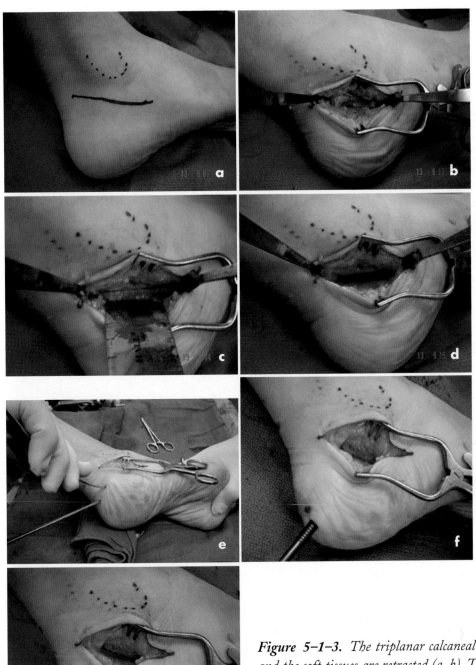

Figure 5–1–3. *The triplanar calcaneal osteotomy. The incision is marked, and the soft tissues are retracted (a, b). The wedge is cut and removed (c, d), and then a guide pin is inserted into the proximal tuberosity only to function as a lever to pull the tuberosity into position while the second guide pin is advanced across the osteotomy and fixed with a cannulated screw (d–f). Note the final position of the calcaneus with lateral and cephalad translation (g).*

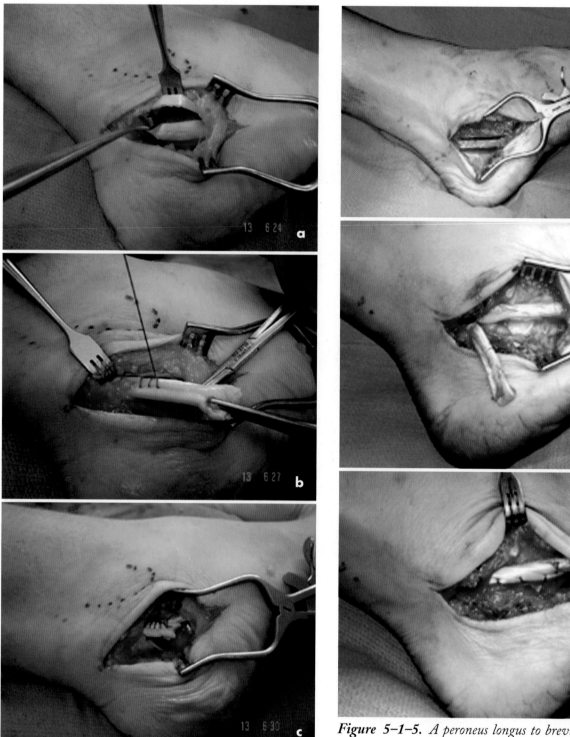

Figure 5–1–4. *The peroneus longus and brevis tendons are separated (a), the longus tendon is cut just under the cuboid and tensioned (b), and a running whip suture is used for the tenodesis (c).*

Figure 5–1–5. *A peroneus longus to brevis tendon transfer was performed in conjunction with a biplanar calcaneus osteotomy (a). Note the slightly longer incision needed to perform the transfer and the repair (b, c).*

peroneal transfer, the plantar flexion of the first ray is clearly weakening, and this weakening has to be considered when the osteotomy is performed to prevent overcorrection and ultimate shift of weight to the second metatarsal. The other issue is whether the forefoot cavus deformity is global or limited to one or two metatarsals. Invariably, the first metatarsal is in equinus, and this osteotomy is what I most commonly use.

An incision is made on the dorsal medial aspect of the first metatarsal extending to the metatarsal cuneiform joint. The periosteum is stripped, and the extensor hallucis longus tendon is retracted laterally. The osteotomy is performed 1 cm distal to the articulation in metaphyseal bone. This osteotomy can be performed in two ways: In one, a closing wedge is used, which has the obvious advantage of preserving a plantar cortical hinge for stability. In the other, a vertical osteotomy is performed; then the dorsal, proximal, and cortical rim is impacted into the metaphysis. This procedure has the advantage of correcting the deformity but also limits the amount of shortening on the first metatarsal (Fig. 5–1–6).

The dorsal wedge resection osteotomy is performed with a vertical cut perpendicular to the axis of the metatarsal more proximally but is not completed, and I preserve about 3 mm of bone on the plantar metatarsal. The second cut is made approximately 4 mm distal to this at an angle of 15 degrees. If more bone is resected originally, overcorrection may occur, and a transfer of pressure may be created to the second metatarsal.

Once the bone wedge has been resected, the first metatarsal is pushed up dorsally, and the plantar surface of the forefoot is palpated with the foot in maximal dorsiflexion. More bone can be shaved through the osteotomy itself until a correct amount of the wedge has been resected. The easiest way to secure this osteotomy is with a dorsally applied two-hole plate. Once the amount of bone to be resected has been verified, the plate is applied on the proximal cortex, and then the metatarsal is pushed up into dorsiflexion. While the corrected position is maintained, the second screw is inserted. I use fully threaded cancellous screws for fixation. This procedure is a stable osteotomy, and depending on additional procedures performed, patients may begin weight bearing in protective boots 2 weeks after surgery.

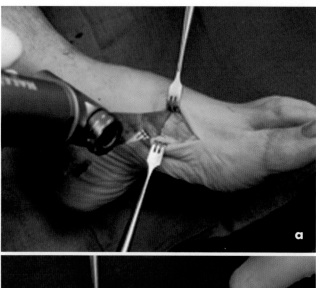

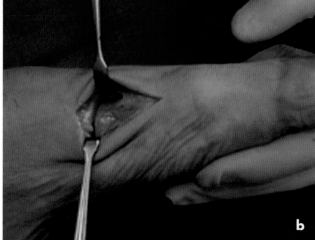

Figure 5–1–6. *The first metatarsal osteotomy is shown with a saw cut oriented vertically to the plane of the metatarsal (a) and with plantar depression of the proximal metatarsal and impaction into the metaphysis (b).*

Midfoot Osteotomy

The midfoot osteotomy is a complex procedure that requires careful preoperative planning. Ideally, the osteotomy is based at the apex of the deformity on the foot, which may correspond to the navicular or the cuneiforms. The osteotomy can be performed with the removal of a biplanar, dorsally based wedge or with a single bone cut. If a single uniplanar cut is made, the distal foot is then impacted and rotated into the cancellous bone of the midfoot as the forefoot is elevated (Fig. 5–1–7).

An incision is made in the midline of the foot extending from the ankle joint distally through the

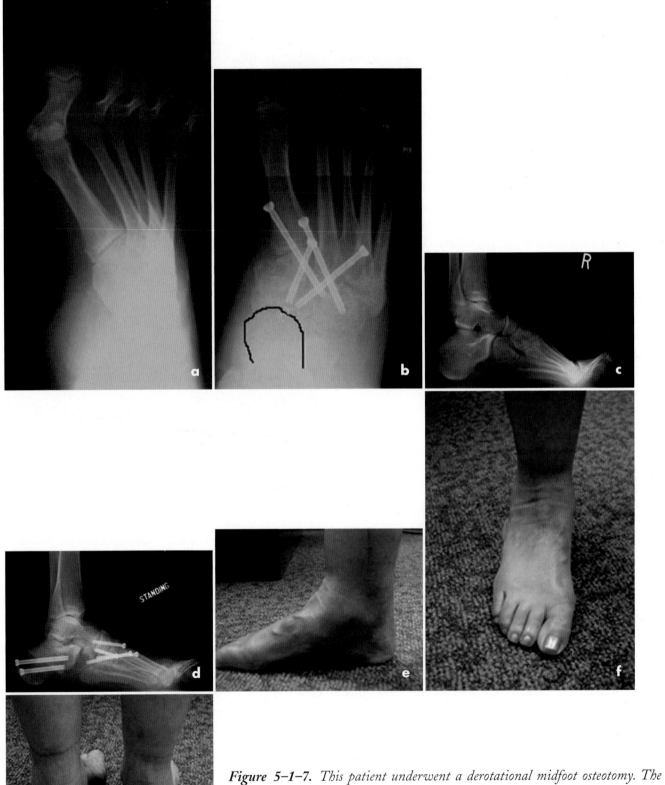

Figure 5-1-7. *This patient underwent a derotational midfoot osteotomy. The apex of the osteotomy was in the cuneiforms and extended as a uniplanar cut into the cuboid. Note the derotation of the midfoot on the anteroposterior x-ray films (a, b) and improvement in the calcaneus pitch angle (c, d). The final appearance of the operated right foot is noted (e–g).*

midmetatarsal. This is an extensile excision, and one must not compromise the length of the incision because skin retraction and wound dehiscence is a potential risk of a shorter incision. The superficial and deep peroneal nerves are retracted laterally and medially, and a plane is developed underneath the neurovascular bundle, which is then elevated with subperiosteal dissection medially. It is usually necessary to cut the extensor hallucis longus brevis tendon to gain access to the dorsal aspect of the midfoot. The entire dorsal central aspect of the midfoot is now stripped with a large broad periosteal elevator. The midfoot is now marked fluoroscopically so that the starting point of the osteotomy is noted. The plane of correction depends entirely on the shape of the foot. I try to exit the osteotomy in the cuboid laterally and in the medial cuneiform medially, but this procedure depends on how much rotation and angulation are necessary. The least amount of shortening of the foot takes place with a uniplanar osteotomy without removal of a dorsally based wedge. If wedge osteotomies are performed, then both the medial and lateral limbs of the osteotomy meet at an apical point, usually over the middle cuneiform. Frequently, most of the cuneiform has to be resected. The base of the osteotomy is dorsal, and it will then be varied to some extent according to the shape of the foot. As the osteotomy moves further laterally, less bone is resected, and the correction is obtained more by dorsal elevation of the lateral border of the foot with rotation than through wedge correction (Fig. 5–1–8).

Planning the osteotomy with transparencies preoperatively is useful. Transparent paper is applied to the lateral x-ray (XR) film of the foot, and the position of the wedge is located. Cut outs are then made in the shape of the foot, and then the osteotomies are performed on the transparencies. With these transparencies, the size and location of the wedge are determined. Predicting the amount of rotation or correction is difficult with these uniplanar templates, but they provide a good idea of the size of the wedge of the dorsal or dorsomedial wedge if a midfoot osteotomy is going to be performed.

A saw is used to perform the osteotomy. If the dorsal position of the apex is in the middle lateral cuneiform joint, the medial exit point is usually at the base of the medial cuneiform. The anterior tibial tendon attachment must be reflected and retracted medially. The osteotomy is then shaped such that the medial limb is taken at about an 8-mm wedge at approximately a 15- to 20-degree angle of the dorsal plane of the midfoot. If there is any adduction deformity in addition to the cavus, then a biplanar wedge is removed. Bone is resected both dorsally and medially, and this resection removes more of the medial cuneiform itself. If a global cavus of the midfoot is present, then the base of the osteotomy dorsally extends from the center of the foot medially at much the same distance as between the osteotomy limbs. The first lateral osteotomy cut is made extending toward the cuboid from the middle or lateral cuneiform, and then the second osteotomy cut is made at a much smaller angle so that the apex is in the cuboid without removing much of the cuboid at all. It is far easier to perform the lateral correction by dorsally translating the cuboid and then rotating it slightly to elevate the base of the fifth metatarsal.

Once the wedges have been resected, the forefoot is then dorsiflexed until good contact between the dorsal bone surfaces is present. The advantage of this osteotomy is that further contouring can be performed, just like with any wedge osteotomy, until sufficient bone has been removed and the forefoot corrected relative to the hindfoot. Fixation of the osteotomy is possible with screws; a dorsal plate; or large, smooth, or threaded pins that are inserted percutaneously. Using pins in this location is sometimes easier because of the plane of the osteotomy and the small bone segments between each articulation. Staples are also possible provided adequate bone on each side of the osteotomy is present, which is not usually the case. Frequently, I insert large pins from the medial and lateral portion of the foot from distal to proximal and then remove them at 6 weeks once ambulation begins. Patient healing of these osteotomies is generally good; however, any incomplete healing of one portion of the osteotomy does not seem to influence the outcome of the procedure.

Occasionally, the apex of the deformity is more distal at the level of the tarsometatarsal joint. Jahss described a truncated wedge arthrodesis of the tarsometatarsal joint for this type of deformity. This procedure is technically easy to perform, but arthrodesis of all of the joints is difficult to obtain. As with the wedge osteotomy previously discussed, more bone is removed medially than laterally. In fact, it is rare that a wedge is removed from the cuboid

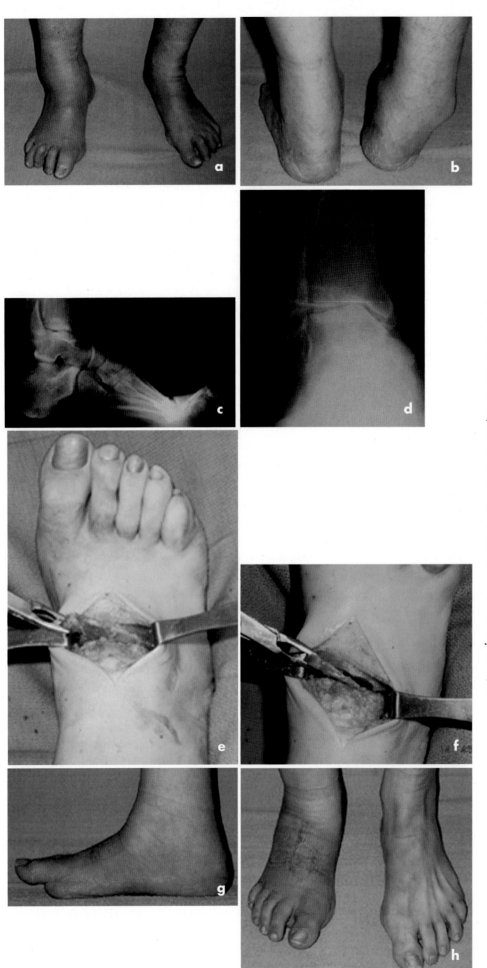

Figure 5–1–8. This severe unilateral deformity of the foot and ankle (a–d) was corrected with an osteotomy of the midfoot and calcaneus. The osteotomy of the midfoot was performed as a derotational biplanar wedge resection, and the medial column was elevated more than the lateral column was (e, f). The varus deformity of the ankle joint was not associated with pain, and although there was a natural tendency for the talus to drift back into varus into the erosion in the distal tibia, the talus did not require correction. The forefoot remains clawed, and the toes are not touching the ground and need to be addressed with subsequent surgery (g, h).

metatarsal articulation. I do not favor this procedure because it relies on arthrodesis of the medial and middle columns of the tarsal metatarsal joint for satisfactory outcome. Furthermore, it is rare that there is any cavus deformity at the metatarso-cuboid joints, and it is preferable and far easier to perform an osteotomy through the cuboid. Such an osteotomy maintains whatever motion is present in the lateral column joints. Fixation of the dorsal wedge arthrodesis from the medial and middle column can be performed with staples, pins, or screws. As with the other wedge procedures, maintaining the plantar aspect of the joint intact at the hinge on which to obtain some axis for the compression dorsally is useful.

Resection of the Fifth Ray

Some feet require resection of the fifth metatarsal. If one looks at a lateral XR film and the fifth metatarsal is depressed relative to the position of the first metatarsal,

then regardless of the manner in which the osteotomy is performed, the fifth ray is inferior to the plane of the cuboid and cannot be rotated sufficiently or translated dorsally to alleviate the plantar pressure. Patients with these feet have tremendous callosity under the base of the fifth metatarsal and absent peroneus brevis muscle function. These are frequently associated with the more severe forms of hereditary sensory motion neuropathy. Although many of the patients still have sensation, the deformity of fifth metatarsal can be painful. Nonetheless, for better correction to be obtained with a more plantigrade foot, ostectomy of the fifth metatarsal is a good procedure. This can be done in conjunction with any additional necessary procedure (Fig. 5–1–9).

The incision that is used for the calcaneal osteotomy, peroneal tendon procedure, or triple arthrodesis is extended, or an additional incision is made from the base of the fifth metatarsal distally along the course of the dorsal shaft of the metatarsal. A saw cut is made

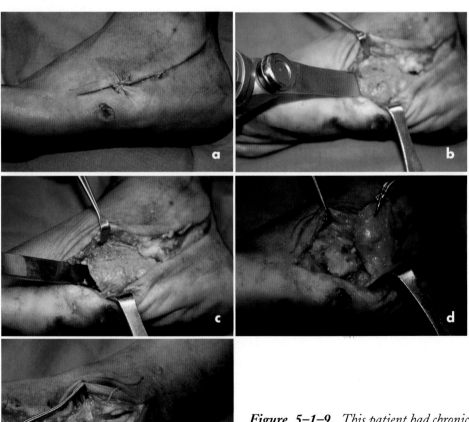

Figure 5–1–9. *This patient had chronic pain under the fifth metatarsal base associated with prior osteomyelitis. In addition to a calcaneus osteotomy and peroneal tendon procedures, resection of the base of the fifth metatarsal was performed. The incision is noted (a), the bone was removed with a saw (b–d), and the peroneal tendon reconstruction was performed (e).*

obliquely in the shaft of the fifth metatarsal in two planes so that the starting point of the osteotomy is dorsal and slightly lateral (Fig. 5–1–9*b*). In this way, the plane of the osteotomy is made so that no bone prominence remains on the plantar lateral weight-bearing surface. The bone is grasped after the osteotomy, and the metatarsal base is grasped with a clamp rotated on its pedicle and is then cut sharply by detaching the short plantar ligament and the remnant of the attachment of the peroneus brevis tendon. The peroneus brevis tendon can be detached distally because it is nonfunctional. If peroneus longus to brevis tendon transfer is performed, however, then the longus tendon needs to be securely attached to the base of the remnant of the brevis tendon and to the fascia overlying the cuboid. At the completion of the ostectomy, the hypertrophic callous needs to be paired with a large blade. Softening the callous with a moist sponge for some time before it is cut is helpful because this is usually extremely hard tissue.

Posterior Tibial Tendon Transfer

The technical details of the posterior tibial tendon (PTT) transfer are in the section on tendon transfers. However, for completeness, the procedure is again demonstrated here in the setting of a cavovarus deformity associated with hereditary motor and sensory neuropathy (Charcot-Marie-Tooth [CMT] syndrome). The tendon transfers do not differ from the PTT transfers; however, the incisions must be planned more carefully when calcaneal and midfoot osteotomies are performed simultaneously (Fig. 5–1–10).

Correction of Multiplanar Deformity

Correction of multiplanar deformity is probably one of the more difficult procedures to perform. Not only is the structural deformity associated with bone deformation in multiple planes, but also joint contractures and muscle imbalance are added. As previously noted, the approach to correction of this type of deformity involves both structural bone alteration, in conjunction with adequate muscle, and soft tissue balancing. Frequently, patients with this deformity have undergone multiple prior operations (commonly, a triple arthrodesis performed when the patients were adolescents). In addition to deformity, ankle instability and ankle arthritis are also present. Throughout this chapter, I have noted the desire to avoid arthrodesis of the cavus foot wherever possible.

Realistically, such avoidance is impossible with severe multiplanar deformity, and arthrodesis is commonly performed in addition to osteotomy and ostectomy. Figures 5–1–11 and 5–1–12 show multiplanar and cavus foot deformities.

Techniques, tips, and pitfalls

1. Avoid arthrodesis wherever possible.

2. I balance the hindfoot, making sure that I slightly weaken the strong inversion and strengthen eversion. This procedure can be made with a PTT transfer through the interosseous membrane to correct an equinocavovarus deformity or posteriorly to augment a weak or absent peroneus brevis muscle.

3. A plantar fascia release invariably needs to be performed, and this should be done before a calcaneal osteotomy because the calcaneus cannot be manipulated into valgus while the fascia is tight.

4. Calcaneal osteotomy is performed in a biplanar or triplanar manner according to the pitch angle of the calcaneus. This is done through closing wedge laterally, then shifting the calcaneus farther laterally, then allowing the calcaneal tuberosity to slide slightly cephalad, and improving the pitch angle if necessary.

5. Always be on the lookout for an unstable ankle in the setting of a cavus foot. This varus deformity of the hindfoot creates an added load on the ankle and on the lateral aspect of the fifth metatarsal. Stress manipulation with radiographs should be performed preoperatively or intraoperatively.

6. Be aware of the triad of a varus heel, ankle instability, and a stress fracture of the fifth metatarsal.

7. In the setting of rigid varus deformity with hypertrophy of the base of the fifth metatarsal and thickened callosity, even with good correction of the hindfoot, this prominence under the base of the fifth metatarsal persists. This is due to inferior subluxation of the fifth metatarsal under the fourth metatarsal, which can only be

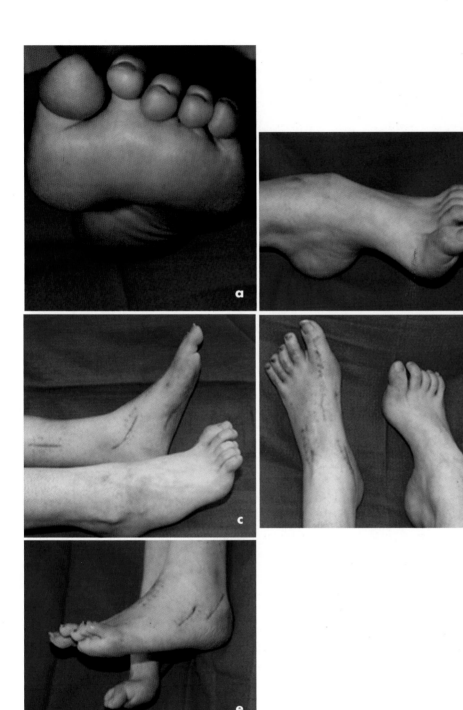

Figure 5–1–10. *Preoperative (a, b) and postoperative (c–e) clinical photographs after correction of deformity caused by hereditary sensorimotor neuropathy. This was corrected with a posterior tibial tendon transfer into the cuboid and calcaneus, a first metatarsal osteotomy, a plantar fascia release, and a percutaneous Achilles tendon lengthening. Note the marked improvement in the length of the foot when compared with the length of the opposite right foot, which still requires correction.*

corrected to a derotational osteotomy of the entire midfoot. Even with this osteotomy, the first metatarsal sometimes is still prominent. For this reason, in a correction of a rigid cavus deformity with a fifth metatarsal prominence, I am reclined to resect the base of the fifth metatarsal completely. Resection of the proximal third of the metatarsal recreates a smooth lateral weight-bearing surface of the foot. Gen-

erally, the peroneus brevis muscle is not functioning at all, and these rigid cavus deformities are usually directed by arthrodesis. Therefore the function of the peroneus brevis muscle is not as relevant.

8. I generally stabilize and correct the hindfoot first and stage correction of the forefoot deformity. Many procedures have to be performed, particularly when the deformity is severe.

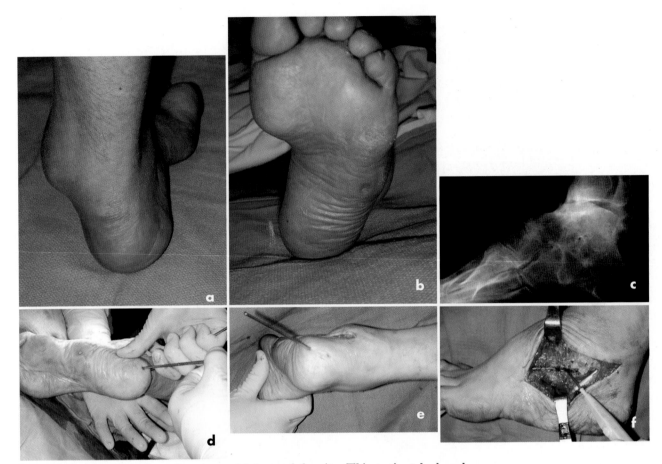

Figure 5–1–11. *Correction of severe multiplanar deformity. This patient had undergone a prior triple arthrodesis for correction of neuromuscular deformity with poor outcome. Note the varus deformity, in the heel, and a severe cavus with fixed deformity of the midfoot (a, b). On the lateral x-ray film, note that there are two deformities, each with a separate apex in the hind-foot: one in the calcaneus and the other in the midfoot (c). The calcaneus osteotomy was per-formed first (d, e). Note the manipulation of the heel with one guide pin changing the varus and the pitch angle, whereas the other is introduced for fixation. The transverse tarsal osteotomy was next performed by marking out the axis of the plane of the hindfoot with the electrocautery (f).*

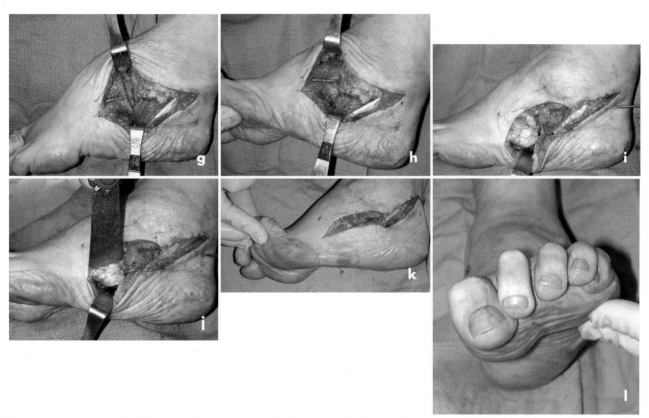

Figure 5–1–11, cont'd. *This axis of the plane of the hind foot marked with the electrocautery is used as a guide to correction once the wedge osteotomy had been performed (g) and the foot was derotated (h). At the completion of the hindfoot osteotomies, the base of the fifth metatarsal was still too prominent and was excised (h, i). The effect of the hindfoot on the first metatarsal can be seen more easily, planning the osteotomy of the medial column (j–l).*

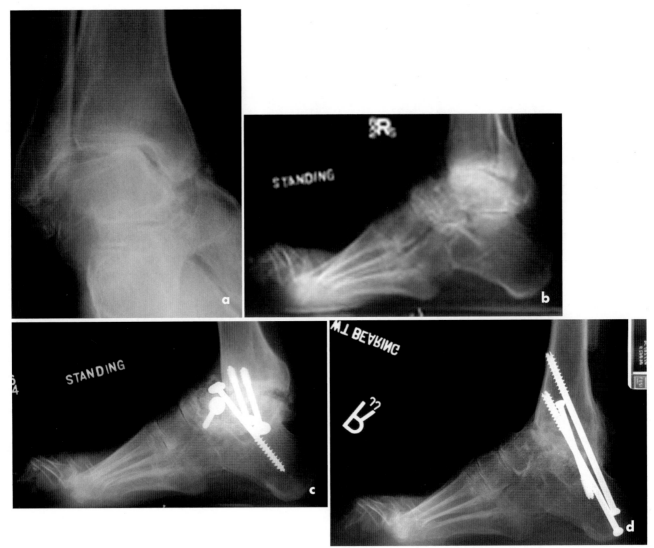

Figure 5–1–12. *This severe cavus deformity associated with flexible ankle varus deformity was due to hereditary sensory motor neuropathy (a, b). The ankle was not painful. The patient was lost to follow-up and underwent an attempted pantalar arthrodesis unsuccessfully. Ideally, because the ankle was not symptomatic to begin with, derotational osteotomies of the hindfoot could have been performed. The patient returned for subsequent treatment, and staged correction was planned, starting with a tibiotalocalcaneal arthrodesis with rotational wedges performed (c, d). Although a cavus midfoot remains, further surgery was postponed because the patient was comfortable with an orthosis.*

Suggested Readings

Giannini S, Ceccarelli F, Benedetti MG, et al: Surgical treatment of adult idiopathic cavus foot with plantar fasciotomy, naviculocuneiform arthrodesis, and cuboid osteotomy. A review of thirty-nine cases. J Bone Joint Surg 84-A:62–69, 2002.

Olney B: Treatment of the cavus foot. Deformity in the pediatric patient with Charcot-Marie-Tooth. Foot Ankle Clin 5:305–315, 2000.

Sammarco GJ, Taylor R: Combined calcaneal and metatarsal osteotomies for the treatment of cavus foot. Foot Ankle Clin 6:533–543, vii, 2001.

Wulker N, Hurschler C: Cavus foot correction in adults by dorsal closing wedge osteotomy. Foot Ankle Int 23:344–347, 2002.

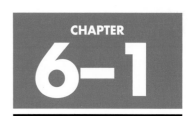

Correction of Paralytic Deformity

Anatomy and Principles of Tendon Transfers

The correction of foot and ankle deformity by means of a correctly performed tendon transfer can be satisfying for both the surgeon and the patient. The goal of any tendon transfer is to create a stable, functioning, and plantigrade foot, and this goal applies to every tendon transfer performed for paralysis because the correction of deformity, the improvement of function, and the establishment of a plantigrade foot are essential.

From a simplistic perspective, any muscle (tendon) that passes anterior to the ankle joint axis functions as a dorsiflexor, and conversely, any tendon passing posterior to the axis of the ankle is a plantarflexor. This is important because the peroneal and posterior tibial tendons (PTT) are plantarflexors of the ankle, although their function is primarily thought of in terms of inversion and eversion. If a tendon lies centrally, in the axis of a joint, it exerts little influence on the motion of that joint. Conversely, the greater the distance a tendon lies from a joint axis, the more it exerts a greater force across the joint because of the longer lever arm. Where a tendon lies is relevant, for example, in the use of the PTT transfer through the interosseous membrane. The transfer is performed subcutaneously, and the tendon is not passed inferior (deep) to the retinaculum because this would decrease power.

The anterior tibial muscle lies almost directly on top of the subtalar joint axis; therefore it has little influence over hindfoot inversion or eversion, although it has an accessory function of inversion by virtue of its insertion on the foot. At times, however, the anterior tibial muscle can become a primary invertor of the foot, for example, in the absence of a posterior tibial muscle. The Achilles tendon lies posterior to the ankle joint axis and provides the primary plantar flexion strength for the ankle. It also normally lies slightly medial to the subtalar joint axis and therefore is a weak invertor of the subtalar joint. This effect is negated in patients who have a long-standing absence of the posterior tibial muscle, where the peroneal tendons then pull the heel into valgus, potentiated by the valgus force of the Achilles tendon insertion. In these patients, the position of the Achilles tendon and thus the force of the gastrocnemius muscle have to be normalized by a medial translational osteotomy of the calcaneus in addition to any tendon transfer performed.

The posterior tibial and peroneal tendons form a force couple around the ankle that controls hindfoot inversion and eversion. The PTT lies posterior to the ankle joint axis and medial to the subtalar axis. It therefore plantarflexes the ankle and inverts the hindfoot, in contrast to the peroneal tendons, which plantarflex the ankle and evert the hindfoot. Paralysis of a component of this force couple allows overpull of the antagonist, and this overpull results in varus or valgus malalignment. Although the balance of inversion and eversion may depend on the relationship between the peroneus brevis muscle and the posterior tibial muscle, the accessory inversion of the anterior tibial muscle and the eversion of the peroneus longus muscle (and the gastrocnemius-soleus muscle outlined earlier) must be considered.

When any tendon transfer is planned, the following must be considered: the relative muscle strengths and tendon excursion of every functioning muscle, no matter how weak it may appear; the positioning of the tendon to be transferred relative to the rest of the foot; the proper tensioning of a transferred tendon; and the pull-out strength necessary to secure the tendon transfer. Optimally, a tendon transfer should approximate the strength and excursion of the motor unit it is trying to replace, but this can be rarely accomplished with a single tendon. Therefore expecting the extensor hallucis longus (EHL) muscle to replace the anterior tibial muscle, or the flexor digitorum longus muscle to replace the posterior tibial muscle is unrealistic. Such a replacement can be difficult if not impossible when an attempt is made to compensate for paralysis of the strongest muscles, such as the gastrocnemius-soleus muscle, where multiple tendon transfers may be required.

Also, it is important to consider that most muscles will lose a grade of power when transferred, particularly if the transfer is not phasic (a tendon that is primarily a flexor and is transferred to function as an extensor). The same does not hold, however, for the PTT, which functions primarily as an invertor and secondarily as a plantarflexor of the ankle. If this tendon is transfer-red behind the ankle to the peroneal muscles to augment eversion, it is not functioning at a mechanical disadvantage because it has been kept posterior to the ankle axis. It is always preferable to use a muscle that is phasic because less "reeducation" of the muscle is required, rehabilitation is facilitated, and less strength of the muscle is lost in the transfer. Typically in a PTT transfer performed through the interosseous membrane to the dorsum of the foot for correction of a flaccid paralysis, one grade of muscle strength is lost. This loss of muscle strength becomes more important when nonphasic muscles are used, for example, the use of the peroneal muscle to substitute for absent ankle dorsiflexion when no alternative tendon is available for transfer. However, the peroneal muscle does not need to pass

through the interosseous membrane (as the PTT transfer does), and they can be passed more directly over the fibula to the anterior foot. Although this is a nonphasic transfer, less strength is lost than when a PTT transfer is used because of minimizing the change in direction of the tendon transfer.

The question often arises as to how tight a tendon transfer should be when secured to the bone. If it is fixed at maximal elongation, the tendon transfer acts more like a tenodesis, although it always stretches out. However, if it is fixed in its relaxed state, it cannot generate adequate tension to pull effectively. Generally, I prefer to insert the tendon under more tension than relaxation because some stretching out of the muscle always occurs. Finally, if transferred underneath a retinaculum which functions as a pulley, this increases the effective tendon excursion (range of motion). However, this transfer brings the tendon closer to the ankle or subtalar axes and diminishes the lever arm and the subsequent strength of the transfer. The opposite holds true for a subcutaneous position of the tendon transfer. Although excursion is decreased, motor strength is maximized because of the greater distance from the axes and the resulting greater lever arm. In general, a tendon is always transferred in a subcutaneous position.

Wherever possible, I perform a transfer using a tunnel with a bone tendon–bone interference fit of the tendon. This ensures excellent apposition of the tendon in the tunnel with little tendency to pull out of the bone. This transfer is important with respect to rehabilitation because weight bearing and passive range-of-motion exercises may begin once the sutures are removed, and the strengthening and reeducation that were initiated earlier may start. Rehabilitation is essential regardless of the type of transfer, although this is easier to accomplish if the transferred tendon is in phase with the muscle it replaced.

Principles and Timing of Tendon Transfers

Recovery of muscle function may occur for up to 1 year after nerve injury, and although an electromyogram (EMG) may have diagnostic benefit, repeat clinical examination during this time is more helpful. Although some muscle recovery may occur up to 2 years after injury, I generally perform the transfer after 1 year. This is particularly relevant when the foot is gradually deforming because of an imbalance in muscle forces about the ankle. The foot must be protected after nerve injury or trauma to prevent progressive deformity, which only makes the reconstructive procedure more difficult, if not impossible. A flexible equinus deformity is far easier to correct than a fixed equinovarus deformity, which may require, in addition to the tendon transfer, hindfoot and forefoot osteotomy to ensure a plantigrade foot.

When patients are evaluated for possible tendon transfer, ascertaining whether they have a static or a progressive deformity is important. Wherever muscle imbalance is present, deformity of the foot will eventually occur, and this is exacerbated if the muscles used for the transfer itself are involved in the paralytic process. Correction of the foot to a plantigrade position is always possible, even in a patient with a progressive deformity such as Charcot-Marie-Tooth disease. However, once the foot is plantigrade and balanced, even if further weakening of the muscles occurs, the foot generally remains plantigrade. Fixed deformity of either the foot or the ankle cannot be corrected by tendon transfer alone, although the transfer may be integral to the success of surgery. For example, in a patient with a rigid hindfoot in equinovarus, a triple arthrodesis may be chosen for correction. Although this may initially correct the deformity, if posterior tibial muscle function remains in the absence of peroneal strength (or vice versa in an equinovalgus deformity), deformity may recur, and a tendon transfer should be incorporated into the treatment plan (Fig. 6–1–1).

Any fixed deformity of the hindfoot must be corrected before a tendon transfer is performed, passive motion across the joint that the tendon transfer acts on must be adequate, and muscles that are in phase are preferable if available.

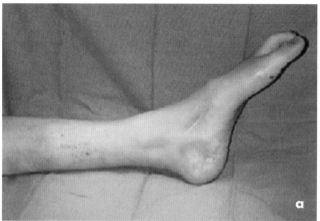
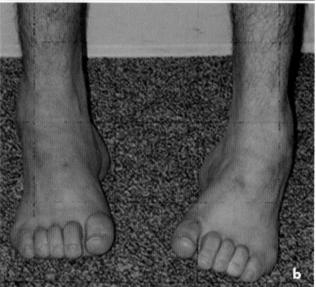

Figure 6–1–1. *These two feet, both with foot drop, appear differently. In this patient the foot is in equinus (a), and in this patient, the foot is in equinovarus (b). These appearances affect the position of the insertion for a tendon transfer and the need for hindfoot osteotomy.*

Techniques, tips, and pitfalls

1. The transferred tendon must have adequate power and excursion. A tendon transfer should approximate both the strength and excursion of the musculotendinous unit it wishes to replace. If it does not, it is unlikely that the transfer will provide adequate power to correct the deformity. This is especially true because most tendons lose one grade of power after being transferred. A musculotendinous unit being considered for transfer optimally should have a grade of 4/5 strength or better.

2. The line of pull should be direct, and there should be no acute angulation of the transferred tendon. This will maximize the effectiveness of the transferred musculotendinous unit. The

force vector generated by the transfer should not be weakened by undesirable angles or turns around the foot and ankle. This weakening is a common problem with the use of the PTT transfer through the interosseous membrane, and an acute angle must be avoided. This will also decrease the likelihood of the tendon getting stuck with scar or contracture.

3. Tendon transfers should be fixed in bone. This allows direct action of the tendon on the skeletal structures without a soft tissue intermediary. Tendon-to-bone healing may also be more reliable than tendon-to-tendon healing, especially in cases with underlying tenodesis or atrophy.

4. A tendon transfer cannot correct fixed deformity around the foot and ankle. This should be done either by arthrodesis or by osteotomy before restoring the lost motor function. Questions then arise about when to fuse and when to perform osteotomies. A triple arthrodesis is a good procedure for correction of deformity, but for correction of neuromuscular problems, osteotomies are preferable, and a triple arthrodesis should be reserved for salvage. An arthrodesis does not guarantee that a deformity will not recur, especially if the neuromuscular condition is progressive. In these cases, tendon transfer to balance the opposing force couples is essential to prevent recurrence after arthrodesis. Similarly, tendon transfer cannot correct soft-tissue contractures, and these should be released or lengthened to allow adequate passive motion of the joint. An example of this is gastrocnemius-soleus muscle contracture in long-standing foot drop. When the PTT is transferred through the interosseus membrane, lengthening the Achilles tendon to provide at least 10 degrees of passive ankle dorsiflexion intraoperatively is essential.

Posterior Tibial Tendon Transfer

I use a four-incision technique for a PTT transfer to restore ankle dorsiflexion. The operation can be done with the patient under regional or general anesthesia and positioned supine. The first incision is made medially from the level of the talonavicular joint to the medial cuneiform to harvest the PTT. The sheath is opened longitudinally, and the insertion of the tendon is exposed. An osteotome is used to remove a small osteoperiosteal flap including the attachment of the PTT to the navicular joint (Fig. 6–1–2*a*). If possible an additional strip of tendon with periosteum is harvested distal to the navicular joint. The end of the tendon is then tagged with a 2-0 suture to facilitate transfer (Fig. 6–1–2*b*), and the PTT sheath is split longitudinally posterior to the medial malleolus to make passage of the tendon easier (Fig. 6–1–2*c*).

The second incision is made medially along the calf approximately 15 cm above the level of the ankle. This corresponds to the location of the musculotendinous junction. Dissection is carried down through the subcutaneous tissue to expose the underlying fascia that is incised longitudinally, and the posterior tibial muscle is then palpated while pulling on the distal tendon stump (Fig. 6–1–2*d*). The muscle and tendon are then pulled proximally with a finger or a curved clamp (Fig. 6–1–2*e*). The tendon should be kept moist with a saline-soaked sponge for the remainder of the procedure. Try to maintain the musculotendinous junction without tearing the muscle. The less the amount of fraying that occurs, the less likely scarring will develop as the tendon passes laterally.

The third incision is made on the opposite side of the leg just anterior to the fibula and slightly distal to the second incision. The incision is deepened through the subcutaneous tissue, and the superficial peroneal nerve is identified and protected. The muscles of the anterior compartment are retracted medially to expose the interosseus membrane, and a 2-cm window of the interosseus membrane is excised. Be careful of the underlying neurovascular bundle that is no longer protected by the PTT muscle belly. A blunt elevator can be used to gently push aside any soft tissue structures deep to the interosseus membrane. The PTT tendon is "lined up" on the lateral leg to identify the optimal angle of passage through the interosseous space (Fig. 6–1–2*f*).

A large, curved clamp is then passed lateral through the interosseous window to grab the tendon or suture medially. The clamp must be held directly against the posterior surface of the tibia to avoid neurovascular injury.

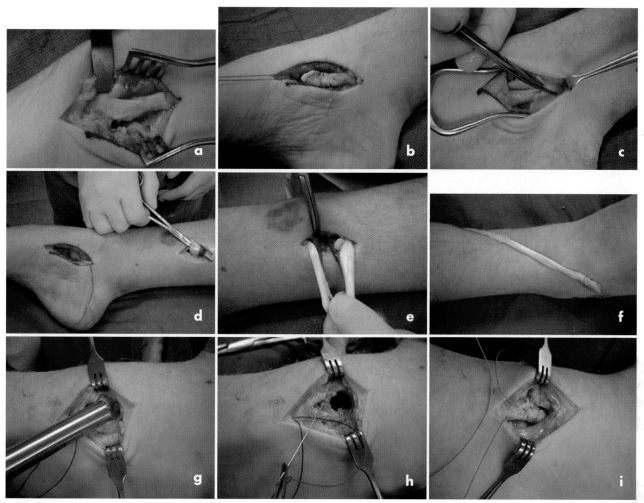

Figure 6–1–2. *The steps in a posterior tibial tendon (PTT) transfer.*

The suture is grasped, and the PTT is passed from the deep posterior compartment to the anterior compartment. Optimally the PTT muscle belly should traverse the window in the interosseus membrane rather than the tendon to avoid adhesions.

The fourth incision is then made over the dorsum of the midfoot. Generally, it is attached somewhere between the middle and lateral cuneiform, but this attachment depends on the deformity and the strength of the remaining muscles. The soft tissues and branches of the superficial peroneal nerve are dissected and protected. The extensor tendons are then retracted and the periosteum is incised over the lateral cuneiform. A long curved clamp is passed subcutaneously from this incision to the incision over the anterolateral aspect of the leg. The suture ends are grasped, and the PTT is then passed into the incision overlying the foot. The lateral cuneiform is prepared with a gouge or trephine that

removes a plug of bone corresponding to the diameter of the tendon (Fig. 6–1–2*g*). The plug is removed and the tendon is advanced into the tunnel by passing the suture ends out the plantar aspect of the foot with a long straight needle (Fig. 6–1–2*h*). If a suture anchor is used for fixation, this should be inserted into the cancellous bone on the side of the tunnel before the tendon is inserted. While the ankle is held in 10 degrees of dorsiflexion, the transfer is tensioned almost at maximal elongation. If necessary, a percutaneous Achilles tendon lengthening should be performed to achieve this dorsiflexion. The sutures attached to the anchor are then used to secure the tendon into the tunnel (Fig. 6–1–2*i*). The bone plug harvested with the gouge may then be replaced into the tunnel beside the tendon for further fixation (Fig. 6–1–3).

A well-padded posterior splint is applied postoperatively for 2 weeks. After suture removal, a cam boot or short-leg

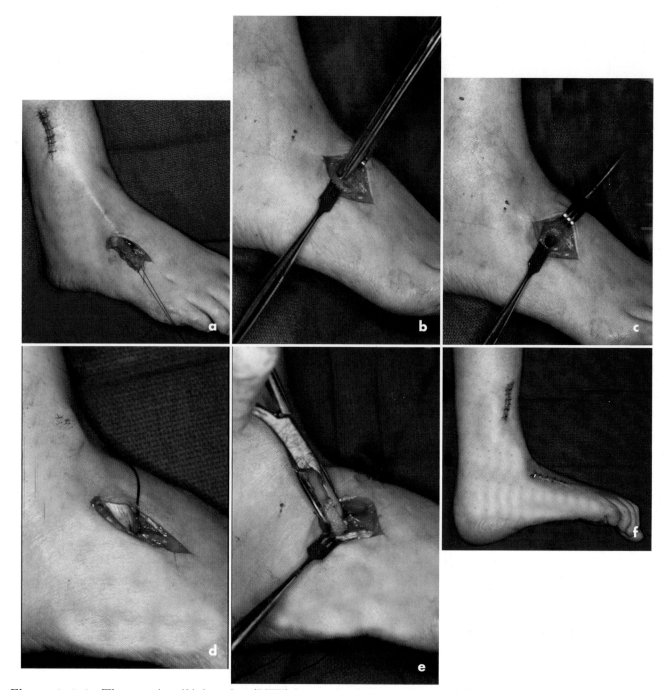

Figure 6-1-3. *The posterior tibial tendon (PTT) is passed subcutaneously to exit into the dorsal foot incision (a). A 6-mm trephine is used to remove a plug of bone from the lateral cuneiform (b, c). The PTT is passed through the bone tunnel with a straight needle out the plantar skin (d), and the bone plug is replaced as an interference fit against the tendon (e). Note the final position of the foot in slight dorsiflexion, with marked flexion of the toes as a result of a tenodesis effect on the long flexor tendons (f).*

walking cast is applied. If no lengthening of the Achilles tendon is performed, then a boot can be used instead of a cast, and active and passive exercises can begin at 2 weeks. At 6 weeks adhesion of the tendon to the bone tunnel is adequate to discontinue immobilization. A night splint is used for 3 months postoperatively. Physical therapy is initiated at 6 weeks to retrain the PTT to become an ankle dorsiflexor. This may take several months.

A modification of the PTT transfer has been proposed as a "Bridle procedure," which combines a standard PTT transfer with anastomosis of the tibialis anterior muscle and an anteriorly rerouted peroneus longus muscle. The procedure is carried out in an identical fashion to that stated earlier with the exception that when the PTT is brought into the anterior compartment, it is routed through a longitudinal slit in the anterior tibial tendon (ATT). An additional longitudinal skin incision is made posterolaterally behind the fibula to expose the peroneus longus tendon. The peroneus longus tendon is transected approximately 5 cm above the tip of the lateral malleolus. The distal limb is retrieved from under the superior and inferior peroneal retinaculum distally and subcutaneously rerouted in front of the fibula into the third incision, described previously. Here it is anastomosed to the PTT transfer, along with the tibialis anterior muscle with nonabsorbable sutures. The proximal stump of the peroneus longus tendon is then sutured to the peroneus brevis tendon. I have no personal experience with this modification of the PTT transfer and have not encountered the presumed problems of balance of the foot that supposedly is the advantage of the bridle procedure.

Tenodesis of Extensors to Tibia (Stirrup Procedure)

Sometimes a patient does not have any available tendon to use for a transfer, and arthrodesis is neither desirable nor necessary. For these patients, the foot drop may be easily controlled during the day with an ankle foot orthosis. Household ambulation may, however, be markedly improved with a tenodesis procedure. This procedure has been used in patients who have flaccid paralysis of all lower leg muscles, usually as a result of polio or low-level myelomeningocele. This procedure can help limit the need for use of a brace and is an alternative to pan-talar fusion (Fig. 6–1–4).

The incision is made in the distal third of the leg. The tibialis anterior, flexor hallucis longus (FHL), and flexor digitorum longus muscles are identified and placed on tension to dorsiflex the ankle 10 degrees. If this dorsiflexion is unattainable, then a percutaneous Achilles tendon lengthening is performed. The periosteum of the tibia where the tenodesis is planned is roughened with an osteotome to encourage tendon adhesion to the bone. The tendons are then divided and tagged with nonabsorbable sutures. The ankle is positioned in 10 degrees of dorsiflexion with the metatarsophalangeal joints held in neutral. A staple is used to affix the tendons to bone while tension on the tendon ends is maintained. The remaining sutures are then passed through a drill hole in the tibia and sutured back into the ends of the transferred tendons.

Patients are allowed to weight bear immediately in a walking boot or cast. This can be discontinued 4 weeks postoperatively. This tendon transfer may stretch out over 2 years but can be easily tightened again if necessary. Other tenodesis procedures may be considered, depending on the proximity and function of adjacent phasic muscles (Fig. 6–1–5).

Nonstandard Tendon Transfers

The traditional transfers, in particular the PTT transfer for paralytic equinus deformity, have been discussed in this chapter. However, some patients have variations of equinus deformity for which the traditional tendon transfer is not feasible, and other methods must be used. If no PTT function is present, then, in order of preference, I would use the common digital extensors (EHL or extensor digitorum longus [EDL] tendon), the peroneal tendon, or even the FHL tendon. If the EHL or the EDL tendon is used, an arthrodesis of the interphalangeal (IP) joints should be performed simultaneously (Fig. 6–1–6). The tendon is then passed proximally into the midfoot and positioned accordingly. Cutting the tendon distally is not necessary, nor is it ideal to insert the tendon into the metatarsal necks, as previously described, but the maximal mechanical advantage, which is obtained when the tendon is transferred into the base of the metatarsals or cuneiforms, should always be sought (Fig. 6–1–7).

The need for a peroneal transfer is not that uncommon when the PTT tendon or other functioning muscles of

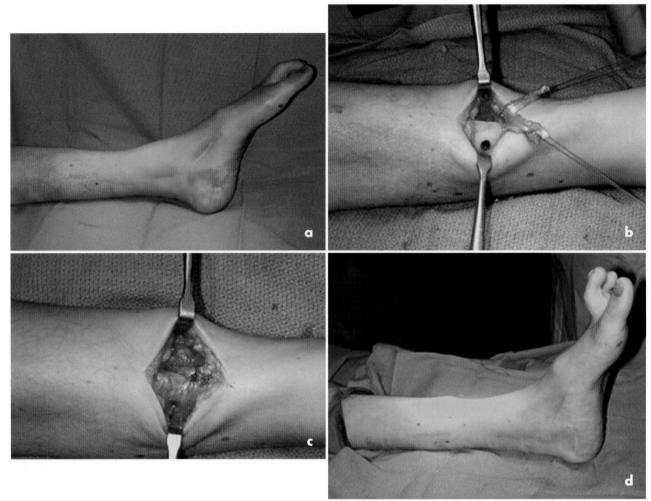

Figure 6–1–4. *In a patient with flaccid paralysis with no tendons available for transfer at all (a), a tenodesis can be performed by attaching the tendons to the tibia. For the foot to be maintained plantigrade, the extensor tendons must be included in addition to the anterior tibial tendon (ATT). One or two drill holes are made in the tibia, and the tendons are pulled through across the tibia and then tied anteriorly (b, c). Although the foot is in neutral position, note that the hallux is below the level of the lesser toes (d), which could be averted with the extensor hallucis longus (EHL) tendon in the tenodesis procedure.*

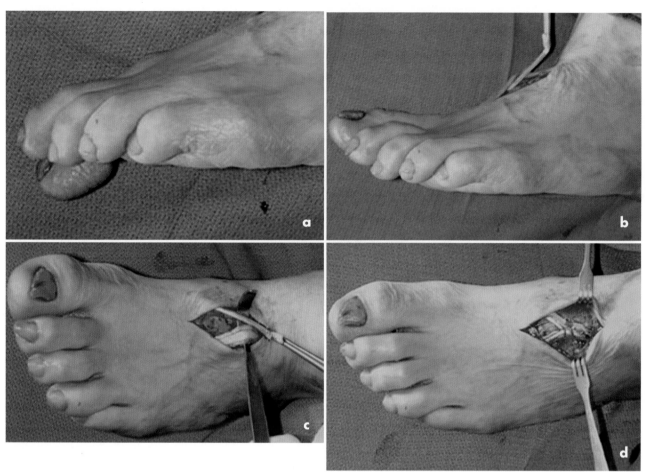

Figure 6–1–5. *Paralysis of the extensors may be patchy, and in this patient with diabetes, a peripheral mononeuropathy of the extensor hallucis longus (EHL) tendon caused a drop hallux deformity. The remaining toes functioned well (a). As an alternative to transferring a functioning tendon into the hallux, a tenodesis of the EHL tendon to the extensor digitorum longus (EDL) tendon under appropriate tension may be used (b–d).*

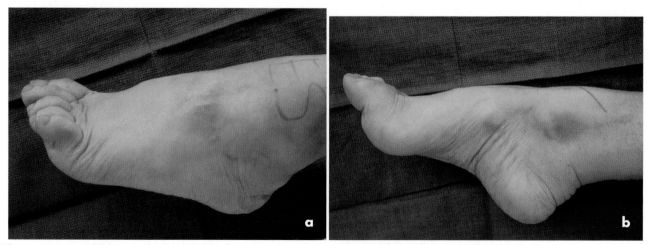

Figure 6–1–6. *This cavoequinus deformity was associated with severe fixed claw toe deformities and a foot drop, but no functioning posterior or anterior tibial muscles were available for transfer. A triple arthrodesis had been performed 20 years previously (a, b).*

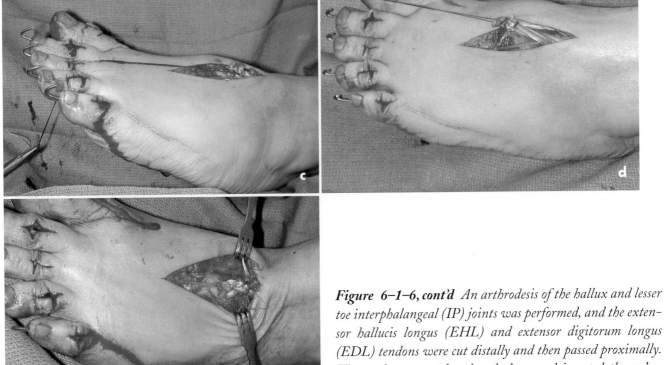

Figure 6–1–6, cont'd An arthrodesis of the hallux and lesser toe interphalangeal (IP) joints was performed, and the extensor hallucis longus (EHL) and extensor digitorum longus (EDL) tendons were cut distally and then passed proximally. The tendons were then bunched up and inserted through a trephine hole into the middle cuneiform secured by a suture anchor and the bone from the trephine tunnel (c–e).

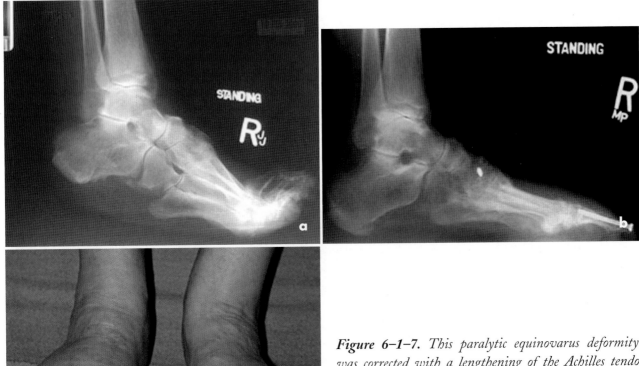

Figure 6–1–7. This paralytic equinovarus deformity (a) was corrected with a lengthening of the Achilles tendon; a transfer of the posterior tibial tendon (PTT), hallux, and lesser toe interphalangeal (IP) fusions; a transfer of the extensor hallucis longus (EHL) and extensor digitorum longus (EDL) tendons to the midfoot; and a transfer of the peroneus longus to the peroneus brevis tendon (b, c).

dorsiflexion are absent. Both peroneal tendons are cut percutaneously on the lateral side of the foot, and then the peroneal retinaculum is released. The sheath is completely opened, and the peroneal tendons are transferred anterior to the fibula. The attachment is similar to that described previously for the PTT. Because no other functioning muscle is present, the tendons are always inserted in the middle of the foot into the lateral cuneiform (Figs 6–1–8 to 6–1–10). An osteotomy of the calcaneus (with medial translation) usually has to be performed simultaneously to correct the hindfoot valgus, which is invariably present.

An interesting transfer is the use of the FHL tendon to correct equinus deformity. This is, of course, a nonphasic transfer, but the FHL tendon may be used if all else fails or if there is no alternative muscle to use. Many surgeons are familiar with its use to augment or substitute for a deficient gastrocnemius muscle or to augment a chronic rupture of the Achilles tendon. When the FHL tendon is used this way, the transfer is phasic, unlike the FHL tendon's use to substitute for a paralytic equinus deformity. It does work, although not with the same strength as the PTT would under similar circumstances.

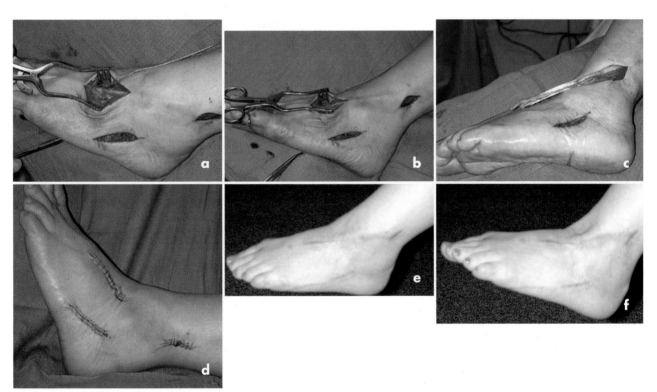

Figure 6–1–8. *This patient had paralysis of both the anterior and posterior tibial muscles after a spine injury. However, the peroneal tendons were functioning, and these were transferred to the dorsum of the foot anterior to the fibula to attain dorsiflexion. Both tendons were harvested through the inferior lateral incision and then pulled out proximally through a second incision (a, b). The tendons were transferred into the middle cuneiform after they had been passed subcutaneously (c, d). The active plantar flexion (e) and dorsiflexion (f) 2 years after surgery.*

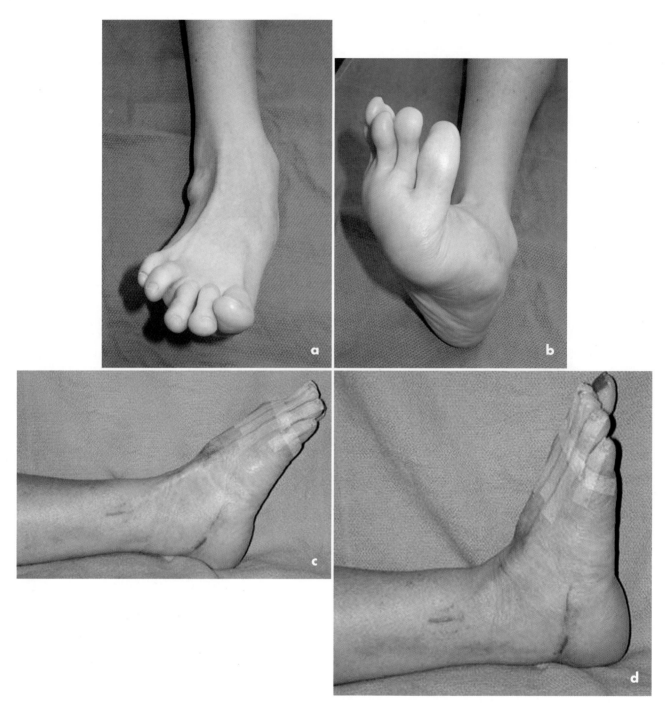

Figure 6–1–9. *This patient had little functioning dorsiflexion, with a marked equinovalgus deformity of the foot (a, b), and a single incision was used laterally to perform a triplanar osteotomy of the calcaneus and harvest the peroneal tendons for transfer into the middle cuneiform. The active plantar flexion and dorsiflexion 6 weeks after peroneal tendon transfer and calcaneus osteotomy (c, d).*

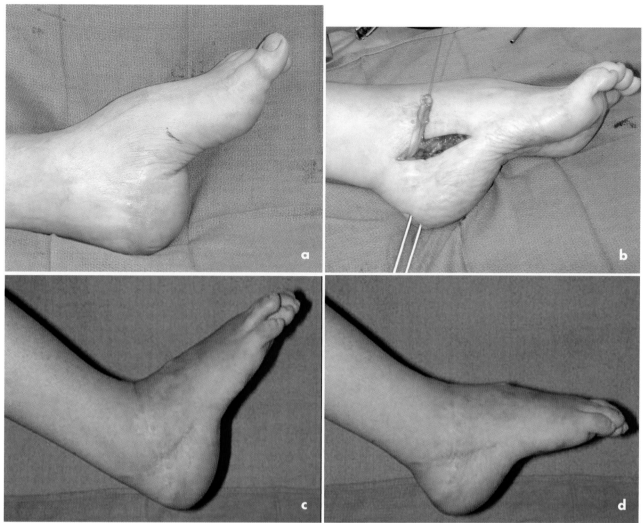

Figure 6–1–10. *Equinovalgus deformity was present in this patient with no functioning posterior tibial tendon (PTT) or anterior tibial tendon (ATT) muscle (a). In addition to a transfer of the extensor hallucis longus (EHL) and extensor digitorum longus (EDL) tendons, a peroneal transfer was planned in conjunction with a medial translational calcaneus osteotomy (b). The result at 1 year with active dorsiflexion (c) and plantar flexion (d).*

Suggested Readings

Hsu JD, Hoffer MM. Posterior tibial tendon transfer anteriorly through the interosseous membrane. Clin Orthop Mar–Apr:202–204, 1978.

Miller GM, Hsu JD, Hoffer MM, Rentfro R. Posterior tibial tendon transfer: A review of the literature and analysis of 74 procedures. J Pediatr Orthop 2:363–370, 1982.

Myerson MS. The use of tendon transfers to correct paralytic deformity. In Myerson MS (ed). Disorders of the Foot and Ankle. Philadelphia, WB Saunders, 2000.

Rodriguez RP. The bridle procedure in the treatment of paralysis of the foot. Foot Ankle 13:63–69, 1992.

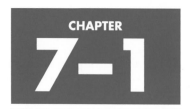

Correction of Flatfoot Deformity in the Child

Pes planus is a common problem, and although predominantly idiopathic, it exists in children who have neuromuscular and other disorders including tarsal coalition and the accessory navicular syndrome. The treatment of flatfoot associated with tarsal coalition is discussed elsewhere (see Chapter 11), and the discussion here is limited to the flexible flatfoot, with or without the presence of accessory navicular syndrome. By and large, the exact same principles of correction of the flatfoot apply to the child as to the adult, and the algorithm of correction for the adult should be followed. Perhaps the most obvious difference is that in children, arthroereisis and osteotomy are emphasized, and arthrodesis is almost completely avoided.

Arthroereisis

The goal of arthroereisis in the child is to properly orient the talus over the calcaneus; the joint is thereby allowed to remodel. This remodeling will hopefully prevent further problems later in life such as degeneration or rigidity of the hindfoot. An arthroereisis implant can be considered as an "internal orthotic device." This procedure has many advantages; most important, however, is the maintenance of motion and the minimal morbidity of this procedure. The indications for correction of adult flatfoot are fairly specific, whereas the indications for arthroereisis of the subtalar joint in the child are broad. For most patients with a flexible flatfoot that results from a rupture of the posterior tibial tendon (PTT), a

reconstruction is performed with a medial translational osteotomy of the calcaneus and a flexor digitorum longus tendon transfer. Treatment results for patients undergoing arthroereisis have been excellent, provided the talonavicular (TN) joint is not significantly uncovered. Once the TN joint sags, particularly on the lateral view, these feet seem to require more correction of the pronation deformity than a medial displacement calcaneal osteotomy can provide. If there is abduction deformity of the foot, with uncovering of the TN joint, then neither the arthroereisis nor the medial displacement osteotomy is likely to be successful. Anecdotally, with arthroereisis in the adult flatfoot, more of the talocalcaneal deformity is corrected than with the abduction of the transverse tarsal joint. In the adult, the arthroereisis procedure has been performed in conjunction with additional hindfoot procedures (e.g., calcaneus osteotomy, flexor digitorum longus tendon transfer, tarsometatarsal arthrodesis, and Achilles tendon lengthening). In addition, we have also used arthroereisis in the symptomatic elderly patient with refractory sinus tarsi pain associated with a flexible flatfoot regardless of the etiology. The most common approach for surgery on these patients has been to use a minimally invasive procedure to realign the subtalar joint, which avoids a more extensive surgical procedure, and to insert the implant in conjunction with a gastrocnemius muscle recession or a lengthening of the Achilles tendon. Most important, these patients are able to bear weight in a boot within days after surgery.

Surgical Technique: Arthroereisis

An incision is made in the sinus tarsi, approximately 1.5 cm in length. To locate the exact position for the incision, palpate the "soft spot" between the distal tip of the fibula and the anterior process of the calcaneus. The incision is inferior to the intermediate dorsal cutaneous branch of the superficial peroneal nerve and dorsal to the peroneal tendons. A guide pin that functions as a cannula for the arthroereisis dilators and sizers is inserted into the tarsal canal from lateral to medial, pushed through a puncture on the medial foot, and then clamped. The anatomy of the tarsal canal must be understood because the canal is shaped as an oblique cone and passes from anterolateral to posteromedial. The guide pin should therefore be inserted in the same plane as the tarsal canal and not directly medially. A slight resistance to the insertion of the pin can be felt as it traverses the interosseous ligament; then it is pushed through until it is protruding on the medial skin. The clamp on the guide pin prevents loss of position of the guide during repeated insertion of the sizers and trial prostheses. Once the guide pin is secure, the first cannulated trial sizer is inserted to get a feel of the position, location, and size of the tarsal canal. The range of motion of the subtalar joint is carefully assessed with each incremental increase in the size of the dilator. The dorsiflexion of the foot now occurs more directly through the ankle joint, rather than in an oblique direction with a combined motion of dorsiflexion and eversion through the subtalar joint. If too large a prosthesis is inserted, limited motion of the subtalar joint is present. Remember that the goal of this operation is simply to limit excessive eversion of the hindfoot. If the prosthesis is too small, hindfoot valgus persists, and dorsiflexion of the foot persists through the subtalar joint. The appropriate sizer should limit abnormal subtalar joint eversion and allow for a few degrees of remaining eversion only.

For young children, a size 6 or 8 prosthesis is usually sufficient; in adults, a size 10 or 12 prosthesis is normally used. The sizer is withdrawn, a trial implant is inserted, and the position of the implant is checked radiographically. The implant should rest between the middle and the posterior facets, and on the anteroposterior view of the foot. The lateral edge of the prosthesis should be 4 mm medial to the lateral edge of the talar neck. If the position of the implant is incorrect, as noted on the anteroposterior radiograph of the hindfoot, then it is easy to adjust the final position by screwing clockwise or counterclockwise in the sinus tarsi.

The range of motion of the subtalar joint is assessed. The eversion with the foot in neutral dorsiflexion should be particularly noted. The primary goal of correction is to limit excessive subtalar joint eversion. The effect of the implant on the range of motion of the ankle and the position of the forefoot is not as important as the limitation of excessive subtalar eversion. For most patients treated for a flexible flatfoot deformity, insertion of the implant is sufficient to correct the foot. The forefoot should be plantigrade, and no supination of the forefoot should be present after hindfoot correction. If supination is present, an opening wedge osteotomy of the medial cuneiform is an excellent procedure to correct any residual forefoot supination after correction of the hindfoot (Fig. 7–1–1).

Techniques, tips, and pitfalls

1. Sinus tarsi pain may occur after arthroereisis, probably the result of irritation from the prosthesis, impingement of the prosthesis against the posterior facet, or an incorrectly sized prosthesis. This pain may also occur when mild forefoot supination is present. For the forefoot to remain plantigrade, the hindfoot has to evert slightly, and this eversion causes jamming of the arthroereisis.

2. If pain is present postoperatively, a boot is used for 2 to 4 weeks. If pain persists, then a corticosteroid injection is administered into the sinus tarsi.

3. The implant may have to be removed for chronic pain. Removal of the implant may not be associated with a predictable reversal of the foot structure.

4. The range of motion of the hindfoot can decrease after arthroereisis, and although this decrease is not significant, it is not normal.

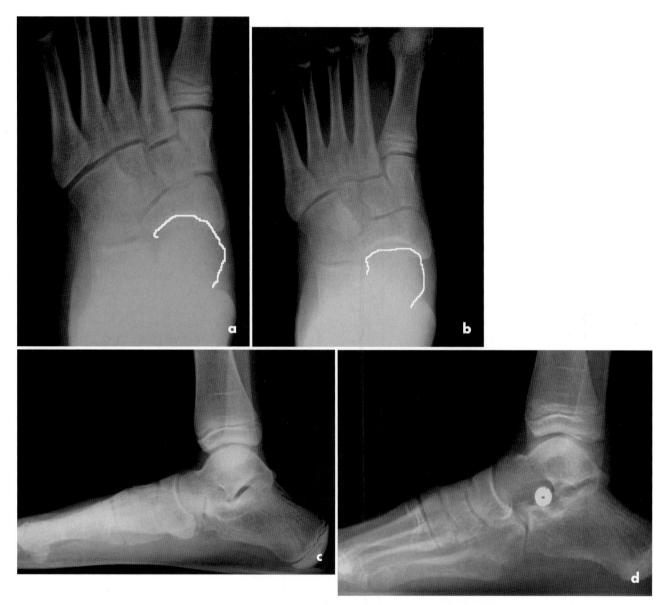

Figure 7–1–1. *Preoperative (a, c) and postoperative (b, d) images of a 9-year-old girl with a painful flatfoot who was treated with an arthroereisis and percutaneous Achilles tendon lengthening. The postoperative images were taken 18 months after surgery. The implant was not painful and was left in.*

Correction of the Accessory Navicular Syndrome

A painful accessory navicular bone is almost always associated with a flatfoot of varying degree. Although this is more prevalent in the child, the same condition can be present in the adult with symptoms resulting from disruption of the synchondrosis. As the synchondrosis is stressed, disruption of the attachment of the accessory navicular bone and thus the PTT occurs with proximal migration of the accessory navicular bone. Elongation of the PTT and an acquired flatfoot then occur. In the child, however, the accessory navicular bone can be painful either as a result of stress on the synchondrosis or from pressure in the shoe as a result of an uncorrected pronated flatfoot. Various degrees of deformity and flexibility of the hindfoot are associated with the accessory navicular bone, and these may also require correction. Generally, I decide on additional surgery according to the location of deformity, and this may consist of medial translational osteotomy of the calcaneus, lateral column lengthening, subtalar arthroereisis, medial cuneiform osteotomy, or Achilles tendon lengthening. Occasionally, if the accessory bone is large, I may use a screw for fixation of a painful os; however, trimming the excess medial bone off the navicular bone is as important as obtaining bone healing. I use a screw in the child or adolescent only if the bone fragment is large, and I want to accelerate healing with bone-to-bone healing. The key to this operation is that because the PTT is not detached from the accessory bone, healing is facilitated.

I use a single utilitarian incision medially and open the PTT sheath. The attachment of the PTT cannot be preserved. The location of the accessory navicular bone varies significantly and must be shelled out completely from the PTT. With the use of a skin hook on the accessory navicular bone, the tendon is then peeled off sharply, and the entire tendon, with the periosteal sleeve, is then preserved. Then, excising the entire accessory navicular bone, including the medial pole of the normal navicula, is necessary. The medial border of the navicula must be flush with the anterior edge of medial cuneiform and the talus so that the TN cuneiform line is corrected. After the ostectomy, the tendon advancement is performed. In the child, the tendon can easily be anchored into the bone with a sharp needle directly into the navicular bone, the cuneiform, or both as the capsuloligamentous tissue is advanced distally. In the adult, reattaching the tendon with a bone suture anchor is easier. There should be moderate tension on the PTT with the foot slightly overcorrected across the midline once the tendon has been advanced. The foot is positioned in slight equinus and varus after the repair, and any additional necessary procedures are now performed. Sometimes, performing either the arthroereisis or the calcaneus osteotomy before excision and advancing the PTT to get a better sense of the tension on the midfoot are easier (Figs. 7–1–2 and 7–1–3).

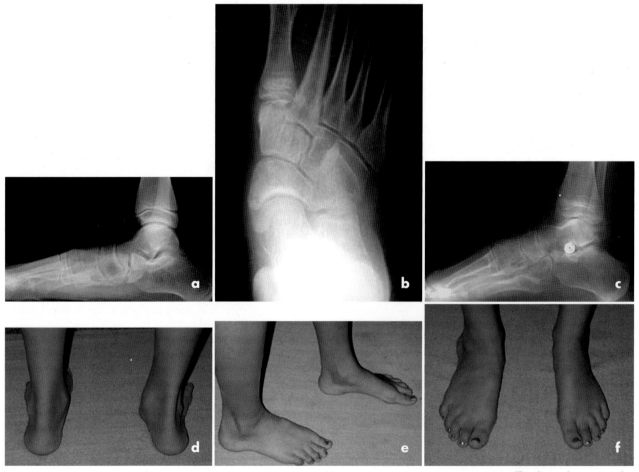

For legend see opposite page

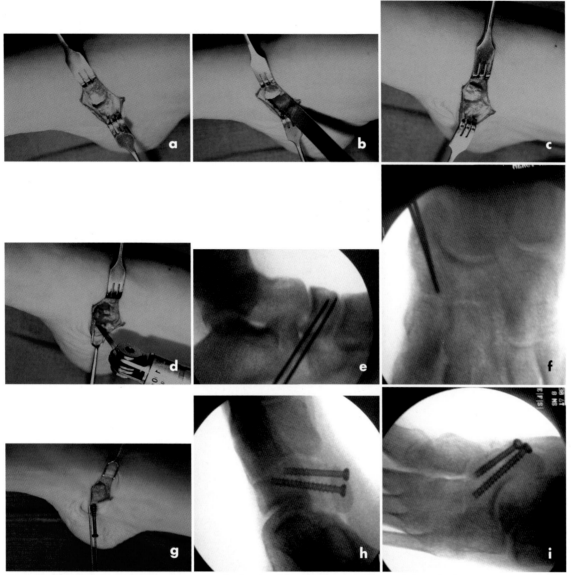

Figure 7–1–3. *The fixation of an accessory navicular in this adolescent athlete. A short incision is used slightly dorsal to the navicular bone to expose the bone. Note the obvious separation of the os naviculare (a). The accessory bone is separated further with an osteotome (b), and then debrided to prepare the bone surfaces (c, d). Cannulated screw fixation is then performed to secure the fragment (e–i).*

Figure 7–1–2. *A 9-year-old girl with a painful accessory navicular syndrome. Note the medial sag of the tavonavicular (TN) joint (a) associated with abduction of the foot (b) and the accessory navicular syndrome that was corrected with the arthroereisis, excision of the accessory navicular bone, percutaneous lengthening of the Achilles tendon, and advancement of the posterior tibial tendon (PTT) (c–f). The foot that was not operated on is shown for comparison purposes.*

Correction of Flatfoot Deformity in the Adult

Nothing elicits controversy as much as the "appropriate" correction of flatfoot. To some extent, this controversy has a lot to do with the many satisfactory operations that are available for correction of similar deformity. Because of the plethora of these surgical alternatives, choosing a procedure does get confusing, and at times a surgeon needs to find an operation that works well and stick with it. This decision does, of course, depend upon the severity of the deformity, the appearance of the foot, and the flexibility of the hindfoot and forefoot. The following is a new classification scheme that has recently been proposed to help with decision making in surgical correction of flatfoot.

The Flatfoot Deformity: Classification

Stage I: Tenosynovitis without Deformity

In stage I disease, the tendon is inflamed or partially ruptured and may or may not be accompanied by systemic inflammatory disease. In either case, deformity is absent or minimal and the overall continuity of the tendon is maintained. Tendon continuity is confirmed on physical examination with an intact single leg heel rise and good resisted foot inversion strength with the foot plantarflexed. Stage I is subdivided into three categories:

A. *Inflammatory disease.* Posterior tibial tendon (PTT) rupture that results from a systemic disease such as rheumatoid arthritis and the other inflammatory arthritides is recognized as a separate

entity. In stage IA, hindfoot anatomy is maintained and the foot alignment is normal. Surgical treatment consists of tenosynovectomy.

B. *Partial PTT tear with normal hindfoot anatomy.* Care for this stage typically begins with a conservative treatment consisting of anti-inflammatory medications and immobilization in a cast, walking boot, or custom brace.

C. *Partial PTT tear with hindfoot valgus.* This is a slight (5 degrees or less) deformity to distinguish it from stage II disease. Although care begins with conservative treatment, this stage may represent a more extensive incipient rupture and should be monitored closely. Surgical treatment consists of a tenosynovectomy and a medial translational osteotomy of the calcaneus.

Stage II: Ruptured Partial Tibial Tendon and Flexible Flatfoot

Stage II disease implies PTT tendon rupture, as evidenced on physical examination by a clinically apparent flatfoot, weakness with inversion of the plantarflexed foot, and inability to single leg heel rise. Stage II disease is subdivided into three categories on the basis of the most salient feature present. Because some patients exhibit several of the following features, some degree of overlap may exist.

A. *Hindfoot valgus.* In stage IIA, once the heel is reduced from valgus to neutral, there is a varying degree of residual forefoot supination. Treatment options for this would include an flexor digitorum longus (FDL) tendon to PTT transfer combined with either a subtalar arthroereisis implant to limit subtalar eversion or a medial displacement calcaneal osteotomy ("calcaneal slide") to reduce hindfoot valgus.

B. *Flexible forefoot supination.* In stage IIB, reducing the hindfoot from valgus to neutral results in forefoot supination because of gastrocnemius muscle contracture. However, the forefoot deformity is flexible; if the ankle is plantarflexed to relax the gastrocnemius muscle, the forefoot supination is corrected. At my institution the surgical recommendations for this would be similar to that for IIA, but with the addition of an Achilles tendon lengthening or a gastrocnemius muscle recession, depending on the cause of equinus.

C. *Fixed forefoot supination.* In stage IIC, because of long-standing hindfoot valgus, adaptive changes have occurred in the frontal plane of the forefoot. Thus, although the hindfoot deformity is supple and reducible to neutral, the forefoot deformity becomes fixed once the heel is held reduced. In other words, when the ankle is plantarflexed while the hindfoot is held reduced, the forefoot remains supinated (Fig. 7–2–1). The operative treatment recommendation for stage IIC is to angulate the medial ray plantarward to correct the fixed forefoot supination and restore a plantigrade foot (in addition to the treatment for IIA or IIB). This is typically accomplished with a dorsal opening wedge osteotomy of the medial cuneiform with insertion of allograft bone.

D. *Forefoot abduction.* This may occur at the transverse tarsal joint (most commonly) or at the first tarsometatarsal (TMT) joint. The first TMT joint instability can be either a primary deformity or a result of TMT joint arthritis. The simplest way to determine this distinction is through examination of the lateral foot x-ray (XR) image for a gap at the plantar joint surface, which is present with primary deformity. Primary deformity of the first TMT joint may also result in secondary hindfoot deformity, including rupture of the PTT. Surgical treatment consists of an FDL tendon transfer combined with a lateral column lengthening procedure such as a modified Evans procedure. At my

institution this is accomplished with a lateral opening wedge osteotomy of the calcaneus 1.5 cm posterior to the calcaneocuboid joint with insertion of allograft bone.

E. *Medial ray instability.* As in stage IIC (fixed forefoot supination), the stage IIE foot retains forefoot supination with reduction of the valgus heel to neutral. This persists even with ankle plantar flexion. This is due to instability of the medial column and may arise from any component within the medial column. It may occur at the talonavicular, naviculocuneiform, or medial cuneiform-first metatarsal joint, or a combination thereof. This situation is similar to IIA; however, after the heel is corrected to neutral, the unstable medial ray will tend to dorsiflex, and this dorsiflexion causes the foot to collapse to pronation and leads to painful subtalar joint impingement. Generally, the treatment used is the same as for stage IID. The addition of medial column arthrodesis (naviculocuneiform or TMT) could be considered. However, this arthrodesis is usually unnecessary for most patients because medial column stability is commonly restored after lateral column lengthening with the addition of an opening wedge osteotomy of the medial cuneiform.

Stage III: Rigid Hindfoot Valgus

Stage III disease is generally associated with a more advanced course of tendon rupture and deformity and is typically characterized by rigid hindfoot valgus. Forefoot deformity may also be present, and it usually consists of rigid forefoot abduction.

A. *Hindfoot valgus.* Treatment usually consists of triple arthrodesis.

B. *Forefoot abduction.* Treatment also consists of triple arthrodesis, but in certain cases lateral column lengthening with a bone block arthrodesis of the calcaneocuboid joint may also be required to fully adduct the forefoot back to neutral.

Stage IV: Ankle Valgus

Stage IV disease occurs after chronic tendon rupture and is associated with deltoid ligament rupture and medial ankle instability, leading to ankle (tibiotalar) joint valgus

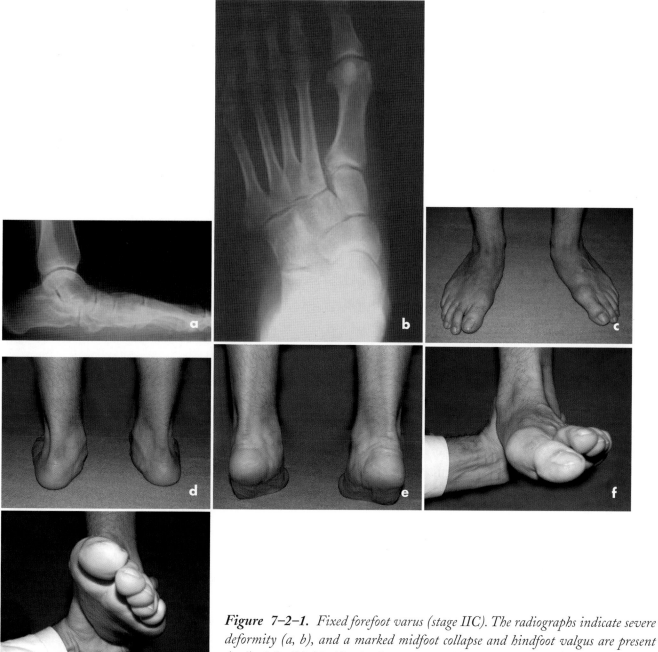

Figure 7-2-1. *Fixed forefoot varus (stage IIC). The radiographs indicate severe deformity (a, b), and a marked midfoot collapse and hindfoot valgus are present (c, d). A flexible hindfoot is also present and is noted on when the patient is standing on tiptoe (e). Note the position of the foot while the heel is held in valgus (f) and then when the heel is reduced to neutral and fixed forefoot varus is present (g).*

deformity. It often occurs in the setting of previous triple arthrodesis. Several variants of this condition have been seen; it may be associated with or without ankle instability and arthritis and a flexible or rigid hindfoot.

A. *Flexible ankle valgus.* In this setting, reconstructing ankle deformity with medial-sided ankle procedures is appropriate. This condition is relatively rare.

B. *Rigid ankle valgus.* This is the more common presentation of stage IV disease. In stage IVA, the ankle valgus deformity is mostly rigid and is almost irreducible. Nonoperative treatment consists of an ankle orthosis such as a custom Baldwin or Arizona brace, and operative treatment is with ankle arthrodesis (in the setting of prior triple arthrodesis), pantalar arthrodesis, tibiotalocalcaneal arthrodesis, or talectomy with tibiocalcaneal arthrodesis.

Tenosynovectomy

Indications

A tenosynovectomy is indicated in patients who have inflammatory changes in the PTT but do not have deformity. Usually the need for tenosynovectomy is early on in the course of the disease process as the tendon is beginning to tear. However, some patients have an inflammatory tenosynovitis associated with a seronegative spondyloarthropathy. These patients also have tenosynovitis and must be approached slightly differently. A tenosynovectomy is indicated after failure of nonoperative care, whatever that happens to consist of. Generally this would be a period of immobilization either in a boot or a cast followed by some sort of brace or orthosis. Along with a tenosynovectomy, a decision has to be made whether to correct any (mild) deformity of the hindfoot.

If one assumes that tenosynovitis represents the early stage of rupture of the PTT, then one can also assume that some hindfoot deformity is likely to be present. This usually consists of valgus of the heel, slight pronation at the midfoot, and contracture of the gastrocnemius-soleus muscle. Therefore in these patients the performance of a medial translational osteotomy of the calcaneus, along with the tenosynovectomy, may be prudent. Certainly, this would be a good idea if minor fissuring indicative of early rupture were present and were associated with the tenosynovitis. This is, however, not usually necessary where the tenosynovitis is associated with a seronegative inflammatory disorder. In patients with this disorder, the tenosynovitis develops as part of a spondyloarthropathy and enthesopathy, and deformity occurs much later on after complete rupture of the tendon. The goals of the tenosynovectomy are to decrease pain and to remove any of the inflammatory tissue that may hasten the rupture. Then the foot should be rested until healing takes place.

Surgery

An incision is made posteromedially along the length of the tendon, and the retinaculum is opened completely.

Occasionally, the tenosynovitis is a result of a stricture or stenosis of the retinaculum immediately behind the medial malleolus. This creates an hourglass deformity to the tendon with obvious deformity and inflammatory change in the tendon visible. Once the retinaculum has been opened, the tendon is inspected. The inflammatory change is not always that obvious and is frequently on the posterior surface of the tendon and tendon sheath. The tendon must then be rotated to inspect the posterior surface. I find that skin hooks are the easiest way to do this by flipping the tendon around to inspect the posterior surface. The inflammatory tissue is then removed from the tendon sheath and the tendon itself, and either dissection scissors or a knife blade is used in this procedure. Rubbing the tendon vigorously with a sponge also facilitates removal of this inflammatory tissue. Finally, the tendon should be inspected for any tears, which, as stated, are usually on the posterior surface (Fig. 7–2–2).

If a tear is identified, it is repaired with a running suture of monofilament absorbable suture. I use a 2-0 suture and bury the knot and then run the suture along the length of the tendon, imbricating the tendon along the way as the repair is performed. I do not repair the flexor retinaculum. In these instances, the tendon will not subluxate provided the foot is immobilized for a few weeks after surgery. Weight bearing can be started as tolerated in a boot, and gentle passive range-of-motion exercises can start after 2 weeks, followed by non–weight-bearing exercise, including swimming and cycling.

The Flexible Flatfoot Deformity

The correction begins with the lateral approach, including calcaneus osteotomy. Once the osteotomy has been completed, the incision is closed, and the patient is turned from the lateral to the supine position to perform the tendon transfer and PTT correction.

Medial Translational Osteotomy of the Calcaneus

This osteotomy is an extremely utilitarian procedure, and although it is included in the section on correction of the flatfoot associated with an FDL tendon transfer, I use the medial translation osteotomy for correction of multiple types of deformities whenever hindfoot valgus is present and when the medial side of the foot needs to be supported. Restructuring the medial column of the

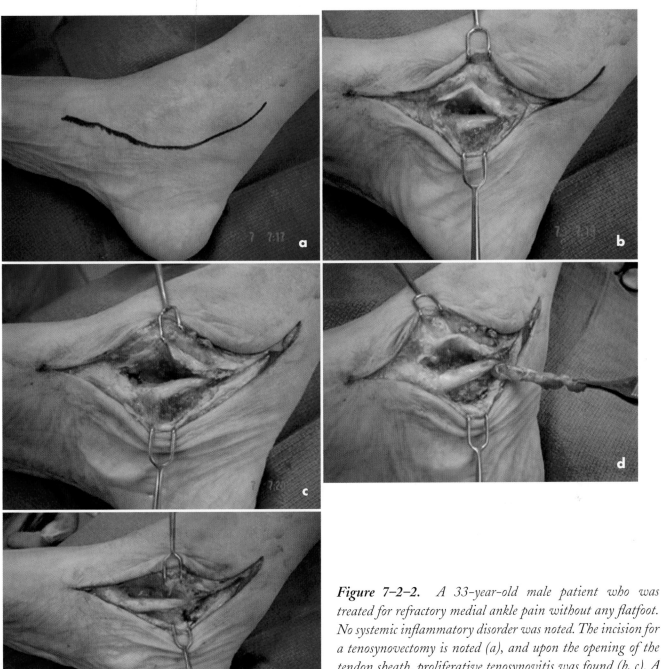

Figure 7–2–2. *A 33-year-old male patient who was treated for refractory medial ankle pain without any flatfoot. No systemic inflammatory disorder was noted. The incision for a tenosynovectomy is noted (a), and upon the opening of the tendon sheath, proliferative tenosynovitis was found (b, c). A tenosynovectomy was performed, and the tendon was noted to be intact with further exploration (d, e). A diagnosis of a seronegative spondyloarthropathy was subsequently made.*

foot, leaving the hindfoot in valgus, is useless. This applies to bone procedures, whether osteotomies or fusions, and is supplemented by tendon transfers. The rationale behind the medial translation is not only the movement of the calcaneal tuberosity medially and therefore the improvement of the mechanical tripod of

the heel with respect to the forefoot, but also the medialization of the insertion of the Achilles tendon relative to the axis of the subtalar joint.

Many clinical and biomechanical studies have supported this osteotomy, with its positive impact on both the foot and the ankle. The osteotomy can be used to improve the mechanics of the tibiotalar joint because medial translation will increase the contact pressure on the medial aspect of the tibiotalar joint when valgus deformity is present in the ankle. The osteotomy can also be added to a triple arthrodesis to improve the mechanical support of the ankle in a stage IV rupture of the PTT in conjunction with reconstruction of the deltoid ligament. This is an extremely reliable operation, and nonunion does not occur. With internal fixation, the tuberosity can be shifted at least 12 mm without any fear of instability or nonunion. Overcorrection into slight varus can occur, albeit rarely.

An incision is made two fingerbreadths below the tip of the fibula in line with the peroneal tendon. The incision is deepened into subcutaneous tissue, and immediately the sural nerve and lesser saphenous vein must be identified and retracted. A retractor is inserted into the tissue, and then once the nerve is retracted, the incision is deepened onto periosteum that is reflected to expose the calcaneus. I try to perform the osteotomy as close to the axis of the subtalar joint as possible. After subperiosteal dissection, two curved soft tissue retractors are inserted on the dorsal and inferior aspect of the tuberosity. The inferior retractor is pushed between the calcaneus and the plantar fascia and serves as a retractor of the soft tissues during the osteotomy. The cut is made perpendicular to the axis of the tuberosity at a 45-degree angle with respect to the calcaneal pitch angle. An osteotome should *not* be used because more control is available with the use of a wide saw blade. A punching action of the saw is used for the osteotomy to feel the perforation as it goes through the medial aspect of the tuberosity. A smooth laminar spreader with no teeth is inserted into the osteotomy site to distract the calcaneus, and the medial periosteum is separated. The medial translation is then facilitated, but cephalad translation is avoided. Once the calcaneus is held in the desired position, which is about 10 to 12 mm of medial shift, it is fixed with one 6.5-mm cannulated screw introduced from inferolateral to anteromedial to enter the harder sustentacular bone. Compressing the overhanging lateral ledge of bone is important because it can cause irritation on the soft tissues and sural nerve. This is a stable osteotomy, and weight bearing can start after 10 days, either in a cast or in a boot, depending on the additional procedures performed (Figs. 7–2–3 and 7–2–4).

Flexor Digitorum Longus Tendon Transfer

The indications for this FDL tendon transfer are a flexible flatfoot and a reducible subtalar joint with minimal forefoot supination. Obesity does not appear to be a contraindication to this procedure, and provided the foot is flexible, the addition of a calcaneal osteotomy to the FDL tendon transfer will support the foot despite obesity. Occasionally, if I am concerned about the ability of the tendon transfer and the osteotomy to support the foot completely, I may add a subtalar arthroereisis to support the subtalar joint. This is particularly helpful in patients who have an increase in the talar declination but have good coverage of the talonavicular joint.

An incision is made medially starting behind the medial malleolus and extending distally toward the medial cuneiform. This incision is deepened to the flexor retinaculum, and the PTT sheath is opened. Frequently, the PTT rupture is partial and longitudinal, and it fissures in the posterior aspect of the tendon and is visible once the tendon is rotated and rolled backwards. In addition to tears of the tendon, the entire capsule-ligamentous complex must be inspected for a defect, tear, or rupture that could involve the deltoid ligament, the talonavicular capsule, or the spring ligament. Each of these much be addressed in addition to the tendon transfer.

I do not leave behind the ruptured posterior tendon, and other than the distal 2 cm, the torn portion of the PTT is excised. If the muscle is still functioning and has some mobility and excursion to it, then a proximal tenodesis should be performed. If a side-to-side tenodesis is done more distally, then bulk and scarring are added. Also, accurately restoring the balance between the transferred FDL tendon and the adjacent redundant PTT is impossible. The entire excursion of the posterior tibial muscle is about 1 cm so that with fissuring and elongation of the tendon, the muscle does not function well. If, at the completion of the flexor tendon transfer, excursion of the PTT is noted, then a side-to-side tenodesis is performed, proximal to the medial malleolus. For this reason, I excise the central segment of the PTT, leaving a distal stump of 2 cm to facilitate the attachment of the FDL tendon for transfer. The proximal stump is cut at the level of the medial malleolus.

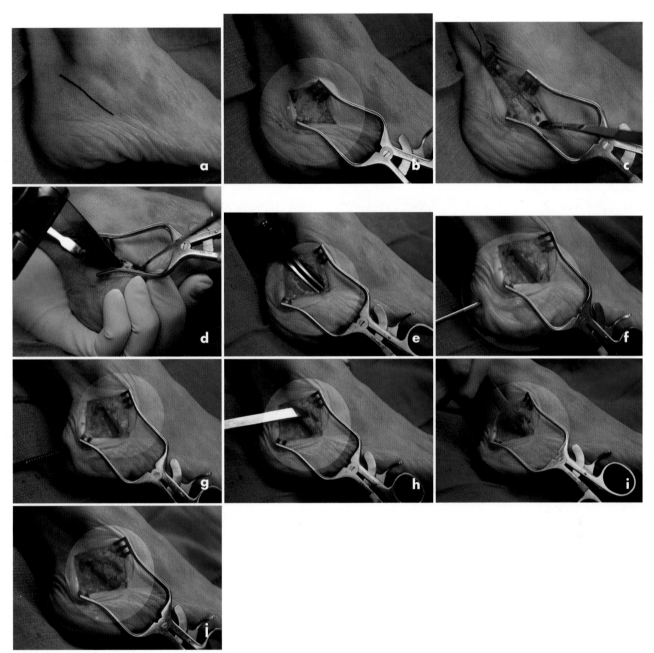

Figure 7–2–3. *The steps in a medial translational osteotomy. The incision is marked out just inferior to the peroneal tendons (a), the sural nerve is retracted inferiorly and the tendons superiorly (b), and the periosteum is reflected as Hohman retractors are used to expose the calcaneus (c). A fan saw blade is used to cut the calcaneus while the opposite hand holds the foot to appreciate the sense of the saw blade as it perforates the medial calcaneus (d). A laminar spreader is inserted lengthways to prevent crushing of the bone (e), the calcaneus is shifted medially by 12 mm in this patient (f), and a cannulated guide pin is inserted followed by a 6.5-mm cannulated threaded screw (g). The dorsal periosteum is elevated, and the overhanging bone is tamped down (i) to smooth out the ledge of bone, which may impinge on the skin (j).*

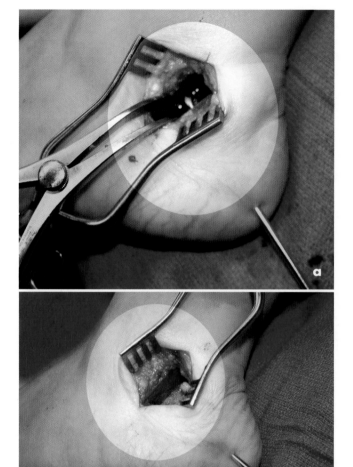

Figure 7–2–4. *Note here how the guide pin for the cannulated 6.5-mm screw is inserted while the osteotomy is distracted (a). This facilitates correct insertion of the guide pin, which is on the lateral aspect of the calcaneal tuberosity inferiorly. In this patient note the slight tilting or gapping of the osteotomy (b). This is not ideal because it creates what amounts to an opening wedge, which may lead to a varus position of the heel.*

Once the PTT has been prepared, the FDL tendon is harvested. The sheath for the FDL tendon lies immediately posterior to the PTT, and the sheath is opened with a knife and is then split longitudinally with scissors. Make no effort to preserve the flexor sheath because the FDL tendon moves into the sheath of the PTT and the sheath of the FDL tendon is split proximally far enough so that the tendon is mobile. The plane of dissection for harvesting the FDL tendon is important and is done by extending the dissection between the

abductor fascia and the medial border of the foot. A retractor is inserted between the abductor fascia and the undersurface of the medial cuneiform and then by gradually putting this on stretch, the dissection is facilitated under direct vision.

The sheath of the FDL tendon must be released up to the junction of the flexor hallucis longus (FHL) tendon at the master knot of Henry, and the tendon is cut under direct vision with scissors. No effort is made to perform a side-to-side tenodesis to the FHL tendon. Sufficient cross-connection functions between the two tendons, and deficit of toe function is not noticed by the patient. A suture is inserted into the tip of the FDL tendon, and the tendon is then passed from plantar to dorsal through a 4.5-mm drill hole. This drill hole is made after subperiosteal dissection on the dorsal medial pole of the navicular bone; the drill should not get inadvertently too close to the medial pole of the navicular bone or to the talonavicular and navicular cuneiform joint. If inadvertent fracture of the medial pole of the navicular bone occurs intraoperatively, the tendon can then be attached with a biointerference screw or a screw with a spiked ligament washer directly into the navicular bone. The use of the drill hole, however, does facilitate early rehabilitation because of the strength of the bone-tendon-bone fixation. Once the drill hole is made, the suction tip is introduced from dorsal to plantar, and the suture on the FDL tendon is withdrawn into the sucker and pulled through the hole from which the tendon can be pulled up dorsally.

The tendon is now tightened maximally to get an idea of where the foot is positioned, with maximal tension on the tendon. The tendon must not be overtightened because overtightening may also tend to cause subluxation of the FDL tendon out of the PTT groove. If the tendon can possibly subluxate, then the retinaculum must be repaired loosely to prevent stenosis and friction with possible abrasion of the FDL tendon. The extent to which the tendon is tightened for the repair partially depends on the weight of the patient and the deformity. The heavier the patient and the more extensive the deformity, the tighter I make the repair. The tendon should not be at what would be considered a physiologic tension, in which the tendon would be somewhere between maximum relaxation and maximum tension. The foot should be positioned beyond the midline medially in inversion because it always stretches out and will assume a more neutral position over time.

Before the sutures are inserted for the FDL tendon repair, the deltoid ligament, talonavicular capsule, and spring ligament must again be inspected, and if a repair on the soft tissue is performed, it should be done before the FDL tendon is tensioned. Usually a 1- to 2-cm strand of FDL tendon passes through the navicular bone, and this can be used to suture the tendon back down onto the stump of the PTT on both the lower and the dorsal surfaces of the tendon. At the completion of the FDL tendon transfer, the excursion of the posterior tibial muscle is again checked with a clamp on the tip of the tendon, and provided a 1-cm excursion is present with a yield point on the pulling of the muscle, a proximal tenodesis is performed. The PTT is grasped, it is pulled as far distally as possible, and then the repair is performed just distal to the musculotendinous junction to the underside of the FDL tendon with a running locking suture of #0 nonabsorbable suture (Fig. 7–2–5).

Rehabilitation after this procedure depends on the extent of additional operations performed. After a straightforward medial translational osteotomy of the calcaneus and flexor tendon transfer, patients can start bearing weight at 2 weeks in a removable walker boot. Exercise, excluding swimming, can be initiated at this time. If, however, a ligament repair is performed (e.g., talonavicular capsule, spring ligament, or deltoid ligament), then the rehabilitation is prolonged, and weight bearing is initiated at 8 weeks to permit full healing of the soft tissues.

Subtalar Arthroereisis

The indications for a subtalar arthroereisis in the adult are different from that in the child because the surgeon has numerous surgical alternatives to choose from. However, the subtalar implant is used specifically for the following reasons for treatment in the adult and in the child: (1) for the heel that remains in valgus after medial translational osteotomy and (2) for any other type of flexible hindfoot corrective procedure. The arthroereisis may not

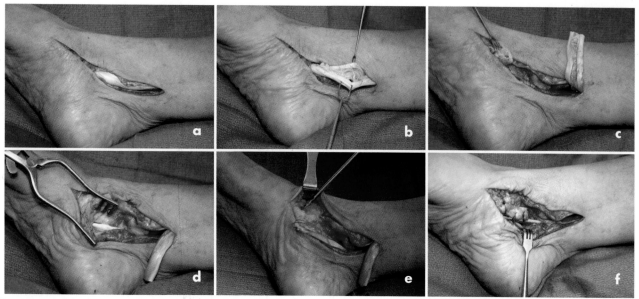

Figure 7–2–5. *The steps in the flexor digitorum longus (FDL) tendon transfer for posterior tibial tendon (PTT) rupture. Note that the tendon appears intact on inspection (a), but the posterior aspect of the tendon is severely torn when it is rotated with the skin hooks (b). The tendon is cut, leaving a 2-cm stump distally (c), and the sheath of the FDL tendon is opened (d). The FDL tendon is cut under direct vision distally, and a 4.5-mm drill hole is made in the navicular joint (e). The FDL tendon is passed through the drill hole from plantar to dorsal and then sutured to the underside of the stump of the partial tibial tendon (PTT) and the dorsal navicular joint (f).*

be required when the talonavicular joint is uncovered, a condition best treated with lateral column lengthening. However, sag of the talus, with an increase in the talocalcaneal angle, and heel valgus are conditions that are most amenable to correction with this procedure. The technique for insertion of the implant is identical to that described previously for use in the child. Generally, I plan to remove the implant between 6 and 12 months, although this removal is often not necessary because the patient is symptom free. In addition to the static correction provided by the arthroereisis, the mechanical support from the prosthesis has a beneficial effect while soft tissue healing is taking place (Figs. 7–2–6 to 7–2–8).

Capsuloligamentous Repair

Repair of the spring ligament is not easy. In the past I have tried to put sutures through this tissue, but it is a thick, strong ligament and does not support sutures well. If sutures are to be used, then they need to be extremely stout, on the order of a #2, nonabsorbable suture material. I do not excise a vertical ellipse from the talonavicular joint to shorten this as part of the repair process, unless a defect is visible in the capsule. If a defect in the talonavicular capsule is significant, then this joint is usually unstable, and the transverse tarsal joint is abducted. This abduction would necessitate a lateral column lengthening procedure to correct the alignment. If severe instability is associated with complete disruption of the spring ligament and talonavicular complex, then an arthrodesis may have to be performed. Generally, once the lateral column lengthening has been performed, then the FDL tendon transfer is sufficient to stabilize the medial column and is added for dynamic correction.

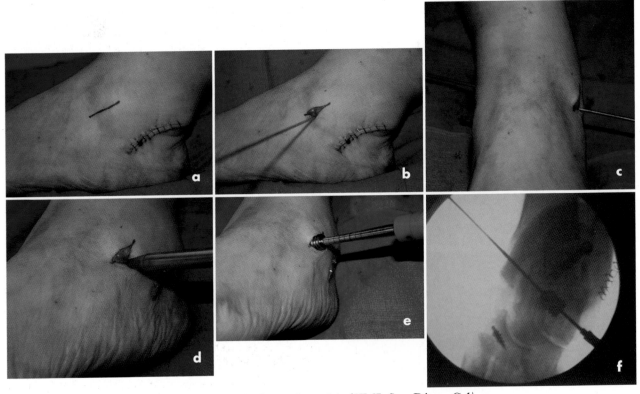

Figure 7–2–6. *The steps for insertion of a subtalar arthroereisis (KMI, San Diego, CA) are shown for this patient for whom a medial translational osteotomy of the calcaneus and an excision of an accessory navicular joint were performed. The incision is marked in the sinus tarsi (a), and a guide pin is inserted obliquely across the tarsal sinus (b) and across the tarsal canal (c). Note the oblique axis of the guide pin, followed by insertion of a broach or probe into the tarsal canal with a dilator (d), insertion of a trial prosthesis (e), and radiographic confirmation of the position of the prosthesis under the lateral talus (f).*

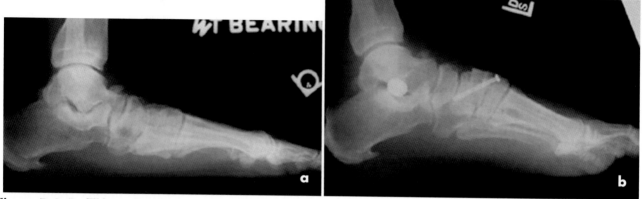

Figure 7–2–7. This patient had an interesting combination of minimal abduction of the transverse tarsal joint, moderate heel valgus, and marked forefoot supination with the heel reduced (a). In addition to the subtalar arthroereisis (KMI, San Diego, CA) and the cuneiform osteotomy, a transfer of the flexor digitorum longus (FDL) tendon was performed to replace the ruptured partial tibial tendon (PTT) (b). A medial translational osteotomy of the calcaneus may have been a good alternative to the arthroereisis.

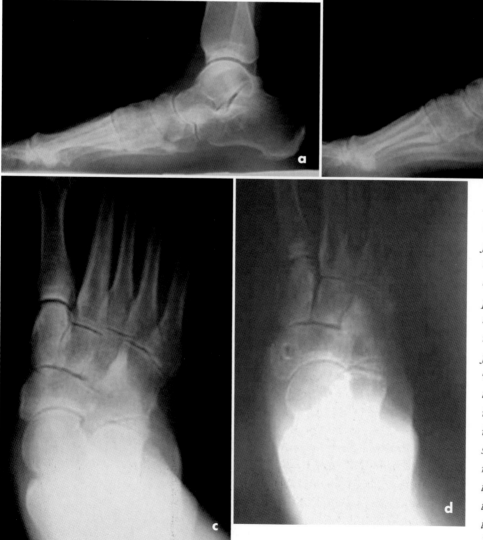

Figure 7–2–8. In this patient, the deformity was corrected with flexor digitorum longus (FDL) tendon transfer and subtalar arthroereisis (b, d). Note on the preoperative images the sag at the talonavicular joint (a) and the uncovering of the talonavicular joint on the anteroposterior (AP) view of about 40% (b). If more than 40% is uncovered, performing a lateral column lengthening is preferable. The arthroereisis seems to be as effective, if not more, than the medial translational osteotomy for correction of the sag of the talus (increase of the talocalcaneal angle on the lateral XR image).

The other option for correction of an unstable spring ligament and talonavicular capsule is the use of a heavy suture anchor inserted into the pole of the navicular tuberosity. Sutures are used to imbricate the talonavicular capsule. This is done in a Y-shaped suture after the capsuloligamentous tissue is pulled down onto the navicular bone (Fig. 7–2–9).

Excision of the Accessory Navicular in the Adult

Symptoms from a painful accessory navicular in the adult are not uncommonly associated with a sudden development of an acquired flatfoot and pain on the medial insertion of the PTT. Unlike the clinical findings of the rupture of the tendon outlined previously, the tendon can easily be palpated on resisted inversion, although the foot remains weak. Pain is located at the insertion of the tendon, and the mass of the accessory navicular is also palpable. For these patients, the principle of correction is no different than that for other ruptures and is determined by the condition and function of the rest of the foot. Although a transfer of the FDL tendon may be necessary in these patients, frequently the PTT is of sufficient strength, only an excision of the bone is required, with advancement of

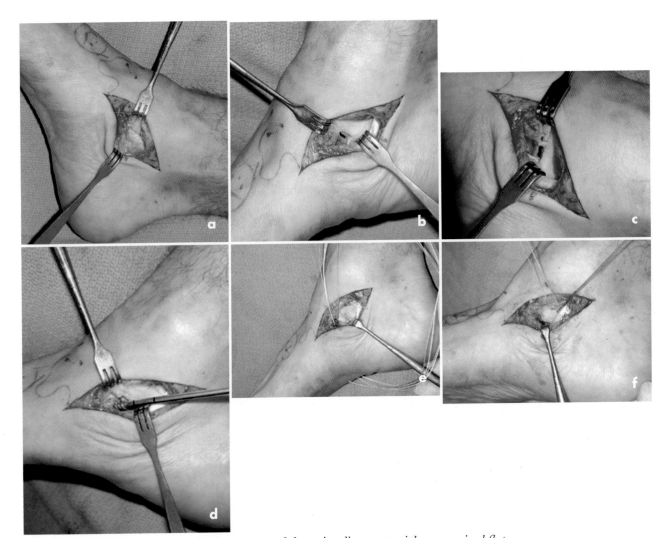

Figure 7–2–9. *This patient sustained a rupture of the spring ligament with an acquired flatfoot deformity. Note the defect in the spring ligament (a–c), which extends up into the inferior aspect of the talonavicular capsule. The edge of the navicular was debrided down to bleeding bone, and the suture anchor was inserted (d, e). These were then inserted as a U-suture to pull the flap down toward the navicular. A medial translational osteotomy of the calcaneus was performed simultaneously.*

the tendon into the navicular. Excising the medial pole of the navicular is important in the adult and in the child because the navicular will be prominent even after excision of the accessory bone. However, in the adult, unlike in the child, the tendon cannot be attached through K-wire holes made in the navicular bone, and a suture anchor is ideally used. The remaining correction with calcaneus osteotomy and additional surgery is performed as required (Fig. 7–2–10).

Techniques, tips, and pitfalls

1. The principle of the calcaneal osteotomy is to shift the tuberosity medially, thereby altering the axis of pull of the Achilles tendon on the hindfoot. As the tuberosity shifts medially, the Achilles tendon is now slightly medial to the axis of the subtalar joint. Therefore plantar

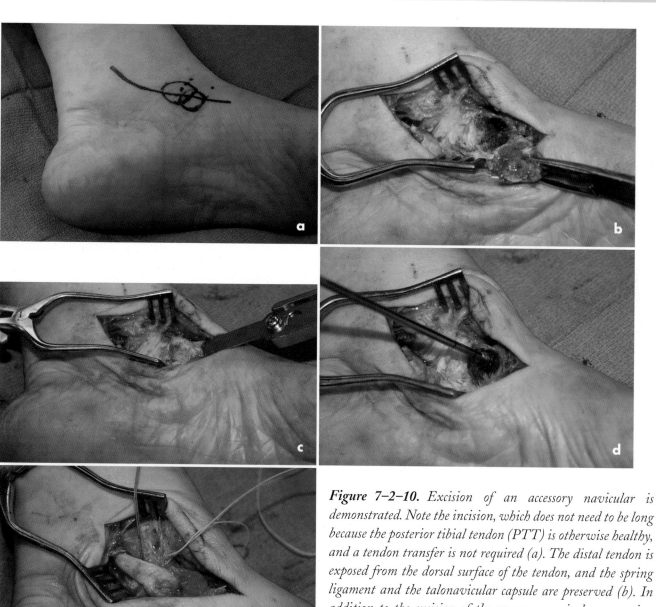

Figure 7–2–10. *Excision of an accessory navicular is demonstrated. Note the incision, which does not need to be long because the posterior tibial tendon (PTT) is otherwise healthy, and a tendon transfer is not required (a). The distal tendon is exposed from the dorsal surface of the tendon, and the spring ligament and the talonavicular capsule are preserved (b). In addition to the excision of the accessory navicular, removing the excess medial pole of the navicular to prevent medial irritation on the shoe is important (c). Once the bone has been removed, the suture anchor is inserted (d), and the sutures are attached to the tendon (e). Note that the sutures are buried under the PTT. A standard sliding knot on the suture is used to advance the tendon down directly on to the raw navicular surface while the foot is held in slight inversion and plantar flexion.*

flexion is facilitated in a neutral position, and the valgus deformity of the heel is not augmented. As long as the osteotomy includes the tuberosity, it probably does not make a difference as to how close to the axis of the subtalar joint the osteotomy is performed. I have seen problems occur when the osteotomy is made too far posteriorly when it does not include enough of the tuberosity of the calcaneus. The pain that occurs is largely the result of an uneven step off on the back of the calcaneal tuberosity.

2. One centimeter is the average amount of medial shift that is used, but the amount can be varied according to the size of the patient and the magnitude of the deformity. In patients with more significant heel valgus and a larger heel, which will tolerate more medialization, I will then shift the calcaneus up to 14 mm. The diameter of the calcaneus at the level of the osteotomy is approximately 30 mm; therefore a shift of 15 mm is easily tolerated and fixation is not compromised.

3. Tamping down the overhanging ledge of bone on the dorsal ridge of the calcaneal osteotomy is important. The effects of this overhanging ridge can be determined by palpation of the bone through the skin. This can be uncomfortable and may need revision if this is not adequately smoothed down at the time of surgery.

4. Neuritis does not seem to be a problem after the osteotomy provided one looks for the nerve and retracts it if it is visible. Usually, however, the nerve is not even visible during the operative procedure.

5. Overcorrection from this osteotomy is rare, but it can occur. If the heel seems to be in slight varus postoperatively, this is probably not arising from overtightening of the tendon transfer medially. I have had to reverse the osteotomy for two patients, and although this reversal does bring the heel back to a better position, the heel is slightly shorter and wider.

6. What should be done when the PTT is intact with minor fissuring but has good excursion? Often, the more minor tears are associated with additional disease on the medial side of the capsuloligamentous complex. Rarely, the tendon is left intact if it appears to be completely healthy. Be careful with this approach because minor fissuring and tearing do lead to functional elongation with a decrease in function.

7. I prefer not to leave the PTT intact when I am doing an FDL tendon transfer. Even if the tendon has moderate tears only, I will cut out a central portion approximately 6 cm. With a 2-cm distal stump left, the stump facilitates the attachment of the flexor tendon, and then the proximal stump can be used for the tenodesis to the FDL tendon.

8. A proximal tenodesis is only performed when a healthy posterior tibial muscle is present with good excursion noted. Performing a tenodesis of any sort to the PTT is unnecessary if the PTT is diseased because this would inhibit the function of the healthy FDL tendon transfer.

9. Looking for additional disease in the capsuloligamentous complex is important. Additional disease ranges from a defect in the deltoid ligament to fissuring and elongation of the talonavicular capsule to a complete rupture of the spring ligament. At times a flexible flatfoot that is associated with a normal PTT and complete disruption of the medial capsuloligamentous complex, which needs repair, may be present.

10. How tight should the FDL tendon transfer be made? I have done this procedure at different tensions believing that one should attach the tendon with the muscle at resting tension to function adequately. However, I am not sure that this is correct. In the patients in whom I have tightened the tendon maximally, the foot does not stay inverted, and gradually some elongation occurs with settling out of the

hindfoot and the arch. Nowadays, I tighten the FDL tendon transfer so that when the sutures are inserted, the foot is about 10 degrees beyond the midline.

11. Preserving a pulley for the FDL tendon is unnecessary. Open up the sheath between the FDL and PTT and reroute this accordingly. Subluxation does not occur.

12. When cutting the FDL, visualize the tendon in the arch of the foot. A plexus of veins is adjacent to the master knot of Henry, and if it begins to bleed, maintaining visualization of the tendon during dissection is difficult.

13. Distal tenodesis between the stump of the FDL and the FHL tendons seems unnecessary. Weakness is not perceived by the patient and is barely discernible even on careful examination.

The Flexible Flatfoot with Fixed Forefoot Supination

Approach to Correction

Although the hindfoot is flexible and the talonavicular joint and the subtalar joints are reducible, when the heel is brought into a neutral position, a fixed forefoot supination is present. In some patients, this is exacerbated as a result of the gastrocnemius muscle contracture. Also, forefoot supination, which is marked with the heel in the neutral position, can reduce as the foot is plantarflexed. In these patients, hindfoot reconstruction is possible in conjunction with a gastrocnemius muscle recession without any action taken toward the medial column instability.

On the other hand, if the forefoot supination persists or is excessive, then it must be addressed. A number of procedures can be used for treatment, all of which rely on structural correction rather than dynamic support on the medial side of the foot. The structural changes must take place at the first TMT joint, the medial cuneiform joint, or the navicular cuneiform joint. To some extent, the location depends on the extent of instability present on the lateral weight-bearing XR image. If the instability is excessive with a gap on the plantar surface, then an arthrodesis of this joint must be considered. This is usually the case with the TMT joint and not the navicular cuneiform joint. I do not focus as much on the navicular cuneiform joint unless arthritis is present. Furthermore, even though instability may be apparent in the medial column joint, invariably the instability is in the talonavicular joint, and I do not think that arthrodesis is warranted in a flexible flatfoot. In these patients, I prefer to perform an opening wedge osteotomy of the medial cuneiform joint. With this osteotomy, the medial column stabilizes, and even though instability may have been present on stress XR film intraoperatively, this will be corrected with medial tension in the foot and the windlass mechanism tightening.

Lateral Column Lengthening

Rarely will I perform an arthrodesis of the calcaneal cuboid joint as part of the lateral column-lengthening procedure. If an indication to perform a lateral column lengthening is present, then this is done with an osteotomy of the calcaneus. In some circumstances, however, arthrodesis with lengthening through the calcaneocuboid joint is preferable. Such a procedure would be used in patients who have a flexible hindfoot, with abduction across the transverse tarsal joint and with 40% or more uncovering of the talonavicular joint and osteopenia. The problem for elderly patients or those with osteopenia is crushing of the cancellous bone in the neck of the calcaneus during the lengthening. If crushing occurs, then the graft collapses, with involution into the cancellous surface.

Patients with arthritis of the calcaneocuboid joint also benefit from arthrodesis. This procedure is not as common because isolated arthritis of the calcaneocuboid joint is not common and arthritis usually implies a rigid hindfoot, in which a triple arthrodesis would need to be performed. However, in this group of patients with severe rigid deformity, a triple arthrodesis is performed including a lateral column-lengthening procedure with a structural graft inserted into the calcaneocuboid joint. I have found that the incidence of arthritis after lengthening osteotomy is minimal and does not warrant the increased risk of performing an arthrodesis of the calcaneocuboid joint. Nonunion of this joint is high despite advances in internal fixation techniques, and malunion seems to be much more of a problem than with osteotomy.

The incision for the lateral column-lengthening osteotomy is made along the dorsal surface of the peroneal tendons, extending from the tip of the fibula to the calcaneocuboid joint. The incision should be slightly more dorsal than lateral because visualizing the neck of the calcaneus from the dorsolateral rather than the lateral direction is easier. Once the incision is deepened onto the periosteum, the peroneal tendons are reflected inferiorly and are retracted through the rest of the procedure. The periosteum on the dorsal surface of the neck must be completely elevated, and the anterior aspect of the subtalar joint must be visualized.

With adequate soft tissue retraction, the neck of the calcaneus is cut with a saw, perpendicular to the axis of the calcaneus and approximately 12 mm proximal to the articular surface of the calcaneocuboid joint. A saw cut is made through both cortices, and the calcaneus is loosened. Inserting a small osteotome to free up the medial cortex is the easiest method. I originally thought that keeping the medial cortex intact might be desirable, but this does not allow significant lengthening of the calcaneus. A lamina spreader is now inserted into the calcaneus. This is a critical step because the foot must be examined while the lamina spreader is inserted under distraction. The spreader should be inserted along the thicker cortical rim of the osteotomy to prevent crushing of the central bone. A radiograph is obtained while the lamina spreader is in place to ensure correct coverage of the talonavicular joint. Usually the calcaneus has been opened approximately 10 to 12 mm. A graft is now fashioned, and I use a structural allograft, either from the iliac crest or from a femoral head. The graft is now cut to shape and inserted. This step is difficult because the lamina spreader gets in the way. Although specially designed lamina spreaders are available for this purpose, the graft must be inserted dorsolaterally without abutting the lamina spreader, which blocks its insertion. However, if the lamina spreader is inserted more inferiorly, it is in soft bone, and can then cause crushing. The graft is tamped into place and must be checked dorsally. The graft tends to be visible from the lateral aspect but not entirely from the dorsal aspect, and some dorsal migration of the graft may occur with abutment up

against the anterior aspect of the subtalar joint. This will cause a painful impingement. Generally, the graft is secured with a fully threaded 4-mm cancellous screw, which is introduced from the anterolateral tip of the calcaneus at the calcaneocuboid joint. If the overhanging bone, which may cause impingement at the anterior aspect of the posterior facet, is still present, it should be trimmed down with a saw. Ideally, the foot should be examined fluoroscopically and then rotated through all planes of examination to ensure correct position of the graft before closure (Figs. 7–2–11 to 7–2–14).

Medial Cuneiform Joint Osteotomy

If any forefoot supination persists after the lateral column lengthening, then the first ray must be plantarflexed. Although an arthrodesis of the first TMT joint may be performed if instability or arthritis is present at that joint, I prefer an opening wedge osteotomy of the medial cuneiform joint for correction. The incision is made over the dorsal aspect of the foot immediately medial to the extensor hallucis longus tendon and lateral to the anterior tibial tendon. This interval is used directly onto the dorsal aspect of the cuneiform joint, which is exposed with subperiosteal dissection. If an incision has been used for a PTT reconstruction, this can be extended distally, although the more dorsally located incision is easier to use.

A guide pin is inserted from dorsal to plantar through the cuneiform and aimed slightly proximally. The position is checked laterally to ensure that the middle of the cuneiform joint has been reached. The saw cut is now made on either side of the guide pin, and as the saw cut is made, the guide pin can then be removed. The cut is made vertically, but the plantar cortex of the medial cuneiform joint should be preserved. The cut is generally in line in the same plane as the second metatarsal cuneiform joint. Rarely, the cut may enter into the edge of this joint. Once the cut is complete, a lamina spreader is inserted dorsally after the cut has been pried open with an osteotome. The graft size used here is not as large as that for the lateral column lengthening. Usually, a 6-mm graft is sufficient. This is a triangular or trapezoidal graft that should be wider dorsally than on the plantar surface in both planes. Insertion of the graft is difficult with the lamina spreader in place. Either the

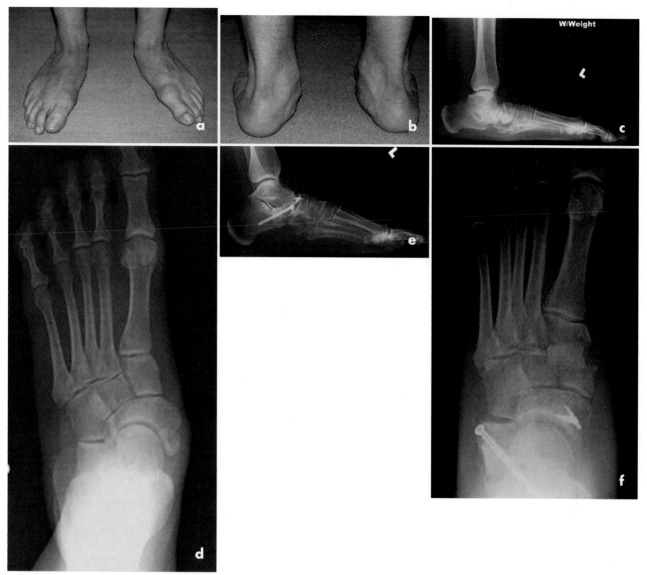

Figure 7–2–11. *This is an example of a severe but flexible flatfoot associated with a painful insertion of the posterior tibial tendon (PTT) (a, b). A marked sag of the talus and a moderate abduction of the forefoot, with a symptomatic accessory navicular joint, are present (c, d). They were corrected with a lateral column lengthening and an opening wedge osteotomy of the medial cuneiform joint, combined with advancement of the posterior tibial tendon (PTT) (e, f). In a patient who has pain and an acquired flatfoot associated with an accessory navicular joint, the tendon is usually normal in quality provided treatment is initiated early enough before degeneration of the tendon occurs. In this patient, after excision of the accessory navicular joint, the tendon was advanced and secured with bone suture anchors. The apparent slight overcorrection on the anteroposterior (AP) view is the result of an x-ray (XR) image taken immediately postoperatively in the non–weight-bearing position.*

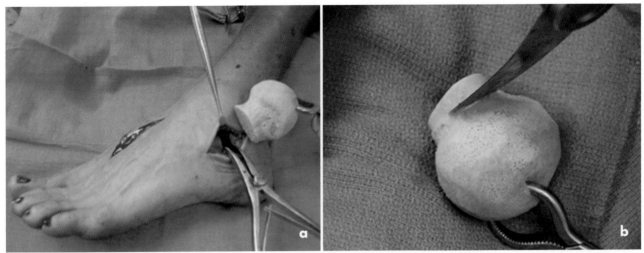

Figure 7–2–12. *The femoral head allograft is demonstrated for use in the lateral column lengthening (a, b). Note the trapezoidal shape that is cut with the saw and a smooth laminar spreader holding the osteotomy apart.*

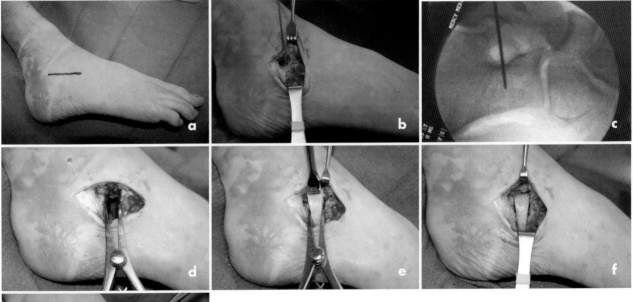

Figure 7–2–13. *The steps in the lateral column lengthening osteotomy of the calcaneus. The incision is marked out slightly dorsal to the axis of the calcaneus to facilitate insertion of the graft from a dorsally directed position (a). The position for the osteotomy is noted with a guide pin (b), which is checked fluoroscopically (c), and should be no less than 1 cm proximal to the joint. The osteotomy is opened with a smooth laminar spreader (d), and the trapezoid-shaped graft is inserted with a tamp (e, f) and secured with a 4-mm cannulated screw (g).*

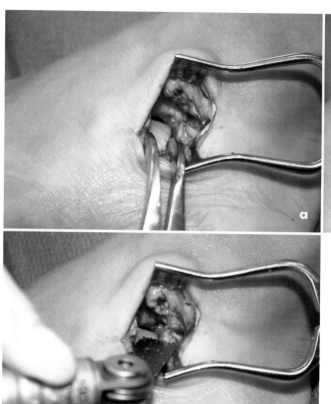

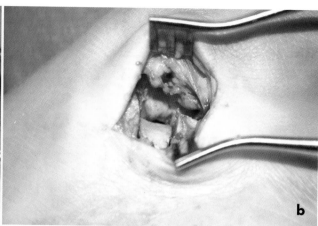

Figure 7–2–14. *When the graft for a lateral column lengthening is inserted, the position of the graft must be checked. Note that the laminar spreader is below the level of the graft (a), which is countersunk into the osteotomy (b). However, a ridge of bone from the host calcaneus is abutting against the anterior edge of the posterior facet, which is then trimmed with a saw (c).*

lamina spreader needs to be opened maximally to facilitate insertion of the graft, or the graft needs to be between the margin of the lamina spreader, which can then be removed. This ought to forcibly plantarflex the first metatarsal by dorsiflexing the hallux during this maneuver of graft insertion. The graft should be tamped down flush with the margin of the cuneiform joint and then checked fluoroscopically. This is a generally stable press fit bone graft, and if fixation is necessary, I use one threaded 4-mm cancellous screw from the dorsal surface at the level of the metatarsal cuneiform joint aiming proximally (Fig. 7–2–15).

Techniques, tips, and pitfalls

1. The key to the lateral column lengthening is to avoid crushing of the calcaneus. Crushing can be prevented by carefully inserting the lamina spread on the dorsolateral aspect of the calcaneus right at the junction of the neck and avoiding the soft cancellous bone.

2. Once the graft is inserted, removal of the laminar spreader is not always easy. Ideally, if the incision is more dorsal and less lateral, then the graft can be inserted and directed vertically, and removal of the laminar spreader from the lateral side of the incision is easier.

3. The graft should be trapezoidal and wider laterally and dorsally. The greatest change in the position of the joint of the graft, however, should be directly lateral.

4. Be careful of the position of the graft once insertion is complete. Obtaining a good lateral XR image of the foot intraoperatively is important. A complication that occurs is impingement between a slightly dorsally subluxated graft and the anterior aspect of the subtalar joint. The problem occurs because the most lateral aspect of the graft appears to

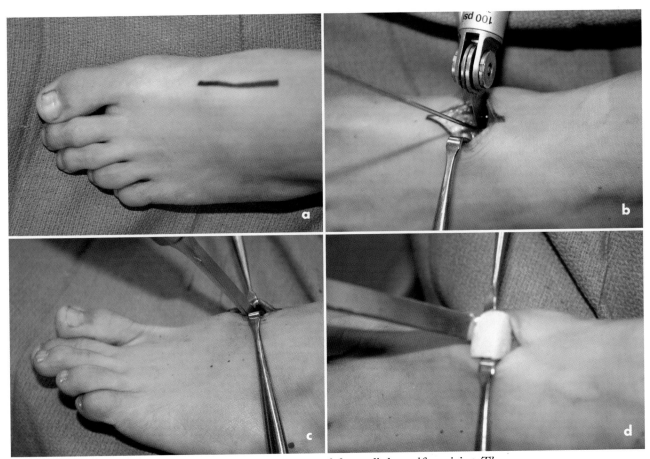

Figure 7–2–15. *The steps in the opening wedge osteotomy of the medial cuneiform joint. The incision is made dorsally, medial to the extensor hallucis longus tendon (a). A guide pin is inserted into the cuneiform joint, and the position is used fluoroscopically to determine the location of the bone cut, which was made proximal to the pin in this case (b). Inserting a laminar spreader and the graft simultaneously is difficult. The osteotomy is wedged open with an osteotome (c), and the graft is tamped into place behind the osteotome (d).*

be in perfect position, whereas the more medial graft is dorsally subluxated. The posterior facet must be visible at completion of graft insertion.

5. The combination of the lateral column lengthening and an opening wedge osteotomy of the medial cuneiform is extremely useful for correction of a flexible flatfoot, which is associated with a fixed forefoot supination.

6. The purpose of the lateral column lengthening is to correct the coverage angle of the talonavicular joint. Rarely, the heel remains in valgus despite the lateral column lengthening,

and the medial translation of osteotomy of the calcaneus can be performed simultaneously.

7. Failure of the lateral column lengthening occurs as a result of bone impingement in the sinus tarsi when the graft is extruded. This extrusion may not, however, occur postoperatively and is a result of incorrect placement of the graft intraoperatively. This must be checked visually to ensure that no impingement is present up against the undersurface of the posterior facet.

8. If the lamina spreader crushes the graft or crushes the calcaneus, the graft will sink into the center of the neck of the calcaneus and will

not provide structural support. The bone graft should rest on the cortical rim and should not sink into the center of the calcaneus. If there is a tendency for crushing of the center of the calcaneus with the lamina spreader, the calcaneus will need to be held open in a slightly distracted position with a plate. An H plate is ideal for this repair. In this instance, a structural graft is not as important because the plate maintains the position of the calcaneus.

9. Before the cut is made on the calcaneus, insertion of a guide pin transversely across the neck of the calcaneus is helpful to ensure the correct position. The cut tends to be too close to the calcaneocuboid joint, and the guide pin should be adjusted until one is about 10 to 12 mm proximal to the articular surface.

10. The lateral column lengthening may be performed at the calcaneocuboid joint. As previously noted, this procedure is not my preference because most of these can be performed through the neck of the calcaneus without the loss of motion that is so commonly present at the calcaneocuboid joint. Nonetheless, this remains a reasonable alternative for correction in the appropriate patient (Fig. 7–2–16).

Management of Deltoid Ligament Instability

A standardized repair of a ruptured deltoid ligament for a degenerative tear associated with a stage IV flatfoot does not work. Many variations of this repair have been attempted including end-to-end repair, a vest-over-pants repair, and advancement of the ligament up into the medial malleolus. All of these repairs tend to stretch out after a while because of the inherent degenerative nature of the local tissue. From a mechanical standpoint, this condition is vastly different from a lateral ankle ligament reconstruction, for which an anatomic repair (Broström repair) works well. Histopathologically, the deltoid ligament is different, and when associated with degeneration, this simply stretches out again, possibly compounded by the mechanical deformity and the

preexisting changes associated with the rupture of the PTT.

The reconstruction of the deltoid ligament is performed with a hamstring allograft, and from a technical perspective, this reconstruction is similar to that for the lateral ankle ligament. Autogenous tissue may be used, but I would refrain from using the local tissue because even the remaining stump of the PTT failed when I tried to use it. The hamstring allograft is attached with a biointerference screw system. In the past I have also used a screw with a spiked ligament washer to anchor this into both the talus and the calcaneus. From a technical standpoint, however, obtaining correct tension and fixation on the calcaneus with a biointerference screw is far easier.

An incision is made medially extending along the course of the ruptured PTT from 4 cm proximal to the malleolus toward the navicular joint. Adjunctive procedures, which may include a triple arthrodesis, a medial calcaneal osteotomy, or an FDL tendon transfer, are performed as required. The medial neck of the talus is exposed. If the talonavicular capsule and the spring ligament are still intact, they should be preserved, and the incision on the talar neck should be made with a puncture without disruption of the talonavicular joint capsule. The drill hole is made with a cannulated guide pin, and the position of the pin is checked fluoroscopically. The guide pin should start at the medial neck of the talus and be aimed toward the posterolateral body. A blind end tunnel technique is used, the hamstring allograft is now harvested, and the correct length of the tendon is prepared. Either heavy nonabsorbable braided (Dacron) or fiber wire suture can be used for the tip of the tendon. The drill hole is made to 17 mm. The 5-mm biointerference screw is used, and the tendon is advanced into the blind end tunnel. A suture is used to tie down the tendon against the edge of the talus.

A 4.5-mm drill hole is made anteriorly to posteriorly in the medial malleolus, and because the PTT is not present, the exit point of the drill does not have to be carefully made. The tendon is advanced and pulled through the tunnel with a sucker tip technique and is either attached to the inferior body of the talus or the calcaneus, depending on the stability of the subtalar

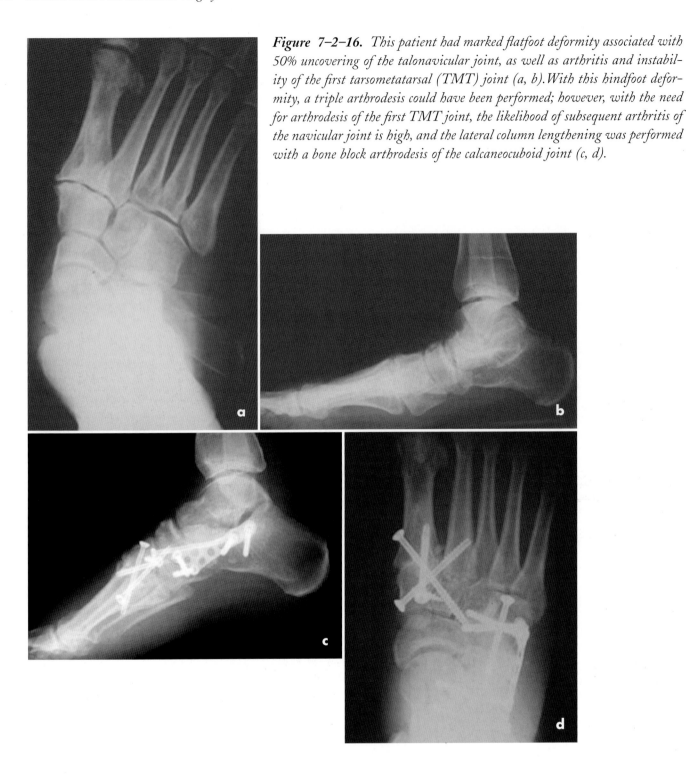

Figure 7-2-16. *This patient had marked flatfoot deformity associated with 50% uncovering of the talonavicular joint, as well as arthritis and instability of the first tarsometatarsal (TMT) joint (a, b). With this hindfoot deformity, a triple arthrodesis could have been performed; however, with the need for arthrodesis of the first TMT joint, the likelihood of subsequent arthritis of the navicular joint is high, and the lateral column lengthening was performed with a bone block arthrodesis of the calcaneocuboid joint (c, d).*

joint. If a triple arthrodesis has been performed, this technique is not as important at which point the tendon is attached. If, however, the subtalar joint is mobile and a calcaneal osteotomy is performed, then the attachment point is preferably into the inferior body of the talus. The problem with attachment of the tendon to the calcaneus is the type of incision used that requires retraction of the neurovascular bundle. Attachment is possible through a single incision by identifying and then retract-ing the neurovascular bundle inferiorly, but considerable retraction is involved to get the graft down onto the calcaneus. Making a separate incision more inferiorly over the calcaneus and then tunneling the tendon graft deep to the neurovascular bundle are preferable.

Unlike the talar blind end tunnel, a through and through tunnel is used in the calcaneus to maximize tension on the tendon graft. Ideally the exit point on the lateral side of the foot should be in the calcaneus because pulling the graft through on the lateral side of the talus, which is protected and covered by the overhanging fibula posterolaterally, is difficult. The drill hole is made in the posterior tuberosity of the calcaneus with a cannulated guide pin with a sleeve for the drill bit to protect the soft tissues. The suture is attached to the tendon, which is measured so that no more than 2 cm of tendon passes through the tunnel. If the tendon is longer, sufficient tension on the lateral aspect of the calcaneus cannot be

generated when the tendon is pulled on. The suture is passed through the calcaneus with a straight needle and is pulled out laterally, avoiding the sural nerve. While tension is being applied to the tendon, the foot is positioned in neutral dorsiflexion, and stability on forced passive eversion or valgus stress on the ankle is noted. The biointerference screw is inserted in a standard fashion, and a larger diameter screw is used for the calcaneus depending on the quality of the bone (Figs. 7–2–17 to 7–2–20).

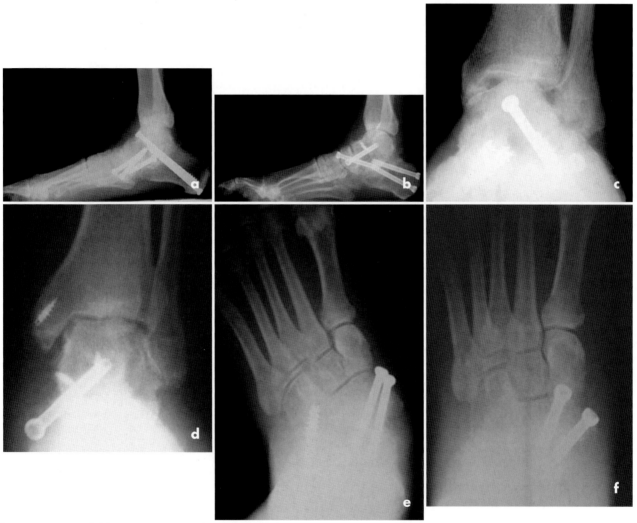

Figure 7–2–17. *This is an example of a severe rupture of the deltoid ligament associated with a chronic rigid flatfoot after attempted triple arthrodesis (a, c, e). This was corrected with a medial translational osteotomy of the calcaneus, a revision of the transverse tarsal arthrodesis with a medially based biplanar wedge resection, and a deltoid ligament reconstruction. The latter was performed with a hamstring allograft attached with suture anchors and passed through a drill hole in the medial malleolus (b, d, f). The final result was a plantigrade foot and ankle. Although arthritis of the ankle persists, it is tolerable, and no further treatment has as yet been provided.*

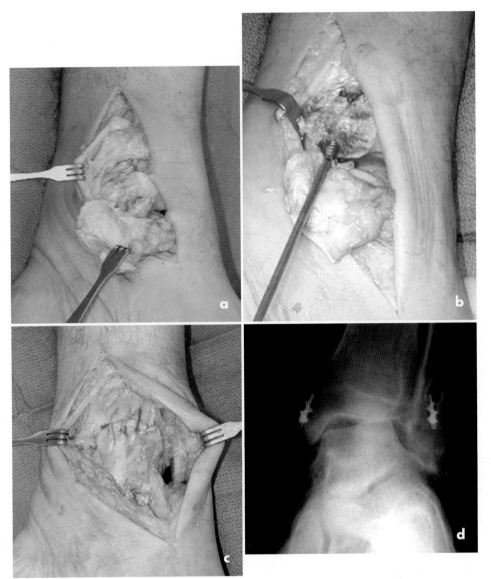

Figure 7–2–18. *This is a good example of what does not work in the setting of chronic flat-foot associated with a deltoid ligament tear. This was a flexible flatfoot with complete tear of the deltoid ligament and medial ankle instability. Note the large flap created from scar on the medial ankle and the visible joint visible (a). The malleolus was debrided and an anchor was inserted, followed by repair and almost immediate failure (b, c, d). The quality of the degenerated tissue medially is just not good enough to support the medial ankle.*

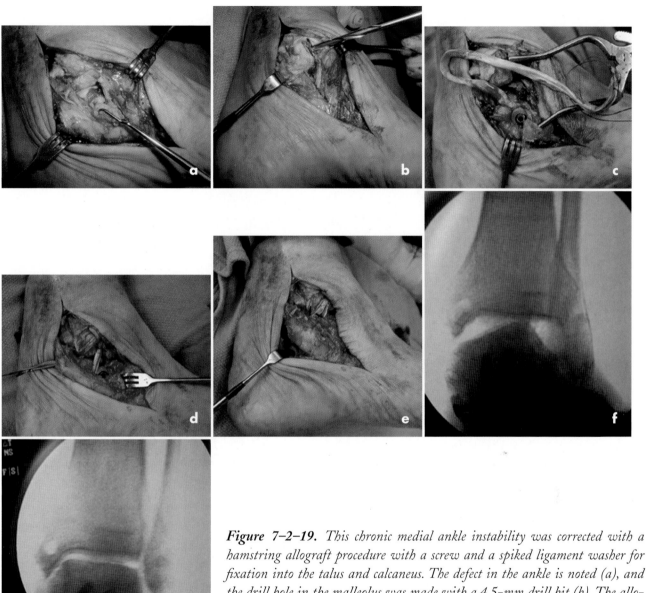

Figure 7–2–19. *This chronic medial ankle instability was corrected with a hamstring allograft procedure with a screw and a spiked ligament washer for fixation into the talus and calcaneus. The defect in the ankle is noted (a), and the drill hole in the malleolus was made with a 4.5-mm drill bit (b). The allograft is passed and anchored onto the talus and then secured with a second washer into the calcaneus (c, d). The redundant tissue from the medial ankle is used to suture over the tendon reconstruction (e). Valgus stress is applied before and after the tendon reconstruction (f, g).*

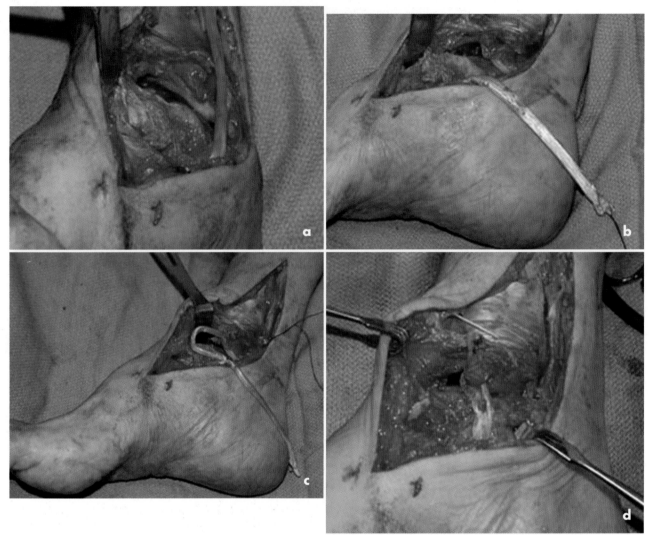

Figure 7-2-20. *In this patient with chronic flexible deformity associated with deltoid instability, a hamstring allograft was used for the reconstruction. Note the attachment of the graft to the talar neck with a suture anchor and the marked instability of the ankle (a, b). A drill hole is made in the medial malleolus, and the tendon is then attached to the calcaneus (c, d).*

Suggested Readings

Bohay DR, Anderson JG. Stage IV posterior tibial tendon insufficiency: The tilted ankle. Foot Ankle Clin 8:619–634, 2003.

Chu IT, Myerson MS, Nyska M, Parks BG. Experimental flatfoot model: The contribution of dynamic loading. Foot Ankle Int 22:220–225, 2001.

Giannini BS, Ceccarelli F, Benedetti MG, Catani F, et al. Surgical treatment of flexible flatfoot in children a four-year follow-up study. J Bone Joint Surg Am 83-A(Suppl 2, Pt 2):73–79, 2001.

Giannini S, Ceccarelli F, Vannini F, Baldi E. Operative treatment of flatfoot with talocalcaneal coalition. Clin Orthop Jun(41):178–187, 2003.

Greisberg J, Hansen ST Jr. Sangeorzan B. Deformity and degeneration in the hindfoot and midfoot joints of the adult acquired flatfoot. Foot Ankle Int 24:530–534, 2003.

Kadakia AR, Haddad SL. Hindfoot arthrodesis for the adult acquired flat foot. Foot Ankle Int 8:569–594, 2003.

Kelly IP, Nunley JA. Treatment of stage 4 adult acquired flatfoot. Foot Ankle Clin 6:167–178, 2001.

Kann JN, Myerson MS. Intraoperative pathology of the posterior tibial tendon. Foot Ankle Clin 2:343–355, 1997.

Myerson MS. Adult acquired flatfoot deformity: Treatment of dysfunction of the posterior tibial tendon insufficiency. Instr Course Lect 46:393–405, 1997.

Myerson MS. Adult acquired flatfoot deformity. Treatment of dysfunction of the posterior tibial tendon [abstract]. J Bone Joint Surg Am 78A:780–792, 1996.

Myerson MS, Corrigan J. Treatment of posterior tibial tendon dysfunction with flexor digitorum longus tendon transfer and calcaneal osteotomy. Orthopedics 19:383–388, 1996.

Myerson MS, Corrigan J, Thompson F, Schon LC. Tendon transfer combined with calcaneal osteotomy for treatment of posterior tibial tendon insufficiency: A radiological investigation. Foot Ankle Int 16: 712–718, 1995.

Neufeld SK, Myerson MS. Complications of surgical treatments for adult flatfoot deformities. Foot Ankle Clin 6:179–191, 2001.

Nyska M, Parks BG, Chu IT, Myerson MS. The contribution of the medial calcaneal osteotomy to the correction of flatfoot deformities. Foot Ankle Int 22:278–282, 2001.

Pinney SJ, Van Bergeyk A. Controversies in surgical reconstruction of acquired adult flat foot deformity. Foot Ankle Clin 8:595–604, 2003.

Toolan BC. The treatment of failed reconstruction for adult acquired flat foot deformity. Foot Ankle Clin 8:647–654, 2003.

Trnka HJ, Easley ME, Myerson MS. The role of calcaneal osteotomies for correction of adult flatfoot. Clin Orthop Aug:50–64, 1999.

Zaret DI, Myerson MS. Arthroerisis of the subtalar joint. Foot Ankle Clin 8:605–617, 2003.

Nerve Entrapment Syndromes

Tarsal Tunnel Syndrome

A tarsal tunnel release is performed for intractable refractory pain, burning, tingling, and numbness on the plantar and medial aspect of the foot. These symptoms can be associated with aching in the foot; aching in the leg; cramping; and vague sensations of soreness, fatigue, and burning with or without activities. In addition to the common recognized causes of tarsal tunnel syndrome, which include hyperpronation of the foot, a valgus hindfoot, stress or pressure on the tibial nerve as a result of a mass-occupying effect, varicosities, or trauma, many patients do not have an identifiable cause for their symptoms.

Before starting an operation, I routinely perform electrophysiologic testing. Although a normal test result does not contraindicate the performance of surgery, having confirmation of the clinical condition from an electromyogram (EMG) and through nerve conduction studies is certainly useful. The approach to tarsal tunnel release must include an extensile incision that extends distally over the abductor hallucis muscle. The most frequent error in performing a tarsal tunnel release is to ignore the compression that occurs deep to the abductor hallucis muscle. The more proximal portion of the tibial nerve under the laciniate ligament is rarely the source of compression other than for patients who have lesions, masses, or varicosities in the tarsal tunnel immediately behind the medial malleolus.

The incision is deepened through subcutaneous tissue, and in the more proximal area of the tarsal tunnel the flexor retinaculum is perforated and opened proximally. Rarely, an entrapment is in the more proximal aspect of the tarsal tunnel behind the malleolus. The flexor retinaculum (laciniate ligament) is inspected and released slightly more distally to the level of the medial malleolus, and the nerve is inspected. I do not perform a neurolysis and have not found that this is necessary for the success of the tibial nerve release. The less the nerve itself is irritated, the better the prevention of epineural scarring. The key to the operation involves the identification of the bifurcation of the nerve into the medial and lateral plantar nerves. The nerve is traced distally after release of the laciniate ligament, and then the abductor hallucis muscle is gently pulled distally. Using a retractor is the best way to identify the deep fascia directly underneath the abductor muscle. Once the fascia is identified, then the lateral plantar nerve is released by completely splitting the deep fascia under direct vision while retracting the abductor muscle distally. Once the dorsal more proximal aspect of the fascia is released, this step is reversed, and the abductor muscle is identified distally at the inferior margin of the muscle and then is pulled proximally. In this way, the entire deep fascia has definitely been released. Occasionally the superficial fascia on the abductor muscle is thick, and it also needs to be released to pull the abductor muscle in both directions.

Once the deep fascia of the underlying abductor muscle has been released, a decision can be made about whether to extend the incision more distally, if, for example, additional entrapment of the lateral plantar nerve or the first branch of the lateral plantar nerve, in conjunction with the heel pain syndrome, is present. The medial plantar nerve is released in a similar fashion, again under direct vision as it courses deep to the abductor hallucis muscle but slightly more anteriorly. The abductor muscle is pulled plantarward, the fascia is identified, and the split is made immediately below the flexor digitorum longus tendon. Palpation with the tip of the scissors distally is needed to be sure that the retinacu-

lum has been completely released. Any bleeding should be controlled before skin closure (Figs. 8–1–1 and 8–1–2).

I have found that this incision is prone to inflammation and dehiscence unless the foot is immobilized for a short time. I use nylon sutures in the skin and immobilize the ankle in a splint or short nonarticulated boot for 2 weeks until the sutures are removed and then allow full weight bearing as tolerated in a boot. Physical therapy and rehabilitation are important to the recovery after this procedure and should be initiated as soon as tolerated.

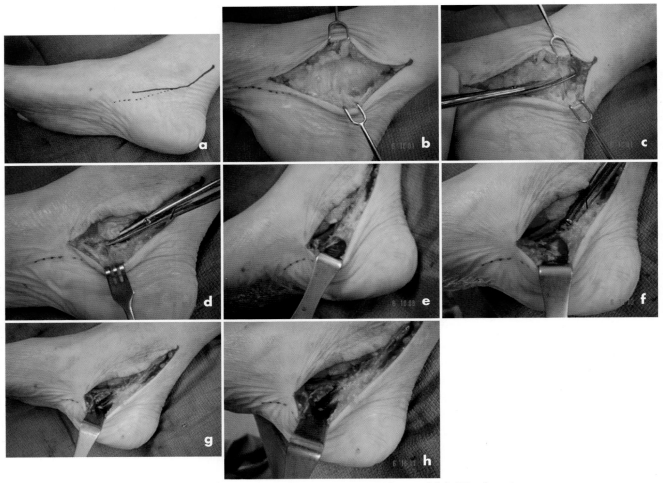

Figure 8–1–1. *The incision for the extensile release of the tarsal tunnel is noted (a). The dotted line represents an alternative extensile approach to the plantar aspect of the foot for a more complete nerve release. The retinaculum is exposed (b) and is released with a sharp scissors (c). A hemostat is then passed under the deep retinaculum into the medial plantar canal tunnel (d). The medial plantar nerve is completely released (e), and the abductor fascia is exposed by pulling down on the abductor muscle with a large retractor (f) to release the lateral plantar nerve completely (g, h).*

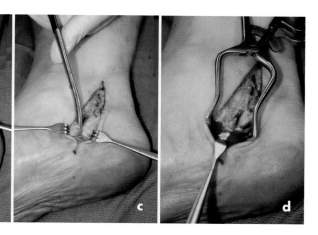

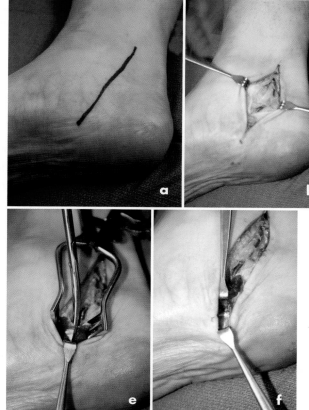

Figure 8–1–2. The tarsal tunnel incision is marked out for this patient with nerve symptoms only. Note the more vertical incision (a) and the appearance of the neurovascular bundle after release of the flexor retinaculum (b). The distal retinaculum is split to expose the branching of the medial and lateral plantar nerves (c). Note the abnormally large abductor hallucis muscle belly, which in this patient may have been the cause of the nerve entrapment. The muscle is swept off the deep fascia (d) and is released with scissors to free the lateral plantar nerve under the muscle (e). The muscle is then pulled forward, and the deeper course of the lateral plantar nerve is released under direct vision (f).

Techniques, tips, and pitfalls

1. The incision must be extensile and include the distal more plantar aspect of the foot.
2. Performing an epineurolysis is unnecessary.
3. In the presence of venous stasis and varicosities, tying off these veins, which are engorged around the nerves, is preferable.
4. I prefer to tie off these veins rather than use electrocautery, which may cause further fibrosis and scarring.
5. The key to the operation is successful release of the deep fascia under the abductor muscle, which overlies the separate medial and lateral plantar nerves. Once the abductor muscle has been reflected and the superficial abductor fascia has been cut, then the muscle must be retracted to identify the deep fascia, which usually is the source of entrapment around the lateral plantar nerves.
6. The foot must be immobilized postoperatively. Although immobilization does not seem necessary, for some reason, I have identified a much larger percentage of postoperative wound complications than normal with tarsal tunnel release. This may have something to do with the quality of the tissue, prior corticosteroid injection, and mild venous stasis. Immobilization is advisable.
7. As with other nerve procedures, physical therapy, massage, and desensitization are helpful once the sutures have been removed. Weight bearing can start at that time.

Neurectomy and Nerve Burial

Neurectomy and nerve burial may be performed in conjunction with additional procedures for correction of midfoot or hindfoot deformity, the most common of which is a subtalar arthrodesis after a calcaneus fracture when a sural neurectomy is performed. The incision varies according to the presence of prior incisions, the location of the neuroma, and the type of additional operation performed. From a vertical incision made posterior to the peroneal tendon sheath, the nerve is identified and inspected. The nerve must be traced from proximal to distal; that is, from the healthy to the abnormal portion of the nerve. Identifying a discrete neuroma is difficult because it is usually encased in scar. The neuroma is frequently caused during prior surgery and is not mobile, particularly if it is under the prior incision. The sural nerve should be traced more distally, until either the scar or a definite neuroma is identified. The nerve is dissected further distally, and if there is no further continuity with the main body of the nerve, it is transected, including the neuroma.

The nerve is now clamped and the tip of the nerve is cauterized either with the electrocautery or with phenol. More proximally, the nerve is passed with a clamp and a 4-0 suture deep to the peroneal tendons or musculature, depending on the level in the leg. Simple resection

of the neuroma is never sufficient. Burial in a muscle may work but recurrence seems to be high, and burying the nerve in bone is preferable. The key is sufficient length on the nerve so that with movement of the leg and contracture of the peroneal muscles, there is no tension on the nerve. Burying the nerve in bone is difficult because the nerve does not easily stay in position. Two small 2.5-mm unicortical drill holes are made through the fibula perpendicular to each other and about 1 cm apart. The nerve is positioned at one end of the bone tunnel, and the suction is applied to the other drill hole to suck the nerve deep into the hole in the fibula. This drill hole technique seems to be the most effective means of burying the nerve inside the fibula. Once the nerve has been passed into the fibular hole, the epineurium can be sutured onto the periosteum. The ankle should be taken through full dorsiflexion and plantar flexion to ensure that there is no traction on the nerve and that the ankle is freely mobile in the posterior aspect of the limb but encased in the fibula itself (Fig. 8–1–3).

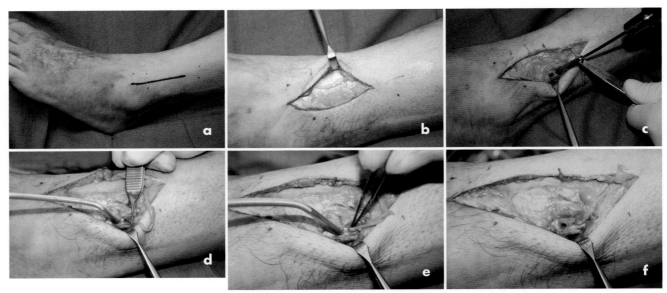

Figure 8–1–3. *The steps in resection of a superficial peroneal nerve with burial into the fibula in a patient after a severe crushing injury to the foot with post-traumatic scarring of the nerve (a). The incision is made in the distal leg and deepened through subcutaneous tissue to find the nerve (b). Two unicortical drill holes are made in the fibula at a 45-degree angle to each other with a 2.9-mm drill bit (c). The nerve is then placed at the edge of one of the drill holes, and the sucker tip is placed at the second hole (d, e), which sucks the nerve into the hole to bury in without tension (f).*

Occasionally after certain types of injuries, including crush injuries, a neurectomy may not be necessary, and a nerve release after removal of the ligament or tendon may be sufficient (Fig. 8–1–4). This applies commonly, for example, in the dorsum of the foot, where the deep peroneal nerve is irritated by the extensor hallucis brevis tendon and an osteophyte from the base of the first or second metatarsal is usually a result of arthritis. Removal of the osteophytes, with release of the extensor hallucis brevis tendon, is sufficient to treat this nerve irritation.

Management of Interdigital Neuroma

General Principles

For the management of all primary and most revision neuromas, I use a dorsal approach. This incision is centered over the affected web space if a single web space neuroma is excised. If both the second and third web space nerves are to be excised, then the incision is centered over the third metatarsal. Removing both web space neuromas through a single incision is easy; two incisions should not be used because two incisions lead to unnecessary retraction, scarring, and the potential for wound compromise. The decision whether one web space or both web spaces is to be approached clearly depends on the clinical evaluation.

Diagnosis and Treatment

Neither magnetic resonance imaging (MRI) nor ultrasound is useful in the management of primary neuroma excision. Although ultrasound can certainly be used in the management of difficult cases to differentiate scar from nerve enlargement in revision procedures, I have

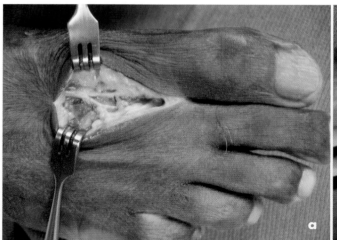
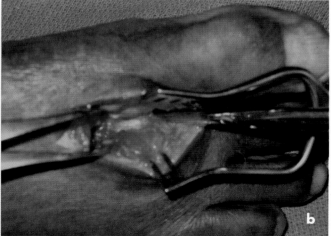
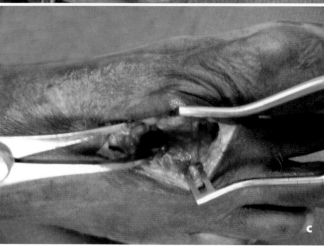

Figure 8–1–4. A first web neuroma involving the common plantar digital nerve was present in this patient after a crush injury to the forefoot. After exposure of the dorsal web space, the branches of the deep peroneal nerve were identified (a). A laminar spreader was inserted into the web space, and the deep transverse metatarsal ligament was identified and cut (b). The nerve was identified, and after release of the deep metatarsal ligament was noted to be intact, a neurectomy was not performed (c).

not found any role for it in the primary case at all. If in doubt, the use of 1 mL of lidocaine in the affected web space given sequentially is usually diagnostic. If I am still in doubt, then I excise the nerve in the most symptomatic web space and then release the deep metatarsal ligaments in the adjacent web space, inspect the nerve, and then excise the nerve if this, too, appears enlarged. The only problem with excision of both the second and third web space nerves is the development of far more numbness in the third toe, which extends slightly proximal to the toe and can also include the third metatarsal fat pad. Although treatment of interdigital neuritis has been reported successfully and has been performed with the release of the deep transverse metatarsal ligament and as either an open or endoscopic procedure, I have not had positive results with this procedure. In fact, 9 years ago I started a prospective randomized study on nerve excision and release of the deep transverse metatarsal ligament. The study was abandoned when most of the patients for whom the release of the deep transverse metatarsal ligament was performed were already returning with more symptoms and requiring further treatment.

The Standard Neurectomy

The standard dorsal neurectomy performed with a dorsal longitudinal incision has a length of 3 cm. I do not use a short incision and prefer to expose and identify the entire nerve. A lamina spreader is inserted between the lesser metatarsals and placed on stretch, and the soft tissue is released off the dorsal surface of the deep transverse metatarsal ligament. A curved incision is now inserted from distal to proximal directly across the deep transverse metatarsal ligament, and the ligament is split. I prefer not to use a cutting motion with the scissors to prevent any inadvertent injury to the nerve that lies immediately below it. Once the ligament is split, it is easy to hook the nerve with a curved hemostat clamp, pull the nerve up into the web space, and then trace it distally to the bifurcation. The nerve is clamped distally and cut distal to the bifurcation. The nerve is elevated out of the web space, and then the small plantar cutaneous branches of the main interdigital nerve are also cut to prevent recurrent neuroma formation. The nerve is then traced as far proximally as possible, lifted out from between the interosseous musculature, and cut as far proximally as possible. I do not

attempt to bury the nerve in the muscle, because I have not found that this improves the rate of success (Fig. 8–1–5).

Revision Neurectomy

The approach to revision neurectomy is slightly different, and as noted, I generally use a dorsal incision even for revision. This is by far the least traumatic approach, and a scar is avoided on the plantar surface of the foot. Although the nerve is always identifiable, finding the nerve with the dorsal approach can take longer because the nerve stump is frequently stuck to the undersurface of the metatarsal, the volar plate, and the soft tissue. This dorsal approach should always be used in a revision when a previously attempted neurectomy has been performed through a short incision. Frequently, in these cases, the nerve lies under the scarred deep transverse metatarsal ligament in the center of the web space, and this procedure is easy to perform. Unfortunately, results of revision neurectomy, whether performed through a dorsal or plantar approach, are not uniformly good. In fact, any revision should be approached with caution because excellent results are uncommon. A plantar incision can be made either transversely or longitudinally, and both incisions have proponents. I only use a plantar foot incision when a prior plantar incision has already been used and exquisite sensitivity is present in the skin, associated with a positive Tinel's sign as opposed to the more typical nerve pain that is in the web space. If a plantar incision is used, I prefer to use a transverse incision and not a longitudinal one that has a greater risk of causing irritation adjacent to the metatarsal heads. The problem with the plantar incision is the potential for wound healing problems, scarring, and then difficult skin and orthotic management. With weight bearing, during toe-off, the fat pad is pulled forward and the incision has to be at least 1 cm proximal to the weight-bearing surface of the metatarsal.

Dorsal Approach to Revision Neurectomy

A revision neurectomy is performed as stated through a dorsal incision, and the deep transverse metatarsal ligament that is always reconstituted is again split. The lamina spreader is used, and the nerve has to be found more proximally. Sometimes, using a curved hemostat is

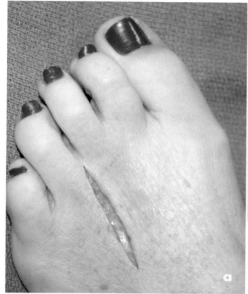

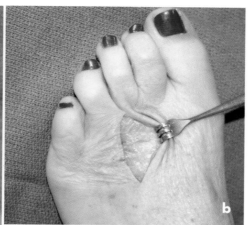

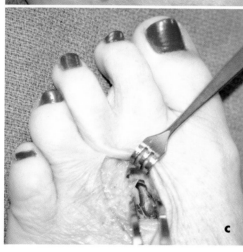

Figure 8–1–5. *Both the second and third interdigital nerves were approached with this incision that was centered over the third web space (a). Note that with skin retraction (b) and insertion of a laminar spreader into the second web space, the third web space can be well visualized (c).*

easier; it sweeps underneath the metatarsal or deep to the interosseous muscle and tendon to try to find the nerve more proximally where it is still normal. Once the nerve has been identified, it can be traced distally where the stump neuroma is identified and removed. I try to identify any cross connections that may be present between the recurrent neuroma and the normal interdigital nerve in the adjacent web space.

If a plantar incision is used, a tourniquet is used, and the incision is made transversely and as proximally as possible. The nerve is not easily identifiable and lies in the web space in fatty tissue between the flexor tendons. If the flexor tendon is indeed identified, then the dissection is too deep. Usually once the retinaculum is incised, the fatty tissue pouches outward, and the nerve must be

identified in this tissue. I find it helpful to identify all the nerves before excising the pathologic structure. If a revision is being performed from a prior plantar incision, then an extensile approach to the plantar foot is used to trace the interdigital nerve back to the more common trunk of the lateral plantar nerve. Neurectomy is performed in a standard fashion, and here it is probably preferable to apply phenol to the tip of the stump of the cut nerve, which can then be buried in the musculature without any tension.

Suggested Readings

Gondring WH, Shields B, Wenger S: An outcomes analysis of surgical treatment of tarsal tunnel syndrome. Foot Ankle Int 24:545–550, 2003.

Lau JT, Daniels TR: Effects of tarsal tunnel release and stabilization procedures on tibial nerve tension in a surgically created pes planus foot. Foot Ankle Int 19:770–777, 1998.

Lau JT, Daniels TR: Tarsal tunnel syndrome: A review of the literature. Foot Ankle Int 20:201–209, 1999.

Raikin SM, Minnich JM: Failed tarsal tunnel syndrome surgery. Foot Ankle Clin 8:159–174, 2003.

Sammarco GJ, Chang L: Outcome of surgical treatment of tarsal tunnel syndrome. Foot Ankle Int 24:125–131, 2003.

Skalley TC, Schon LC, Hinton RY, Myerson MS: Clinical results following revision tibial nerve release. Foot Ankle Int 15:360–367, 1994.

Stamatis E, Myerson MS: Treatment of recurrence of symptoms after excision of an interdigital neuroma. J Bone Joint Surg Br 86:48–53, 2004.

Total Ankle Replacement

Overview

The successful outcome of the Agility total ankle replacement (DePuy, Warsaw, Ind.) is determined not only by careful preoperative planning, but also by the anticipation of potential intraoperative complications. The surgeon should maximize postoperative range of motion, ensure adequate fixation of the implant to prevent late subsidence, and correct all preoperative foot and ankle deformities that create an unfavorable mechanical environment for the prosthesis. The decision as to when to perform ankle replacement as opposed to arthrodesis or allograft osteoarticular graft replacement is beyond the scope of this book. Nonetheless, this decision is based not only on traditional concepts, such as activity, age, weight, and daily activities, but also on the type and extent of arthritis, involvement of the subtalar and other hindfoot joints, the existing range of motion of the ankle and other joints, and patient expectations (Fig. 9–1–1). Because the ankle replacement has a higher rate of failure than arthrodesis (from a technical perspective only), both the surgeon and the patient must confront the outcome and expectations, including the possibility for failure, realistically.

The Incision

I use a single anterior incision that is supplemented by a second small lateral incision for insertion of the plate for the syndesmosis arthrodesis (Fig. 9–1–2). This lateral incision can be extended distally when a lateral ligament reconstruction is performed. A posterolateral incision is required in cases where the fibula lies more posterior to the tibia than normal, as is seen in patients with post-traumatic arthritis with a fixed fibula malunion or in patients with a congenital equinovarus deformity. If two incisions are used, the skin bridge must be at least 6 cm wide.

The anterior incision must protect the sheath of the anterior tibial tendon and should be made slightly lateral to the tendon (Fig. 9–1–3). If the retinaculum tears, inserting a suture in it early is preferable, rather than repairing the retinaculum after surgery to maintain the tendon in the sheath. The retinaculum must be closed to prevent bowstringing of the tendon and to minimize the potential for disaster if a wound dehiscence occurs postoperatively. The central aspect of the incision directly over the ankle is at the most risk for subsequent wound dehiscence.

Exposure of the Joint

Minimize skin tension by retracting either in a medial or lateral direction simultaneously. Finger retraction may be preferable, whereas simultaneous retraction of both sides of the incision should be avoided. The superficial peroneal nerve must be identified, carefully retracted laterally, and protected throughout the procedure, particularly when the cut on the talus is made. Visualizing

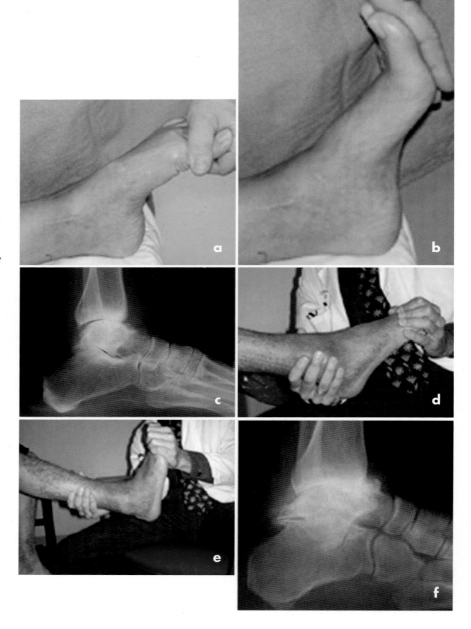

Figure 9–1–1. The range of motion of the ankle is important in decision making and may have no bearing on the x-ray (XR) appearance. For example, this patient has no ankle motion at all, but moderate arthritis appears on XR film (a–c). This patient may be a better candidate for an ankle arthrodesis than another patient with excellent motion but with a far worse XR, for whom a replacement is ideal (d–f).

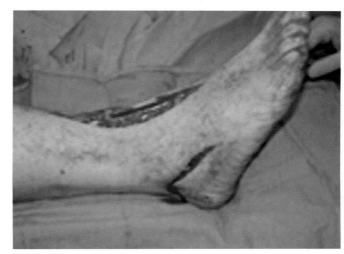

Figure 9–1–2. The lateral second incision was used to perform a simultaneous subtalar arthrodesis. If a plate is applied to the fibula, the incision can be extended proximally, or the plate can be inserted through the anterior incision with the screws inserted percutaneously.

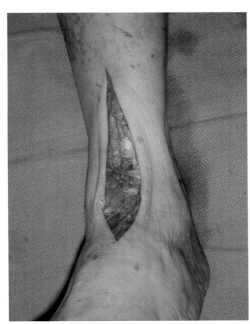

Figure 9–1–3. *A single midline incision is used for exposure. Protecting the anterior tibial tendon and maintaining the extensor retinaculum that covers the tendon are essential.*

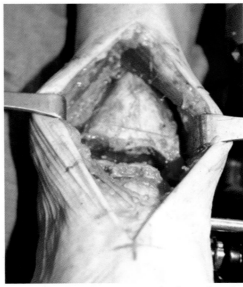

Figure 9–1–4. *The joint exposure is through a single anterior incision, and with lateral retraction, the syndesmosis is easily visible. All osteophytes are removed before preparing the syndesmosis and applying the fixator.*

the nerve during the exposure is easy by wiping the superficial tissues aside with a sponge. The deep peroneal nerve lies in a deeper plane and is the easiest to identify more proximally over the distal tibia with a large periosteal elevator. Retract the entire bundle medially or laterally, depending on which seems to create less tension. Exposure of the medial malleolus is easier than the distal fibula, and both must be completely visualized. A problem may arise with exposure of the distal fibula at the talofibular articulation. The distal fibula is more difficult to visualize, and the tibiofibular articulation is best exposed with movement of the ankle until the joint is probed with a periosteal elevator (Fig. 9–1–4). If hypertrophic osteophytes are present, a synovectomy and debridement of these osteophytes will facilitate improved exposure, including a sense of the position and plane of the talofibular joint. Performing an extensive ostectomy or cheilectomy of the anterior distal tibia to improve visualization of the joints is often helpful.

Preparation of the Syndesmosis

It is easier to expose and debride the syndesmosis before planning the bone cuts. Once the fibula has been loosened, the syndesmosis exposure is facilitated by the insertion of a laminar spreader just proximal to the joint,

and the debridement can be extended more distally to the ankle joint. Common errors are to debride a portion of the anterior fibula and to ignore the posterolateral inclination of the distal fibula. This is a particular problem with post-traumatic arthritis, in which the margin of the anterior aspect of the talofibular joint is poorly defined. I start with an ostectomy of the anterior and lateral distal tibia using a chisel, followed by a thorough decortication. All soft tissue and loose bone that may impede syndesmosis arthrodesis must be removed. Following the contour of the fibula and tibia distally with a periosteal elevator, inserting the elevator into the syndesmosis, and twisting it around 90 degrees to facilitate insertion of a laminar spreader into the syndesmosis are useful (Fig. 9–1–5). The biggest problem here is failure to adequately debride the fibula out of concern for a fracture of the fibula, a problem that can be ignored because a plate is routinely applied to the fibula for syndesmosis fusion (Fig 9–1–6).

Application of the External Fixator

Applying the fixator once the joint has been completely exposed is preferable and helpful when deformity is corrected. The fixator is used to correct deformity with insertion of the pins into the talus and calcaneus in the

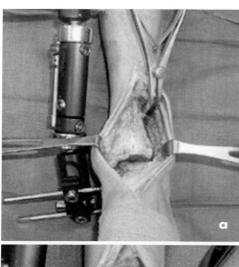

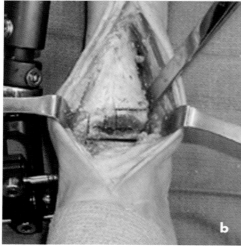

Figure 9–1–5. The syndesmosis is prepared after insertion of a laminar spreader between the tibia and fibula, with more care taken distally at the talofibular junction (a). Note that an osteotome is placed into the syndesmosis to protect it at all times when the tibial cuts are made to prevent inadvertent fibula fracture (b).

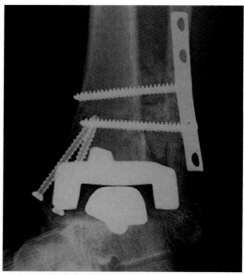

Figure 9–1–6. The syndesmosis is prone to failure in this patient. The fibula has been pushed out too far laterally. Either a smaller prosthesis could have been used, or a better cut could have been made into the fibula to obtain improved lateral coverage.

plane of the hindfoot and to realign the ankle with either a varus or valgus deformity. The fixator is not, however, used to maintain this corrected position because the extent of deformity correction cannot be determined if the fixator is in distraction. The problem with correction of varus deformity is that the ankle returns to the varus position once the fixator is removed, and planning the final soft tissue release without the fixator attached is better. Insertion of the talar pin can be a problem for patients who have a flattened talus after partial avascular necrosis (AVN) or trauma, and the pin should not interfere with the cut on the talus. The ankle should be distracted to remove 4 to 5 mm of bone from either side of the joint, but the amount of distraction that should

be applied is difficult to determine. It is worse to under-distract, and thereby remove too much bone, but the novice surgeon tends to over-distract the joint and remove too little bone. This procedure results in "over-stuffing" the joint with components. Try to establish the position of the talus relative to the tibia with the ligaments at the appropriate tension. It is always possible to remove a little more bone from the talus later on if the joint appears tight, and range of motion is diminished after insertion of the trial components (Fig. 9–1–7). Although the distractor can be used to correct preoperative alignment of the hindfoot, the talus sometimes remains tilted into either varus or valgus even after distraction. Here it is best to insert a small osteotome into the joint to equalize the direction of the bone cut on the talus. For example, with preoperative valgus, laxity of the deltoid is present. Instead of equal distraction of the joint, the talus tilts into more and more valgus, and the talus must be cut in the plane of the dome and not in the plane of the valgus.

Sizing of the Implant

Patient weight should be offset by the expected size of implant to be used. A heavy patient with a large joint who needs a size 6 implant would be expected to have fewer

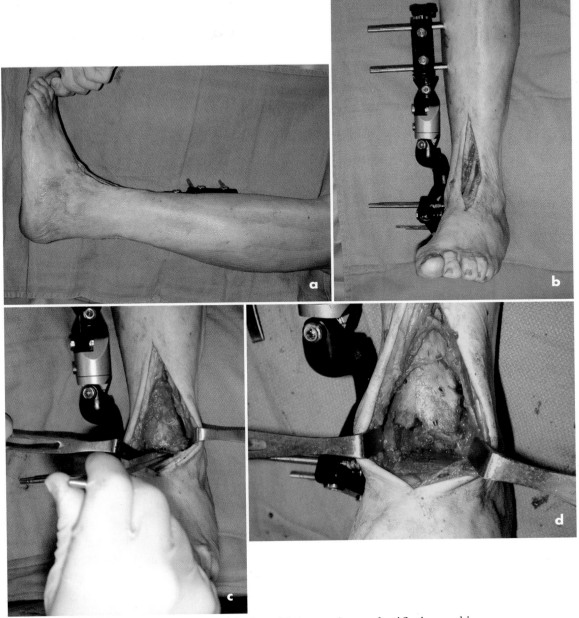

Figure 9–1–7. *The external fixator is applied with the ankle in maximum dorsiflexion and is locked in place (a, b). The tension on the distraction is determined by inserting an osteotome into the joint and making sure that 1 to 2 mm of "give" remains. This length indicates that the ankle ligaments are at a functional length (c, d).*

complications with subsidence and wear than would an obese patient of the same weight with a small ankle requiring a smaller implant. In general, the exact prosthetic template should be inserted. In patients with severe ankle ankylosis after trauma, an acceptable range of motion may not be attainable, and this risk can be minimized to some extent by downsizing the prosthesis (but not at the expense of the size/weight ratio). A smaller-

sized prosthesis increases the potential for malleolar impingement and subsidence, but with improved range of motion possible. A larger prosthesis has an increased size of the base plate for support under the tibia preventing subsidence but pushes the fibular aside and increases the potential for syndesmosis nonunion, as well as decreasing motion. Measure the prosthesis size preoperatively off the radiographs but do not adhere rigidly to

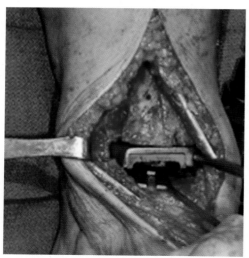

Figure 9–1–8. *A reasonable "fit" of the tibial trial, but either the fit is too far medially or too much bone has been removed from the fibula laterally. The fibula space can be filled with graft, or a larger component can be inserted by recutting the tibial component fin. Note also that the talus-cutting guide is in the center of the talus. Shifting the cutting guide to fit the center of the joint is a common error.*

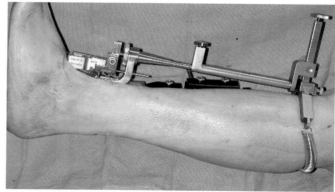

Figure 9–1–9. *The cutting block and alignment guide have been incorrectly attached here. Note the slope on the tibial alignment guide. This will lead to an incorrect cut on the tibia, with a resection that is more anterior than posterior, followed by a likelihood of anterior subsidence of the tibial component.*

this sizing and leave some flexibility for changing the size intraoperatively. Frequently, making a change in the size of the prosthesis at some point during surgery becomes necessary (Fig. 9–1–8).

Planning the Bone Cuts

The bone cuts for implantation of the tibial component require resection of the inner one third of the medial and the lateral malleolus. Before making these cuts, be sure that nothing will block the saw (e.g., prior hardware). Leaving hardware in wherever possible is preferable to prevent fracture. The medial malleolus presents a particular problem because the removal of screws creates a stress riser that is prone to intraoperative fracture. If there is concern about the viability of the medial malleolus, insert a temporary guide pin into the malleolus before making the bone cuts to help prevent fracture. The screws that can give the worst problem are those in the anterior tibia that are either buried or stripped. They block the correct bone cut, and worse, when an attempt is made to remove them, the small chunk of bone that often comes out with it leaves a bone void. Application of the alignment guide is an important step, and the guide must be well aligned with the tibia. If tibia vara

or other torsional deformities of the leg are present, then the hip–knee–ankle axis should be the guide, and the cord from the electrocautery can be extended along the limb to gauge the correct position of the alignment guide (Fig. 9–1–9). The correct positioning of the cutting block is the most important phase of the joint replacement. It should not be performed visually, and it must be done with careful fluoroscopic monitoring to ensure optimal alignment. With the ankle viewed from the anteroposterior position, the correct view of both malleoli is not present simultaneously, and the ankle needs to be rotated around fluoroscopically to ensure perfect alignment of the cutting block. Use a free saw blade in both the tibial and talar slot to ensure the correct plane of the cut on the lateral fluoroscopic image. Always move the cutting block as close to the tibia as possible before initiating the cuts to prevent inadvertent angulation of the saw blade (Fig. 9–1–10).

If the positioning is correct, the question always arises as to how much bone to resect from the tibia, talus, and malleoli. This step cannot be emphasized enough, because resecting too much bone may result in malleolar fractures, as well as subsidence and malalignment. Although the amount of bone resected from the tibia and talus should normally be equal, this standard should not be rigidly adhered to and it is determined by the quality of the bone. For example, where a flat talus is present, less bone may be taken from the talus and proportionately more from the tibia. Although the

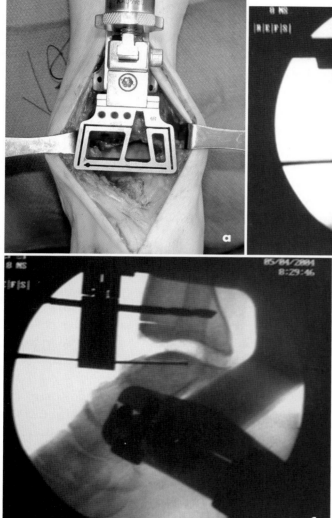

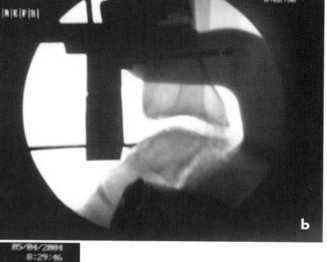

Figure 9–1–10. *The position of the cutting block (a) is critical. Because the entire limb cannot be examined under fluoroscopy, care must be taken to ensure that the cuts will be perpendicular to the axis of the limb and the weight–bearing surface of the foot. Note that in the fluoroscopic views (b, c), the foot is not correctly positioned and is in equinus. The cut should be projected posteriorly on the lateral view to determine how much bone will be resected. In this case, the foot was dorsiflexed, and the cut on the talus was corrected.*

cutting block is generally centered over the tibia, at times it may have to be shifted more medially, to compensate, for example, for fibular deficiency or hindfoot deformity. Proximal displacement of the cutting block results in more tibia resected, impingement of the gutters, and the likelihood of subsidence into softer metaphyseal bone.

Positioning the cutting block in the horizontal and sagittal plane to line up the mediolateral and vertical position is easily facilitated by fluoroscopy. Correction of any rotation of the block that would place the cut in either varus or valgus is not as easy to determine, even with fluoroscopy because a full image of the leg is not present. Because fluoroscopy does not help, correction is much more difficult, and the position of the patella, the ante-

rior tibia, and the floor should be relied on. If a patient has tibia vara, ignore the position of the cutting block relative to the tibia and focus on the hip-knee-floor axis. Before securing the cutting block with the guide pins, make sure that the threaded wheel has been opened to leave enough room to move the tibial component proximally *or* distally. This ensures that last minute adjustments can be made to the position of the tibial bone cut, even after the cutting block has been secured.

Making the Bone Cuts

Pay attention to the position of the posteromedial soft-tissue structures, in particular the posterior tibial tendon, when making the medial malleolar cut and the flexor hallucis longus tendon with the cut on the posterior aspect of the tibia. The posterior tibial tendon is frequently visualized with the medial malleolar cut and therefore any postoperative symptoms of the posterior tibial tendon that occur should not be surprising. Assuming that the cutting block has been positioned vertically and that no external rotation is present, no difference in the thickness of the medial malleolar cut should exist (Fig. 9–1–11). Make a last-minute check to ensure that this cut is indeed going to be vertical. If the cutting block is externally rotated, the saw cut will not be perpendicular to the tibia, and the posteromedial tibial component will protrude on the posterior tibial tendon. Cutting less initially is always preferable; then gradually remove more bone with a reciprocating saw

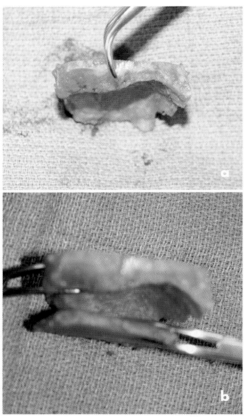

Figure 9–1–11. *The cut on the tibia in both of these ankles appears incorrect. Although more bone was cut laterally, this was the result of a varus ankle deformity in which the erosion on the medial tibia was created by the intra-articular varus (a). Note, however, that the cut on the talus (b) is planar, which is correct. One must not try to compensate for a varus ankle by adjusting the plane of the talus cut.*

until completed. When the posterior tibial cut is made in cases of post-traumatic arthritis, removal of the posterior lip of the tibia is difficult. The tibia can be prominent posteroinferiorly, and the flexor hallucis and peroneal tendons may be scarred down to the underlying bone. Do not rip out the bone with a rongeur but slowly remove the hypertrophic osteophytes. The cut on the fibula should be perpendicular and include one third and, at the most, one half of the fibula. A problem arises at times when the fibula is posteriorly translated with the cut because excessive bone may be resected because of this aberrant position that is encountered after trauma or from congenital equinovarus conditions (Figs 9–1–12 and 9–1–13).

Fracture

A fracture of either malleolus must be recognized and fixed. Fractures of the fibula must not be ignored, but because a plate is routinely applied to the fibula to increase the rate of syndesmosis fusion, these fractures are less of a problem, and one can be as aggressive with the syndesmosis debridement as is necessary. If a fracture does occur intraoperatively, it should *always* be secured with internal fixation because the malleoli are required for the stability of the prosthesis. Fracture of the medial malleolus creates more of a problem and is usually caused by carelessness with sizing or positioning of the tibial component or inadvertent manipulation of the ankle or the external fixator. Lateral malposition of the tibial component can occur when an attempt is made to minimize the medial bone cut. Because the fin is precisely positioned on the cutting jig, if the cuts are carefully planned and the correct prosthesis size is selected, lateral translation malposition should not occur. Be prepared to change the size of the prosthesis, particularly to downsize as needed, even after the cuts have been made, and back fill with small amounts of bone graft if required.

Perhaps the most common error that causes fracture of the medial malleolus is due to an oblique (not vertical) cut of the medial malleolus so that when the tibial component is inserted, the posterior margin of the component abuts against the obliquely cut medial malleolus. This cut is caused by slight external rotation of the cutting block. If fracture of the medial malleolus occurs, screw fixation can be challenging because not much

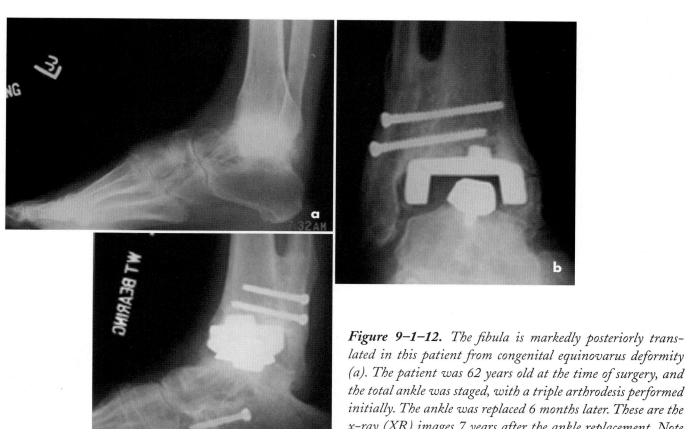

Figure 9–1–12. *The fibula is markedly posteriorly translated in this patient from congenital equinovarus deformity (a). The patient was 62 years old at the time of surgery, and the total ankle was staged, with a triple arthrodesis performed initially. The ankle was replaced 6 months later. These are the x-ray (XR) images 7 years after the ankle replacement. Note insufficient coverage of the fibula but a well-incorporated component without loosening (b, c).*

room is available for fixation adjacent to the medial tibial component. However, fixing the fracture is always possible, whether with cannulated screws or with K-wires or a tension band construct.

Of all the intraoperative complications, few are as troubling as a fracture of the talus. Ensure that the cutting block is correctly positioned on the lateral fluoroscopic view, and the foot must be forced upward into neutral dorsiflexion before the talar cut is made so that the posterior cut on the talus does not encroach on the posterior facet of the subtalar joint. Obviously, if the foot is in any plantar flexion, this increases the likelihood that the cut on the talus will be incorrect. If the patient is a suitable candidate for joint replacement and the talus looks as if it is going to be a problem, it may be preferable to stage the surgery and first perform a subtalar arthrodesis. If a fracture does occur, the safest procedure is to perform a subtalar arthrodesis to stabilize the talus.

Syndesmosis Arthrodesis

A successful arthrodesis of the syndesmosis is imperative to the outcome of this ankle replacement. Adequate preparation of the syndesmosis with stable fixation is important but not necessarily sufficient to ensure arthrodesis. I routinely use a four-hole one-third tubular plate on the fibula using two screws for fixation, stabilization, and compression of the syndesmosis. Through the anterior central incision, a periosteal elevator is used to expose the anterior aspect of the fibula up to a level 6 cm above the joint line. A rongeur is then used, and after removal of the anterior tibiofibular ligament, it is inserted into the syndesmosis. This step is performed considering the orientation of the syndesmosis level, which lies slightly obliquely to the coronal plane from anterolateral to posteromedial. After the rongeur is gently twisted and the tibia is levered, the syndesmosis is gradually loosened. Then a lamina spreader is inserted

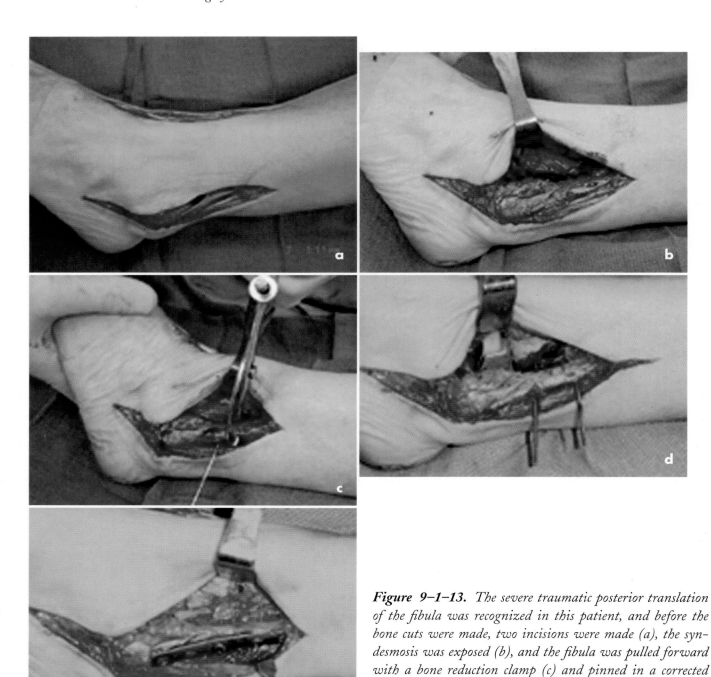

Figure 9–1–13. *The severe traumatic posterior translation of the fibula was recognized in this patient, and before the bone cuts were made, two incisions were made (a), the syndesmosis was exposed (b), and the fibula was pulled forward with a bone reduction clamp (c) and pinned in a corrected anterior position (d). Once the implants were in place, the fibula was plated over the cannulated guide pins (e).*

proximally to the ankle joint level at the interosseous space, and the syndesmosis is further distracted. Flexible chisels are used for decortication and roughening of the bony surfaces up to 2 cm proximal to the tibiofibular groove (Fig. 9–1–14).

Nonunion of the syndesmosis seems to be increased with inadequate bone debridement and excessive periosteal stripping on both sides of the fibula when two incisions are used, with inadequate compression of the fibula into the prosthesis, and when the fibula is pushed away from the tibia when the tibial component is inserted (Fig. 9–1–15). If the fibula is pushed laterally, remove the prosthesis, and cut 3 mm more bone from the fibula. Once the tibial component fits against the medial distal fibula correctly, the plate is inserted

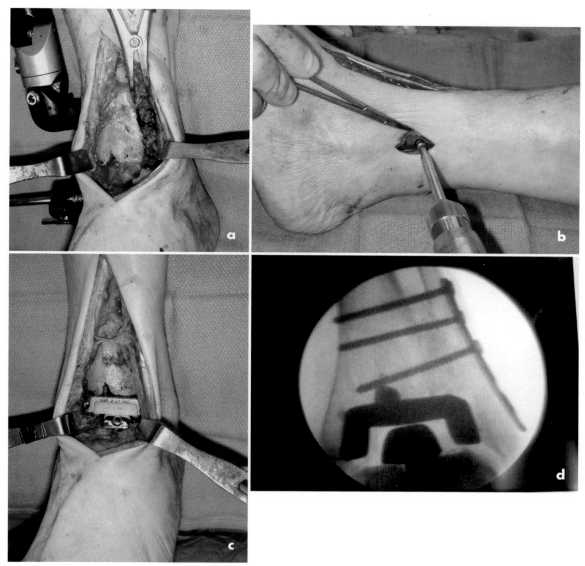

Figure 9–1–14. *The syndesmosis is carefully prepared by inserting a laminar spreader (a), aggressively debriding the margins of the fibula and tibia, and then inserting screws through a four- or five-hole plate under power (b). The power insertion of the screws compresses the fibula against the tibia and the lateral aspect of the tibial component (c, d).*

through a separate lateral 2-cm incision. Cancellous bone graft from the resected tibia and talus is inserted to fill the area of the tibiofibular groove before the plate is compressed, and two fully threaded cancellous screws purchasing all four cortices are used, positioned just above the fin of the tibial component. The screws are inserted with power, and considerable compression across the total length of the syndesmosis should be noticed, in particular into the lateral tibial component. Try to insert the screws as parallel to the joint line as possible to increase the likelihood of compression.

Correction of Deformity

Planning the strategy for the correction of a *varus* ankle deformity is probably the most difficult part of any ankle joint replacement. A wide spectrum of deformity ranges from a slightly deformed ankle joint with minimal soft tissue contracture to a severely deformed cavovarus foot and ankle with lateral ligament and peroneus brevis muscle insufficiency, which should not be corrected with ankle replacement. Depending on the severity and the nature of the deformity, the following must be

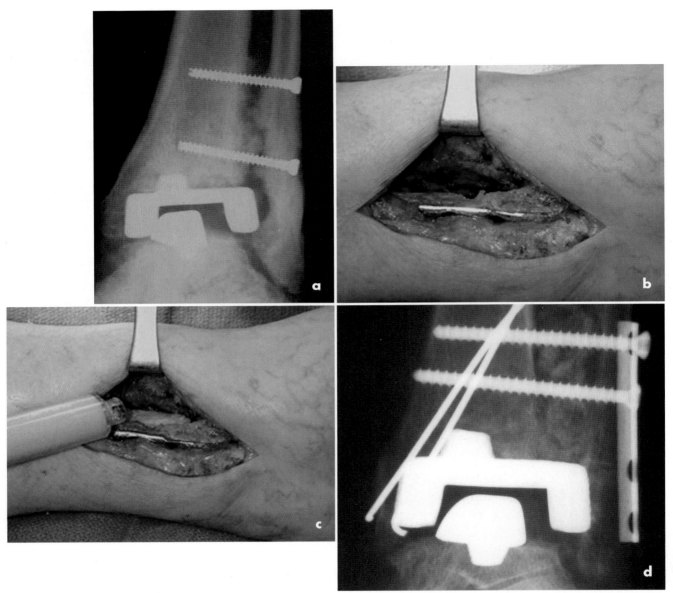

Figure 9–1–15. *Nonunion of the syndesmosis occurred in this patient. Note the lateral and valgus subsidence of the tibial component that is loose (a). A complete joint revision, with two incisions, and allograft bone grafting were performed, in addition to injection of demineralized bone matrix (EBI, Parsippany, NJ) (c) and plate fixation (d). Note the intraoperative occurrence of an undisplaced fracture of the medial malleolus, which was fixed with K-wires. All malleolar fractures must be fixed regardless of displacement.*

examined: the contracted deltoid ligament, the contracted posterior tibial muscle, lateral ankle ligament insufficiency, motor deficit of the peroneus brevis muscle, focal bone loss on the medial aspect of the distal tibial articular surface, the varus heel, the plantarflexed first metatarsal, and a medially displaced Achilles tendon. Inserting the prostheses parallel to the ground is imperative, and adequate soft tissue balancing and complete ankle and hindfoot alignment are necessities. The cut of the talus must be rectangular and not triangular because the latter cut leads to an oblique cut of the talus and recurrent deformity.

Correcting varus deformity that is associated with bone loss on the medial distal tibial plafond is easier because the perpendicular positioning of the cutting block

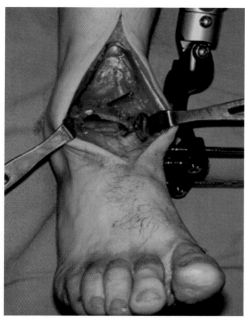

Figure 9–1–16. *Varus ankle deformity must be approached with cuts made in the axis of the limb and not according to the deformity of the tibiotalar joint. If the distractor does not realign the joint to the correct axis, then a small osteotome should be inserted medially to push the talus inferiorly before the cut is made. This is followed by correct release of the deltoid.*

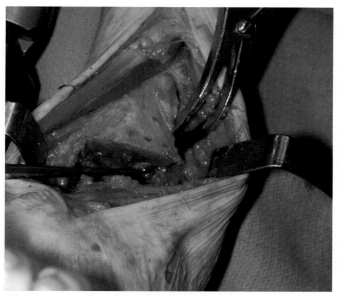

Figure 9–1–17. *After the bone cuts, a large defect was noted in the distal tibia as a result of a valgus deformity of the talus. This was debrided with a curette and filled with bone graft before insertion of the components.*

relative to the limb axis always removes slightly more bone from the lateral than the medial distal tibia. Once the bone cuts have been made, the fixator is loosened, and the varus deformity of the ankle is corrected with a deltoid ligament release through the joint (Figs 9–1–16 to 9–1–18). The deep portion is initially released, and then while a valgus force is applied to the ankle, the other portions are palpated and sequentially released. At times, a second incision should be made posteromedially to perform a fractional lengthening of the posterior tibial muscle at the musculotendinous junction. After an adequate medial release the lateral ligaments are usually loose, the ligaments are redundant, or the ankle is unstable, and a ligament reconstruction must be performed. The easiest method for lateral ligament reconstruction is to use half of the peroneus brevis tendon that is passed under the plate and over one of the screws. The tendon is pulled around the screw, and then the plate is compressed against the tendon, which is then sutured onto itself (Fig. 9–1–19). The lateral gutter osteophytes must be debrided to allow rotation of the talar body in the mortise. Once the realignment is complete and the ankle

stable, a decision is made as to the necessity for a calcaneus osteotomy (Fig. 9–1–20). The decision is best determined by looking at the foot from below and checking the axial alignment.

A *valgus* ankle deformity is potentially associated with combinations of a contracted lateral ligament, deltoid ligament insufficiency, a valgus heel, a laterally displaced Achilles tendon that acts as a hindfoot evertor, a shortened and deformed fibula due to chronic impingement, and spring ligament and posterior tibial tendon rupture. Although the pathologic anatomy is different, the same treatment philosophy applies for the correction of the valgus as with the varus deformity (Fig. 9–1–21). The external fixator will worsen the valgus deformity as distraction is applied, and an osteotome or laminar spreader should be inserted into the lateral joint space to balance the talar cut. With severe valgus deformity, a joint replacement should not be performed because the deltoid ligament is completely torn, severely stretched, and irreparable. Joint replacement can be considered after flatfoot correction and a deltoid reconstruction, but I would wait at least 6 to 12 months to ensure that the deltoid reconstruction has been successful (Fig. 9–1–22).

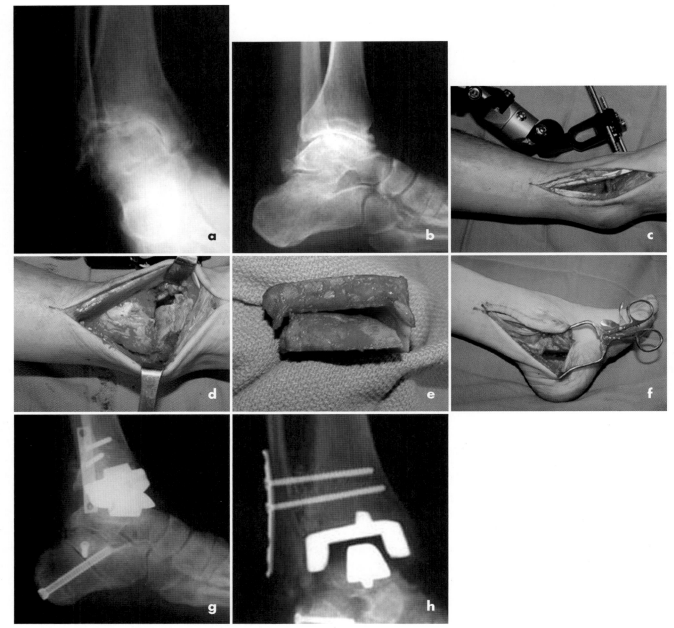

Figure 9–1–18. *This varus ankle deformity was corrected with replacement calcaneus osteotomy and a peroneus brevis tendon augmentation of ankle instability. Note the varus in the hindfoot as a result of chronic ankle instability and of erosion of the medial tibia (a, b). The external fixator was applied with the distal pins inserted perpendicular to the axis of the talus and calcaneus (c, d). Once distraction was applied and the deltoid ligament was released, the alignment improved. Note the size and geometry of the bone removed with a defect in the medial tibial plafond as expected from the x-ray (XR) film (e, f). Before insertion of the prosthesis, the fixator was removed to ensure adequate tensioning and release of the deltoid ligament. The early postoperative XR films are shown, and the foot is not weight bearing. Note that the position of the talus is not ideal because it is slightly anterior to the lateral process of the talus (g). The tibial component is well aligned with respect to the limb axis (h).*

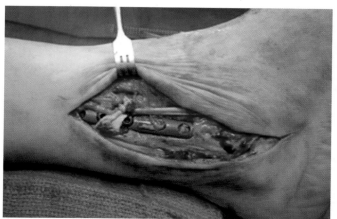

Figure 9–1–19. *Ankle instability must be checked after every replacement but, in particular, when any preoperative varus is present. This should be determined manually, and then if any tilting of the talus is noted, a peroneal augmentation should be performed. The peroneus brevis tendon is split, and the anterior half of the tendon is passed under the plate around one of the screws and tensioned. The plate is then compressed against the tendon, which is then sutured back onto itself.*

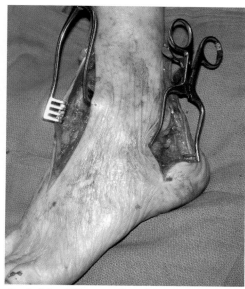

Figure 9–1–20. *When performing a calcaneus osteotomy, ensure that the skin bridge is sufficiently wide. The incision for the osteotomy is usually extended proximally to add the ankle ligament stabilization with half of the peroneus brevis tendon under the plate.*

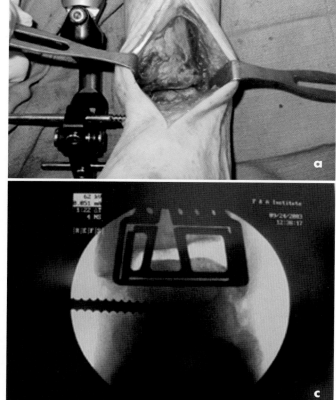

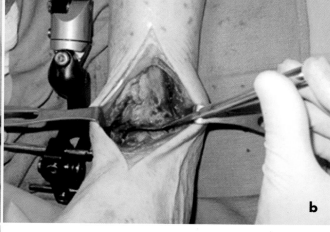

Figure 9–1–21. *Valgus ankle deformity is easier to correct if the deformity is in the distal tibia rather than in the foot. Note the relatively normal appearance of the ankle (a), and the correction to a neutral position with an instrument is inserted laterally (b). The jig is applied in the correct position with the talus well aligned. Note the increase in bone to be removed medially off the tibia (c).*

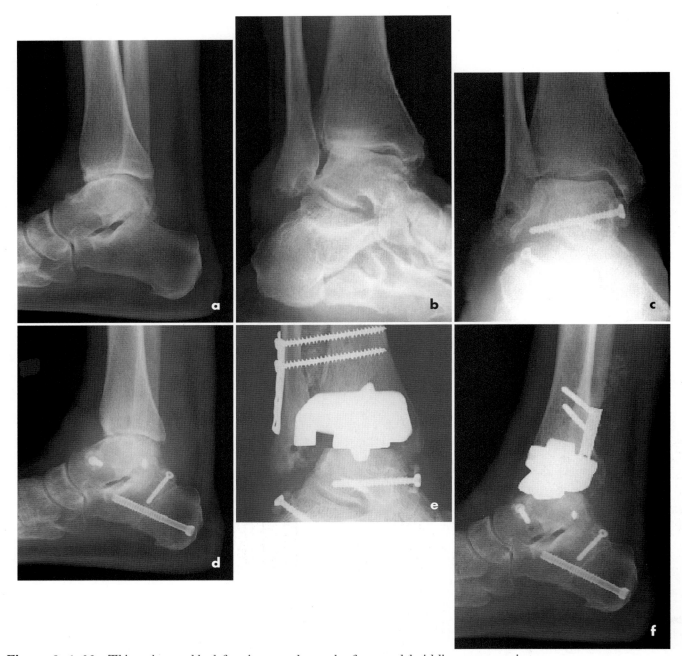

Figure 9–1–22. *This valgus ankle deformity was the result of a torn deltoid ligament associated with a mild flatfoot (a, b). Ankle replacement cannot be performed unless the foot is plantigrade and deltoid stability is present. As part of the flatfoot correction, which included a transfer of the flexor digitorum longus (FDL) tendon, a calcaneus osteotomy, and a medial cuneiform osteotomy, a staged deltoid reconstruction was performed with a hamstring allograft (c, d), followed by the ankle replacement 6 months later (e, f).*

Additional Procedures

Wherever possible, I perform additional operations simultaneously. To avoid the stiff fibrosis of the soft tissues after staged procedures, I prefer to perform an isolated talonavicular or subtalar arthrodesis at the same time as the ankle replacement, provided the arthrodesis is performed for arthritis and not for bone loss. A triple arthrodesis is also performed as a staged procedure approximately 6 months before the ankle to correct more severe hindfoot and midfoot deformities and to create a plantigrade foot. This restores more normal bone anatomy and minimizes incorrect cuts, especially on the talus. A triple arthrodesis must be staged 6 months apart, and the incision for the talonavicular joint arthrodesis must be made more anteriorly so that this can subsequently be incorporated into the incision for the ankle replacement (Fig. 9–1–23). Two long 3.5-mm screws are used for the subtalar arthrodesis and are inserted from the anterior neck of the talus posteroinferiorly into the calcaneus. If there is subtalar or talar bone loss, and subsidence of the talar component into the subtalar joint is anticipated, the surgery should be staged.

Maximizing Range of Motion

One of the most critical factors affecting the postoperative range of motion is any preexisting ankle stiffness or equinus contracture, which is often the case with post-traumatic arthritis. In patients with this arthritis, obtaining a satisfactory range of motion is more difficult, despite aggressive mobilization of the soft tissues (see Fig. 9–1–1). In particular, avoid over-distraction of the joint because this leads to inadequate bone removal, overstuffing of the joint, and inevitable stiffness. Adequate removal of any scar tissue and of hypertrophic osteophytes from the gutters is important, including a champfer cut on the talus followed by application of bone wax to the cut talus surface. After the cuts have been completed and the appropriately sized trial prosthesis has been inserted, the range of motion of the ankle joint should be assessed before insertion of the final prosthesis. This assessment helps determine if there is any residual bony impingement or stiffness, and, if necessary, a thicker (plus 2 mm) polyethylene component is used to avoid impingement. If limited dorsiflexion is still present, then a percutaneous lengthening of the Achilles tendon with a triple hemisection step-cut technique is used. If the desired range of motion (usually a lack of dorsiflexion) has not been obtained, then the components are removed, and provided sufficient bone is present, an additional 2 mm of the talus can be shaved off to create some "slop" in the joint. Before any additional bone cut is made, the talus must be checked fluoroscopically to ensure that the posterior subtalar joint is not compromised. Any further cuts on the talus must therefore be made with the ankle fully dorsiflexed. If motion is still limited, consider downsizing the prosthesis size if possible, provided that it adequately covers the cortical rims of talus and distal tibia and provides sufficient clearance of the malleoli from the talar body.

Management of Complications

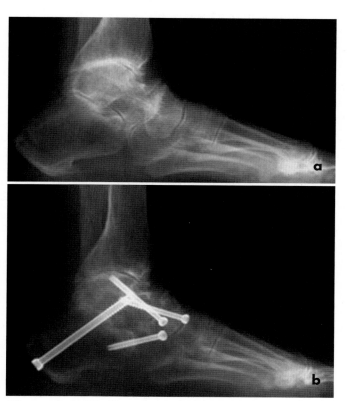

Figure 9–1–23. *Pantalar arthritis must be staged with the triple arthrodesis performed first (a, b) and the ankle replacement about 6 months later, once complete wound healing is present.*

To some extent, many of the complications have been covered in the previous section on preoperative and intraoperative planning. I look at these complications in three phases. The first occurs early and is the result of wound healing problems. To a large extent, these problems have been eliminated through careful patient selection; through preoperative treatment of dysvascularity; through careful handling of the soft tissues; and by application of Symphony (Ace/DePuy, Warsaw, Ind.), a platelet-rich plasma harvested from the patients' own centrifuged serum, onto the subcutaneous tissues immediately before skin closure.

The second phase of problems becomes apparent early on when abnormality in the alignment of the prosthesis and lack of healing of the syndesmosis arthrodesis are apparent. Because these are obvious, the question then is how aggressive should a surgeon be with correction of malalignment or delayed union of the syndesmosis. One of the more concerning problems is the potential for nonunion of the arthrodesis of the tibiofibular joint. Fusion of the syndesmosis correlates with stability of the tibial component and has the greatest influence on the outcome of the replacement. Conversely, nonunion or delayed union results in a statistically significant increase in tibial subsidence rates and ballooning lysis at the interface between the bone and the tibial component. A solid fusion mass between the distal tibia and fibula should be radiographically evident by the third postoperative month. Because we have added a one-third tubular plate over the lateral fibula to compress the syndesmosis and have routinely sprayed the Symphony platelet-rich plasma onto the bone graft at the syndesmotic arthrodesis site, the fusion rate has diminished but still occurs. I have not found that continued immobilization or external bone stimulation has much effect after the fourth month on stimulating the fusion to mature. Therefore if the arthrodesis is symptomatic and evidence of lucency is present, then a persistence of the nonunion beyond 6 months necessitates a revision of the arthrodesis with supplemental cancellous bone graft and demineralized bone matrix. If nonunion is noted incidentally after 1 year and the prosthesis is stable, and no inflammation is present, then I suggest that the arthrodesis should remain as is.

If deformity of the ankle or foot persists and the prosthesis is not aligned, then a different issue exists. I have tried to help these patients initially with shoe modifications and even a brace. These are rarely sufficient in the long term, and revision of the prosthesis must be performed. When revision is performed, frac-

ture and wound healing are potential complications, and attention to detail is essential. Generally, I assume that the prosthesis was not originally implanted correctly or that a problem exists with the soft tissue balance around the ankle. The surgeon must start over and must use the external fixator to achieve the correct tension on the ankle, correct the implant malalignment, and establish the correct balance. This revision may necessitate bone grafting, a differently sized implant, use of a larger polyethylene tray, a revision talar component, or even a custom implant. In addition to bone grafting, I sometimes maintain the external fixator in place for 6 weeks to control subluxation or instability (Fig. 9–1–24). As with all revision procedures, removal of the implant can be difficult because of bone ingrowth, and fracture must be prevented through carefully prying loose the prosthesis with a small curved osteotome (Fig. 9–1–25). The third set of problems occurs later in the evolution of the prosthesis, with implant subsidence, bone overgrowth, cyst formation, and infection. Even minor overgrowth of bone around the medial and lateral margins of the prosthesis results in painful impingement. Symptomatic impingement may be managed by local injection of hydrocortisone. If this modality fails, open or arthroscopic resection can be performed to remove the excess bone. During this procedure, champfer cuts should be used for a good marginal resection of bone on either side of the talus. More significant subsidence, particularly of the talar component, creates a whole different set of problems, which may necessitate arthrodesis of the subtalar joint, possibly with custom implants (Fig. 9–1–26). Severe subsidence requires either complete prosthetic revision or conversion to an ankle arthrodesis (Fig. 9–1–27). The latter procedure must be performed with bulk allograft, and if at all possible, the subtalar joint should be preserved. Cyst formation usually implies microparticle wear. Revision of the polyethylene component may be necessary, in addition to bone grafting (Fig. 9–1–28). Finally, although it is extremely rare, late infection after ankle arthroplasty does occur and is managed according to the type of organism in the infection, the timing of the diagnosis of the infection, and staged revision as required (Fig. 9–1–29).

In the future, revision of more complex deformities is likely with the Agility ankle replacement. The

Text continued on p. 250

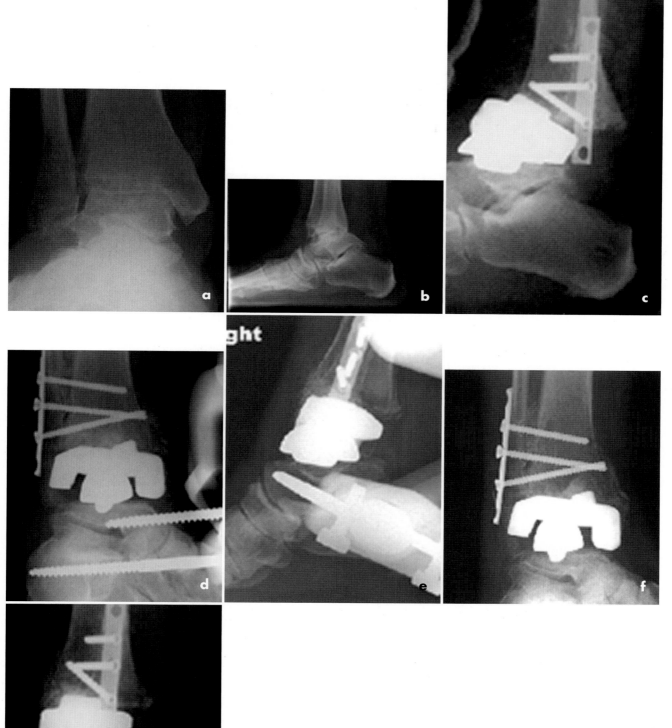

Figure 9–1–24. *This was an extremely difficult problem to resolve, and one that fortunately rarely occurs. This patient had posterior translation of the ankle pre-operatively but no varus or valgus instability, which was checked preoperatively (a, b). During surgery, the position of the tibial component was difficult to maintain, and unexpected crushing of the anterior plafond was noted. The foot was immobilized in a cast, and despite what appeared to be adequate intraoperative position, anterior subluxation of the joint occurred immediately postoperatively with further anterior bone erosion (c). This was immediately revised with a cancellous bone graft, but the only way to maintain the position of the joint reduction was with an external fixator (d, e), which was removed at 8 weeks. The x-ray (XR) images at 1 year after the replacement (f, g).*

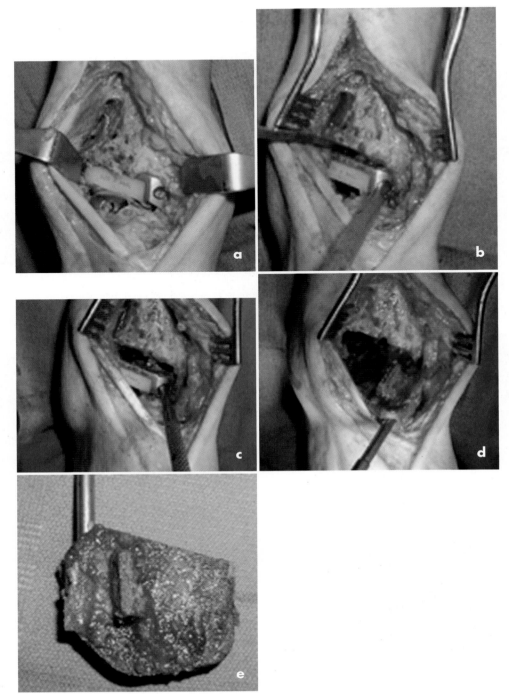

Figure 9–1–25. *A revision arthroplasty was performed for this patient for valgus malalignment and subsidence, with bone overgrowth and pain. Note that because the prosthesis is surrounded by bone and soft tissue, removal of the components was difficult (a). A 0.5-cm curved osteotome was used to pry open the prosthesis (b), which was then carefully removed (c, d). Note the bone ingrowth into the tibial component (e).*

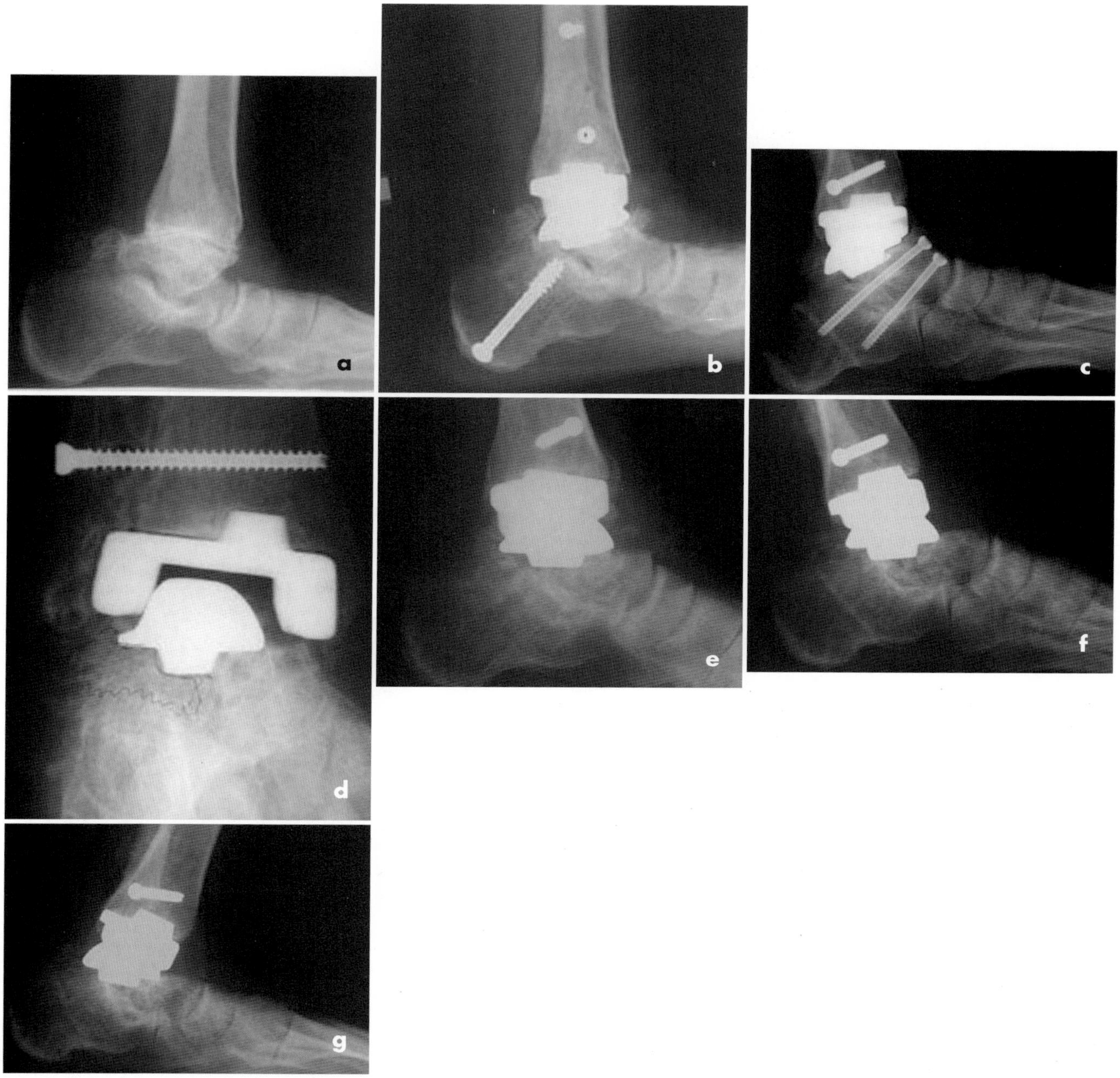

Figure 9–1–26. *A complication with total ankle replacement associated with flatfoot that was preventable. Note the flatfoot with the change in the talar declination angle (a). The total ankle replacement was performed in conjunction with a medial translational osteotomy of the calcaneus and a transfer of the flexor digitorum longus (FDL) tendon, but with failure. Note the subsidence of the talar component into the subtalar joint (b). Unless the talar declination is corrected before replacement, the talar cut enters posteriorly, too close to the subtalar joint. The deformity was corrected with a staged subtalar arthrodesis followed by revision of the replacement 6 months later. Note further subsidence into the subtalar joint in the interim despite subtalar arthrodesis (c). Revision was successful, and a revision talar component was used with no further subsidence (d, e). Note that range of motion remains good 5 years after this revision procedure (f, g).*

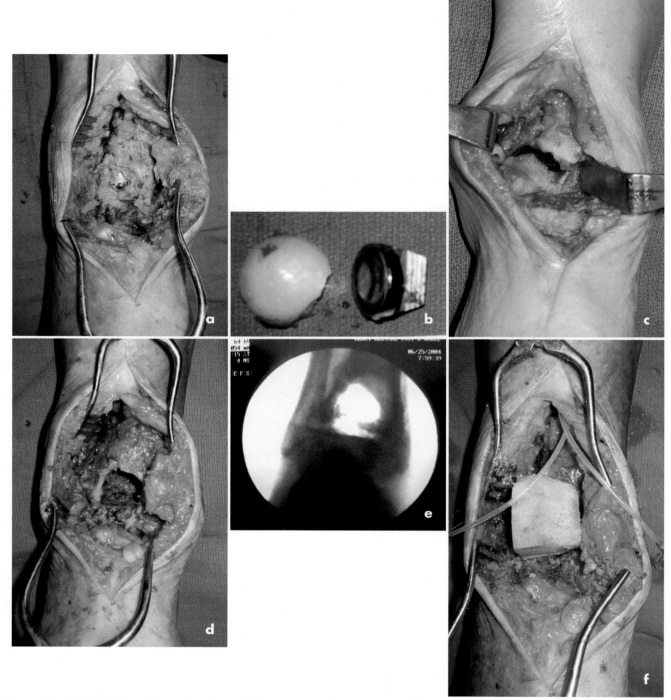

Figure 9–1–27. *This ankle was implanted 25 years ago and was removed for subsidence and pain (a, b). The cement was removed (c), and a sizeable defect in the distal tibia was left (d, e). A femoral head allograft was contoured with a saw directly on top of the defect (f), and then it was impacted into the hole with a mallet and infused with Symphony platelet-rich plasma.*

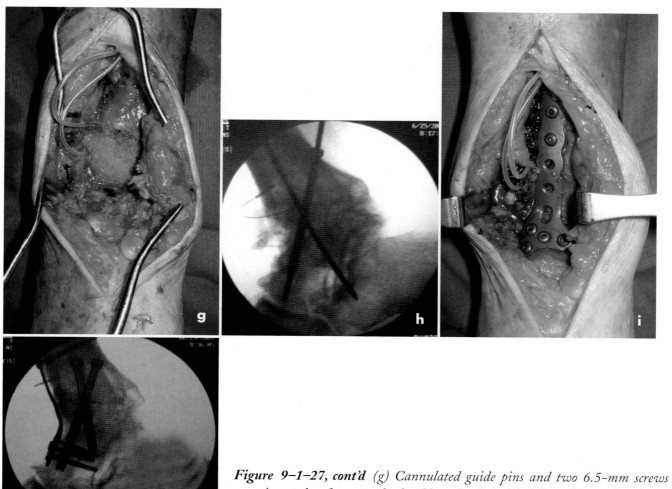

Figure 9–1–27, cont'd *(g) Cannulated guide pins and two 6.5-mm screws were inserted as for a standard ankle arthrodesis (h), followed by application of a humeral plate (DePuy, Warsaw, Ind), which was contoured over the anterior surface of the distal tibia and talus (i, j).*

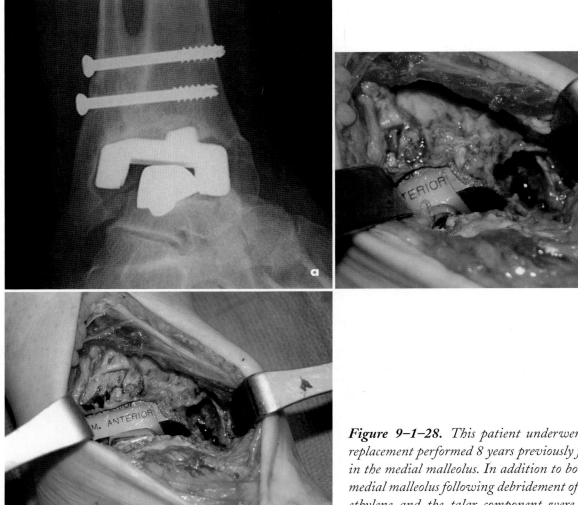

Figure 9–1–28. *This patient underwent revision of the replacement performed 8 years previously for cyst formation in the medial malleolus. In addition to bone grafting of the medial malleolus following debridement of the cyst, the polyethylene and the talar component were revised, and the margins of the talus were trimmed with champfer cuts.*

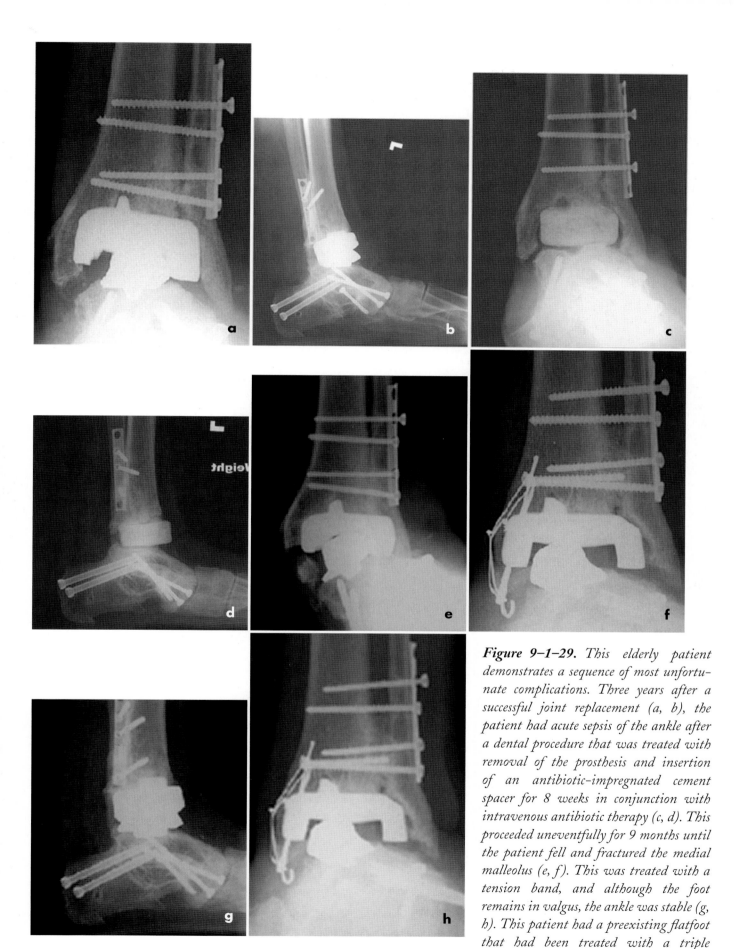

Figure 9–1–29. *This elderly patient demonstrates a sequence of most unfortunate complications. Three years after a successful joint replacement (a, b), the patient had acute sepsis of the ankle after a dental procedure that was treated with removal of the prosthesis and insertion of an antibiotic-impregnated cement spacer for 8 weeks in conjunction with intravenous antibiotic therapy (c, d). This proceeded uneventfully for 9 months until the patient fell and fractured the medial malleolus (e, f). This was treated with a tension band, and although the foot remains in valgus, the ankle was stable (g, h). This patient had a preexisting flatfoot that had been treated with a triple arthrodesis, and continued stresses on the medial ankle will be likely.*

indications are limited for revising an ankle arthrodesis and converting it to an ankle replacement. Technically, this operation is feasible but must only be performed in the setting of intractable pain and limitation of activities as an alternative to a below-the-knee amputation. Usually, patients who require these revisions have arthritis of adjacent joints (Fig. 9–1–30), and further arthrodesis of these joints of the foot are not going to realistically improve function. Clearly, the preservation of joint anatomy, in particular the fibula with the initial arthrodesis, makes the conversion to an ankle replacement technically feasible. Although this is not a plea for preservation of the fibula during the primary arthrodesis procedure, it makes sense to maintain the anatomy and not to "burn any bridges." This concept can also be applied to patients treated for a nonunion of an ankle

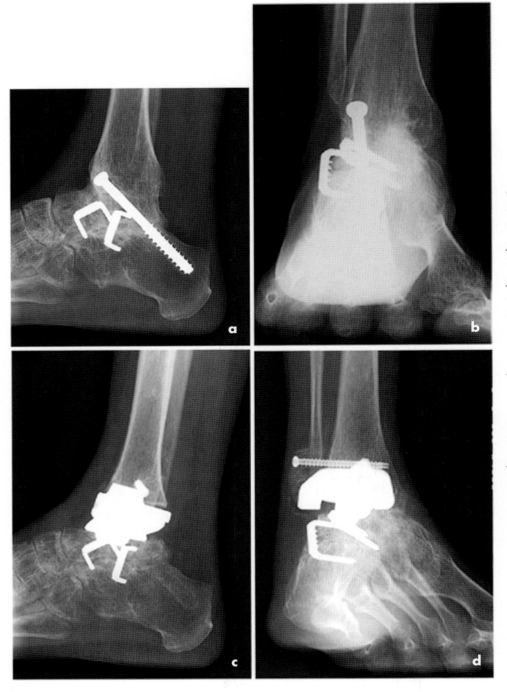

Figure 9–1–30. This patient had undergone multiple prior operations for management of post-traumatic ankle arthritis. The patient had severe midfoot pain, and as an alternative to a below-the-knee amputation, this conversion to an ankle replacement was selected (a, b). This was not an easy procedure given the absence of the fibula, but the block of bone removed for the tibial component was then turned around and secured with one screw to support the prosthesis laterally. The x-ray (XR) images 2 years after the arthroplasty (c, d).

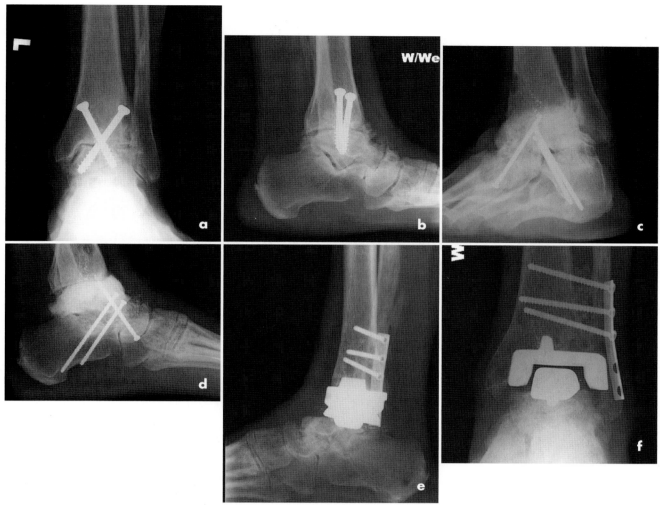

Figure 9–1–31. *This patient presented for treatment of a failed ankle arthrodesis with nonunion and pain in both the ankle and subtalar joints (a, b). As an alternative to revising the ankle with a more extended arthrodesis, this arthrodesis was converted to a total ankle replacement. Because of the bone loss, the latter could not be performed as a single-stage operation and was initiated with a subtalar and talonavicular arthrodesis with cement inserted into the ankle as a temporary spacer (c, d). This was performed and converted 5 months later to a total ankle replacement (e, f).*

arthrodesis, for which conversion to a total ankle replacement can be considered (Fig. 9–1–31).

Suggested Readings

Alvine F. Total ankle replacement. In Myerson MS (ed): Foot and Ankle Disorders. Philadelphia, WB Saunders, 2000.

Easley ME, Vertullo CJ, Urban WC, Nunley JA. Total ankle arthroplasty. J Am Acad Orthop Surg 10:157–167, 2002.

Mroczek KJ, Myerson MS: Perioperative complications of total ankle arthroplasty. Foot Ankle Int 24:17–22, 2003.

Myerson MS, Miller SD. Salvage after complications of total ankle arthroplasty. Foot Ankle Clin 7:191–206, 2002.

Stamatis ED, Myerson MS. How to avoid specific complications of total ankle replacement. Foot Ankle Clin 7:765–789, 2002.

Valderrabano V, Hintermann B, Nigg BM et al. Kinematic changes after fusion and total replacement of the ankle: part 1: Range of motion. Foot Ankle Int 24:881–887, 2003.

Osteotomy of the Tibia and Fibula

Indications

Indications for the supramalleolar osteotomy are numerous and include preservation of limb alignment, correction of deformity, and joint preservation. Supramalleolar osteotomy can also be a staged procedure that leads up to other operations, including total ankle replacement. Osteotomy is performed for correction of a malunion of a distal tibia fracture with or without ankle joint arthritis to beneficially alter or decrease the contact pressures on the degenerated cartilage with mechanical realignment. Osteotomy can be used for preservation of limb alignment as a prelude to a total ankle replacement. One of the prerequisites for a successful total ankle replacement is a balanced mechanical axis of the foot with respect to the lower leg, and a supramalleolar osteotomy works well as a staged procedure for the appropriate patient (Fig. 9–2–1).

The goal of osteotomy in the treatment of ankle arthritis is to shift the loads and redistribute stresses to a part of the ankle joint that is not involved in the degenerative process. The redirection of forces around the tibiotalar joint can be approached either above or below the ankle with osteotomy of the tibia or calcaneus. If either subtalar or supramalleolar deformity is present, the increased stresses on the tibiotalar joint may increase the likelihood of failure. The same concepts of realignment of the tibia apply to malunion after ankle arthrodesis. With the ankle joint fused in equinus, a leg length discrepancy is present because the involved leg is lengthened. This leads to a genu recurvatum thrust on the knee joint, an uneven gait pattern, and increased stress concentration across the midfoot. With the ankle fused in dorsiflexion, repetitive calcaneal impact and stress concentration on the heel pad during the heel strike phase leads to chronic heel pain and gait impairment. Varus malunion of the ankle fusion causes the patient to walk on the lateral side of the foot. This inverted position of the subtalar joint increases the rigidity of the transverse tarsal joints with substantial increase in stress concentration and subsequent degenerative changes and pain (see Fig. 9–2–1). Additionally, stress is increased under the fifth metatarsal head or base, and patients may have painful calluses or sustain stress fractures.

Valgus malunion generates increased stresses along the medial aspect of knee and hindfoot joints. In such a valgus position, the foot becomes more flexible and this results in flatfoot posture. For all of these deformities, a revision of the ankle arthrodesis malunion is required but not at the level of the ankle itself. On the basis of the mechanical axis, a supramalleolar osteotomy is recommended. Correction of ankle valgus deformity in patients with a ball-and-socket ankle joint deformity due to an extensive tarsal coalition is best accomplished with a closing wedge supramalleolar osteotomy. Valgus instability of the ankle always seems to accompany the ball-and-socket ankle joint deformity. The correction of the valgus hindfoot deformity associated with the ankle

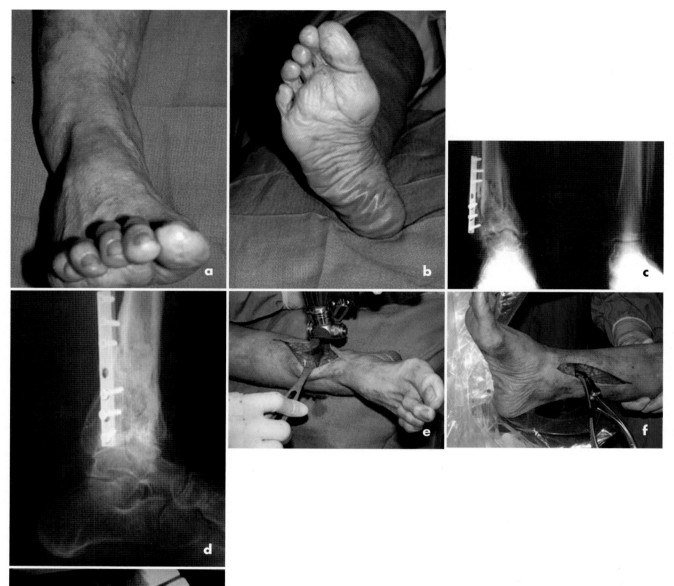

Figure 9–2–1. *A 57-year-old female patient with good but painful ankle motion who did not want an ankle arthrodesis performed. Otherwise she was a good candidate for a total ankle replacement and was prepared to undergo a staged procedure. She already had trauma to the ipsilateral tibia with shortening, and the clinical and radiographic appearance is noted (a–d). Because of the shortening of the limb, an opening wedge tibial osteotomy with structural allograft was performed. Note the use of a saw to cut the tibia (e) and the insertion of a laminar spreader under fluoroscopic control to position the plafond perpendicular to the tibia (f, g).*

instability is best accomplished with a closing wedge medial osteotomy of the distal tibia for realignment, and stabilization of the hindfoot. To this, additional procedures may be considered, including medial sliding translational calcaneus osteotomy to improve the mechanical axis of the subtalar joint (Fig. 9–2–2).

I perform supramalleolar osteotomy as often as possible to preserve hindfoot alignment in cases of deformities due to neuroarthropathy or avascular necrosis of the distal tibia. Correction of neuropathic deformity with distal tibia osteotomy is an excellent alternative to a more extensive hindfoot and ankle arthrodesis,

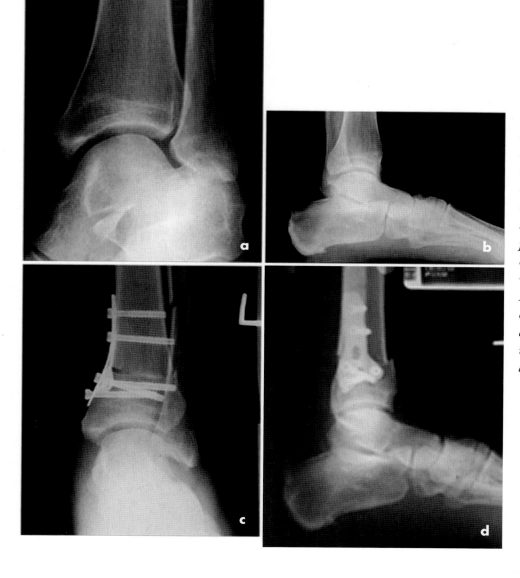

Figure 9–2–2. This ball-and-socket ankle joint deformity caused by a talonavicular coalition was associated with typical hindfoot valgus, subfibular impingement, and pain (a, b). This deformity was corrected with a medial closing wedge supramalleolar osteotomy. Note the marked improvement of the axis of the tibiotalar-calcaneal alignment (c) and the improvement in the height of the arch of the foot (d).

particularly in the setting of neuroarthropathy. Wherever possible, arthrodesis should be avoided in patients with Charcot deformity to prevent added stresses on the remaining hindfoot joints (Fig. 9–2–3).

Preoperative Planning

The opening wedge osteotomy has the advantage of avoiding leg shortening, but delayed union or nonunion may occur. Although the leg length change may not seem significant if only 1 cm of shortening is performed with the wedge resection osteotomy, the length does become significant if an opening wedge osteotomy is performed with a 1-cm graft, when the height differential is almost 2 cm once the graft has healed. If there are skin-related problems (previous incisions with scar formation or prior infection) or any potential for vascular compromise, a closing wedge must be performed. The closing wedge osteotomy has a major disadvantage of limb shortening, and although the osteotomy has been reported to not promote quicker bone healing, my experience is different. By using wedge modifications, a surgeon can correct biplanar deformities. For example, a recurvatum-varus deformity can be corrected either with

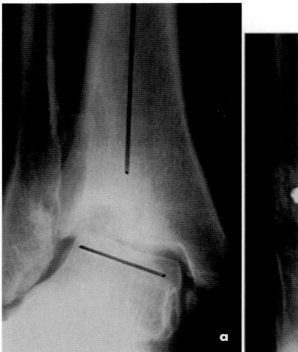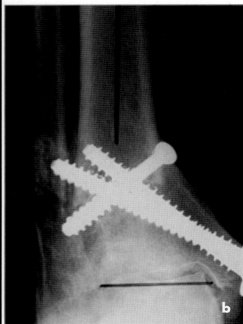

Figure 9–2–3. *This patient had severe diabetic neuroarthropathy with valgus deformity and early ulceration over the medial malleolus (a). Although an arthrodesis of either the ankle or hindfoot could have been performed, a medial closing wedge supramalleolar osteotomy was performed to preserve motion (b). Note that the goal of surgery was accomplished, although a secondary medial translational deformity of the foot was created. The deformity was, however, asymptomatic.*

a posterolaterally based closing wedge osteotomy or with an anteromedially based opening wedge osteotomy. The size of the wedge is determined by drawing the desired correction angle on the preoperative radiographs, measuring the wedge size on a template, and taking magnification into account.

Measuring the center of rotation of angulation (CORA) of the deformity is important. The CORA is located at the intersection of two lines representing the mechanical axes of the proximal and distal segments of the deformity. A closing or opening wedge osteotomy at the level of the CORA leads to complete realignment of the foot and ankle. If the osteotomy is made proximal or distal to the CORA, the center of the ankle translates relative to the mechanical axis of the tibia and creates an unnecessary shift of loads and a clinically obvious zigzag deformity (Fig. 9–2–4).

The osteotomy line should be translated and angulated so that a secondary translational deformity is not created when the osteotomy is intentionally made at a different level than the CORA. A simple example of this is with correction of an equinus malunion of an ankle arthrodesis. In this deformity, the position of the forefoot is fixed relative to the axis of the tibia. The simplest (but not

the best) method of correction is to remove an anterior-based wedge from the distal tibia and close the osteotomy while maintaining the posterior cortex intact as a greenstick-type maneuver. The problem with this type of correction is that the foot has been translated anteriorly relative to the tibia, and with this position of the foot, the mechanical limb axis is no longer aligned or efficient for ambulation.

Bear in mind the extent of compensation that can be achieved by the ankle and subtalar joints after correction. Deformities in the coronal plane are well compensated by the subtalar joint, and deformities in the sagittal plane are well compensated by the ankle joint. For example, a varus deformity of the tibia is compensated by eversion of the subtalar joint. In cases of chronic deformity the subtalar joint may then become stiff. This stiffening is important to recognize before the bone correction; otherwise, the foot ends up in a deformed position after full correction of the distal tibial deformity. If the subtalar joint is very stiff, this correction is not always possible. For the foot to be kept in a plantigrade position, the tibia may have to be undercorrected. Undercorrection is not ideal, and to keep the foot plantigrade, I use a biplanar calcaneal osteotomy or even a triple arthrodesis for correction.

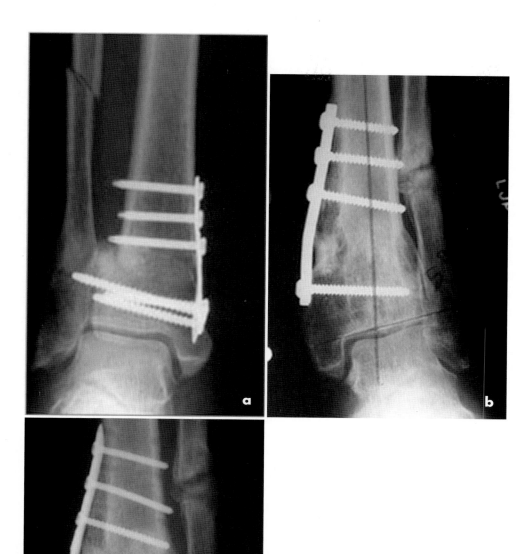

Figure 9–2–4. *The x-ray (XR) images demonstrate incorrect correction of a closing wedge lateral supramalleolar osteotomy (a). Note that the ankle joint is correctly aligned with respect to the floor, but the center of the talus has been translated laterally relative to the axis of the tibia. The valgus deformity in a different patient with post-traumatic arthritis (b) was corrected with a medial closing wedge supramalleolar osteotomy (c), and the center of rotation of angulation (CORA) of the ankle was maintained (c).*

Surgical Technique

For the correction of a varus deformity of the tibia or a varus tibiotalar joint, I prefer a medial opening wedge osteotomy, and I use an anteromedial and a small lateral incision (for the fibular osteotomy). Which cut is made first is a matter of preference, but leaving the fibula intact provides some stability while the tibial cut is completed. When the deformity is minimal, then a greenstick cut of the tibia is made, with the hope that a fibular osteotomy may not need to be performed. This greenstick cut markedly increases the stability of the cut, and the tibia can be opened with a lamina spreader to the desired amount. The advantage of this is that the tibia does not move around after the cut is made, and movement may compromise stability.

The opening wedge osteotomy is performed 4 to 5 cm proximal to the medial malleolar tip (see Fig. 9–2–1). Once the skin incision is made, minimal periosteal stripping that is sufficient only to complete the osteotomy is performed. Make the cut on metaphyseal bone, instead of on the tibia arbitrarily, and have secure fixation. I apply the selected periarticular plate to the distal tibia, ensure that sufficient space is maintained to obtain fixation with three screws distally, mark the osteotomy, and complete it. I keep periosteal stripping to a minimum when the bone cut is made perpendicular to the tibia with a broad oscillating saw, and I preserve the opposite cortex and periosteal sleeve to act as a fulcrum for the opening wedge and to enhance stability. If translation and rotation are also necessary, then the opposite cortex must be cut to allow the distal segment to move. The fibular osteotomy is performed with the lateral incision at the same level as that for the tibial osteotomy, although this location is not critical. A wedge osteotomy of the fibula can be performed if marked angular deformity is present and when a closing lateral wedge of tibia is performed. Although the graft may be harvested from the ipsilateral iliac crest, I prefer to use tricortical structural allograft from a femoral head. Once the osteotomy has been performed, a lamina spreader is inserted to gradually distract the osteotomy to the desired level. This is checked fluoroscopically. The structural bone graft provides immediate mechanical support, with little likelihood of collapse even after resorption, which occurs during revascularization. Some structural integrity remains during the process of

bone graft incorporation to allow the graft to withstand loads. After the deformity has been corrected, the osteotomy is provisionally fixed with K-wires through the periarticular plate, which is applied to the tibia at this time. The alignment is assessed with fluoroscopy. I have found that the periarticular titanium plates (DePuy Ace, Warsaw, Ind) provide excellent stability, contouring, and a low profile alternative to bulkier plate devices. The plate permits the insertion of three screws in the distal segment, and I use fully threaded 4-mm titanium cancellous screws. In the proximal cortex, 3.5-mm titanium cortical screws are used. Fixation of the fibula is variable, although I usually apply a three-hole plate.

The identical concept applies to correction of a valgus deformity in which shortening of the fibula is present. An opening wedge lateral osteotomy of the tibia should be performed instead of a closing wedge medial osteotomy. The reason is that although a closing wedge osteotomy will correct the alignment of the ankle joint, it will not address the shortened fibula, and the mechanics of the ankle will continue to be abnormal (Fig. 9–2–5). By and large the closing wedge osteotomy technique is used when the skin condition is not ideal and when limb shortening is not an issue. The varus deformity is corrected through a single lateral approach over the fibula. After the lateral part of the tibia has been exposed and the osteotomy level has been determined, a K-wire is inserted to the tibia perpendicular to the mechanical axis. A second K-wire is inserted parallel to the ankle joint line intersecting the first K-wire, ideally at the apex of the deformity (Fig. 9–2–6). Once the pins are in place, their position is checked with fluoroscopy, and if the position is satisfactory, the pins can be used as a guide to make the tibial cuts. Adding a medial incision is unnecessary because the tibia can be fixed with percutaneous cannulated screws or a two-hole plate over the lateral anterior cortex. The latter works well if the medial cortex of the tibia is preserved; the plate can act as a tension device.

The closing wedge osteotomy is frequently used to correct valgus deformity of the distal tibia or ankle. The same incision is used as that for a medial opening wedge osteotomy. For these cases, the fibula usually has to be cut and is done so generally at the level or slightly proximal to the tibial osteotomy (Fig. 9–2–7). The key to this osteotomy is to maintain a slight cortical bridge on

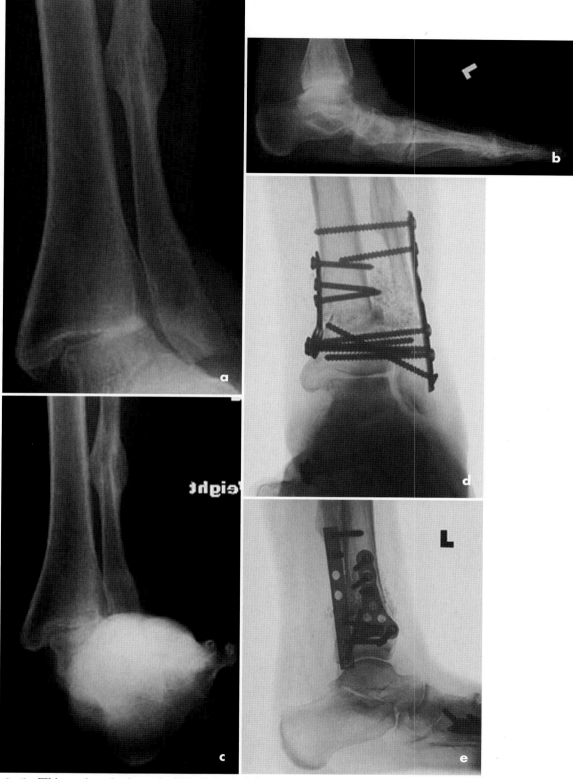

Figure 9–2–5. *This patient had a painfully deformed foot and ankle associated with flatfoot, followed by a stress fracture of the fibula, which worsened the preexisting flatfoot. The patient already had a painful contralateral foot after a pantalar fusion, and an arthrodesis of this ankle was not thought to be ideal (a–c). An opening wedge osteotomy of the tibia and fibula was performed through a lengthening of the fibula and the tibia with a structural allograft, and then an arthrodesis of the tibiofibular syndesmosis was created (d, e). The alternative would have been to have used a closing wedge medial osteotomy, and this decision was based on the skin condition, the length of the limb, and issues pertaining to the likelihood of bone healing and vascularity.*

Figure 9–2–6. A closing lateral wedge supramalleolar osteotomy combined with ankle ligament reconstruction was performed in this 60-year-old patient for management of varus deformity of the hindfoot and ankle, associated with ankle instability. Despite evidence of arthritis on the x-ray (XR) film (a–c), the patient had minimal pain. Despite the slight improvement in the appearance of the alignment of the ankle joint, arthritis is still present (d). Attempting correction of the ankle with a supramalleolar osteotomy is unrealistic when a defect is within the distal tibial articular surface. Stability was present for this patient, and 4 years later, a total ankle replacement was performed.

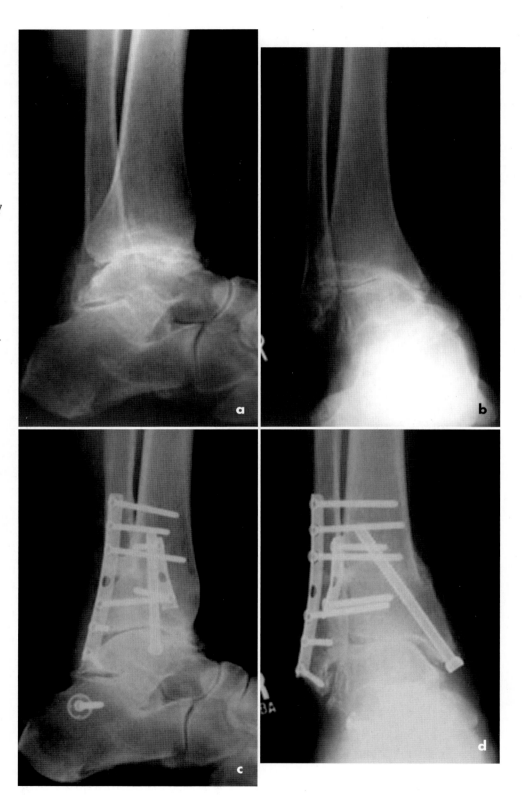

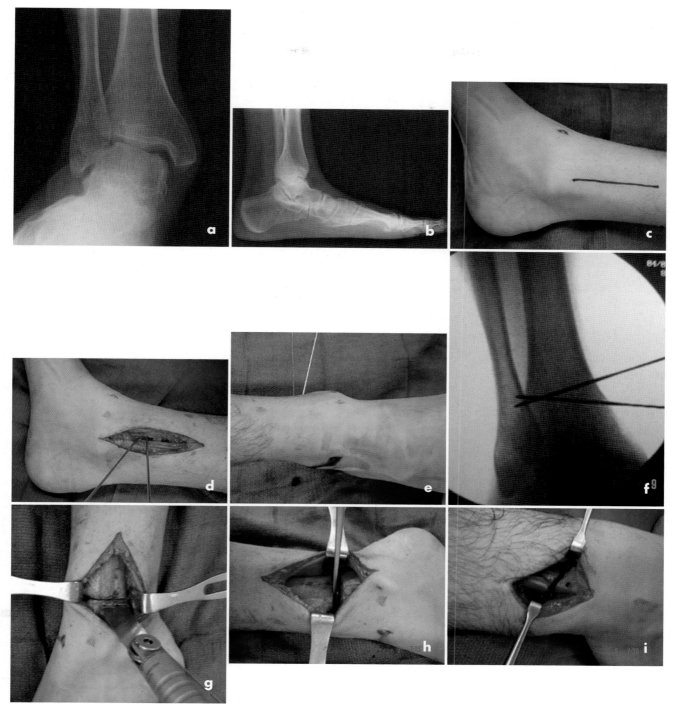

Figure 9–2–7. *A medial closing wedge supramalleolar osteotomy was performed in this 17-year-old patient for management of premature lateral physeal closure that caused severe subsequent valgus of the ankle associated with a flatfoot (a, b). The incision is marked out (c), followed by insertion of two guide pins, one perpendicular to the tibia and the other parallel with the articular surface of the tibia (d–f). The pins should meet at the lateral border of the tibia, and the osteotomy should preferably not cut through the lateral tibia. A greenstick-type fracture should be created first with a saw, then with an osteotome (g). For the tibial alignment to be maintained over the center of the talus, the tibia had to be slightly translated laterally, and an oblique osteotomy of the fibular had to be performed (h, i).*

Continued

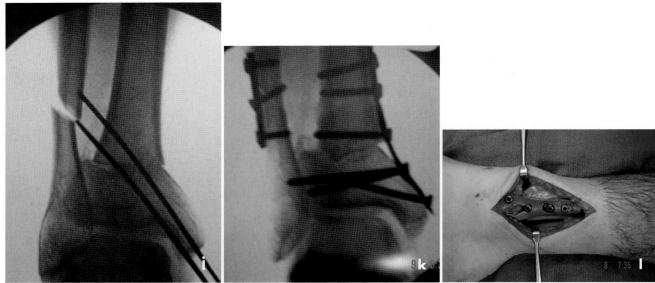

Figure 9–2–7, cont'd. *Guide pins were then inserted across the tibial osteotomy, and the position was confirmed fluoroscopically (j). Note the lateral translation of the distal tibia relative to the axis of the talus. A lateral notch is in the distal tibial osteotomy where the distal segment interdigitates (k). A medial periarticular plate was applied (DePuy, Warsaw, Ind) (l), followed by application of a one-third tubular plate on the fibular.*

the lateral tibia that will markedly facilitate correction and maintain alignment. If a secondary translational deformity is created by the osteotomy, then the lateral cortical bridge will have to be cut to shift the tibia laterally (see Fig. 9–2–7). The guide pins for the osteotomy are inserted perpendicular to the axis of the tibia and parallel with the ankle joint, and the cut is made either inside or outside the guide pins according to the amount of bone to be resected. Additional pins are inserted after removal of the bone wedge to hold the position of the osteotomy, which is checked fluoroscopically, and in particular to ensure that the alignment is correct in both the coronal and sagittal planes. A periarticular plate (DePuy, Warsaw, Ind) is applied to the tibia (Fig. 9–2–7k), and the stability is checked because an additional lateral plate or crossed cannulated screws may be used as required. If the tibia is shifted laterally to avoid a secondary medial translational deformity, the osteotomy of the fibula will have a gap, and it should be fixed with a two- or three-hole one-third tubular plate.

Ankle Osteoarticular Allograft Replacement

This procedure is indicated for patients with end-stage arthritis and for whom either an arthrodesis or total ankle replacement is not ideal. Generally, patients are unsuitable candidates for these procedures because of their age, activity level, weight, and desire for continued mobility of the ankle. The most significant aspect of planning this operation involves the potential for failure. Certainly, a primary ankle arthrodesis has a recognized success rate from a technical standpoint that should be greater than 95%. If one resorts to a secondary ankle arthrodesis after failure of an osteoarticular allograft replacement, clearly this success rate is due less to the need for a structural allograft. The other options after failure are to repeat the graft procedure and to perform a total ankle replacement. These procedures are much easier, assuming that the appropriate indication for an ankle replacement is met.

Tissue typing is not involved with this procedure, and although immune antibodies are discernible with laboratory testing, no rejection of the graft occurs. If failure does occur, it is due to fracture or failure to heal the bone graft at the talus graft interface. Late failure has not yet been dealt with because this procedure is still in its infancy and we only have 2 to 4 years of experience with these osteoarticular grafts. A most important aspect of planning surgery involves the correct sizing of the graft. Correct sizing is critical to successful outcome, and the graft must fit perfectly. Although size matching is necessary, if the graft is a few millimeters too small, the fit

nonetheless works because the "fit" occurs between the articular surfaces of the tibia and the talus, not between the host surface area. However, if the graft is too large, it will not fit at all, and for the graft to be inserted, the fibula has to be sprung apart from the syndesmosis. Although this procedure is technically feasible, it will clearly not lead to a desirable outcome over the long term.

The incision is identical to that for total ankle replacement with an anterior central midline incision over the ankle. Once the joint has been exposed and denuded of all juxta-articular osteophytes, the cutting block for the agility ankle is inserted on the tibia. The sizing of the cutting block is not important, but the position on the medial side of the joint is critical. Judging the position of the cutting block according to the lateral side of the ankle, which is not cut, is unimportant. The position of the block must be verified carefully fluoroscopically, and minor adjustments must be made until the block is positioned to remove approximately one half of the medial malleolus and 8 mm of the distal tibial surface.

The cut is initiated, and the only difference between this cut and the total ankle cut is that the syndesmosis and the fibula is preserved. With this cut, protection of the fibula is difficult, unlike like that in a total ankle replacement, because no osteotome can be inserted through the syndesmosis. For this reason, I cut only the anterior lateral tibia and then complete this under direct vision with an osteotome while protecting the articular surface of the fibula. Sometimes the fibular articular surface is abnormal because of articular wear or deformity, such as shortening or external rotation. I do not normally disturb the fibula, although clearly for some cases, an osteotomy of the fibula may be required to restore length and correct rotational deformity simultaneously. Once the cutting block is correctly positioned, the cuts are made in a standard manner as for total ankle replacement with the exception of the anterolateral tibia, which is only perforated. The bone is then carefully pried off the tibia, while fracture of the medial malleolus is avoided. The remaining lateral tibia is then removed in segments with a small osteotome until the entire joint is visible (Fig. 9–3–1).

The talar cut is made freehand with removal of an 8-mm thickness in the center of the dome of the talus. Making the cut more distally into the neck of the talus is sometimes advantageous, but the advantage depends to some extent on the local anatomy. The more distal cut facilitates screw insertion into the neck of the allograft (Fig. 9–3–2).

The tibial graft is then sized, and the cutting block is applied to the tibia fluoroscopically. All soft tissue is debrided off the margins of the tibia (Fig. 9–3–3). The same precise cut is made on the donor graft with removal of the same amount of tibia, particularly medially. I have no problem removing an excessive amount of bone off the distal tibia and then shaving this to a perfect cut once the size match is confirmed on the

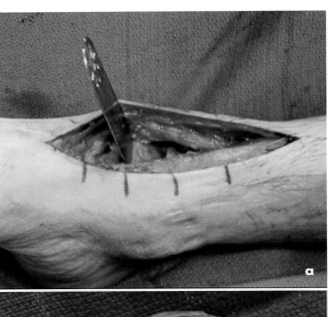

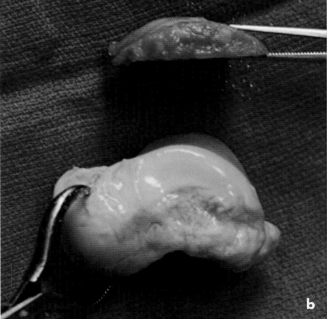

Figure 9–3–2. The talus is partially cut about 4 mm, and a free saw blade is inserted into the bone cut, which is then checked fluoroscopically. This checking is similar to that for a total ankle replacement cut on the talus (a). The talar graft is sized according to the bone resected and is cut freehand (b).

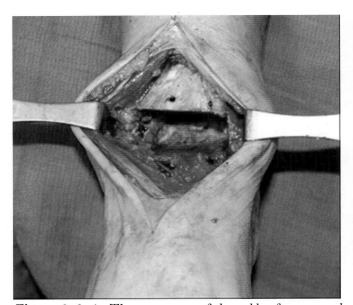

Figure 9–3–1. The appearance of the ankle after removal of the tibia and talus. Except for the preservation of the fibula, the cut on the tibia and medial malleolus is similar to that for total ankle replacement.

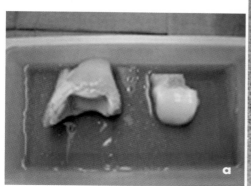
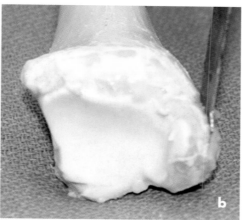

Figure 9–3–3. The graft is carefully preserved during the operation and is then cleaned of all soft tissue before the bone cuts are made (a, b).

patient. However, making one precise cut on the tibial allograft is easier (Fig. 9–3–4). The tibial graft rarely fits perfectly because of the anatomic constraints of the anterior and posterior ankle and the position of the fibula posterolaterally. Generally, therefore, the tibial graft has to be cut so that it is 6 to 8 mm wider anteriorly than posteriorly. The graft is then slotted into place, and minor adjustments can be made to ensure a perfect fit.

The cut on the talar allograft is made freehand, again to the size of the ankle. Cutting sufficient talus to prevent fracture is important. If I had to err in one direction or another, I would remove a smaller amount of host tibia and more of the talus than the other way around. The tibia always incorporates and heals rapidly in contrast to the talar dome. The position of the graft must now be checked fluoroscopically. The talus needs to be centered, under the tibia, and the graft tends to position itself perfectly with forced passive dorsiflexion of the ankle as the talus finds its resting position under the tibial articular surface. The tibial graft is then secured with the two 4 mm screws (DePuy, Warsaw, Ind.), and the talus can be fixed with a bioresorbable pin, which is inserted through the anterior aspect of the articular surface of the talus. Alternatively, if more talus is cut from the graft, then some of the neck of the talus may be present through which the screws can be inserted.

The tibial graft tends to open slightly posteriorly, but this gap does not seem to be a problem because it fills in during healing. If the tibia is not in good apposition,

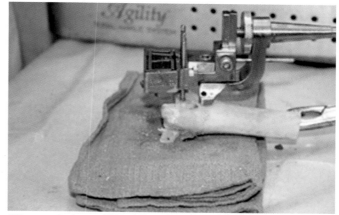

Figure 9–3–4. The tibia is cut through the cutting block of the Agility ankle replacement (DePuy, Warsaw, Ind.).

then this gap may be backfilled with cancellous graft, although this is clearly not ideal because a good size match to begin with is preferable (Fig. 9–3–5). A slight posterior gap is sometimes a result of an incorrect plane of the tibial cut on the allograft, but it does not seem to present a problem. It may also occur as a result of the plane of screw insertion from the anterior aspect of the graft into the posterior tibia, and to avoid this, I have changed the plane of the screw insertion from the anterior tibia superiorly into the posterior aspect of the tibial graft inferiorly (Fig. 9–3–6).

Weight bearing is delayed for approximately 8 weeks. Starting range-of-motion exercises as soon as they can be tolerated is important, and once the incision is healed, water activities with fins are encouraged. One of the marked advantages of this procedure is the

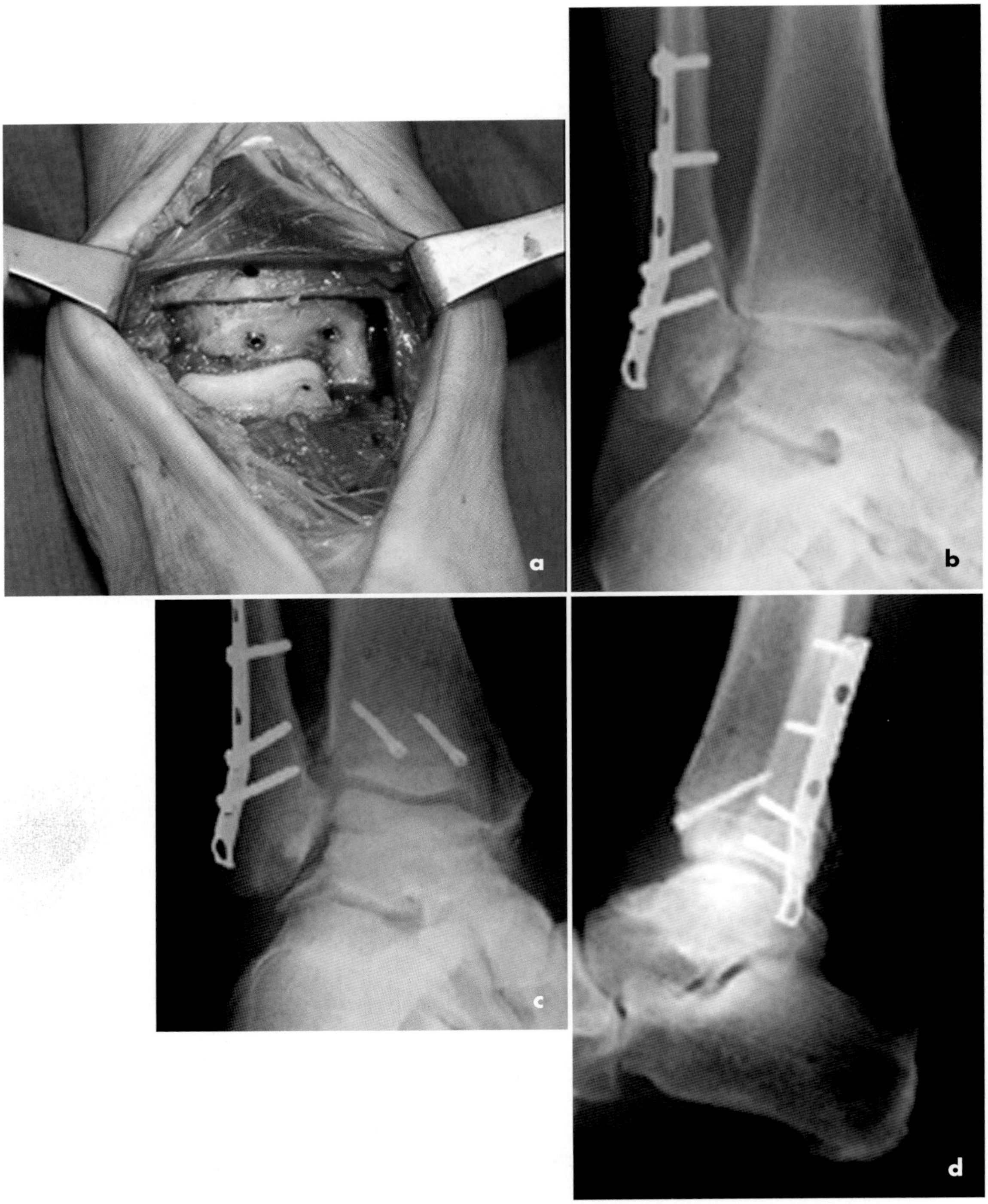

Figure 9–3–5. *Note the good apposition of the tibia with respect to the talus and the poor fit medially, where a gap is noted (a). This gap was filled with cancellous graft. The preoperative (b) and postoperative radiographs (c, d) show a complete filling in of the defect medially.*

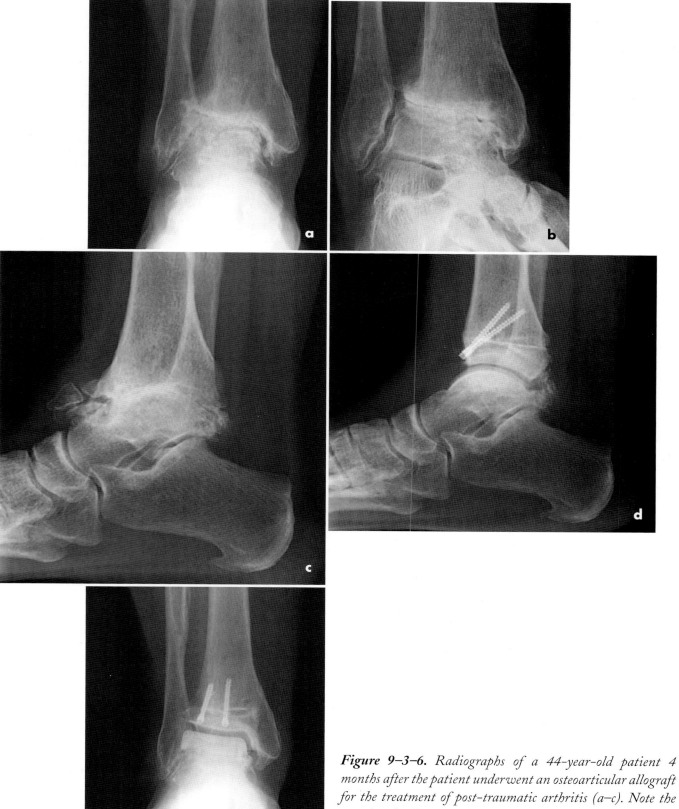

Figure 9-3-6. *Radiographs of a 44-year-old patient 4 months after the patient underwent an osteoarticular allograft for the treatment of post-traumatic arthritis (a–c). Note the complete healing and incorporation of the tibial graft, and although healing of the talus graft is noted, bone density remains abnormal (d, e).*

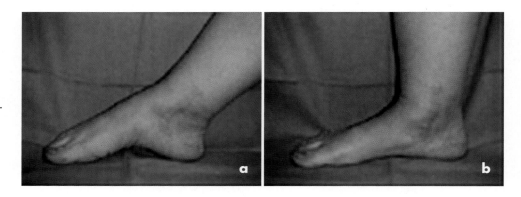

Figure 9–3–7. The range of motion following an osteoarticular allograft 2 years after surgery is noted in plantar flexion (a) and with standing (b).

tremendous and rapid improvement in both symptoms and motion that patients report. This improvement has been far quicker, more satisfying, and more encouraging for the patients and has allowed the surgeons to see how these patients have fared, particularly in the short term.

Range of motion improves dramatically, and for patients with severe post-traumatic arthritis for whom an ankle replacement does not yield good motion, this procedure is associated with a far better recovery of motion (Fig. 9–3–7).

Reconstruction of Malunited Ankle Fractures

The premise for reconstruction of a malunited ankle fracture is based on joint preservation. Frequently, the joint may appear to be irreparable with articular wear and erosive changes on the medial or lateral plafond. However, even with these more advanced cases, restoring the alignment of the ankle is worthwhile. Most of these cases involve a malunion, a nonunion, or both of the fibula. Occasionally, the medial malleolus or posterior tibia is also involved in this malunited fracture and requires simultaneous correction. Lateral weight-bearing x-ray (XR) images of the ankle and a computed axial tomography (CT) scan are helpful to plan the reconstruction. The CT scan is not necessary, but it does aid in determining the rotation of the fibula that needs to be performed.

A decision needs to be made whether arthroscopic debridement of the joint is to be performed simultaneously. Debridement is unnecessary unless I suspect a posterior and inaccessible chondral defect that is not going to be visible with arthrotomy. Arthrotomy is routinely performed medially because the malunited fibula is generally associated with a lateral translational deformity of the talus. The hypertrophic tissue between the medial malleolus and the talus must be excised from the medial gutter for the reposition of the talus. Surprisingly, minimum amounts of tissue in the medial gutter can actually block the correct medial shift of the talus back into the mortise.

A vertical incision is made medial to the anterior tibial tendon directly over the anterior notch of the medial ankle over a 2-cm length. The incision is deepened through the joint. Then the capsule is incised, and the hypertrophic synovium, capsule, and scar are excised completely from the medial gutter. The insertion of a rongeur is useful; it should be turned around 180 degrees to ensure that the medial gutter is completely free and that the talus is mobile. The medial gutter will again be checked subsequently for correction of the fibula as the talus is pushed over medially.

An extensile excision is now made laterally directly over the fibula, frequently corresponding to the original incision that was made. Existing hardware is removed. The key to the operation now is to obtain the correct length and rotation of the distal fibula. These are easy to judge by virtue of the bimalleolar axis, which should be measured out and planned preoperatively on the basis of the contralateral normal ankle. However, correction of the external rotation, which is usually present, is not as easy. If healing of the fibula is complete, then an osteotomy has to be performed. This should be done at a level so that adequate fixation can be applied distally. Usually, I apply a seven-hole plate on the fibula to ensure at least three screws distally, and the osteotomy should be made proximal to this. The ideal lateral plate is a specially designed fibular plate (DePuy Ace, Warsaw, Ind.), which is a combination of a one-third tubular plate and a dynamic compression plate (DCP) designed to fit over the fibula.

The plane of the fibular osteotomy can be either exactly transverse or oblique. The advantage of a transverse osteotomy is that lengthening of the fibula is far easier to obtain with this type of osteotomy. This is particularly the case if the fibula is short and needs to be lengthened with a lamina spreader. If a transverse osteotomy in the fibula is made, structural interpositional bone graft should be used, provided, of course, that shortening of the fibula is present. Occasionally, external rotation of the fibula is present without shortening, and an internal rotational osteotomy is performed without lengthening (Fig. 9–4–1).

The alternative is to lengthen the fibula with an oblique osteotomy and to slide the fibula more distally. The better bone contact may obviate the need for an interpositional bone graft. With either type of osteotomy, the syndesmosis needs to be taken down to facilitate the actual lengthening. The tissues surrounding the fibula are stripped, the periosteum is com-

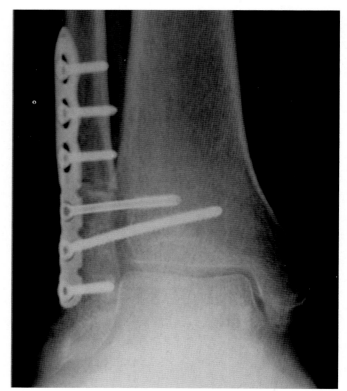

Figure 9–4–1. *An internal rotational osteotomy was performed for this malunion of the fibula without shortening, and no bone graft was used.*

pletely elevated, and then the fibula is mobilized on its distal pedicle. If a transverse osteotomy is made, a lamina spreader is inserted in the osteotomy site, the fibula is distracted, and then provisional fixation is obtained from the fibula into both the talus and the distal tibia to lock the fibula at the correct length (Fig. 9–4–2).

The position of the fibula is then checked fluoroscopically. Axial lengthening is easier to obtain without internal rotation, but some rotation is usually required. For control of the length and rotation, a bone reduction clamp should be applied to the distal fibula while it is lengthened with the lamina spreader. Then the clamp should be internally rotated to facilitate insertion of the guide pins into the fibula to hold it in position (Fig. 9–4–3).

If an oblique osteotomy is preferred, then the plane of the osteotomy should be made over a length of about 2 cm, with the cut beginning proximal lateral, then going to distal and medial, and ending proximal to the joint. The fibula is stripped of soft tissues in the same manner, and then the plate is applied to the distal fibula. With the plate in position, a screw is then inserted into the fibula, proximal to the plate, and then a lamina spreader is positioned between this screw and either the plate or one of the more distal screws to facilitate the lengthening. Internal rotation is performed in a similar manner with a bone reduction clamp, and then the fibula needs to be held in position with guide pins. As noted, this type of lengthening does not always require a structural or interpositional bone graft. Nonetheless, the plane of the osteotomy is such that once the distal fibula is internally rotated, apposition of the osteotomy site is not perfect, and some form of cancellous grafting may be required.

Depending on the magnitude and associated deformity, and the bone quality, I often include the syndesmosis in the fixation and occasionally attempt an arthrodesis of the syndesmosis, facilitated with debridement with a burr (Fig. 9–4–4). If an arthrodesis is not performed, then at the very least, multiple screws will be used from the fibula across into the tibia to provide more rigid and stable fixation (Fig. 9–4–5).

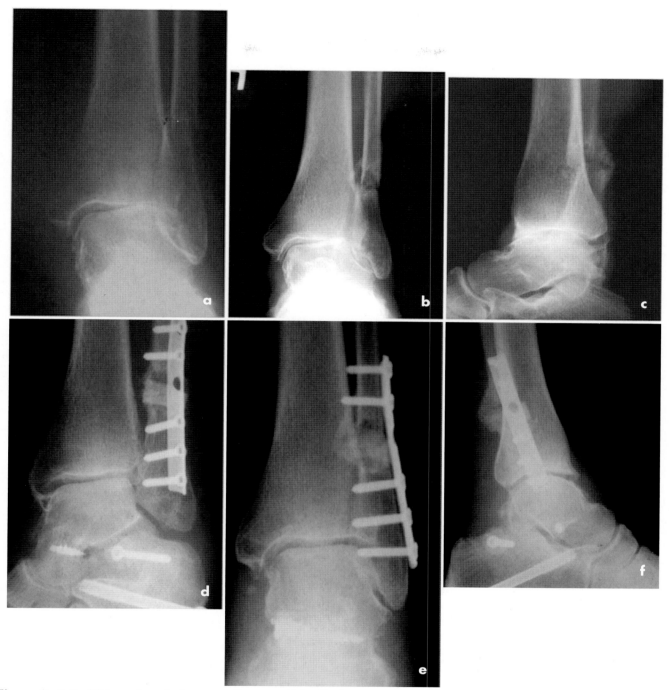

Figure 9–4–2. *This patient had a stress fracture of the fibula as a result of a valgus ankle deformity (a). Over a short period, despite immobilization, a nonunion developed with further deformity occurring (b, c). This nonunion was treated with a lengthening osteotomy of the fibula with interposition bone graft, a medial translational osteotomy of the calcaneus, and a deltoid ligament reconstruction with a tendon allograft (d–f).*

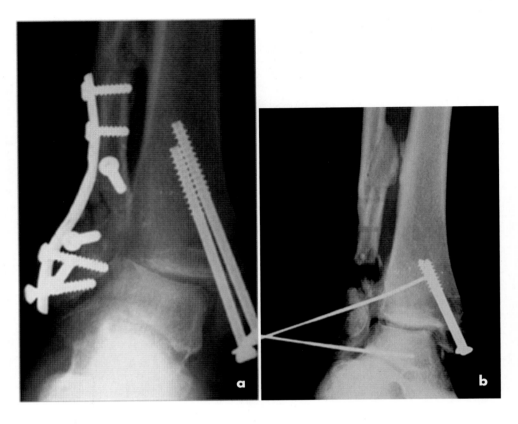

Figure 9–4–3. Despite the severity of this deformity, reconstruction is worthwhile (a). In this patient, revision of both the medial and lateral ankle was performed after debridement of the medial joint gutter. Note that the fibula is then held in position with guide pins, and the alignment is checked (b).

Figure 9–4–4. A burr can be used to prepare the syndesmosis for arthrodesis after stabilization with a plate and screws.

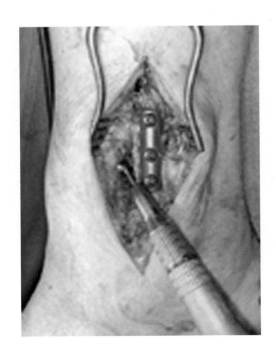

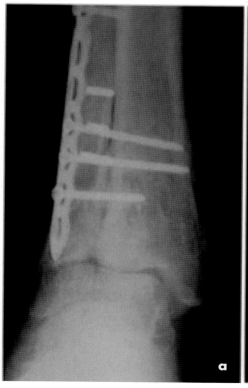
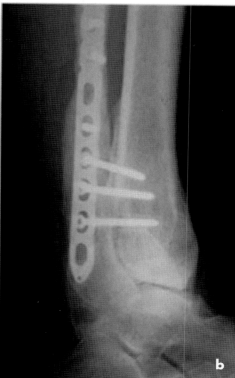

Figure 9–4–5. *A lengthening osteotomy of the fibula was performed with a sliding oblique osteotomy, followed by stabilization of the syndesmosis with three lag screws (a, b).*

Techniques, tips, and pitfalls

1. Correction of malunion is worth the effort despite marked deformity. The ankle seems to be forgiving with respect to deformity in some patients, and corrective osteotomy provides pain relief despite the appearance of arthritis.

2. The length of the fibula and its rotation must be restored. Internal rotation is usually necessary to correct malunion of the fibula.

3. Rarely, if the deformity is significant, then a slight medial closing wedge osteotomy of the tibia may be performed, in addition to the lengthening osteotomy of the fibula (Fig. 9–4–6).

4. If a malunion of the medial malleolus is present, it, in addition to the fibular osteotomy, needs to be addressed. This may involve either an ostectomy of the medial malleolus or an osteotomy (Fig. 9–4–7). If an ostectomy is performed, this usually detaches the superficial deltoid ligament, which can be reattached through K-wire holes in the malleolus. Rarely will the deep deltoid ligament be disrupted with this ostectomy (Fig. 9–4–8).

5. If the deformity of the medial joint cannot be corrected, the lateral side of the ankle should be corrected, particularly if a nonunion is present (Fig. 9–4–9).

6. I use adjunctive bone grafting, either a cancellous graft or a supplement with demineralized bone matrix, for the syndesmosis.

7. Some injuries necessitate an osteotomy of the medial malleolus, the fibula, or even the anterior distal tibia. These osteotomies have been covered in the approaches to the ankle in the section on osteochondral injury. However, a window can be removed from the distal tibia to perform the bone grafting in patients who have avascular necrosis of a segment of the distal tibia. The window can be made in a number of ways, preserving the articular surface or incorporating the articular segment into the window. The window is made large enough, however,

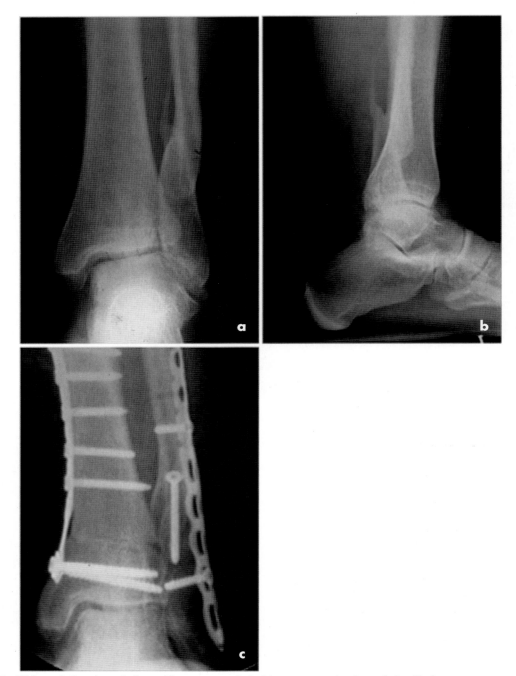

Figure 9–4–6. *Valgus deformity of the ankle accompanied this severe malunion of the fibula with shortening (a, b). A closing wedge osteotomy of the tibia was performed simultaneously with the osteotomy of the fibula (c).*

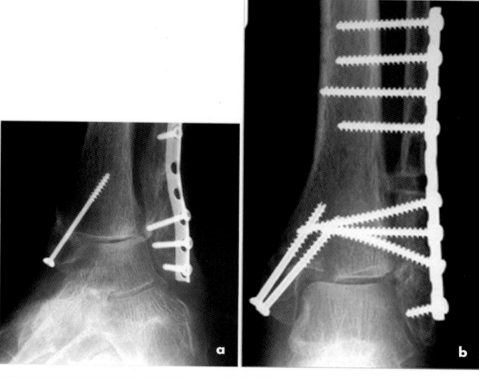

Figure 9–4–7. This malunion involved both malleoli, which were corrected with medial and lateral osteotomies (a). Although a step off persists medially, the alignment of the ankle was much improved (b).

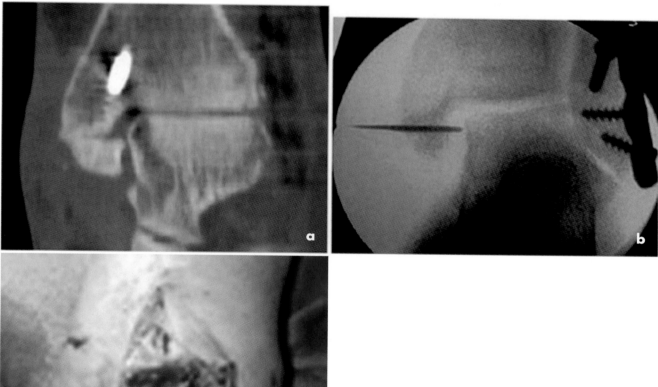

Figure 9–4–8. This malunion of the medial malleolus was noted best on computed axial tomography (CT) scan (a). During the operation the level of the malleolar ostectomy was marked fluoroscopically (b), and the tip of the malleolus was excised (c).

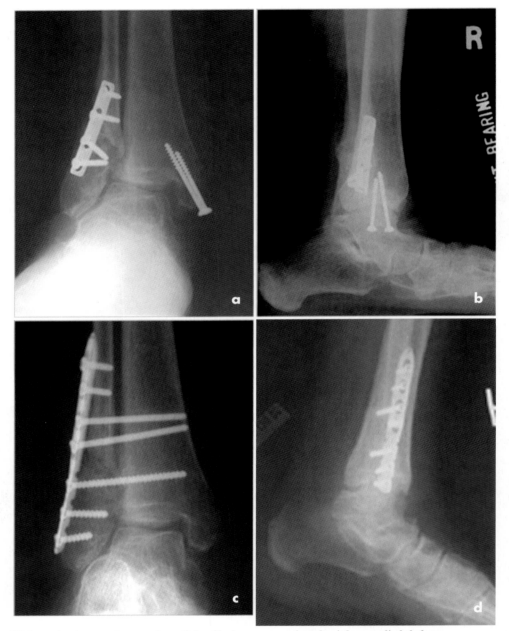

Figure 9–4–9. *This malunion and nonunion of the fibula was associated with a medial defect of the plafond that could not be corrected (a, b), and the revision focused on the correction of alignment of the fibula only (c, d).*

so that it can be replaced with screws (Fig. 9–4–10).

8. An osteotomy of the tibia and fibula can be performed in some individuals with post-traumatic malunion and deformity, and the medial malleolus malunion can be ignored (Fig. 9–4–11).

9. A ring fixator may provide optimal correction for supramalleolar deformity following malunion, particularly in the presence of neuropathy (Fig. 9–4–12).

Text continued on p. 281

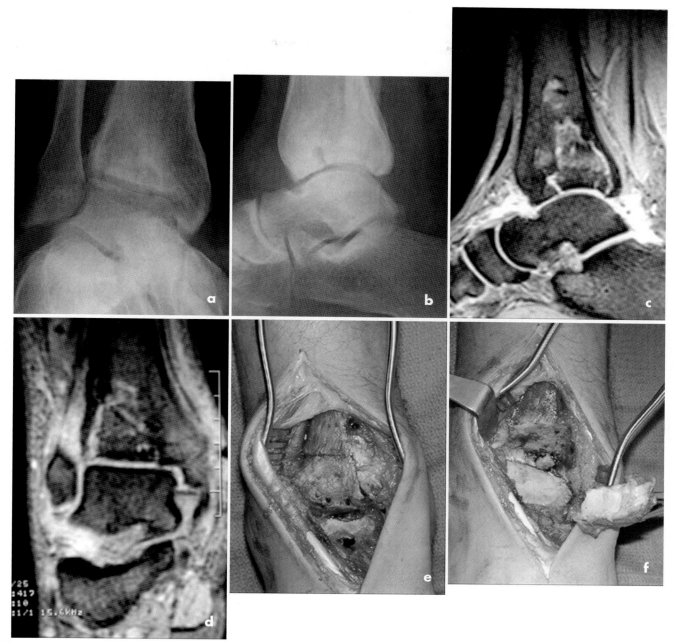

Figure 9–4–10. *This deformity of the distal tibia was associated with osteonecrosis following trauma (a–d). An anterior approach to the ankle was used to perform the arthrotomy and osteotomy of the distal tibia, with a window made in the supramalleolar region (e–f).*

Continued

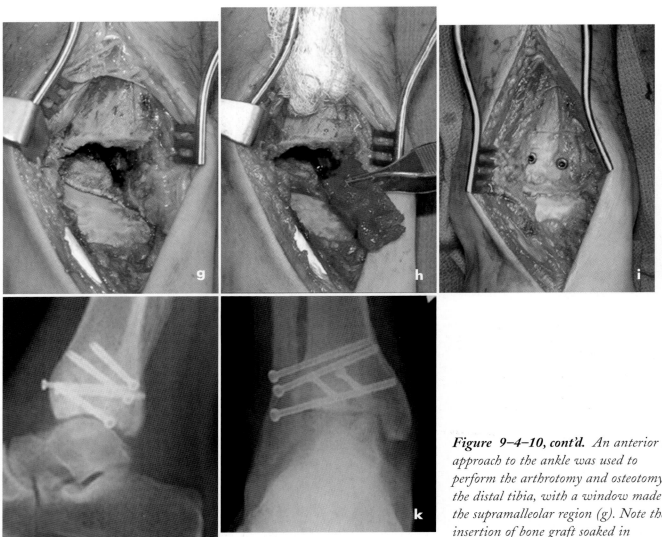

Figure 9–4–10, cont'd. *An anterior approach to the ankle was used to perform the arthrotomy and osteotomy of the distal tibia, with a window made in the supramalleolar region (g). Note the insertion of bone graft soaked in Symphony (DePuy, Warsaw, Ind.) (h), followed by replacement of the tibial window with cannulated screws (i–k).*

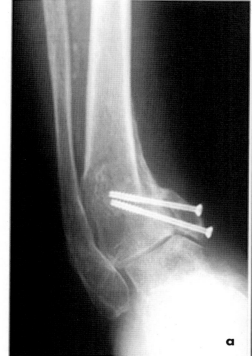

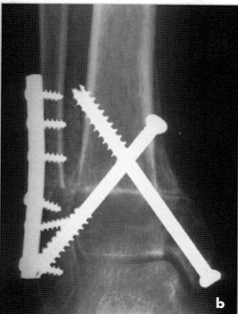

Figure 9–4–11. *Despite the marked deformity present, this patient with neuropathy was prepared to accept the shortening required to perform a lateral closing wedge osteotomy of the tibia and fibula for this severe malunion (a). Note that despite the malunion of the medial malleolus, alignment is acceptable (b).*

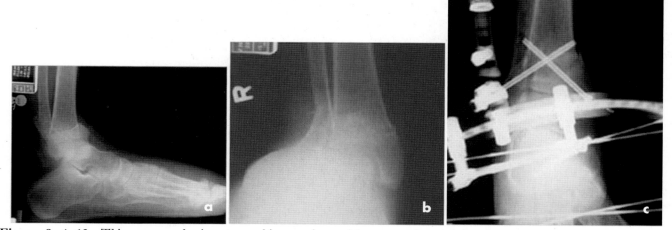

Figure 9–4–12. *This severe malunion occurred in a patient with neuropathy, peripheral vascular disease, and skin ulceration (a, b). In addition to a ring fixator (DePuy Ace, Warsaw, Ind.), percutaneous cannulated screws were used to add stability (c).*

Continued

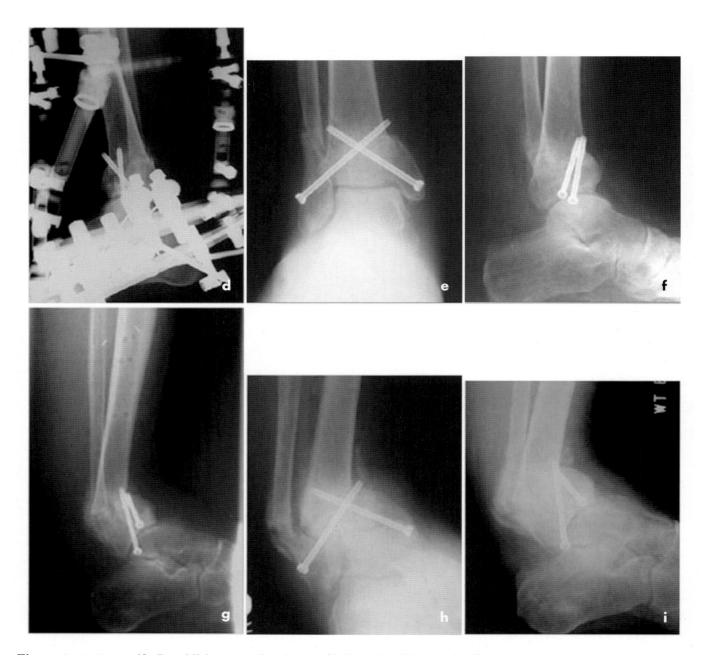

Figure 9–4–12, cont'd. *In addition to a ring fixator (DePuy Ace, Warsaw, Ind.), percutaneous screws were used to add stability (d). The fixator was removed at 4 months (e, f), but despite immobilization, further deformity ensued (g, h) and became even worse over the next month (i).*

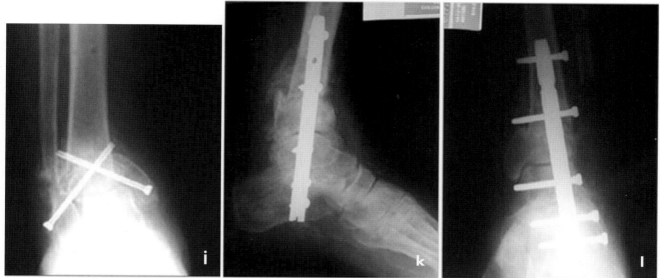

Figure 9–4–12, cont'd. *Deformity became worse over the next month (j). Finally, an intramedullary rod was used to perform a tibiotalocalcaneal arthrodesis (VersaNail, DePuy, Warsaw, Ind.) (k, l).*

Suggested Readings

Paley D, Herzenberg JE. Applications of external fixation to foot and ankle reconstruction. In Myerson MS (ed): Foot and Ankle Disorders. Philadelphia, WB Saunders, 2000.

Stamatis ED, Cooper PS, Myerson MS. Supramalleolar osteotomy for the treatment of distal tibial angular deformities and arthritis of the ankle joint. Foot Ankle Int 24:754–764, 2003.

Stamatis ED, Myerson MS. Supramalleolar osteotomy: Indications and technique. Foot Ankle Clin 8:317–333, 2003.

Steffensmeier SJ, Saltzman CL, Berbaum KS, Brown TD. Effects of medial and lateral displacement calcaneal osteotomies on tibiotalar joint contact stresses. J Orthop Res 14:980–985, 1996.

Takakura Y, Takaoka T, Tanaka Y, et al. Results of opening-wedge osteotomy for the treatment of a posttraumatic varus deformity of the ankle. J Bone Joint Surg Am 80:213–218, 1998.

Takakura Y, Tanaka Y, Kumai T, Tamai S. Low tibial osteotomy for osteoarthritis of the ankle. Results of a new operation in 18 patients. J Bone Joint Surg Br 77:50–54, 1995.

Tarr RR, Resnick CT, Wagner KS, Sarmiento A. Changes in tibiotalar joint contact areas following experimentally induced tibial angular deformities. Clin Orthop Oct(199):72–80, 1985.

Ting AJ, Tarr RR, Sarmiento A, et al. The role of subtalar motion and ankle contact pressure changes from angular deformities of the tibia. Foot Ankle 7:290–299, 1987.

Disorders of the Achilles Tendon

Insertional Achilles Tendinopathy, Retrocalcaneal Bursitis and Haglund's Syndrome

In this chapter tendinopathies are discussed from a practical standpoint as insertional or not insertional. To some extent, the nonoperative treatments are similar and involve rehabilitation with isokinetic strengthening, physical therapy modalities with stretching, orthotic support, and anti-inflammatory medication. Once nonoperative methods have failed, the next decision to be made has to be the type of incision used to approach insertional tendinopathy. I make this decision according to the extent of the underlying disease, the presence of tendon degeneration, and the location of maximum tenderness. If osteophytes are present on the posterior central aspect of the heel, then I use a central splitting incision of the posterior Achilles tendon and calcaneus. This incision works well, and the entire broad plate of the osteophyte can be removed. Use of this Achilles splitting incision is advantageous because it allows direct visualization of the disease and ease of dissection of the torn portion of the tendon with removal of the osteophyte. However, this invasion is associated with a more prolonged recovery.

If the pain is not posterocentral, the incision should be made medially or laterally because the irritated or torn portion of the tendon may not be visible from the central or posterior splitting incision. If no large osteophyte is present in the posterior calcaneus and thickening and degeneration of the tendon are diffuse, then a medial or lateral incision is made to debride the retrocalcaneal space and decrease the impingement of the calcaneus against the Achilles tendon (Figs 10–1–1 and 10–1–2).

The operation is performed with the patient under local anesthesia and in a prone position. A 4-cm vertical incision is made directly over the tendon extending toward the junction of the plantar heel skin. The incision is deepened through the tendon, which is split longitudinally, and the incision is deepened directly onto bone, even inferiorly. The central portion of the tendon is the location of maximum degeneration, and this can be exposed either through a vertical ellipse or by a split of the tendon and its separation with a retractor. The enlarged osteophyte is visible below the central portion of the degenerated tendon, and this is excised with an osteotome. The dorsal posterior surface of the calcaneus must be smoothed down to remove any irritation on the anterior aspect of the Achilles tendon insertion. The tendon must be repaired with a running locking suture. If significant degeneration and tearing of the tendon are noted and the tendon could be separated off the calcaneus, then a suture anchor can be used to help with the reattachment of the tendon. Usually, however, this is not necessary because wide bands of the tendon, inserted both medially and laterally, prevent rupture. Removal of up to one third of the central aspect of the tendon does

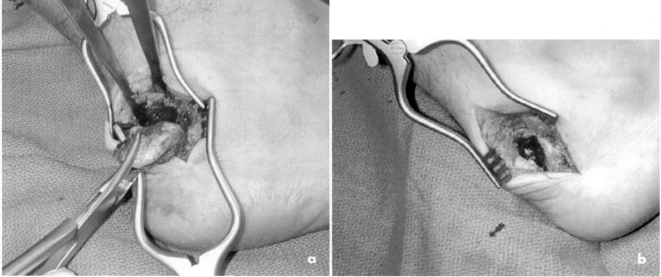

Figure 10–1–1. A small lateral incision is sufficient to treat the postero-supero-lateral impingement (Haglund's syndrome), which was used in this patient to excise the bone mass superolaterally (a, b).

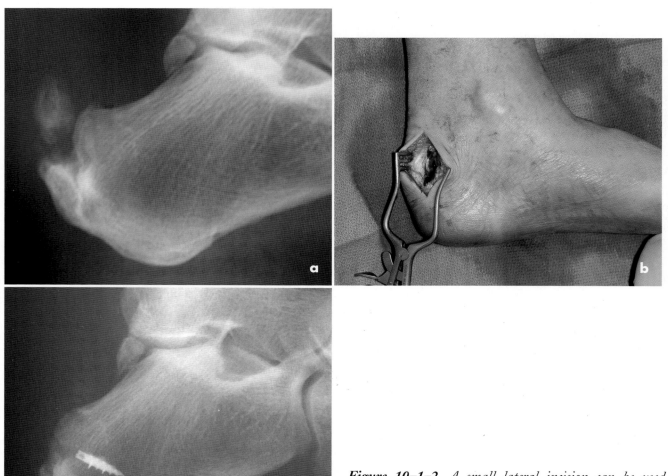

Figure 10–1–2. A small lateral incision can be used to debride chronic insertional tendinopathy successfully (a–c). The bone was excised through this lateral incision, and the anchor was inserted to hold the lateral border of the tendon attached.

not disrupt its attachment whatsoever, and possibly up to one half of the tendon insertion can be detached (Fig. 10–1–3).

The only concern that I have with this condition (whether or not it is related to the use of the central splitting incision) is the length of the recovery time. These patients can take up to 1 year to completely recover and return to full function. The advantages of the central splitting incision are the direct access to

the degenerative disease and the removal of the hypertrophic osteophytes, and it is unclear whether it is the disease or the approach used that is responsible for this delayed return to full painless activity.

Surgeons need to be careful with the healing of central splitting and other incisions that are used to expose the distal Achilles tendon. Healing invariably occurs uneventfully, provided the foot is held immobilized to prevent formation of a hypertrophic scar. This could be

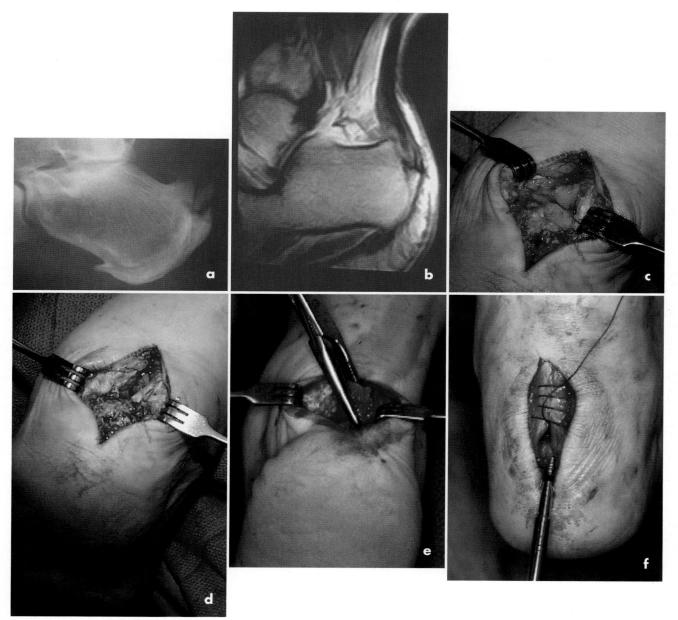

Figure 10–1–3. For patients who have pain with bone buildup directly centrally in the posterior tendon (a, b), a central splitting incision may be used. The skin is incised, the tendon is split, the bone mass is removed, and the tendon is repaired as presented (c–f).

catastrophic; and if it forms directly over the heel, the scar causes problems with shoe wear. The foot must therefore be immobilized postoperatively until full wound healing is present. Rehabilitation of the Achilles tendon is important with strengthening, modalities, heel elevation, and orthotic arch support. Generally, I will use a removable range-of-motion walker boot for approximately 6 to 8 weeks after surgery, allowing plantar flexion but blocking dorsiflexion to facilitate physical therapy and treatment.

This condition of insertional tendinopathy should be distinguished Haglund's syndrome and retrocalcaneal bursitis. In patients with these conditions the bursitis occurs as a result of enlargement of the dorsal superior lateral aspect of the calcaneus. The dorsolateral tuberosity causes impingement against the lateral insertion of the Achilles tendon, and retrocalcaneal bursitis develops. If the bursitis is refractory to nonoperative treatment, then this is approached through a short dorsolateral incision just anterior to the Achilles tendon (Fig. 10–1–4). The incision is deepened through subcutaneous tissue, the retrocalcaneal bursa is excised, and the insertion of the Achilles tendon and the enlarged posterolateral bone is exposed. Only a lateral ostectomy

Figure 10–1–4. Swelling was present and associated with boggy tender inflammation in the retrocalcaneal space (a, b). The tendon was viable, and minimal bone impingement was noted after the bursectomy and ostectomy, which were performed from a lateral incision (c, d).

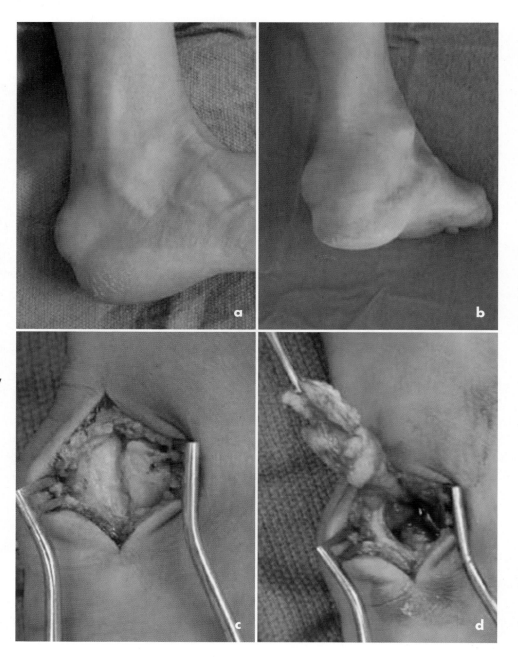

is performed because a more medial extension of the ostectomy is unnecessary (see Fig. 10–1–1). In the event that bilateral bone prominence is present, then I prefer to use two incisions. Strictly speaking, the latter condition is not true Haglund's syndrome, but this anatomic variant does occur.

Haglund's syndrome is commonly associated with retrocalcaneal bursitis, but the retrocalcaneal bursitis may indeed be present without a lateral bone prominence. The bursa is irritated as a result of impingement between the Achilles tendon and the posterior dorsal surface of the tuberosity, which causes the inflammatory change. If surgery is required, the bursa is excised along with any bone prominence as previously described.

Alternative incisions may be used to correct insertional tendinopathy, including an extended J-incision. The advantage of this type of incision is that it gives complete access to the entire insertion of the tendon. I use this incision for more severe diffuse insertional tendinopathy when I do not think that I can access the entire tendon from through either a central splitting incision or bilateral incisions. In patients with this incision, the tendon is completely detached from its insertion, the offending bone is debrided, the retrocalcaneal space is denuded, and then the tendon is reattached with a suture anchor (Fig. 10–1–5).

In addition to the debridement of the insertion of the tendon with bursectomy and ostectomy, the Achilles tendon needs to be repaired for management of severe insertional tendinopathy with loss of the integrity and function of the Achilles tendon (Fig. 10–1–6). Generally, the tissue is insufficient or of such a poor quality that a simple debridement cannot be performed. The management of these more severe forms are discussed in the following section about noninsertional tendinopathy, which consists of resection of the insertion of the Achilles tendon with either a flexor hallucis longus (FHL) transfer or an Achilles tendon allograft (Fig. 10–1–7).

Management of Noninsertional Tendinopathy

The questions involved with surgery for noninsertional tendinopathy are where and what to debride, how much to debride, and then how to do the repair. If this is

considered a degenerative hypovascular condition, approaching this with excision of the degenerated tendon and hoping for a repair process with improved tendon function make sense. However, these are easier said than done. Although this remains a clinical diagnosis, I like to use magnetic resonance imaging (MRI) preoperatively to locate the maximum point of degeneration.

As an alternative to an open invasive procedure for the treatment of the Achilles tendon, multiple percutaneous tenotomies can be made in the tendon as described by Mafulli. This procedure is indicated for patients in whom nonsurgical care has failed but in whom a more extensive reconstruction is not thought to be necessary or appropriate. If these percutaneous tenotomies fail, then a more major reconstructive procedure, as described here, is performed. The percutaneous tenotomies create a hypervascular response, which theoretically facilitates tendon healing. The other possible explanation for the success of this procedure is a slight elongation of the Achilles tendon, which may occur as a result of the longitudinal tenotomies.

With the patient under local anesthesia, a #15 knife blade is introduced posteriorly, and multiple slits on the tendon are made. The knife blade is inserted perpendicular to the axis of the tendon, and then the foot is passively dorsiflexed while the knife blade is pushed up against the tendon proximally. A second and third incision is made percutaneously with the foot moved distally while the knife blade is pushed in toward the distal aspect of the tendon. The tenotomy incisions can be closed with absorbable sutures, although none are really necessary.

After these procedures, the Achilles tendon swells, and this swelling may be even more significant than had it been associated with the degenerative tendinopathy. This swelling is the result of a hypervascular reaction with fibrosis and is to be expected. These patients will continue to have symptoms for 3 to 6 months after this procedure, but most can perform activities, including exercise, comfortably by that time (Fig. 10–1–8).

The reconstructive procedure for debridement of tendinopathy is made with a more extensive incision that is based medially over a length of about 6 cm. I prefer to

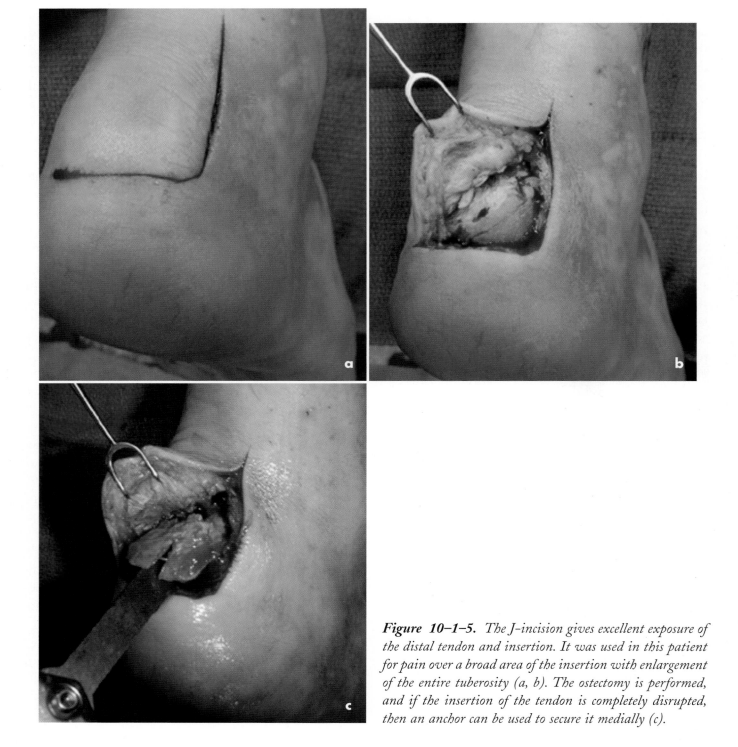

Figure 10–1–5. *The J-incision gives excellent exposure of the distal tendon and insertion. It was used in this patient for pain over a broad area of the insertion with enlargement of the entire tuberosity (a, b). The ostectomy is performed, and if the insertion of the tendon is completely disrupted, then an anchor can be used to secure it medially (c).*

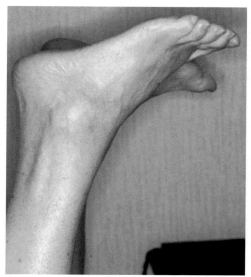

Figure 10–1–6. *Note the loss of dynamic plantar flexion on the affected foot as a result of chronic insertional tendinopathy with loss of the length of the Achilles tendon.*

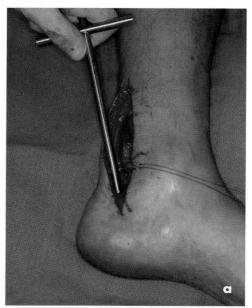

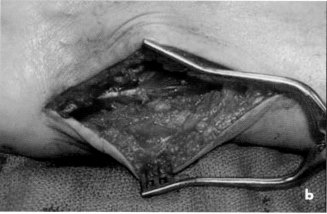

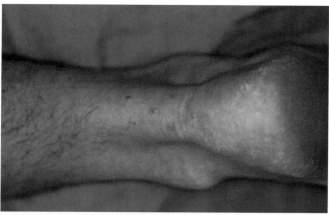

Figure 10–1–8. *Multiple punctures (percutaneous longitudinal tenotomies) of the Achilles tendon were used in this patient to treat a chronic degenerative tendinopathy as described originally by Mafulli.*

avoid a lateral incision to prevent any inadvertent injury to the sural nerve. The incision is deepened onto the paratenon, which is inspected and may need to be debrided or excised if thickened or inflamed. Removal of the paratenon is followed by inspection of the tendon. Grossly identifying the area of tendon degeneration is not easy. In patients with severe tendinopathy, with fusiform thickening of the tendon, the bulge in the tendon may be visible. The tendon is incised longitudinally and the yellowish, mucinoid degenerative intrasubstance portion of the tendon is excised. I excise a vertical ellipse of tendon, removing approximately 50% of the cross-sectional diameter of the tendon in the area of the maximum fusiform degeneration. Knowing where to start and stop with this debridement is difficult because no clear demarcation exists between the healthy and diseased tendon. With excision of the tendon, repair is performed with a running 2-0 absorbable suture, and the knot is tied inside the tendon to prevent any friction subcutaneously (Fig. 10–1–9).

Figure 10–1–7. *This patient had severe insertional tendinopathy with complete loss of the function of the Achilles tendon, with gradual weakening and eventual partial rupture. There was little functional Achilles tendon distally, and because of the severe degeneration after tendon debridement, the flexor hallucis longus (FHL) tendon was transferred into the calcaneus with a trephine to make a 5-mm tunnel for passage of the tendon (a, b).*

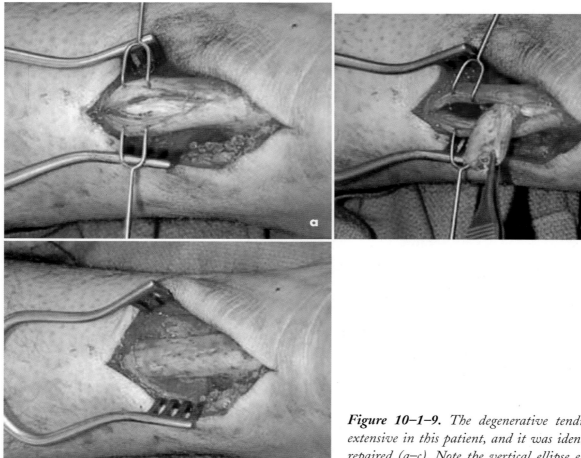

Figure 10–1–9. *The degenerative tendinopathy was not extensive in this patient, and it was identified, excised, and repaired (a–c). Note the vertical ellipse excised (b) and the repair with a buried running suture (c).*

With more advanced degeneration, particularly that involving the more distal insertion, there has been recent interest in the use of the FHL tendon to augment or replace the degenerated portion of the Achilles tendon. The rationale behind this procedure is to bring the muscle belly of the FHL tendon adjacent to the avascular Achilles tendon, thereby facilitating a process of healing by proximity. The addition of the FHL tendon also unloads the Achilles tendon and supposedly increases push-off strength (see Fig. 10–1–7). Although this is an operation that certainly has its merits, I think that one may be "robbing Peter to pay Paul." Certainly, if the Achilles tendon is totally disrupted and irreparable, then the addition of autogenous tissue, including the FHL tendon, may have merit. However, harvesting the FHL tendon is not without morbidity and even though patients tolerate the loss of flexion of the interphalangeal joint, this is definitely noticeable with weakness of the hallux, particularly when patients are barefoot.

The FHL tendon transfer is performed through a vertical incision made immediately anterior to the Achilles tendon. A curved incision along the path of the FHL tendon behind the medial malleolus is not necessary because the tendon is easily harvested through a vertical incision. The incision is deepened through subcutaneous tissues, and then the interval between the neurovascular bundle and the FHL tendon is used to identify and harvest the tendon. The incision of the flexor retinaculum and the anterior retraction of the tibial neurovascular bundle expose the deep fascia over the FHL tendon, and the retinaculum is split distally with scissors. The tendon in the arch of the foot does not need to be harvested because a long piece of FHL tendon is unnecessary. Once the retinaculum over the FHL tendon is open, I grasp the muscle with a retractor and then cut the tendon at the level of the sustentacular tunnel under direct vision. Usually a stump of about 2 to 3 cm of tendon that is distal to the musculotendinous junction is present, and that is all that is needed for the tendon transfer. The tendon

is anchored into the calcaneus with a trephine hole technique. An 8-mm trephine hole is made from the dorsal aspect of the tuberosity and extends down inferiorly. The entry point for this hole is made posteriorly at the insertion point of the Achilles tendon (Fig. 10–1–10).

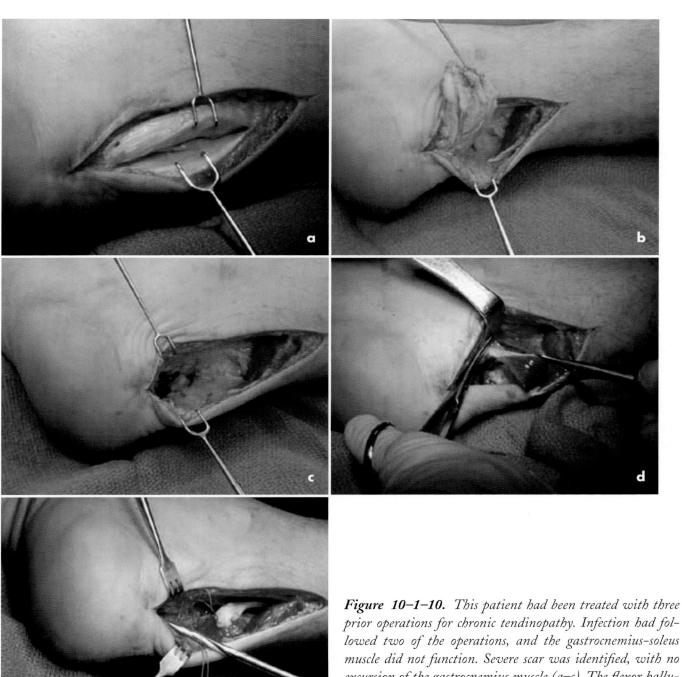

Figure 10–1–10. This patient had been treated with three prior operations for chronic tendinopathy. Infection had followed two of the operations, and the gastrocnemius-soleus muscle did not function. Severe scar was identified, with no excursion of the gastrocnemius muscle (a–c). The flexor hallucis longus (FHL) tendon was harvested and transferred into the calcaneus for salvage (d, e). Note that the FHL tendon is cut just distal to the musculotendinous junction (d).

The bone plug is withdrawn, and the tendon is now advanced into the tunnel using a straight needle and suture, which are pulled out through the plantar aspect of the heel. If the tendon is too long, then the tension cannot be set correctly on the transfer in the bone tunnel. I pull the suture out through the heel, and then by pulling on the suture with the foot in maximum equinus, I get a sense of the resilience of the transfer with the foot in passive dorsiflexion. Some tension to this should exist when the foot is in about 20 degrees of equinus (e.g., for repair of a ruptured Achilles tendon). Usually, the musculotendinous junction is at the margin of the bone tunnel superiorly. The tendon is then secured to the bone with a suture anchor supplemented by the bone plug, which is placed back in the tunnel to give a good bone/tendon/bone interference fixation. The foot should be left in equinus during bandaging and rehabilitation.

Should the remaining gastrocnemius muscle be used to supplement the flexor tendon transfer? If this transfer is performed for severe degenerative tendinopathy, then a choice can be made about excising the entire degenerative portion of tendon, usually the distal 6 cm of the tendon. If a strip of the Achilles tendon is left behind, the correct tension can be maintained on the gastrocnemius muscle, assuming that a contracture is not present. The problem with leaving behind diseased tendon of this nature is that pain may continue as a result of the degenerative process. Because revascularization of some sort is relied on for healing, a portion of this tendon can be left behind with the FHL muscle belly lying up against it. Suturing the FHL muscle to the Achilles tendon stump is not easy because this is usually at the level of the musculotendinous junction and the best that can be obtained is small 4-0 sutures to tack down the FHL muscle through its musculotendinous junction onto the Achilles tendon.

As an alternative to the FHL tendon as a local autogenous graft, I have used an Achilles tendon allograft with a bone block attached to the calcaneus for management of degenerative tendinopathy. If the disease process to the Achilles tendon is that extensive, the alternative of an allograft tendon, as opposed to an autogenous tendon transfer, remains an option. However, the use of the allograft does not "burn any bridges" because the FHL tendon transfer can always be performed at a later date should the allograft fail.

The Achilles allograft procedure is performed through a vertical incision made centrally down the back of the leg onto the posterior aspect of the calcaneus. If any Achilles tendon is present, this is excised, and a healthy portion is left behind proximally to which the graft is attached. The Achilles allograft bone is now fashioned into a block, which will fit into the posterior aspect of the calcaneal tuberosity. Once the insertion of the Achilles has been debrided, excised, and removed, then a slot is cut out of the posterior calcaneus to facilitate insertion of the block of the allograft. I generally use two fully threaded cancellous 4.0-mm screws for fixation. Once this slot is accomplished, the key to success of this operation is the tension on the repair (Fig. 10–1–11).

The repair never seems to have enough equinus tension. Because this repair is performed with the patient in the prone position, I bend the patient's knee and flex the foot down into maximum equinus and pull proximally on the allograft tendon into equinus. Only while tension on the graft is maintained can the repair be performed. A running nonabsorbable #2 whip suture is inserted on either side of the allograft on the undersurface of the indigenous Achilles tendon. If only the distal portion of the Achilles tendon is involved and excised, an end-to-end repair, rather than a vest over pants repair, can be considered, but this depends on the integrity and quality of the host Achilles tendon. Not surprisingly, healing takes longer than with a primary end-to-end repair.

The foot is immobilized in equinus in a removable boot for approximately 10 weeks, during which time active and passive range-of-motion exercises in the equinus position are performed, including swimming. Swimming is an excellent exercise for rehabilitation and can be done early on, approximately 3 to 4 weeks after repair once the incision is healed. The use of fins is encouraged for swimming in a pool, and a block to dorsiflexion can be constructed out of Orthoplast splint molded to the anterior ankle.

Management of Paratendinitis

Paratendinitis is a condition that is different from the degenerative tendinopathies. This is an inflammatory condition typically occurring in athletes, and usually associated with hyperpronation of the foot in conjunction with a mild gastrocnemius muscle contracture

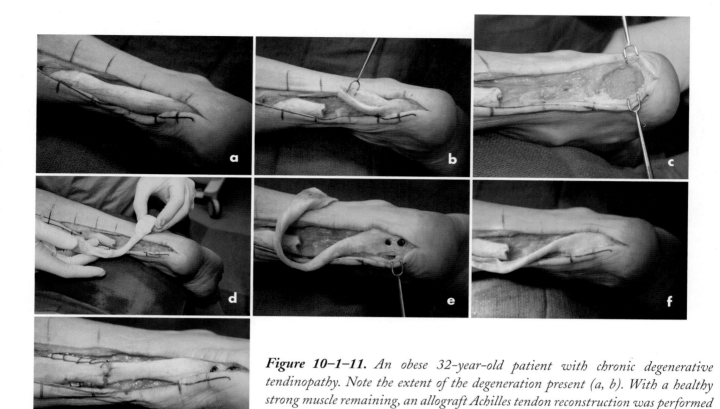

Figure 10–1–11. *An obese 32-year-old patient with chronic degenerative tendinopathy. Note the extent of the degeneration present (a, b). With a healthy strong muscle remaining, an allograft Achilles tendon reconstruction was performed with excision of the degenerative tissue (c), preparation of the bed in the calcaneus (d), attachment of the graft with cancellous screws (e), and positioning the graft under tension with the repair in equinus (f, g).*

(Fig. 10–1–12). The usual nonsurgical methods of treatment, including contrast bathing, physical therapy, orthotic arch support, and gastrocnemius muscle stretching, are usually sufficient to alleviate symptoms. If the paratendinitis is persistent, then a brisement of the paratenon is performed with 3 cc of lidocaine. The needle is inserted just underneath the paratenon, advanced into the tendon, and then backed off so that it lies indirectly under the paratenon. Injection of the anesthetic not only confirms the diagnosis and the correct location of the needle, but also elevates the inflamed, scarred paratenon off the tendon and works sufficiently enough that it should be tried before surgery.

The surgical procedure involves a short incision on the medial aspect of the tendon over a length of 2 cm. The subcutaneous tissue is elevated, and then the paratenon is identified and incised. The paratenon is then elevated off the Achilles tendon and stripped by excising the superficial anterior sheath of the paratenon medially, dorsally, and laterally as one sleeve (Fig. 10–1–13). The

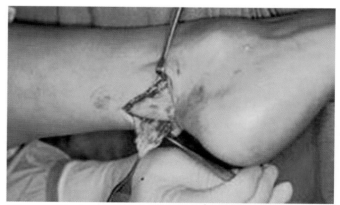

Figure 10–1–12. *The typical appearance of the inflamed paratenon that was removed in this patient.*

deep ventral surface of the Achilles tendon is left intact to leave the blood supply undisturbed. The foot should be immobilized for a short period to prevent any hypertrophic scar formation, and then therapy with cross training and modalities used in rehabilitation of the boot immobilization can proceed for approximately 3 weeks.

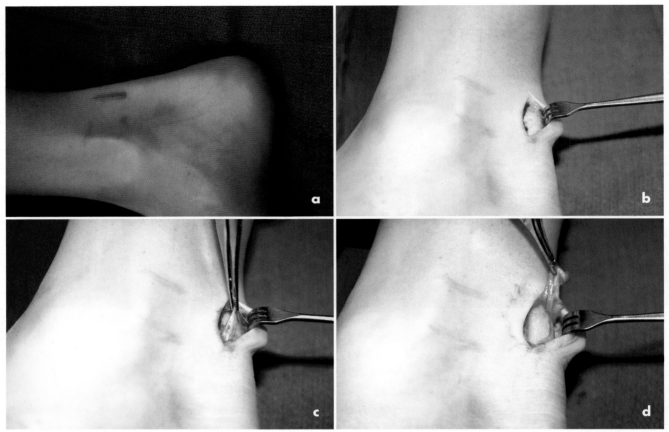

Figure 10–1–13. *The incision is marked out for excision of the paratenon (a), it is deepened through subcutaneous tissue (b), and the paratenon is incised and clamped (c). The stripping is gradually performed by retracting the paratenon over the superficial (anterior) tendon, leaving the deeper surface undisturbed (d).*

Acute Rupture of the Achilles Tendon

Over the years, we have seen cycles of operative and nonoperative management of the Achilles tendon come and go. Certainly in this age, operative management of the Achilles tendon seems to be the ideal treatment to rapidly rehabilitate the patient and restore maximum function of the limb in the absence of weakness and the potential for rerupture. Although nonoperative treatments are still advocated, the correct anatomic position of the tendon is impossible to obtain with them, and elongation of the musculotendinous unit occurs with limb weakening.

Given the goals of treatment, which are to maximize limb function with a minimal morbidity and rapidly return the individual to isokinetic strength, some form of surgical treatment is necessary. The surgeon must decide which type of surgical correction is ideal, including the extensile open or percutaneous methods. Regardless of which procedure is actually used, the goal of all procedures is identical: ensure that the repair is performed with the tendon in an anatomic position. This is certainly attainable with all methods, provided the tendon ends are inspected (i.e., a true percutaneous method of treatment is not used).

Perhaps the most significant change to my approach to these ruptures has been to make sure that the foot is positioned in more equinus than I anticipate will be necessary. Traditionally, I had prepped out both limbs into the operative field to check the dynamic resting position of the contralateral limb and compared it with the ruptured Achilles tendon so that as the sutures were being tightened, the position of the feet were noted and the tension on the repair was adjusted accordingly. Although these methods are useful, they only provide a guide as to the resting position of the foot. The problem is that some stretching out of the Achilles tendon always occurs during the recovery process and this seems to be regardless of the type of immobilization and rehabilitation used. Many surgeons have moved away from rigid immobilization of the limb to a functional rehabilitation program, which includes weight bearing and motion of the foot. The motion is protected in plantar flexion, and a blocked dorsiflexion ensures that stretching out does not occur. It is far worse and more debilitating to have a foot that dorsiflexes excessively because power will never be restored.

Finally, there are additional concerns regarding the types of incisions used and the potential for wound breakdown and sural neuritis. The open extensile approach permits maximum exposure to the tendon, but a greater likelihood of wound breakdown. Although breakdown does not occur frequently, nonetheless, this is of sufficient concern that modified incisions and mini approaches with modified percutaneous approaches have been developed. The problems are not only the length of the incision, but also the location, the tension on the skin from the repaired tendon, and the vascular dermatomes.

The ideal incision does not disrupt the dermatomal blood supply, which has been noted by Attinger to have a watershed in the center of the limb so that an incision based centrally on the tendon has the least likelihood of disrupting this blood supply. The biggest problem with these incisions is that after repair, the subcutaneous tension is considerable because the retinaculum does not hold the tendon in its anatomic position and tension is present on the skin from the repaired tendon. This tension can be lessened by positioning the foot in equinus, and it can easily be seen intraoperatively. If you dorsiflex the foot once the repair is done, the skin will have considerably more tension during skin closure. A fasciotomy of the deep compartment has been described for when an extensile incision is used, which increases the transverse cross-sectional diameter of the posterior leg and facilitates closure without tension. This fasciotomy is easy to perform, and once the tendon has been exposed, the deep posterior compartment becomes visible, the fascia is incised, and then the fascia is split vertically both proximally and distally with scissors. Fasciotomy is not necessary when mini open

approaches and modified percutaneous approaches are used for repair.

I now rarely use an extensile incision for repair and prefer a modified approach using the Achillon system (Wright Medical Technology, Inc., Arlington, Tenn). This modified percutaneous method of treatment is reliable and is able to appose the frayed tendon end in the desired position with minimal exposure of the ruptured tendon. The other approach, which I have used on occasion, is the modified percutaneous approach described by Mafulli.

A short transverse or a longitudinal incision is made, centered on the middle of the leg and based over the rupture. The rupture usually occurs 4 to 6 cm proximal to the insertion, and the incision is made over a length of 14 cm. The incision is deepened through the subcutaneous tissue, and the retinaculum and the peritenon are incised longitudinally (Fig. 10–1–14). The hematoma is evacuated, and the ends of the tendons are identified and delivered into the incision. Usually severe fissuring and fraying of the tendon ends occur. With a skin hook, the tendon ends are then lifted out of the bed, and the deep compartment is identified. An incision is made over the deep fascia with a knife, and then the fascia is stripped longitudinally both proximally and distally with scissors until the entire compartment is visible.

The type of sutures used does not matter as much as the specific location where the suture is inserted and the tension of the repair once suturing is complete. I start with the proximal suture, and a running whip lock suture of #2 braided nonabsorbable material is used. The sutures are locked at each corner, and three to four passes in the tendon are made until each strand of the suture is pulled distally. The entrance point for the suture is *not* where the fissuring of the rupture is noted but is located more proximally (Fig. 10–1–15). Avulsion of tendon strands from the distal stump of the tendon is always present, and with the foot in maximum equinus, the overlapping of these strands can be seen. The same principle applies to the insertion point of the distal strand of the suture. With the knee now bent and the tension applied to both ends of the sutures, maximum tension is applied until the foot is in gross equinus and is then slightly released until the foot remains in about 20

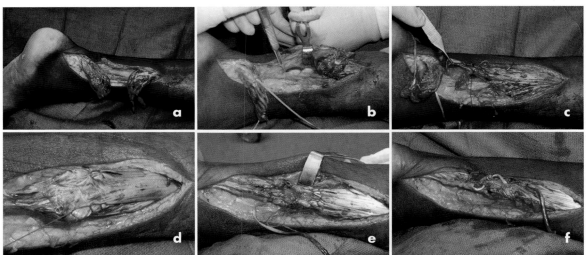

Figure 10–1–14. *An extensile incision used to repair an acute Achilles tendon rupture (a). It is unusual that I use this type of incision nowadays. Once the incision is made, a fasciotomy of the deep posterior compartment is made to facilitate later wound closure (b). The key to this repair is the correct tension of the Achilles tendon and the correct starting point of the suture, which is identified with the strands of tendon overlapping each other (c). A locking whip suture is used with #2 nonabsorbable suture (d), and an additional suture is used on the distal stump for the repair (e). The plantaris tendon was present and used as a weave to reinforce the repair in this patient (f).*

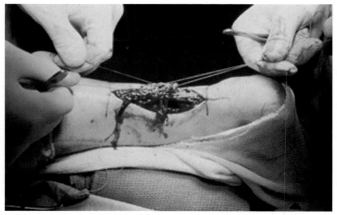

Figure 10–1–15. *In this patient, the sutures in both the proximal and distal tendon ends have been inserted but were not done so correctly because the tendon ends overlap when the suture is tensioned. If the suture is tied in this position, there will be a relative lengthening of the tendon, and strength will never be regained.*

degrees of equinus. As noted previously, I prefer to use more equinus in the repair than seems to be necessary.

Usually one strand of suture material is sufficient for the repair. The knot must be tied posteriorly deep to the Achilles tendon; otherwise, the strands will become markedly irritating if left in a subcutaneous position. The one side of the suture is tied while tension is maintained on the opposite side, and then the second side is used to set the tension on the repair. At the completion of the repair, the foot should be in 20 degrees of equinus, and with gentle pressure on the foot in a plantar direction, the repair should not have a tendency to stretch out.

The mini approach with the Achillon system has been effective. This is an ingenious device developed by Assal and colleagues that minimizes exposure, decreases the incidence of wound complications, and facilitates end-to-end apposition of the tendon, with a modified percutaneous approach. The incision is centered over the rupture and is made over a length of 2 cm vertically, or transversely, in the center of the leg posteriorly. Locating the position of the rupture is important; otherwise, the incision will be off plane and the repair will be more difficult. Once the incision is deepened through subcutaneous tissue, the peritenon is incised transversely and then tagged for later repair. The tendon ends are identified but do not need to be pulled out into the incision. In fact, it is preferable not to deliver the frayed tendon end into the incision and leave the strands of the tendon lying where they are (Fig. 10–1–16).

The fins for the Achillon system are inserted under the paratenon and on the sides of the Achilles tendon and advanced proximally. The percutaneous side pins are now introduced with an attached #2 braided suture in the eye of the guide pin. The sural nerve, which lies slightly more laterally and centrally, depending on where the needles are passed percutaneously, does not appear to be in any danger in this location. The sutures should

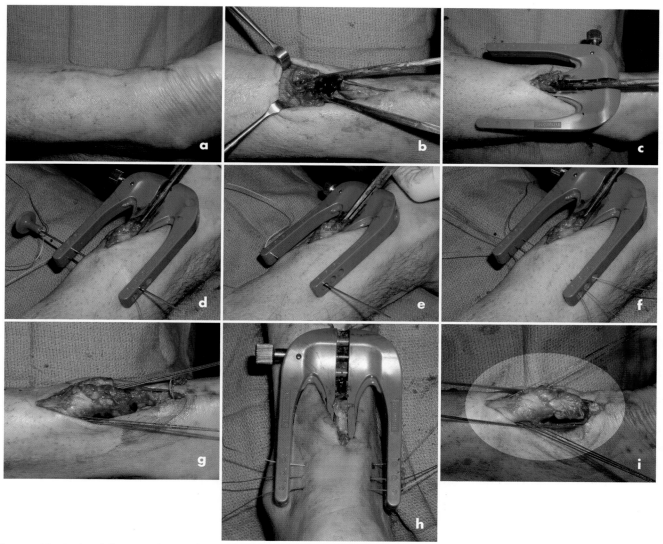

Figure 10–1–16. *The steps for repair of a rupture with the Achillon system. This patient was referred for treatment following rerupture after an extensile approach to repair (a). A smaller incision was used, and the tendon ends were explored (b). The fins of the Achillon device are inserted under the paratenon and on each side of the tendon, which is clamped distally (c). An inserter is used to push each suture pin through the body of the tendon proximally, and three sutures are used (d–f). The Achillon, including the three suture strands, is withdrawn (g); is turned around and inserted distally in the same manner (h); and is then withdrawn proximally as the three sutures are pulled out (i). The repair is then performed under appropriate tension as previously described.*

be passed through the center of the musculotendinous unit. If the needle is advanced too deep, it will be in the muscle itself, which can cut through when the suture is pulled on distally. The six strands of the suture are now lifted out from the incision and clamped while the Achillon device is now withdrawn, and the suture strands are left directly on top of the tendon. The procedure is now reversed, again making sure that the plane of the fins of the Achillon device are lying in the plane of the tendon. Once the sutures are withdrawn from the distal tendon segment, the one side is sutured while the other set of three suture strands is held. With the knee bent, the second set of sutures is now tied and tension is set so as to leave the foot in approximately 20 degrees of equinus. If the suture knot is anterior, it can be irritating, and the suture knot must be tied deep, behind the tendon.

Management of acute avulsion of the Achilles tendon as an acute rupture must be managed differently because the avulsion is associated with degenerative insertional tendinopathy. The distalmost portion of the Achilles tendon is usually fibrillated, necrotic, and partially ossified. Avulsion is usually "clean" in that there is not much fibrillation associated with this tearing, and it is torn out of a sleeve of its insertion. A cavity with synovia is left behind (Fig. 10–1–17).

I occasionally use a hockey stick incision to approach this repair. A central longitudinal incision can also be used, but exposing the entire attachment and performing the debridement of the tuberosity with the hockey stick J-type incision are easier. Once the incision has been deepened down onto bone, the entire remnant of the attachment including the dorsolateral tuberosity is debrided, and then an ostectomy is performed, with removal of the dorsal posterior surface of the tuberosity. This ostectomy is performed similarly to a painful insertional tendinopathy so that there is a raw bleeding surface present for reattachment of the Achilles tendon. The ruptured tendon is now debrided sharply. This tendon cannot be debrided back to a normal, healthy tendon because debridement will shorten it abnormally and prevent reattachment. Instead, the margin is debrided obliquely, with as much of the superficial tendon left intact as possible. Reattachment is performed with suture anchors, with two suture strands attached, and the tendon is approximated to the bone.

Obtaining a firm attachment of the tendon to the bone with a suture anchor is difficult. One of the suture strands is used in a standard fashion with a crisscross sliding suture to try to pull the tendon down distally against the bone. The second suture is used at the loop anterior and superficial to the tendon and then tied deep to the tendon so that the crisscrossing strand pulls the tendon down against the bone.

Reconstruction Chronic Achilles Tendon Rupture

The approach to repair of a chronic Achilles tendon rupture is determined by the size of the gap between the tendon ends, the presence of a functioning (preferably strong) gastrocnemius-soleus muscle, and the age and activity level of the patient. An end-to-end repair is ideal because only this will return to maximum isokinetic strength and, if at all possible, is performed even if the repair necessitates position of the foot in slight equinus. However, retraction of the tendon ends is usually not possible. An end-to-end repair can only be performed when the gap is about 1 to 2 cm because some freshening up of the tendon ends needs to be performed, and by the time this is done, the gap may be an additional 1 cm, which makes the end-to-end repair difficult. The dilemma with this method of repair is the delineation of normal and abnormal tissue. If a rupture is complete with atrophic ends, seeing where the tendon end lies is easy, and after debridement, the repair is performed. However, with many chronic degenerative ruptures, a degenerative scar is present in the center of the tendon, and the scar makes this type of repair implausible.

For patients who have sustained a rupture and who were initially treated nonoperatively, some elongation of the tendon often occurs during healing, with resulting weakness in peak torque, power, and strength. For these patients, although the tendon has healed, it has done so in an elongated position. For these symptomatic patients, excision of a segment of the Achilles tendon, followed by primary end-to-end repair, works well. For this central excision to be performed, the tendon is cut transversely 6 cm proximal to the insertion. Two skin hooks are then placed on either end of the tendon, and the tendon is retracted proximally and distally. With the knee flexed, the overlap of the two tendon ends is measured when the foot is held in 20 degrees of equinus. This

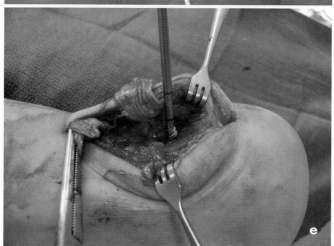

Figure 10–1–17. *Acute rupture occurred in this patient with chronic painful insertional tendinopathy. Note the bone lump at the insertion of the tendon and the degeneration at the tendon insertion (a, b). A small bone avulsion often occurs with this rupture. The posterior tuberosity is shaved to prepare the attachment for the tendon (c, d), which is maintained in position with a suture anchor (e).*

overlap is usually about 1 to 2 cm, and this is the segment that is then cut out, followed by an end-to-end repair as described for the acute rupture.

For a gap in the tendon between 2 and 5 cm, a V-Y tendon advancement works well. If the gap is greater than 5 cm, an adequate excursion of the tendon is difficult to get, and some detachment of the muscle then occurs, decreasing strength. A V-Y advancement is performed by measuring the gap and then doubling the length of the segment of the tendon to be advanced. The base of the V is distal, and the apex is extended proximally all the way up into the musculotendinous junction. The incision starts proximally at the musculotendinous junction at the apex of the V, and then the fascia is sharply cut but the muscle is less intact (Fig. 10–1–18).

If the gap is greater than 5 cm, the V-Y advancement will not likely be sufficient. Although it can still be used,

it is probably insufficient on its own, and a transfer of the FHL tendon is performed in the same manner as described previously for chronic tendinopathy (Fig. 10–1–19). The alternative is to perform an Achilles tendon allograft when no functional tendon is present, and the attachment of the graft is performed in the same manner as described for tendinopathy (Figs 10–1–20 and 10-1-21).

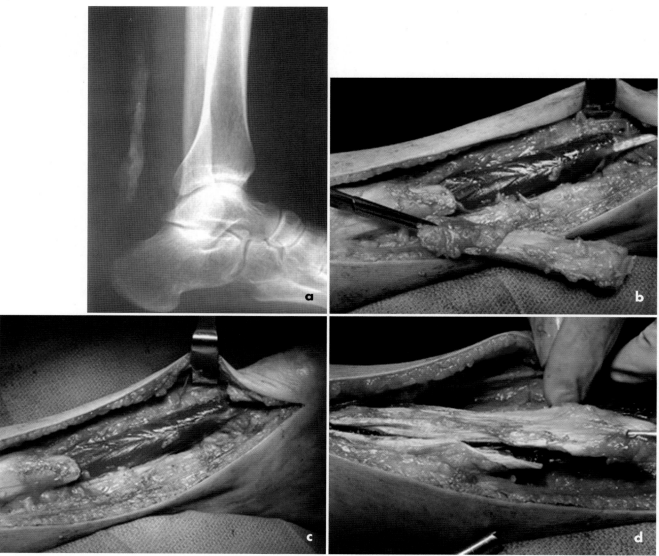

Figure 10–1–18. This patient was a healthy 42-year-old man who had experienced pain in the Achilles tendon for 20 years after a rupture of the tendon was treated nonoperatively. This ossification of the tendon is not usually painful, but although good strength was present in push-off, severe pain was present over the mass of calcified tendon, which was excised (a, b). The muscle was healthy, and although the flexor hallucis longus (FHL) muscle could have been used here on its own, it was supplemented with a V-Y advancement and gained the necessary length for the reconstruction (c, d).

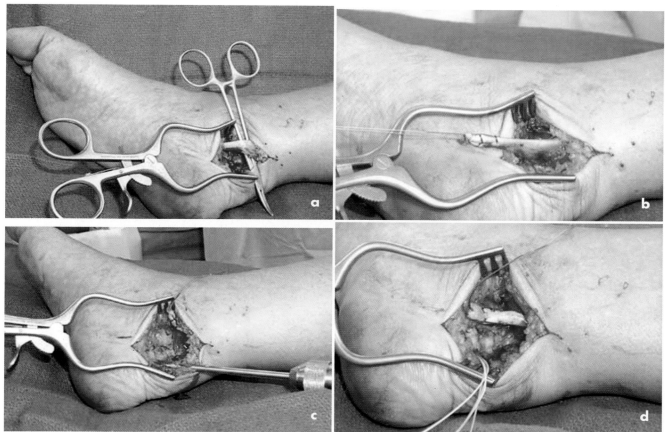

Figure 10–1–19. *This patient had a chronic rupture of the Achilles tendon with a gap of 8 cm, which was reconstructed with the flexor hallucis longus (FHL) tendon transfer. The FHL tendon is identified in the posterior compartment and cut as it enters the retinaculum (a, b). A 4.5-mm drill hole is made in the calcaneus, and a suture anchor is inserted into the calcaneus (c, d). The tendon is then passed through the drill hole and tensioned with the sutures on the anchor.*

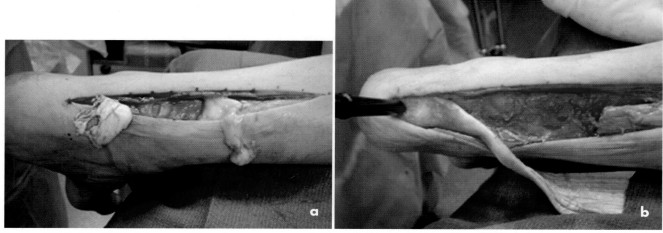

Figure 10–1–20. *This 56-year-old patient was treated for an acute rupture of the Achilles tendon operatively, followed by open wound infection, and ultimate settling down until the point that a flexor hallucis longus (FHL) tendon transfer was performed, followed by repeat wound dehisced. Eight months later, with chronic weakness, an Achilles tendon allograft was performed. Note that the necrosis of the remaining tissue, which was tested at the time of surgery, was noted to be culture and gram stain negative and had no white cells present under high power magnification (a). The allograft was secured to the calcaneus with two screws (b).*

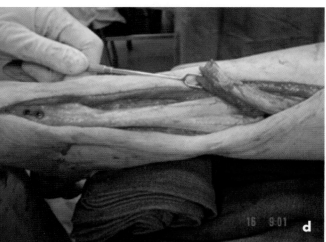

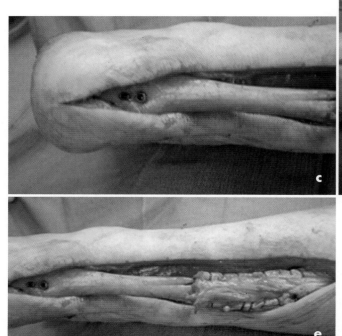

Figure 10–1–20, cont'd *(c) and was then laid under the host Achilles tendon at the musculotendinous junction (d), where it was attached with a #2 running locking suture (e).*

Figure 10-1-21. *The gap in this chronic rupture measured 8.5 cm. Note the presence of the plantaris tendon. The alternatives for treating this chronic rupture are limited. Although a tendon transfer with a flexor tendon such as the flexor hallucis longus (FHL) can be used, the gap is too great for a V-Y advancement alone. In this case, an allograft was used to repair the defect.*

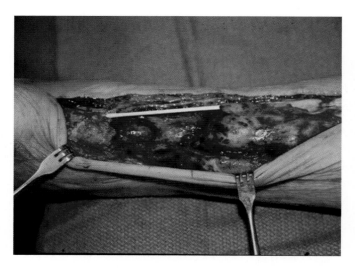

Suggested Readings

Assal M, Jung M, Stern R, et al. Limited open repair of Achilles tendon ruptures. A technique with a new instrument and findings of a prospective multicenter study. J Bone Joint Surg 84:161–170, 2002.

Feibel JB, Bernacki BL. A review of salvage procedures after failed Achilles tendon repair. Foot Ankle Clin 8:105–114, 2003.

Jarvinen TA, Kannus P, Paavola M, et al. Achilles tendon injuries. Curr Opin Rheumatol 13:150–155, 2001.

Josey RA, Marymont JV, Varner KE, et al. Immediate, full weightbearing cast treatment of acute Achilles tendon ruptures: a long-term follow-up study. Foot Ankle Int 24:775–779, 2003.

Kann JN, Myerson MS. Surgical management of chronic ruptures of the Achilles tendon. Foot Ankle Clin 2:535–545, 1997.

Leppilahti J, Lahde S, Forsman K, et al. Relationship between calf muscle size and strength after Achilles rupture repair. Foot Ankle Int 21:330–335, 2000.

Maffulli N, Kader D. Tendinopathy of tendo achillis. J Bone Joint Surg Br 84:1–8, 2002.

Maffulli N, Wong J, Almekinders LC. Types and epidemiology of tendinopathy. Clin Sports Med 22:675–692, 2003.

McClelland D, Maffulli N. Percutaneous repair of ruptured Achilles tendon. J R Coll Surg Edinb 47:613–618, 2002.

Monroe MT, Dixon DJ, Beals TC, et al. Plantarflexion torque following reconstruction of Achilles tendinosis or rupture with flexor hallucis longus augmentation. Foot Ankle Int 21:324–329, 2000.

Mandelbaum BR, Myerson MS, Forster R. Achilles tendon ruptures: a new method of repair, early range of motion, and functional rehabilitation. Am J Sports Med 23:392–395, 1995.

Myerson MS. Achilles tendon ruptures. Instr Course Lect 48:219–230, 1999.

Myerson MS. Disorders of the Achilles tendon and the retrocalcaneal region. In. Myerson MS (ed): Foot and Ankle Disorders. Philadelphia, WB Saunders, 2000.

Myerson MS, McGarvey W. Disorders of the insertion of the Achilles tendon and Achilles tendinitis. J Bone Joint Surg 12:1814–1824, 1998.

Paavola M, Kannus P, Jarvinen TA, et al. Achilles tendinopathy. J Bone Joint Surg Am 84-A:2062–2076. 2002.

Sorosky B, Press J, Plastaras C, Rittenberg J. The practical management of Achilles tendinopathy. Clin J Sport Med 14:40–44, 2004.

Rupture of the Anterior Tibial Tendon

The management of rupture of the anterior tibial tendon (ATT) depends almost entirely on the size of the gap present (Fig. 10–2–1). Generally, ruptures occur in older individuals from degeneration and friction underneath the extensor retinaculum, followed by varying degrees of retraction of the tendon. A small stump of tendon is usually left distally under the retinaculum, and the proximal stump retracts between 2 and 10 cm. The options for correction include an end-to-end repair, transfer of the extensor hallucis longus (EHL) tendon, a tendon graft interposition, or a V-Y lengthening advancement of the proximal ATT. The decision as to which of these is performed depends on the strength of the limb, the presence of an equinus contracture, the presence of any accessory clawtoe deformities as a result of the rupture of the ATT, and additional foot deformities. Even with early prompt diagnosis, degeneration of the tendon is usually present with fraying of the tendon ends and retraction, and augmentation or supplementation of the tendon repair needs to be performed (Fig. 10–2–2).

If fixed clawing of the hallux is present as a result of accessory use of the EHL and extensor digitorum longus (EDL) tendons, then an arthrodesis of the hallux interphalangeal (IP) joint is ideal, and the EHL tendon can be used to augment the repair. If the rupture is of relatively recent onset and the proximal muscle is still healthy and excursion is present, then wherever possible, I try to incorporate this into the repair process. A tendon graft works well in this instance, but it should be supplemented possibly with an EHL tenodesis or transfer to augment the degenerative rupture. Positioning the foot in at least 10 degrees of dorsiflexion at the completion of the repair is important.

The main problem with the final repair is the potential for wound dehiscence. Bowstringing of the repair always occurs, and because the extensor retinaculum is invariably deficient at the completion of the repair, increased pressure from the repaired tendon is on the underlying skin. For this reason, I make the skin incision more lateral than the underlying repair and then raise the skin flap so that with the closure, no pressure from the tendon is on the actual incision. Although bowstringing inevitably occurs, pressure from the tendon repair on the incision itself should be avoided. The other problem that occurs with all repairs is that the foot is slightly over-supinated during the repair process. This oversupination is inevitable as a result of tightening of the repair. This should not present a concern initially, although this has to be watched during the recovery and rehabilitation phase. An Achilles tendon lengthening is frequently necessary to regain adequate dorsiflexion and correct position of the foot during the repair. The repair should have minimal tension, and the foot *must* be passively correctible to at least 10 degrees of dorsiflexion without much resistance. It is preferable to maintain the foot in a cast rather than in a splint immediately postoperatively to hold the foot in dorsiflexion.

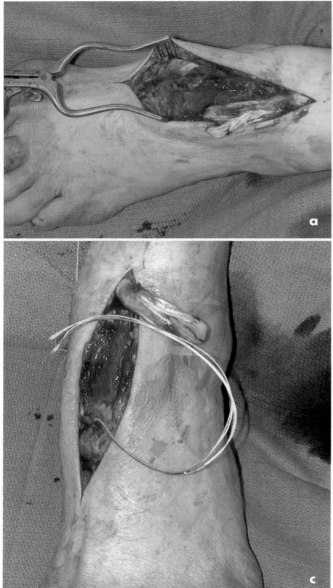

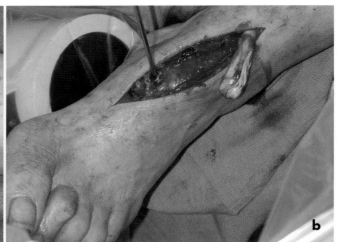

Figure 10–2–1. *The anterior tibial tendon (ATT) rupture occurred in this 68-year-old man spontaneously, which was diagnosed 7 weeks later. Note the proximal splitting in the tendon with retraction to the midfoot (a). The treatment included an arthrodesis of the hallux interphalangeal (IP) joint and transfer of the extensor hallucis (EHL) tendon to supplement the repair of the ATT. These procedures were selected because of preexisting and symptomatic hallux deformity. The medial cuneiform was identified fluoroscopically, and a suture anchor was inserted (b). Once the anchor was inserted, the EHL tendon was attached to the medial cuneiform under tension, and then the EHL tendon was folded back on itself to bridge the gap with the shortened ATT (c).*

An incision is made along the central aspect of the foot at least 1 cm lateral to the position of the ATT and is deepened through subcutaneous tissues, and the nerves are retracted. The skin is retracted medially, the extensor retinaculum is incised longitudinally, and the tendon ends are visualized. Depending on when the rupture occurred, fibrillation and fraying of the tendon with degeneration at both ends are present. Frequently, the extensor retinaculum has to be incised distally to be able to identify the stump of the tendon. The proximal tendon is sutured with a whip suture of nonabsorbable 0-material, and the tendon is then pulled distally. Tension is applied as much as possible to the tendon

for at least 2 minutes to determine the mobility of the muscle and then obtain some relaxation with elongation of the tendon. The biggest problem with this repair is to obtain the correction tension, and unless constant tension is applied at this time, the elongation of the muscle occurs later on with dorsiflexion weakness and a partial foot drop.

If an EHL tendon transfer is to be performed in conjunction with an IP joint arthrodesis, the arthrodesis is performed first. The EHL tendon is then cut distally and pulled distally to lie adjacent to the insertion point of the ruptured tendon. The length is usually sufficient for a double strand of the EHL tendon. The tendon is pulled distally and then secured over the distal stump or the medial cuneiform with a suture or suture anchor. The distalmost portion of the EHL tendon is then pulled back up as a second strand and sutured down onto the proximal ATT under tension (Fig. 10–2–3).

Under usual circumstances, I do not like to harvest a normal, healthy, functioning tendon, and the only time the EHL tendon is used is when a fixed claw hallux deformity is present or if no other tendon tissue is available. Usually, if I need to bridge the gap, I use a hamstring allograft. Two or three tendon strands are used and sutured in a routine manner under tension. A turn down technique of the ATT, as performed occasionally for the Achilles tendon, is not possible here because of the bulk of the tendon in the distal leg and ankle. However, performing a V-Y advancement lengthening

of the tendon is possible, provided the muscle and proximal tendon are healthy. If a V-Y procedure is performed, the incision has to be made about 8 cm more proximally to facilitate exposure of the musculotendinous junction. The V-Y advancement is done in a standard fashion on the basis of the length of the gap present. The length of the V-Y is double that of the tendon gap after debridement of the tendon edges. The apex of the advancement is made in the extensor of the proximal tendon just at the musculotendinous junction and then is cut in a long V distally, with the base exiting at the tip of the stump of the ruptured tendon. Knowing the correct length is important, because the tip of the stump, if chronically ruptured, has to be debrided back to a reasonably healthy tendon. The suture is inserted after debriding the distal tip of the tendon with a lock suture, and then by pulling on the sutures at the tip of the tendon, the V is advanced

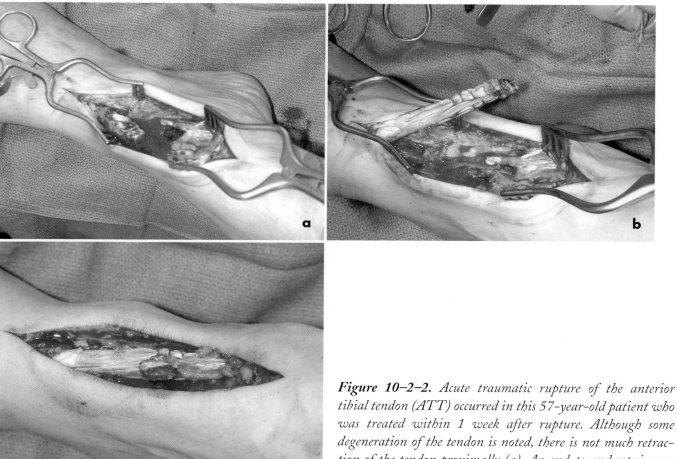

Figure 10–2–2. Acute traumatic rupture of the anterior tibial tendon (ATT) occurred in this 57-year-old patient who was treated within 1 week after rupture. Although some degeneration of the tendon is noted, there is not much retraction of the tendon proximally (a). An end-to-end repair was performed without augmentation (b, c).

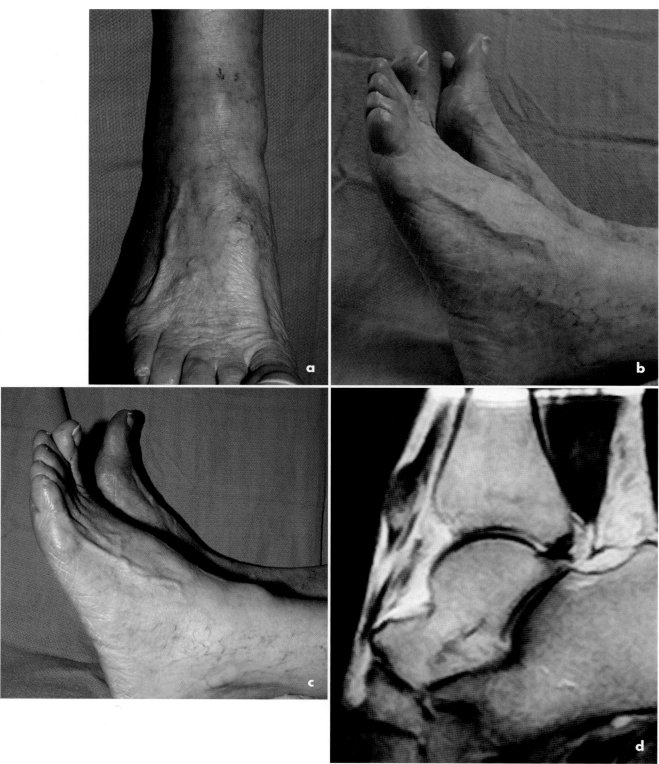

Figure 10–2–3. *A chronic rupture of the anterior tibial tendon (ATT) was present in this 67-year-old man. Note the bulge in the distal leg just proximal to the ankle where the tendon has bunched up (a–d). Note also the talonavicular arthritis, with dorsal osteophytes on the distal talus, which was probably responsible for the attritional tear in this patient.*

to the adjusted correct length. The V-Y limbs are now sutured with a running suture of 0 Ethibond, and then with the foot in maximal dorsiflexion, the repair is performed distally.

Regardless of the type of suture repair, the foot must be immobilized in dorsiflexion of at least 10 degrees and preferably 20 degrees during recovery. A cast is preferable to a postoperative splint, and this is split in the recovery room after surgery. Patients can start weight bearing in the cast at approximately 2 weeks once wound healing is apparent. A boot with a plantar flexion stop is also permissible, but the plantar flexion beyond neutral must be avoided during the recovery process for the first 8 weeks. Aggressive physical therapy with rehabilitation is important once the cast is removed to regain strength.

Suggested Readings

Ouzounian TJ, Anderson R. Anterior tibial tendon rupture. Foot Ankle Int 16:406–410, 1995.

Petersen W, Stein V, Tillmann B. Blood supply of the tibialis anterior tendon. Arch Orthop Trauma Surg 119:371–375, 1999.

Peroneal Tendon Injury and Repair

Repair of Isolated Tears of the Longus and Brevis Tendon

An incision is made along the length of the posterolateral ankle extending along the course of the peroneal tendons behind the fibula. The proximal and distal extent of the incision is determined once the disease is identified after opening the retinaculum. Preserving the extensor retinaculum, particularly at the margin of the distal fibula, is important. If the superior peroneal retinaculum is not adequately preserved, dislocation of the peroneal tendon with recurrent tendinopathy and tearing occur. The tendon is frequently split longitudinally with tears that are intrasubstance and posteriorly located. This is particularly the case when longitudinal peroneal tendon splits are present in conjunction with ankle instability. The decision has to be made whether to repair the split or to excise a portion of the tendon. This decision depends on the size, length, and extent of the split. If I can preserve at least 50% of the tendon, then the split portion may be excised longitudinally. The remaining tendon can be left intact, or, if further splits are encountered, the tendon is tubed with a running absorbable suture (Fig. 10–3–1).

Repair of the peroneus longus tendon is performed identically, unless the tendon is torn directly under the cuboid. The cuboid is the more frequent location for a peroneus longus tendon tear in association with interruption of the os peroneum as the tendon winds underneath the cuboid (Fig. 10–3–2). Occasionally the os peroneum is visible radiographically, and its more proximal location from the undersurface of the cuboid indicates the rupture. Long-standing tears cannot be repaired end-to-end because the retracted portion of the tendon is difficult to repair distally under the cuboid. The same applies to a rupture that occurs in conjunction with the os peroneum because excision of the os peroneum frequently leaves a defect that is greater than 1 cm, which is difficult to repair. However, for a more acute injury, with careful excision of the os peroneum, the shell of the remaining longus tendon can be repaired through creation of a tube out of the tendon as it passes under the cuboid. A decision has to be made, however, whether this is worthwhile (i.e., whether the tendon should be cut distally) and whether a tenodesis should be performed to the adjacent peroneus brevis tendon. This side-to-side tenodesis of the peroneus longus or peroneus brevis tendon is a frequently performed operation in conjunction with a cavus foot deformity (see Chapter 5–1).

As noted previously, the longus and brevis tendons distal to the fibula have a separate sheath, and both tendons should be opened with small scissors. The split in the tendon is identified under the separate retinaculum, and the peroneal tubercle is debrided if enlarged. I use bone wax on the raw abraded surface under the peroneal tubercle once the repair is done.

311

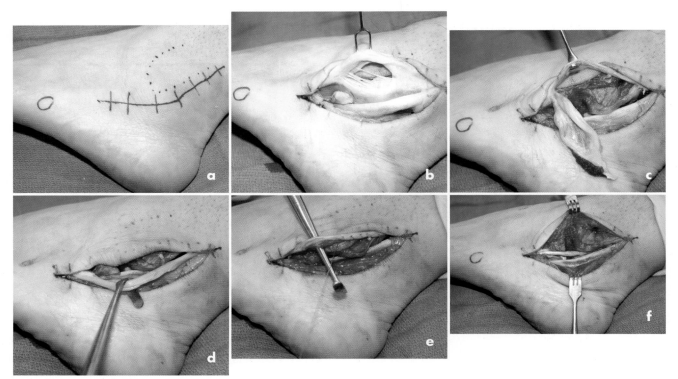

Figure 10–3–1. *This patient had an isolated rupture of the brevis tendon, and the approach is noted (a). Multiple splits in the tendon are noted, and the bulk of the torn tendon was excised (b, c). This excision left approximately one third of the tendon, which was then repaired with a running 2.0 monofilament suture (d–f).*

As with ruptures of both the longus and brevis tendons, the additional pathologic conditions must be addressed. Ankle ligament instability needs to be corrected, and if a varus heel is present, a biplanar or triplanar calcaneal osteotomy should be performed to decrease the force on the heel and protect the repair. It does not make any sense to perform a repair of the peroneal tendon in the setting of heel varus that could lead to recurrent hindfoot instability and recurrent tearing of the tendon (Fig. 10–3–3).

Techniques, tips, and pitfalls

1. It is often not possible to determine ahead of surgery the extent of the tearing of the tendon. Although magnetic resonance imaging (MRI) is useful, it does not play a role in clinical decision making.

2. A rupture of the peroneus brevis tendon is frequently associated with ankle instability, and manual stress testing of the ankle should be performed in conjunction with the repair.

3. If the ankle is unstable and a longitudinal split or tear of the peroneus brevis tendon is present, the split can be extended distally and proximally, and then the anterior limb of the peroneus brevis tendon can be used to perform a reconstruction with the application of a Chrisman-Snook procedure as described in the section on ankle instability (Chapter 12).

4. Rupture of either peroneal tendon occurs commonly in association with an enlarged peroneal tubercle and is particularly prominent in patients with a varus hindfoot.

5. With any repair distal to the fibula, both tendon sheaths must be opened to rule out stenosis as each tendon passes in a separate sheath. In particular, the peroneal tubercle must be debrided if prominent. This tubercle is often the source for isolated stenosis and tearing distal to the fibula.

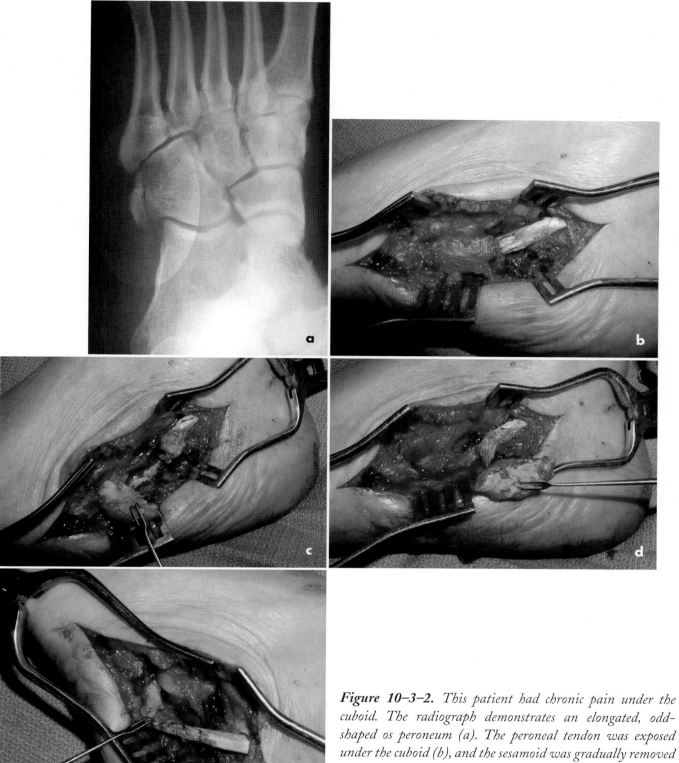

Figure 10–3–2. *This patient had chronic pain under the cuboid. The radiograph demonstrates an elongated, odd-shaped os peroneum (a). The peroneal tendon was exposed under the cuboid (b), and the sesamoid was gradually removed with a small bone hook while the peroneus longus tendon was intact (c, d). The peroneal tendon defect was finally repaired after excision of the sesamoid (e).*

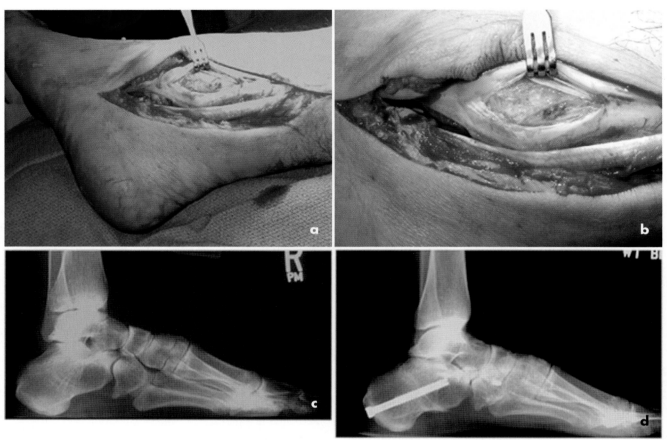

Figure 10–3–3. *This patient was treated for a chronically unstable varus ankle with lateral ankle pain. The split in the peroneal tendon is noted, a common occurrence with an unstable ankle (a, b). The torn portion of the peroneal was extended more proximally and distally, and then the anterior dorsal split portion of the tendon was used to stabilize the ankle with a modified Chrisman-Snook procedure. A calcaneus osteotomy was performed simultaneously, and the preoperative and postoperative lateral x-ray (XR) film is shown (c, d).*

6. Distal tears of the peroneus brevis tendon are not that common. Isolated insertional peroneus brevis tendinopathy does occur in conjunction with varus hindfoot and/or recurrent trauma to the base of the fifth metatarsal.

7. If either the peroneus brevis or longus tendon is completely torn and not salvageable, a decision must be made about the potential use of the remaining tendon. This decision is based on the excursion of the muscle. If, for example, the peroneus longus tendon is completely torn and irreparable but muscle function is still adequate and excursion of the longus tendon is noted, then a tenodesis of the distal stump of the longus tendon is performed to the brevis tendon.

8. Occasionally the enlarged peroneal tubercle may be the source of the tear of the peroneus brevis tendon. This seems to be fairly common in a cavus or varus hindfoot. As the tubercle enlarges, the retinaculum's tightening causes a constriction and thus the rupture. Removing the enlarged tubercle with a chisel followed by bone wax on the roughened bone surface is useful.

Repair of Both the Peroneus Longus and Brevis Tendons

Other than one large report from our institution, rupture of both the peroneus longus and peroneus brevis tendons has rarely been documented. These ruptures are difficult, and combined tears have to be approached as determined by the presence of functioning tendon(s), the mobility of the remaining peroneal musculature, ankle stability, and the position of the heel. Peroneal weakness is often associated with a cavovarus foot, and injury to the tendons of these muscles has a similar effect on the structural balance of the foot. A tear of the peroneus longus tendon with or without a concomitant peroneus brevis tendon tear results in net inversion of the hindfoot by the tibialis posterior muscle. In long-term cases, this scenario results in a fixed varus hindfoot deformity, which must also be corrected.

Although obtaining an MRI preoperatively is helpful, the true extent of the tendon disease is generally revealed only at the time of surgery. The condition of the peroneus longus and brevis tendons should be noted intraoperatively, and when the tendons are ruptured, an estimation is made of the type of rupture and the affected percentage of cross-sectional tendon area. If both tendons are grossly intact, then they are repaired in a standard manner through excision of the longitudinal tear and tubularization of the tendon with a running absorbable braided suture. If one tendon is completely torn and irreparable but the other tendon is considered functional or usable, then a tenodesis is performed proximally, with at the least the musculotendinous tissue or the healthy tendon distal to the muscle for the tenodesis (Fig. 10–3–4). The decision to include a tenodesis should be based on the health of the muscle because no tenodesis should be performed if the muscle excursion of either tendon is absent as a result of scarring or presumed fibrosis. However, if the other tendon was unusable, then a tendon graft or tendon transfer should be considered. If I use a tendon transfer, the flexor digitorum longus (FDL) tendon transfer to the stump of the peroneus brevis tendon or the base of the fifth metatarsal is performed. This transfer is preferable if there is no proximal muscle function or excursion (Figs. 10–3–5 to 10–3–7). If, however, excursion of the proximal muscle is present, a tendon graft (with a hamstring allograft) seems more logical, but it is contraindicated in the presence of muscle fibrosis. Then, the state of

the tissue bed for either the FDL tendon transfer or a tendon graft has to be considered. If active inflammation or fibrosis exists, then either may not function because of the likelihood of scarring and limited tendon excursion. For this reason, either procedure would then be staged with a silicone rod at the initial surgery (Figs. 10–3–8 and 10–3–9). The tendon transfer or graft can be performed at the same sitting if there is minimal scarring. The silicone rod is inserted and attached to the distal stump of the brevis tendon or the base of the fifth metatarsal but is left free proximally. In this way, passive range of motion postoperatively helps form a good synovial-lined tissue bed for the tendon graft or transfer. When the second-stage surgery is performed, a small incision is made proximally to attach the FDL tendon to the silicone rod, which can then be pulled out distally without another long incision. The FDL tendon always provides enough length, and it can be harvested as demonstrated in the following example.

Correcting any deformity of the hindfoot or ankle that could lead to recurrent tendon injury is important. Repair of an unstable ankle must be performed as a planned procedure that is based on preoperative symptoms of instability of the ankle confirmed with stress radiographs. If present, associated hindfoot varus is corrected with a closing wedge biplanar calcaneal osteotomy, and the same incision is used for the peroneal tendon repair as for the osteotomy. Peroneal tendon subluxation or dislocation without ankle instability is treated by a groove-deepening procedure. If peroneal tendon dislocation is present, in addition to ankle instability, then the ankle ligament reconstruction is performed with a modified Chrisman-Snook procedure with the anterior split portion of the peroneus brevis tendon for the reconstruction. The fibula groove is deepened, and the posterior limb of the split tendon, which passes through the fibula, is passed superficial to the remaining peroneal tendon(s) to maintain reduction of the tendon(s). Any tear or redundancy of the superior peroneal retinaculum is repaired (Fig. 10–3–10).

Repair of Dislocation of the Peroneal Tendon(s)

Common to all repairs of a dislocated peroneal tendon is a groove-deepening procedure. Although alternatives have been described, these methods are of historic

Text continued on p. 322

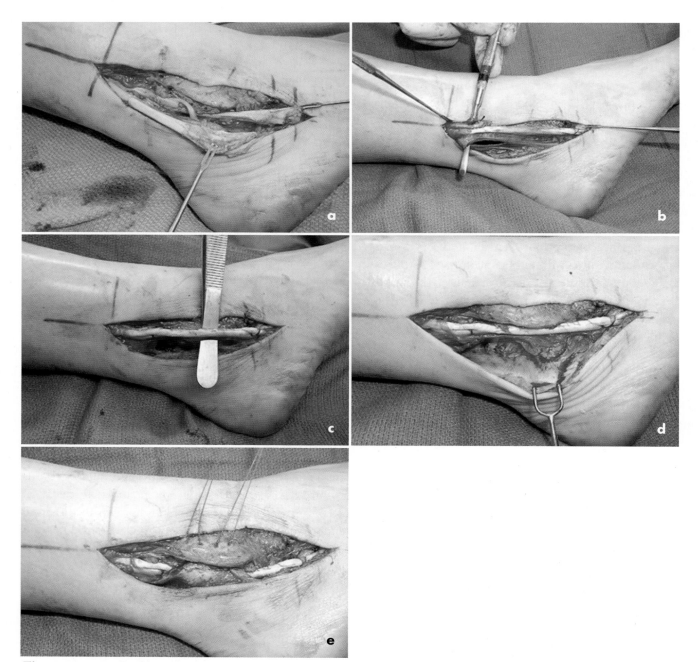

Figure 10–3–4. *In this patient, both brevis and longus tendons were torn; however, the muscles of both tendons still had excursion (a). The torn longus tendon was cut distally and transferred into the stump of the torn brevis tendon distally, and a tenodesis of the longus tendon to the muscle of the brevis tendon was performed proximally (b, c). The fibula groove was deepened (d), and a retinaculum was created from the retrocalcaneal tissue and brought up into the fibula through K-wire holes (e).*

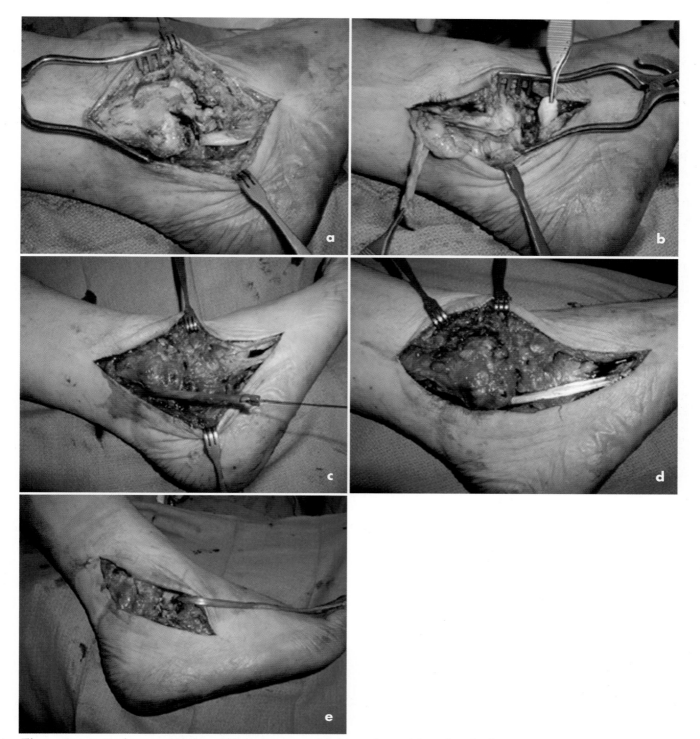

Figure 10–3–5. *Severe ankle instability was present in this patient with no functioning peroneal. Note the appearance on dissection with the scarred stump of the peroneus longus and brevis tendons (a, b). A transfer of the flexor digitorum longus (FDL) tendon was performed and attached to the stump of the brevis tendon (c, d). Then a hamstring allograft was used to perform a reconstruction of the instability (e).*

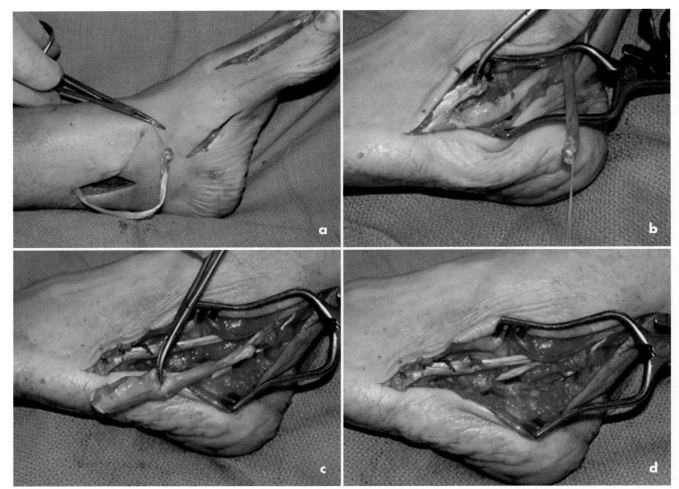

Figure 10–3–6. *An osteotomy of the first metatarsal and calcaneus was performed in addition to transfer of the flexor digitorum longus (FDL) tendon and tenodesis of the torn peroneus longus tendon to repair an unstable ankle. Note the incisions used medially (a), the torn tendons (b), and the transfer of the FDL tendon and the torn longus tendon (c), which was used as a tenodesis to stabilize the ankle (d).*

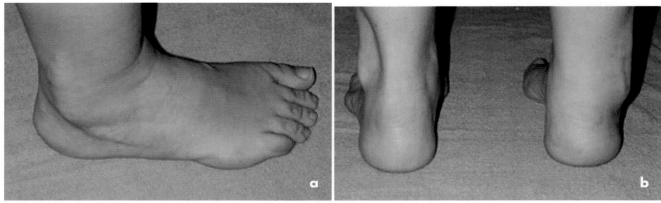

Figure 10–3–7. *This patient had been operated on numerous times for tears of the tendons, neither of which was working. Note the heel varus (a, b).*

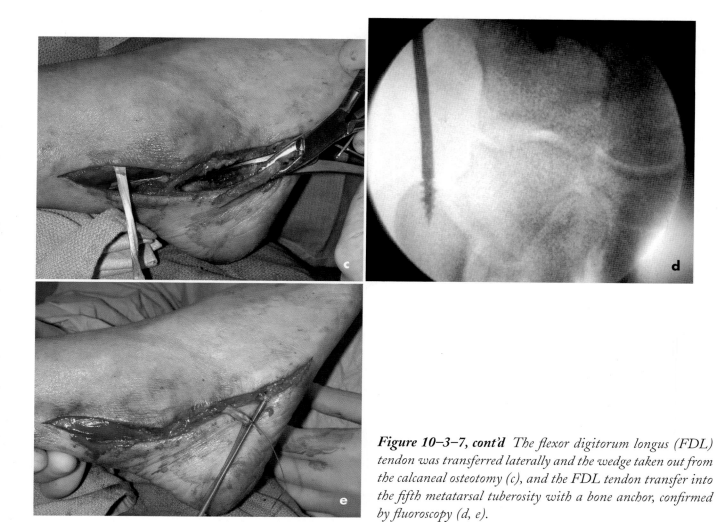

Figure 10–3–7, cont'd *The flexor digitorum longus (FDL) tendon was transferred laterally and the wedge taken out from the calcaneal osteotomy (c), and the FDL tendon transfer into the fifth metatarsal tuberosity with a bone anchor, confirmed by fluoroscopy (d, e).*

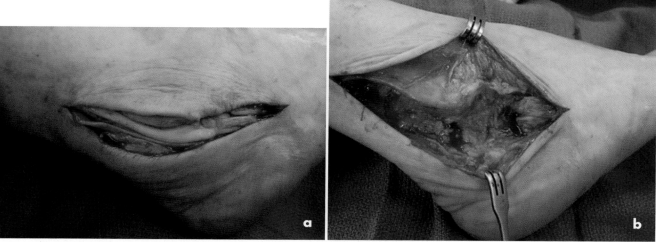

Figure 10–3–8. *Absence of both peroneal tendons was noted here, with severe scarring of the retrofibular space (a, b).*

Continued

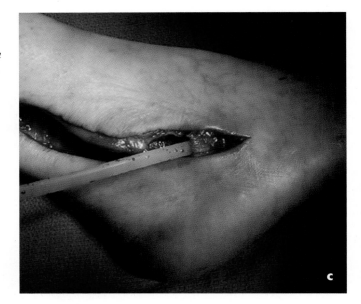

Figure 10–3–8, cont'd A 20-cm silicone rod was attached to the stump of the brevis tendon, but it was left free proximally for staged flexor digitorum longus (FDL) tendon transfer at 6 to 8 weeks. (c). Until the second-stage surgery, active movement of the foot and ankle is encouraged.

Figure 10–3–9. At the second-stage surgery, the flexor digitorum longus (FDL) tendon is harvested (a) and attached to the proximal end of the silicone rod (b), which is then pulled out distally in the synovia-filled tunnel created by the silicone foreign body, and the FDL tendon is attached distally (c, d).

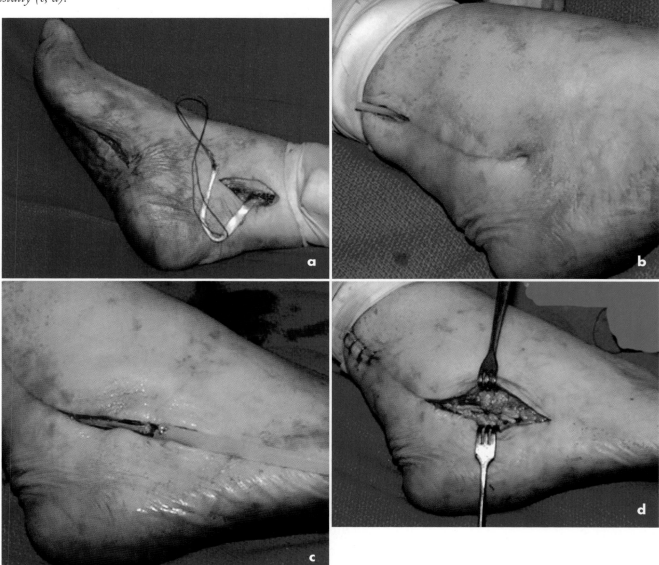

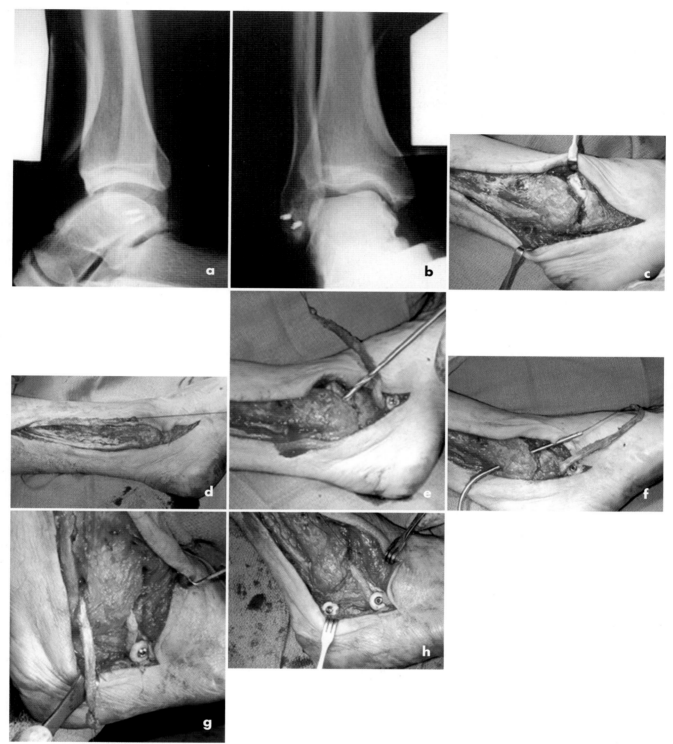

Figure 10–3–10. *This patient had been treated for chronic ankle instability with three prior operations, with persistent instability clinically and noted radiographically (a, b). After the incision, no peroneal tendons were present (c). A slip of the peroneal fascia was harvested (d), it was attached to the neck of the talus under a screw, and a spiked ligament washer and a drill hole were made in the fibula (e). A sucker tip was passed through the fibula to pass the tendon graft (f), which was pulled down and anchored into the calcaneus with a second screw and spiked ligament washer (g, h). At the completion of this procedure, a flexor digitorum longus (FDL) tendon transfer was performed, passing the tendon from the medial side of the foot into the stump of the peroneus brevis tendon laterally to aid dynamic stability of the foot and ankle.*

interest only. Bone block procedures and tendon procedures to hold the dislocated peroneal tendons in place (e.g., with slips of the Achilles tendon) are not nearly as reliable and should not be performed unless under exceptional circumstances. The simplest approach to correcting the dislocation is a deepening of the groove of the posterior fibula, with one method or another, and I prefer to deepen the groove with a large, oval-shaped burr.

The incision for the dislocation must be made carefully, and the tendons must be palpated in the dislocated or subluxated position above the fibula. In this way, the superior peroneal retinaculum can be cut on the fibula itself; then, as the retinacular and periosteal flap is raised off the fibula, the flap serves as part of the soft tissue repair once the groove is deepened. The soft tissue and periosteal flap are raised off the fibula completely, and then the peroneal tendons and the periosteal flap are reflected posteriorly. Some authors recommend a tamp-type procedure where a periosteal flap is raised off the fibula, and then the fibula is tamped down deep in the groove. This procedure can be performed, but the fragment of the bone commonly remains slightly loose and does not adhere to the edge of the fibula adequately. I prefer to perform a simpler deepening of the groove using a burr. Once the groove is created, the distal tip of the fibula should not have a rough edge because of the potential for additional tearing of the tendon as it winds under the fibula. With the foot in dorsiflexion, the tendons should sit behind the fibula without any tendency to subluxate whatsoever. The roughened

groove is smoothed with bone wax, all loose pieces of wax should be removed, and the retinaculum is reattached to the underside of the fibula to prevent any potential for subluxation. This reattachment must be fairly snug; otherwise, the tendons have a tendency to subluxate into a pouch created by the redundant retinaculum. Therefore cutting the retinaculum so it fits directly underneath the trough created by the groove-deepening procedure is frequently necessary. The retinaculum is reattached through K-wire holes. Two pairs of K-wire holes are made so that pairs of sutures can be inserted through the fibula into the retinaculum; then, the retinaculum is pulled in underneath the fibula as noted (Fig. 10–3–11).

Dislocation of the peroneal tendons occurs frequently in association with a fracture of the calcaneus. Dislocation may occur during the impact of the fracture, associated with a fracture of the tip of the fibula. Additionally, dislocation may occur if the calcaneus fracture is treated operatively, in which case the retinaculum may be released to increase exposure and the tendons subluxate. The most common scenario for dislocation is after untreated fractures, with a widened lateral wall of the calcaneus and with abutment against the undersurface of the fibula and eventual dislocation. The approach to correction of these dislocations must be creative because available tissue for the repair may be limited. The principles of reduction, however, remain the same, with a groove deepening, often in conjunction with a modified Chrisman-Snook procedure to hold the tendons in place (Fig. 10–3–12).

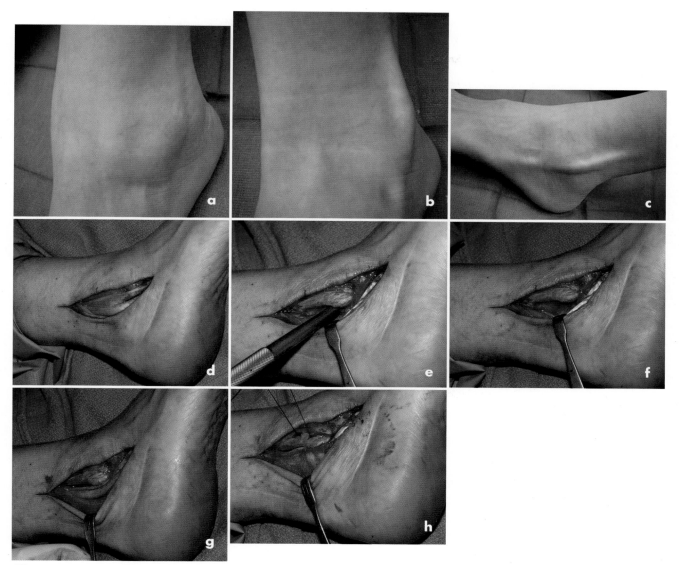

Figure 10–3–11. *This patient had chronic pain resulting from peroneus brevis tendon dislocation. The tendon is reduced (a), and then by rotating the ankle, the patient could voluntarily dislocate the tendons (b, c). The tendon is dislocated with a torn superior peroneal retinaculum, which was reduced by tamping the posterior fibula (d–f). The tendons are now reduced but are maintained in the reduced position through securing the retinaculum with sutures under the fibula (g, h).*

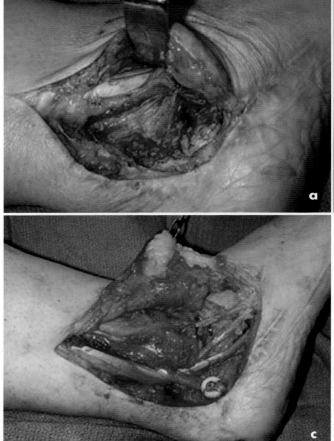

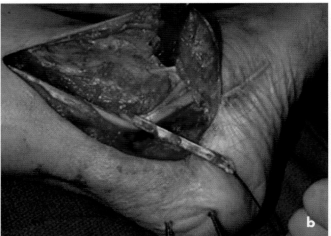

Figure 10–3–12. *Dislocation of the peroneal tendons occurs commonly after untreated fractures of the calcaneus, with widening of the tuberosity. They can also dislocate after open reduction and internal fixation when the peroneal retinaculum is completely released for exposure. In this patient, a calcaneus osteotomy was combined with arthrodesis of the subtalar joint and with peroneal repair. Note here that both of the tendons are dislocated (a) and are corrected with a strip of the peroneus brevis tendon. With a modified Chrisman-Snook procedure, the tendon is attached to the calcaneus with a screw and a spiked ligament washer.*

Suggested Readings

Baumhauer JF, Nawoczenski DA, DiGiovanni BF, Flemister AS. Ankle pain and peroneal tendon pathology. Clin Sports Med 23:21–34, 2004.

Clarke HD, Kitaoka HB, Ehman RL. Peroneal tendon injuries. Foot Ankle Int 19:280–288, 1998.

Krause JO, Brodsky JW. Peroneus brevis tendon tears: pathophysiology, surgical reconstruction, and clinical results. Foot Ankle Int 19:271–279, 1998.

Molloy R, Tisdel C. Failed treatment of peroneal tendon injuries. Foot Ankle Clin 8:115–129, ix, 2003.

Pelet S, Saglini M, Garofalo R, Wettstein M, et al. Traumatic rupture of both peroneal longus and brevis tendons. Foot Ankle Int 24:721–723, 2003.

Tarsal Coalition

Overview

Regardless of the type of tarsal coalition present, once it becomes symptomatic, it rarely resolves with nonoperative care. Although traditional references have been made to treatment with immobilization of the foot to decrease symptoms, this does not usually have long-term beneficial effects. Although this treatment may temporarily decrease the soreness in the foot, the reactive tenderness in the lateral calf musculature, and the generalized lower limb dysfunction and aching, symptoms recur. Rarely therefore, will I apply a cast or boot to a child or adult for definitive treatment purposes. If a marked foot and limb tenderness is present, then this can be used as an initiating form of treatment, while definitive surgical plans are put into effect.

Examination and Decision Making

Examination of a person's foot is useful while the person is standing, walking, sitting, and lying down. When a person with a normal foot is sitting, a natural equinovarus posture is present in the foot as it relaxes. This is not the case with a tarsal coalition because the foot is held in a more rigid position of neutral dorsiflexion with slight valgus. The peroneal tendons are often visible because of ongoing contraction, but true peroneal "spasm" does not occur. The terminology used historically (i.e., as a peroneal spastic flatfoot) is incorrect. The peroneal musculature may be tender and certainly tight

as a result of subtalar joint irritation, but spasm does not occur. The decision for surgery, and in particular the type of surgery, is based on the flexibility of the foot, the presence of arthritis, the type of coalition, and function of the remaining foot (Fig. 11–1–1).

Arthritis of the foot is rare in a child in association with either a subtalar or calcaneonavicular coalition. The beaking of the talonavicular joint appears naturally as a result of traction on the anterior capsule of the ankle on the neck of the talus and does not in any way imply the presence of arthritis. However, arthritis can occur because subtalar arthritis is common in adults with a middle facet coalition. Early arthritis is caused by prior surgery, or it may be associated with extreme rigidity, even in the child. Do not be fooled by the presence of motion in the hindfoot. If the foot is examined carefully, most of this motion is coming from either a transverse tarsal or the ankle joints. True subtalar motion is not normal and is usually absent, particularly with a middle facet coalition. In patients who have severe stiffness, knowing how much true motion is present in the foot and how much the peroneal muscles are limiting subtalar motion is worthwhile (Fig. 11–1–2).

In both the adult and the child, if the peroneal muscles are tight, I will block the peroneal nerve at the fibular neck with a short-acting anesthetic (lidocaine [Xylocaine]) and reexamine the foot. After the peroneal nerve block, the foot is frequently much easier to

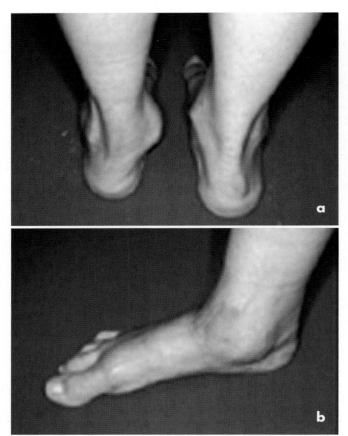

Figure 11–1–1. A middle facet coalition can present as a mass on the medial hindfoot. It was so large that it presented not as a stiff foot but with compression of the tibial nerve and as a tarsal tunnel syndrome in this adolescent patient (a, b).

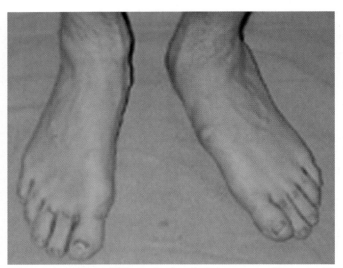

Figure 11–1–2. When the foot is in severe valgus, as this left foot is, the outcome of resection of the coalition without additional surgery is poor. If this hindfoot were reasonably mobile, then regardless of the type of coalition present, once the subtalar joint is more flexible after excision of the coalition, worsening flatfoot will occur.

examine, the rigidity of the hindfoot previously noted is no longer present, and the surgery can be planned correctly. Diagnostic lidocaine blocks of the subtalar joint or the sinus tarsi are not too helpful in these patients. Sometimes the coalition is not visible radiographically, and rarely, even with appropriate imaging, including radiographs, magnetic resonance imaging (MRI), and computerized axial tomography (CAT) scan, the coalition is difficult to visualize. In these patients, a diagnostic block of a longer acting anesthetic would be useful to plan treatment.

Wherever possible, I attempt resection of a coalition rather than an arthrodesis. Certainly in the presence of arthritis of the hindfoot joints, an arthrodesis would be necessary, but in my experience the arthrodesis is overused as a treatment in adults and children. If arthrodesis is performed, a triple arthrodesis is only indicated with extensive deformity, which includes the subtalar and transverse tarsal joints and arthritis. A triple arthrodesis is therefore not required for correction of a middle facet coalition unless additional disease is present in the transverse tarsal joint (Fig. 11–1–3). Rarely will I perform an arthrodesis for a calcaneonavicular coalition, even in adults.

The onset of pain in adults with a calcaneonavicular coalition usually begins after a minor episode of trauma. This condition is the subject of frequent dispute in worker's compensation claims. In these patients, imaging studies clearly show a tarsal coalition, which was previously asymptomatic, and as a result of a minor twist or trauma, the condition becomes symptomatic. Excision of a calcaneonavicular coalition in the adult is still worth the effort. Provided no degenerative changes are present and the foot is not too rigid, attaining surprising mobility and improvement of symptoms from resection is possible. This does not, however, apply to symptomatic subtalar coalition in the adult, which usually requires a subtalar arthrodesis.

According to the literature, a middle facet coalition in a child can be excised if it is less than 50%. I do not agree

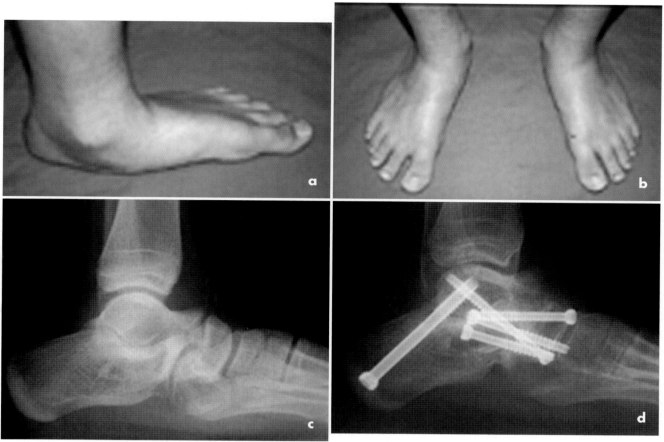

Figure 11–1–3. *This patient was 16 years old at the time of treatment for a rigid middle facet coalition. Note the marked abduction of the midfoot (a) and the pes planus associated with arthritis of the subtalar joint (b, c). Performing a resection was unrealistic, nor could an isolated subtalar arthrodesis correct the deformity. A triple arthrodesis was performed (d).*

with this position, and regardless of the size of the coalition, I perform a resection of the entire coalition. The outcome of resection of the middle facet coalition depends more on the flexibility and deformity of the remainder of the foot. The problem with a complete coalition is not the ability to resect it, but the adaptive changes that have taken place in the subtalar joint and the remainder of the foot over time.

The question then is not whether to resect the coalition, but what additional procedures need to be performed to maintain motion and improve function. These include procedures that are discussed in other parts of this book, including calcaneal osteotomy, subtalar arthroereisis, Achilles tendon lengthening, and medial cuneiform osteotomy. Although most of my experience is with a middle facet or a calcaneonavicular coalition, the more

unusual coalitions, either talonavicular or calcaneocuboid, are also encountered. These present a unique set of problems, including stiffness of the hindfoot, planovalgus deformity, and a ball and socket ankle. The foot is always pronated, the hindfoot is fixed in valgus, and the ankle is in valgus as well.

Resection of a Middle Facet Coalition

An incision is made medially and extends from the undersurface of the medial malleolus distally and beyond the talonavicular joint. The incision is deepened through subcutaneous tissue, veins are cauterized, and the sheath of the flexor digitorum longus (FDL) tendon is opened. This tendon forms the upper boundary of the coalition, and the tendon is retracted dorsally. Inferior to this, the sheath of the flexor hallucis longus (FHL) tendon is now carefully opened and identified. The tendon is retracted inferiorly, and then these tendons mark the boundaries for dissection of the coalition. Elevation of all of the soft tissue, including a large periosteal flap from the sustentaculum, is useful to adequately visualize the bone to be resected. Starting with this bone resection can be intimidating because standard landmarks are usually absent. If necessary, the surgeon can proceed more distally to the talonavicular joint and then work back posteriorly after opening up the joint, but this is not usually necessary.

The sustentaculum is now gradually removed until the scar of the original middle facet is visualized, which is seen slightly more posteriorly. Try to preserve some of the arch of the sustentaculum for support of the FHL tendon when progressing with the debridement. A large pineapple-shaped burr can be used above the sustentaculum, or, use a combination of a rongeur, curette, and chisel, as I do. One way of identifying the location of the anterior aspect of the coalition is to make a lateral puncture in the sinus tarsi and insert a probe, which is then advanced and pushed medially. The exit point of this probe marks the anterior aspect of the coalition. As the bone is gradually debrided, a rongeur is now inserted once fatty tissue is observed on the medial aspect of the sinus tarsi. This represents the apex of the cone of the tarsal canal. Once this can be identified, then the rest of the procedure is much easier because movement of the subtalar joint directs the dissection.

A laminar spreader is inserted into the tarsal canal from the medial side, and then, with gradual distraction, the middle facet and ultimately the posterior facet become visible. Removal of most, if not all, of the middle facet is necessary until the entire posterior facet is visible. Perfect, unrestricted motion of the posterior facet should be present, and it should be checked visually with rotatory motion (Fig. 11–1–4).

Before the resection is started, the foot must be inspected and deformity must be assessed. Some heel valgus with abduction across the transverse tarsal joint is often present, and additional procedures need to be planned carefully. If the hindfoot is left in valgus, medial stress increases, and with the lack of support of the sus-tentaculum, gradual collapse of the midfoot with increasing pes planus can develop. If heel valgus and not midfoot abduction is present, I add an arthroereisis to the excision of the middle facet coalition. This can be done almost under direct visualization because the medial aspect of the subtalar implant is visible and protrudes from the resected portion of the coalition. In addition to slightly inverting the heel, this arthroereisis slightly opens up the posterior facet, and this opening is desirable. I try to leave these implants in for at least 6 months in the child so that as the foot grows, an adaptive change, which is helped with a good orthotic arch support, takes place in the hindfoot.

Excision of the Calcaneonavicular Coalition

An incision is made in the sinus tarsi and extends from the tip of the fibula over toward the base of the fourth metatarsal. The extensor brevis muscle is identified, and it is carefully elevated off the floor of the sinus tarsi and the dorsal surface of the calcaneocuboid joint. Tagging this muscle as it is elevated from the floor of the sinus tarsi is helpful. Once the entire muscle and its proximal periosteal attachment are elevated, a small tag suture is inserted, and this insertion then facilitates further dissection of the muscle off the calcaneocuboid joint (Fig. 11–1–5).

A lamina spreader is inserted into the sinus tarsi and intermittently distracted until the anterior aspect of the subtalar joint is visible. The lateral aspect of the talonavicular joint capsule must be incised until the articular surface is visible because this surface guides the surgeon as to the extent of the dissection. The coalition is not always that easily visible. For this reason, I start at the edge of the calcaneocuboid joint, and using a half-inch straight osteotome, I cut the bone. This piece of bone includes the portion that extends from the calcaneus up to the navicular, but usually there is a large protruding piece, which abuts the talonavicular joint as well. Here, I use either a half-inch or quarter-inch osteotome to remove a rectangular and not a triangular piece of bone.

The coalition extends far medially, and if either a triangular or trapezoidal piece of bone is taken out, the

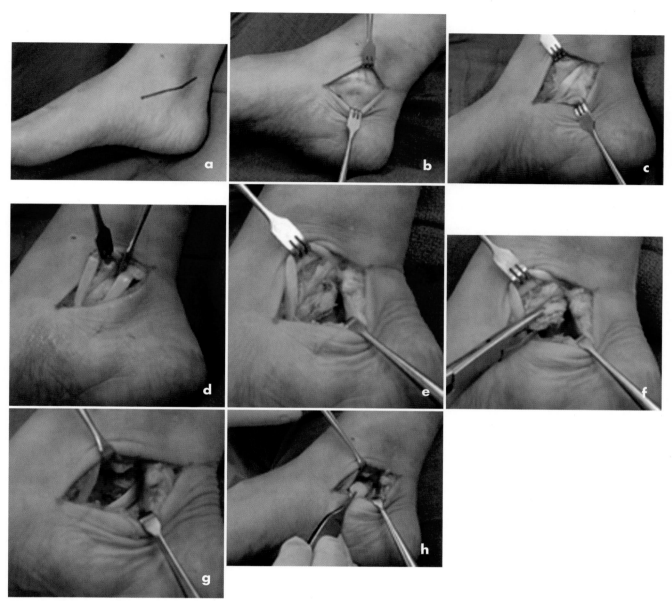

Figure 11–1–4. *The sequence of steps with excision of a middle facet coalition. The incision is marked out (a), subcutaneous dissection is performed (b), and the flexor digitorum longus (FDL) (c) and flexor hallucis longus (FHL) tendons (d) are identified. With the tendons retracted, the coalition is visible (e), and it is gradually removed (f). At the completion of resection of the coalition, the posterior facet is visible, the FHL remains under the sustentaculum (g), and bone wax is applied to the exposed cancellous surfaces (h).*

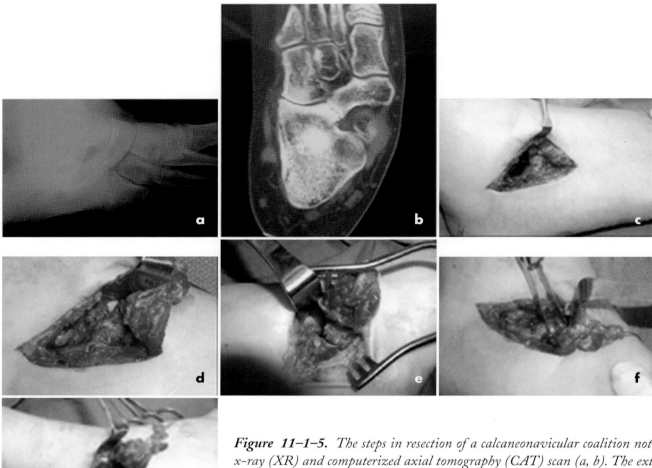

Figure 11–1–5. *The steps in resection of a calcaneonavicular coalition noted on x-ray (XR) and computerized axial tomography (CAT) scan (a, b). The extensor brevis muscle is elevated off the floor of the sinus tarsi (c–e). Note the edge of the talonavicular joint, which demarcates the dorsal margin of the coalition (d, e). Two chisel blades are inserted into the coalition (f), and the position is noted on fluoroscopy before complete excision (g).*

coalition will persist on the medial aspect of the joint complex. Excision of the coalition must be verified fluoroscopically. Check the range of motion of the peritalar joints to ensure that adequate decompression has been performed. Rarely, the foot is still stiff, and possibly a combined calcaneonavicular and middle facet coalition is present. In these instances, a second incision has to be made medially, and the approach should be made as previously outlined. Before concluding this procedure, insert a lamina spreader into the sinus tarsi to open up the subtalar joint itself. The entire subtalar joint should move freely, and the middle facet should be visible and mobile. At the completion of the procedure, I use bone wax on the resected bone surfaces. An alternative technique to prevent either recurrent or heterotopic bone is to insert the extensor brevis muscle into the coalition site. This insertion has the advantage of a large muscle surface being present, preventing bone formation. The disadvantage of this technique is that it leaves a rather substantial hollow on the lateral side of the foot, which may not be cosmetically desirable. Nonetheless, some covering of the bone becomes necessary (Fig. 11–1–6).

Treatment of More Extensive Coalitions

In this section, the approach to correction of an isolated talonavicular coalition, or more extensive coalition of the transverse tarsal joint, is discussed. This may

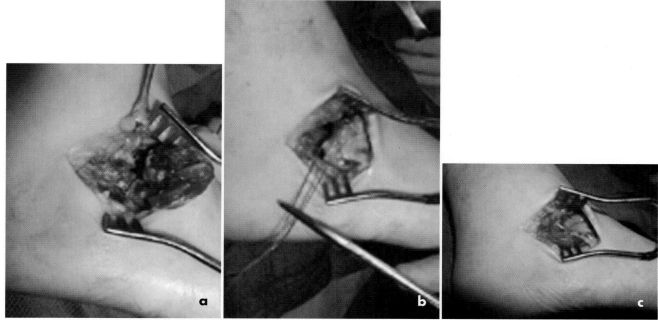

Figure 11–1–6. *The extensor brevis muscle has been elevated (a); tagged with a suture (b); and then, at the completion of the coalition excision, inserted into the void with the tagged suture inserted percutaneously through to the medial side of the foot (c).*

include variants of fibular hemimelia and absence of the fifth ray. The foot is always rigid, is pronated, and has a fixed heel valgus and a flattened calcaneal pitch angle. Patients with such a condition have aching, fatigue, and soreness along the medial arch of the foot with sinus tarsi pain. The goal here is not to create a normally shaped foot but simply to restructure the hindfoot to decrease the abnormal forces on the ankle. Where possible, osteotomies are performed through the coalition, although arthrodesis may have to be performed (Fig. 11–1–7).

The hindfoot osteotomies are performed with a calcaneal osteotomy, which is done in two planes. The calcaneus must be pulled distally and then pushed medially. The Achilles tendon must be lengthened or a gastrocnemius muscle recession must be performed at the same time because the latter is always tight. This biplanar calcaneal osteotomy restores the calcaneal pitch angle and shifts the weight-bearing forces on the ankle slightly medially. The remainder of the procedure depends on the extent of the coalition. If it is extensive, then a transverse tarsal osteotomy can be performed. At times, this can be limited just to the talonavicular coalition or can extend laterally to include the calcaneocuboid coalition as well.

The incision is made in the plane between the anterior tibial and the posterior tibial tendons. The neck of the talus is opened, and with subperiosteal dissection, a guide pin is inserted across the transverse tarsal joint to exit at the level of the calcaneocuboid joint. If only the talonavicular osteotomy is to be performed, then this can exit slightly more posteriorly in the sinus tarsi. The osteotomy is done with the biplanar resection, and a small plantar and medial-based wedge is removed to adduct and plantarflex the arch of the foot. Good correction of the midfoot can be obtained in this manner.

Both children and adults will need 18 months to regain function, to regain strength, and to sense the normalization of the anatomy. Orthotic arch supports are important, and occasionally physical therapy is useful to improve the strength of the limb. If a ball and socket ankle is present, then this is treated simultaneously with a medial closing wedge supramalleolar osteotomy in conjunction with one or more of the procedures outlined here (Fig. 11–1–8).

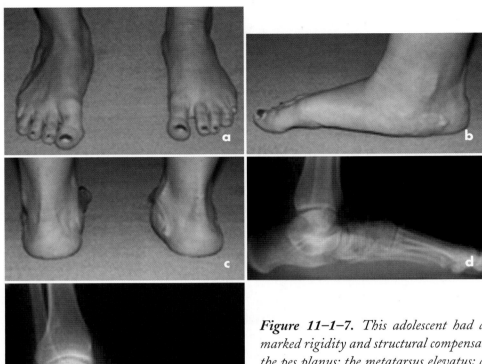

Figure 11–1–7. This adolescent had a severe middle facet coalition with marked rigidity and structural compensation of the midfoot and forefoot. Note the pes planus; the metatarsus elevatus; and the hindfoot valgus (a–c), which was associated with the fixed hindfoot deformity seen on x-ray (XR) (d). This deformity was corrected with a bone block arthrodesis of the subtalar joint to improve the talar declination and the calcaneal pitch. Then, an opening wedge osteotomy of the medial cuneiform was performed to reduce the metatarsus elevatus (e).

Techniques, tips, and pitfalls

1. Range of motion is the key to the success of this operation. If the foot is stiff at the completion of excision of the coalition, it will be permanently stiff after the operation, and arthrodesis would have been a preferable procedure.

2. If an occult double coalition is suspected after resection of the calcaneonavicular coalition and the hindfoot remains stiff, try to open up the subtalar joint with a laminar spreader in the sinus tarsi to completely visualize the middle facet.

3. Excision of the calcaneonavicular coalition must be done by resection of a rectangular piece of bone, not a trapezoidal or triangular piece of bone, because the latter leaves behind part of the coalition medially.

4. Additional procedures are commonly performed in conjunction with resection of either coalition.

5. Having a sense of rigidity of the foot before the start of excision of the coalition is helpful. With a common peroneal nerve block in the office or after administration of a general anesthetic, the foot is manipulated, and the extent of the rigidity (or reactive contracture of the peroneal muscles) can be more appreciated.

6. Resection of the middle facet coalition *can* be performed for extensive (including 100%) coalitions. However, the hindfoot must be mobile after resection; adjunctive procedures should be performed; and postoperative rehabilitation, including orthotic arch supports, should be used vigorously.

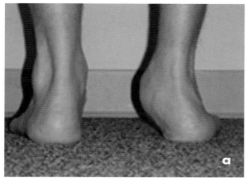

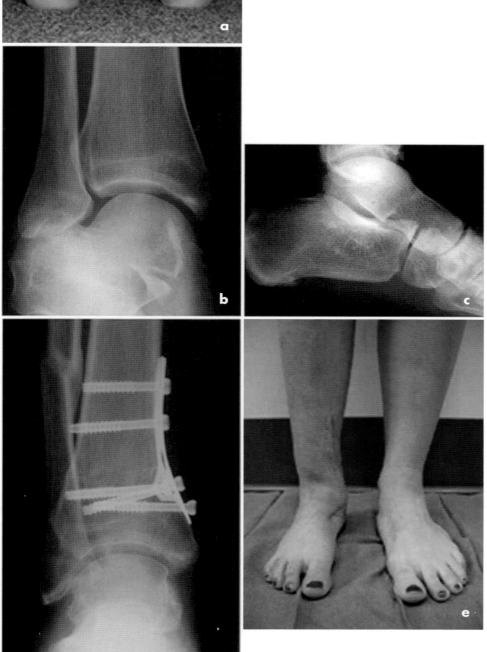

Figure 11–1–8. *This severe hindfoot deformity with a fixed heel valgus (a) and a ball and socket ankle (b) was caused by a talonavicular coalition (c). This was corrected with a medial closing wedge supramalleolar osteotomy, an oblique fibular osteotomy, and a medial translational osteotomy of the calcaneus (d). Note the marked improvement in the tibiotalar axis and the position of the hindfoot (d, e).*

Suggested Readings

Cohen BE, Davis WH, Anderson RB. Success of calcaneonavicular coalition resection in the adult. Foot Ankle Int 17:569–572, 1996.

Drennan J. Tarsal coalitions. Instr Course Lect 45:323–329, 1996.

Richardson EG. Tarsal coalition. In Myerson MS (ed): Disorders of the Foot and Ankle. Philadelphia, WB Saunders, 2000.

Vincent KA. Tarsal coalition and painful flatfoot. J Am Acad Orthop Surg 6:274–281, 1998.

Ankle Instability and Impingement Syndromes

Lateral Ankle Ligament Reconstruction

Before the lateral ankle ligament is reconstructed, the surgeon must consider the type of instability, the presence of pain, and the exact location of symptoms. For example, if a patient has pain associated with instability, either a rupture of the peroneal tendon or another intra-articular disease, including synovitis or an osteochondral injury, has to be considered. Ankle instability on its own does not cause pain. Ascertaining whether symptoms are present when the patient walks on a flat surface or whether they only occur when the patient walks on uneven ground surfaces is important (Fig. 12–1–1). If the patient has symptoms intermittently on flat surfaces, then the need for reconstruction is increased.

The presence of the pain must be distinguished from its location. If the pain is posteriorly located behind the fibula, then I routinely use an open and not a percutaneous approach for the reconstruction. This incision (either an anatomic repair or a modification of the Elmslie procedure) needs to be more posterior, behind the fibula, to facilitate inspection of the peroneal tendons. If the pain is more anterolateral, this can be associated with an anterior capsular impingement syndrome or an intra-articular process, which would warrant further investigation with magnetic resonance imaging (MRI) or a computerized axial tomography (CAT) scan. Sinus tarsi pain should be evaluated for the associated possibility of combined ankle and subtalar

ankle instability, which is unusual, but also the presence of an unrecognized injury to the lateral process of the talus or the anterior process of the calcaneus.

Ordinarily, athletes can have recurrent ankle instability with subtle heel varus. The triad of recurrent ankle sprains, heel varus, and stress fracture of the fifth metatarsal should always be taken into consideration when treatment is planned (Fig. 12–1–2). The patient in Figure 2 represents a good example of failure of treatment if the underlying biomechanical and anatomic process is ignored. A calcaneus osteotomy, in addition to a stronger ankle ligament repair, which may have prevented the subsequent problems, would have been a better correction for the patient. Performing an ankle ligament reconstruction without correcting the heel varus is possible, but the surgery depends on the flexibility of the subtalar joint and additional symptoms.

If, for example, the patient has symptoms while walking on a flat ground surface and heel varus is present, then my inclination would be to correct the calcaneus at the same time. If a patient has undergone prior ankle ligament reconstruction and has recurrent symptoms, I always look for unrecognized heel varus or mild tibia vara as a source for the failure. One question that often arises is whether the opposite foot should be corrected if deformity is present. Most patients with heel varus have this deformity bilaterally. I have not, however, seen any biomechanical problem with correction of the heel

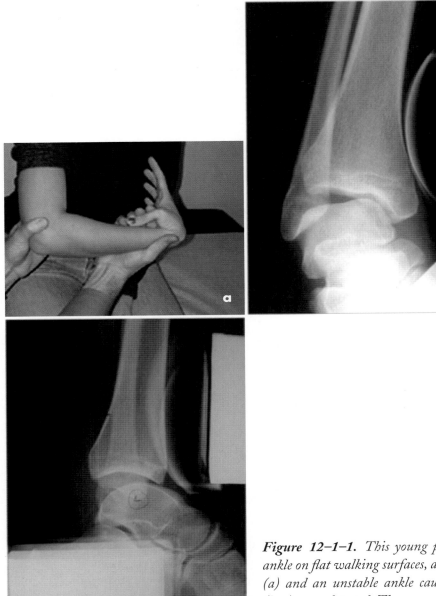

Figure 12–1–1. *This young patient had symptoms of "giving way" of the ankle on flat walking surfaces, and on examination marked generalized laxity (a) and an unstable ankle caused by inversion and anterior drawer stress (b, c) were detected. The generalized laxity must be taken into consideration when treatment is planned.*

varus on one heel alone. Patients seem to adapt to this correction fairly well, and if contralateral symptoms subsequently occur, the correction can be done at a later date.

Usually an orthotic arch support with correct posting is sufficient to alleviate any minor symptoms of heel varus on the asymptomatic ankle. If a calcaneal osteotomy is performed, then this is done in either one or two planes, depending on the pitch of the calcaneus. A lateral closing wedge osteotomy is always performed. Then the

calcaneus can be translated slightly laterally and then shifted cephalad if the calcaneal pitch is markedly increased. For some patients with more severe heel varus associated with ankle instability, a plantar fascia release may need to be performed simultaneously.

The radiographic evaluation should routinely include weight bearing and x-ray (XR) images (Fig. 12–1–3). In addition to routine radiographs, I obtain an MRI picture and a CAT scan as needed on the basis of additional disease present.

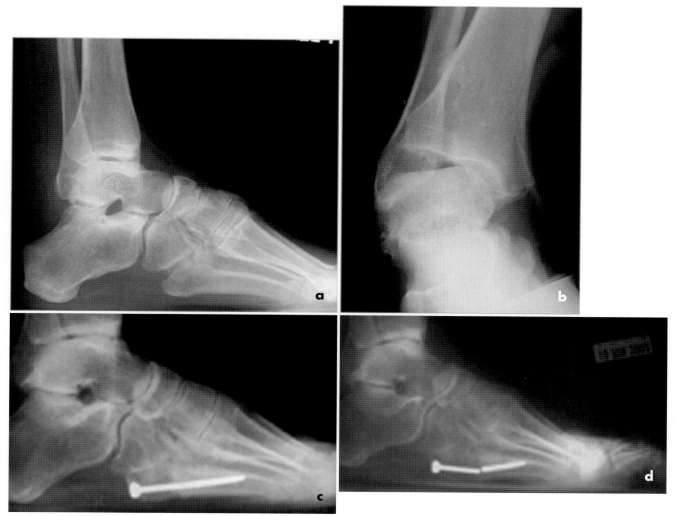

Figure 12–1–2. *This patient complained of intermittent ankle instability without pain. Note the cavovarus configuration of the foot on the lateral weight-bearing x-ray (XR) image (a). Inversion stress XR image showed laxity on inversion stress, and an ankle ligament reconstruction was performed with a Broström procedure (b). Four months later, the patient sustained a stress fracture of the fifth metatarsal. It was treated with percutaneous screw fixation (c), but failure occurred 3 months later (d), along with ultimate recurrence of ankle instability, when he was referred for further reconstruction.*

Assessment of the strength and function of the peroneal tendons in all patients who have recurrent ankle instability is important. Generally, these tendons are weak, and peroneal tendon rehabilitation is essential, even before the ankle ligament reconstruction is started. This facilitates their recovery and restoration with a return to sporting activities. I do not generally obtain an MRI on the ankle even in patients who have peroneal tendon symptoms because the incision is simply modified, as noted previously, and the peroneal tendons are inspected.

Operation Selection

Ankle ligament reconstruction in the high-performance athlete must be approached differently. Never sacrifice the peroneal tendon as part of a reconstructive procedure, and even using a strip of the peroneal brevis tendon is not warranted in the high-performance or competitive athlete. If a patient has gross ankle instability and anatomic repair is not thought to be sufficient, then augmentation of this anatomic repair with a hamstring allograft should be performed. Under these

Figure 12–1–3. Varus and valgus stress was applied to this ankle in a patient with recurrent ankle instability and mild intra-articular ankle pain. Note the lateral ankle instability (a), but on valgus stress (b), a divot or depression was detected in the medial tibial plafond. Even with correct lateral ligament reconstruction, the talus will tend to "fall" back into varus, and the repair will probably fail, with recurrent symptoms of instability.

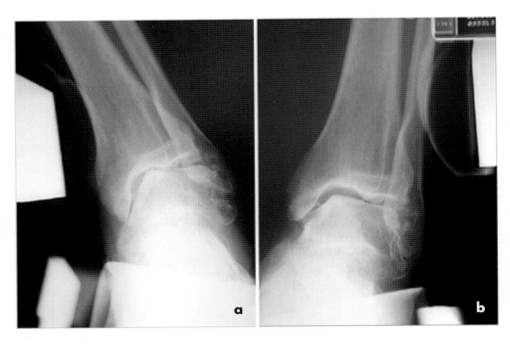

circumstances, my preference is to perform a percutaneous hamstring allograft procedure in these athletes anyway and not to resort to an open procedure.

Use of the hamstring allograft is preferable where possible. Although a hamstring autograft reconstruction has been popularized recently, this reconstruction should be avoided in athletes who run and in those athletes who are involved in ball and racket sports. This reconstruction is particularly relevant in the sprinting athlete in whom terminal flexion torque is compromised if the hamstring is sacrificed.

When should an anatomic repair be performed as opposed to a reconstruction? I am inclined to perform a percutaneous procedure using a hamstring allograft with biointerference screws wherever possible. If this tissue is not available, then two alternatives have to be considered: a modification of either the Elmslie or Chrisman-Snook procedure, or the hamstring procedure with an autograft. Although I routinely used an anatomic repair of the Broström procedure for most reconstructive procedures in the past, this was used with caution in the heavyweight athlete, such as a boxer or body builder, or in the patient with any heel varus, in which case a tendon graft procedure needs to be performed.

Whenever a tendon reconstruction procedure is performed, maintaining the correct kinematics of the ankle,

which is impossible with a slip of the peroneal tendon, is important. For this reason, I prefer to use a free tendon graft. Even with the allograft hamstring procedure, which is currently my preferred operation, attention has to be paid to the entrance and exit points of the graft in the fibula. Note again caution with the use of hamstring autograft in the sprinting athlete, which causes a deficit in terminal flexion torque.

In the patient with intra-articular ankle disease, the timing of the surgery is always a concern. For example, if an osteochondral defect, which requires treatment, is present, how is this operation performed, in addition to ankle ligament reconstruction (Fig. 12–1–4)? In these patients an ankle arthroscopy, in conjunction with the ligament reconstruction, is recommended.

However, the traditional rehabilitation after ligament reconstruction consists of immobilization for up to 6 weeks, which would conceivably have a negative effect on the recovery and rehabilitation after debridement of an osteochondral defect. The traditional rehabilitation with immobilization is really outmoded and should rarely be used. Although immobilization in a boot or brace can be used for comfort purposes, realistically, if fixation techniques are used correctly, immobilization should not be needed at all. After any ankle ligament reconstruction, I let patients start passive range-of-motion exercises at 2 weeks and walk out of the boot

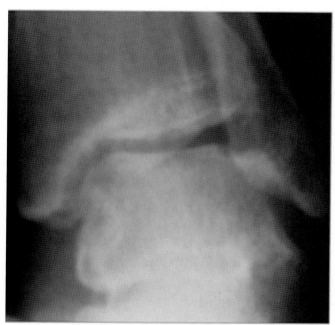

Figure 12–1–4. *This patient underwent treatment of painful ankle instability. Note on stress x-ray (XR) film the instability that is present and the anterolateral defect of the talus. The rehabilitation after surgery must take both diseases into consideration.*

with a stirrup brace, with physical therapy and rehabilitation started as early as possible.

Therefore for most patients, the concept of contrary rehabilitation does not apply. Nonetheless, it is something to consider when combined diseases are addressed. The other issue pertaining to the intra-articular disease concerns the type of reconstructive procedure used. After ankle arthroscopy, interstitial tissue edema is always present with fluid leakage into the soft tissues, and I have found that finding the correct anatomic plane, for example, for reconstruction using a Broström procedure, can be more difficult because of the tissue edema. I do not believe that performing an ankle arthroscopy is necessary in the absence of intra-articular disease or symptoms of ankle pain.

The Broström Procedure

The incision for the Broström procedure can follow the traditional hockey stick or J-type incision, but this is difficult to perform when the peroneal tendon is inspected. As a rule, I use a more longitudinal incision toward the posterior aspect of the fibula, inspecting the peroneal tendon simultaneously and facilitating repair of the calcaneal fibular ligament (Fig. 12–1–5). Accessing the anterior ankle and even extending it to perform an open cheilectomy from a lateral or even a posterolateral incision on the fibula are easy.

Take care to avoid the superficial peroneal nerve in the terminal portion of the incision anteriorly. The soft tissue is reflected and the extensor retinaculum identified as a separate layer before the ankle joint is opened. This extensor retinaculum can be a strong supplement to the strength of the anatomic procedure (Fig. 12–1–6). The inferior root of the extensor retinaculum inserts into the neck of the calcaneus just anterior to the subtalar joint and can be used to stabilize both the ankle and subtalar joints in cases of combined instability.

This extensor retinaculum is not strong enough on its own to correct instability and should be combined with the anatomic procedure described. The incision through the anterior talofibular ligament must be made carefully. Sometimes a bony avulsion is present off the tip of the fibula, and therefore the incision through the ligament must be as close to the fibula as possible. The original description of this procedure included a vest-over-pants repair of the anterior talofibular ligament, which is almost impossible to perform correctly because of the paucity of adequate ligamentous tissue. For this reason, I make the incision through the anterior talofibular ligament as close to the fibula as possible and dissect the ligament off the tip of the fibula. The periosteal tissue is then raised with a small cuff of the remnant of the anterior talofibular ligament off the fibula, and this can then be used to lie over the anatomic repair once the anterior talofibular ligament has been pulled up into the fibula. I generally debride the edge of the fibular with either a rongeur or a small burr to create a bleeding trough for reattachment of the ligament.

The same principle is applied to the calcaneal fibular ligament. Detaching it directly from the fibula is easier than cutting it in the central body of the ligament and attempting a repair of a short ligament. Attachment of the anterior talofibular ligament to the fibula can be done either with a suture anchor or with K-wire holes through the fibula. I prefer the latter technique because these holes can be made in pairs and the suture can be

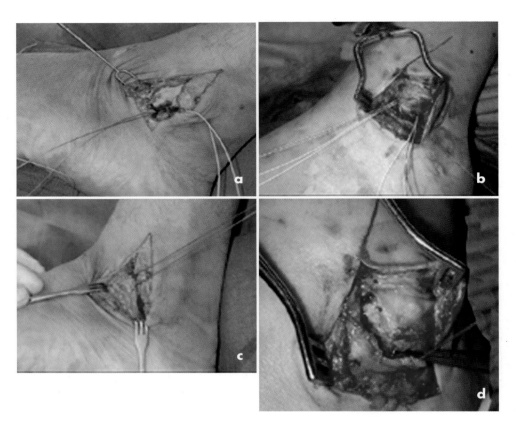

Figure 12–1–5. The Broström procedure with a vertical incision anterior to the fibula. In this patient, suture anchors were inserted into the fibula tip (a) and used to imbricate the anterior talofibular and calcaneofibular ligaments (b, c). The extensor retinaculum is finally used to reinforce the reconstruction as a layer on top of the repaired ligament (d).

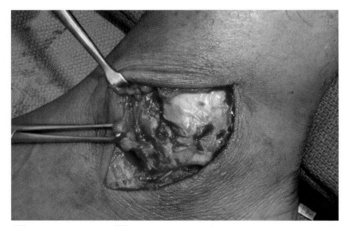

Figure 12–1–6. The extensor retinaculum is shown in the forceps as a separate layer anterior to the talofibular ligament.

inserted through the ligament as a Y-shaped suture, pulled up, and imbricated with the ligament into the prepared trough on the tip of the fibula. Two sets of sutures are used to reattach the anterior talofibular ligament. When tying down the ligament, do not tie the knot over the fibula (Fig. 12–1–7). The knot is invariably prominent, and this can be irritating and painful,

particularly in patients who have thin subcutaneous tissue. The knot should therefore always be tied on the ligament side of the repair, rather than on the bone. I use a nonabsorbable suture, using a stout-tapered needle to pass through the predrilled holes in the fibula.

A similar approach is used for the calcaneofibular ligament. The peroneal tendons must be retracted completely to visualize the calcaneal fibular ligament. If the peroneal tendons are dislocated or are dislocating, then a modification of this repair can be performed by cutting the tip of the calcaneal fibular ligament off the fibula and then reattaching the calcaneofibular ligament on top of, rather than underneath, the peroneal tendons. This is a useful technique that does not seem to cause any problems with the peroneal tendon popping into the ankle or subtalar joints. It is useful to prepare the sutures for both the anterior talofibular and calcaneal fibular ligament before tying off the anterior talofibular ligament. Afterward, the ankle needs to be moved around, and the suture repair on the anterior talofibular ligament should not be disturbed when the calcaneofibular ligament is tied off. The anterior talofibular ligament is tied off first, with the foot in neutral dorsiflexion and slight

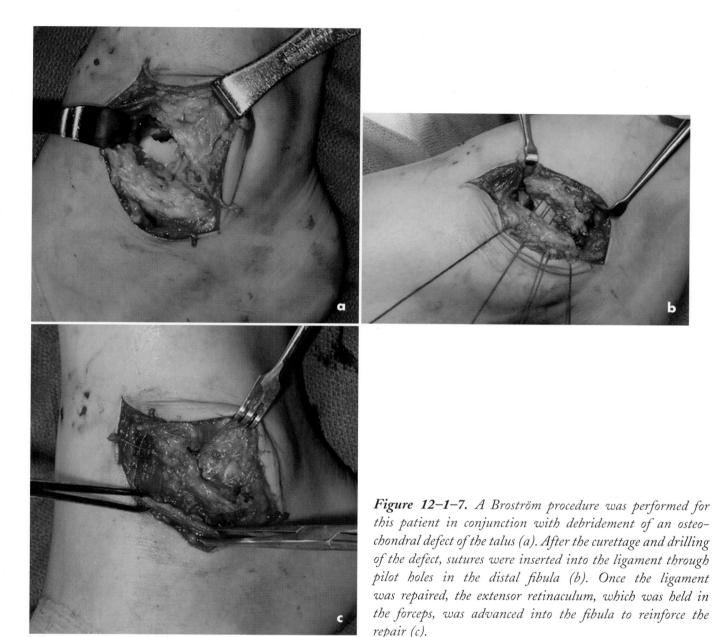

Figure 12–1–7. *A Broström procedure was performed for this patient in conjunction with debridement of an osteochondral defect of the talus (a). After the curettage and drilling of the defect, sutures were inserted into the ligament through pilot holes in the distal fibula (b). Once the ligament was repaired, the extensor retinaculum, which was held in the forceps, was advanced into the fibula to reinforce the repair (c).*

eversion. Overtightening the ligaments with this technique is possible, and the foot should not be in dorsiflexion or forced eversion during this repair. At the completion of the repair of the anterior talofibular and calcaneofibular ligaments, the extensor retinaculum can be pulled up and sutured to the prepared flap of the periosteum and remnant of the anterior talofibular ligament over the fibula. Not all patients have a well-defined extensor retinaculum, and this part of the procedure is not always feasible. These final sutures must be buried; otherwise, they will be irritating. I use

absorbable sutures here for this reason because even with a buried suture, the knot can be irritating.

Modification of the Chrisman-Snook Procedure

The original description of the Chrisman-Snook procedure included a long strip of the peroneus brevis tendon, which was harvested and placed through a bone tunnel in the calcaneus. This is not necessary because a short strip of the anterior half or third of the peroneus brevis tendon is sufficient. The incision is made paralleling the peroneal tendons and extending for no more than 6 cm proximal to the tip of the fibula. The length of tendon that is required can be measured with the cord from the electrocautery, and the length required rarely exceeds about 8 cm (Fig. 12–1–8). The advantage of this procedure is that it can be used in the presence of a severe tear of the peroneus brevis tendon where a split portion of the tendon can be incorporated and used for the ligament reconstruction. Splits in the peroneus brevis tendon are common in combination with recurrent ankle instability, and if these splits are present, this

portion of the tendon is then cut proximally and used for the reconstruction.

Even though the quality of the tendon may not be ideal, it always provides sufficient strength for the reconstruction. The anterior half or third of the tendon is used. Distally, as the tendon is divided, be careful that this does not split down too far along the peroneus brevis tendon. A stay suture can be inserted just distal to the peroneal tubercle to prevent the tendon from splitting down too far. This technique does not even closely reproduce the kinematics of the ankle joint. Nonetheless, it does provide stability and is a reliable procedure for most patients. A 4.5-mm drill hole is made from the tip of the fibula extending posteriorly through the body of the distal fibula and exiting anterior to the peroneal tendons in the posterior half of the fibula. The tendon is passed through the fibular tunnel with a sucker tip technique and then passed over (on top) of the remaining half of the peroneus brevis and the peroneus longus tendons to prevent subluxation of these tendons.

A small portion of the peroneal retinaculum can be left intact with this technique when the anterior portion of the peroneus brevis tendon is harvested to prevent subluxation of the peroneal tendon. Instead of passing the tendon through a complex tunnel in the calcaneus, which is prone to fracture, attaching the tendon to the bone with a screw and a spiked ligament washer is the easiest method. This is inserted at the attachment of the calcaneofibular ligament just inferior to the peroneal tendons. A drill hole, aimed toward the sustentaculum, is made, and the screw and washer are passed through the peroneal tendon, with tension placed in the direction on the tendon to see the point at which the screw is passed through the tendon. The tendon can be split at this point with a hemostat, which simultaneously grasps the screw and pulls it through the tendon. Debriding the lateral cortex of the calcaneus is unnecessary. The tendon seems to adhere well to the periosteal tissue, and when I have had to remove the washer or screw for pain, no redundancy, instability, or loosening of the attached tendon is noted. When the screw is tightened, the foot is held in dorsiflexion and eversion, and simultaneous traction is applied to the peroneus brevis tendon. The stay suture is pulled on while the screw is inserted. Because the washer contacts with the tendon, minor adjustments to the tension of the tendon

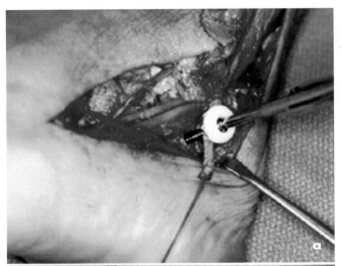

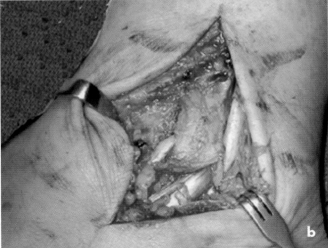

Figure 12–1–8. *The attachment of the transferred split peroneus brevis tendon to the calcaneus with a screw and a spiked ligament washer (a). The final passage of the tendon is shown as it passes through the fibula tunnel and over the remainder of the peroneal tendons (b).*

can be made until fixation is secure. A biointerference screw can also be used instead of the screw and spiked washer. In this case, a slightly longer piece of peroneal tendon would need to be harvested, and the same technique would need to be followed for the free tendon graft as that described for the hamstring allograft procedure. These patients can be mobilized almost immediately after surgery. This is a strong reliable method of fixation. Attachment of one or two sutures to the anterior aspect of the distal fibula is useful, through the old anterior talofibular ligament into the passed tendon with nonabsorbable zero sutures. After 2 weeks of immobilization in a boot or a posterior splint, patients begin ambulation in a removable stirrup brace with eversion strengthening starting at this time.

Percutaneous Hamstring Allograft Reconstruction

Examination of the ankle one more time before proceeding with the reconstruction is useful, with a focus on the planes of instability. The reconstruction is planned, and although a percutaneous approach is used, small incisions are needed for insertion of the graft. The neck of the talus should be marked with a guide pin fluoroscopically, and a small incision of approximately 1.5 cm is made, extending from the lateral aspect of the shoulder of the talar body to the tip of the fibula. In this way, addressing the introduction and passage of the tendon graft through the same incision is possible. The incision is deepened through subcutaneous tissue with a hemostat to avoid any injury to the superficial peroneal nerve during the dissection. The hemostat is probed down onto the bone through the extensor retinaculum.

Technique for Through-and-Through Tunnel in Talus

Although a through-and-through tunnel technique can be performed, I rarely use it and invariably use the blind tunnel technique, as outlined later. The neck of the talus is narrow at this level, and although the graft can be inserted at the level of the neck with a through-and-through bone tunnel for the tendon graft, inserting the tendon directed up into the body of the talus with a blind tunnel technique is easier. If instrumentation is unavailable for bioresorbable interference screws, then an alternative technique with a bone suture anchor

(which is, however, not my preferred procedure) can be used. The operation begins with the insertion of a guide pin for a cannulated 4-mm drill, which is directed across the neck of the talus. The position of the starting point for the drill hole must be checked fluoroscopically and must be made perpendicular to the axis of the neck of the talus. Before the start of the tendon reconstruction, a 3.5-mm bone suture anchor is inserted into the neck of the talus through the edge of the drill hole. A hamstring allograft is now prepared for insertion into the predrilled hole. The tendon is passed percutaneously into the bone tunnel with a tendon passer, which is pulled out through a percutaneous puncture on the medial aspect of the ankle while tension is maintained on the tendon that is held securely in the bone tunnel. The suture from the bone suture anchor is now inserted with a slipknot onto the base of the tendon, which is firmly secured, and the end of the suture is cut.

Talus Blind Tunnel Technique

Because of the size of the talus at the level of the anterior talofibular ligament, insertion of the tendon graft up toward the body of the talus from the anterior lateral shoulder of the talus with a blind tunnel technique is preferable. This technique is easier to perform than the through-and-through tunnel described previously, and instrumentation for insertion of the graft with biointerference screws is helpful. From the same incision, the guide pin from the Arthrex system is introduced. The size of the cannulated drill is determined by the thickness of the graft and the screw to be used. The drill hole is about 1 mm wider than the thickness of the screw to accommodate the tendon, but with tension. I almost routinely use a 5.5-mm drill hole, which is made to a depth of 17 mm (the depth of the drill is easy to read off the guide on the drill). Visualizing the lateral edge of the entry hole into the talus is important when both measuring the depth of the hole and inserting the screw, which must be flush with the edge of the talar cortex. The hamstring allograft is now cleaned, freshened, and trimmed to a thickness of 4 mm along the entire length of the graft. The length must also be measured correctly. Measuring the length of the graft at this stage is far easier because a whip suture is inserted into the end of the tendon for passage through the fibula into the calcaneus and it saves a step if the correct length is cut. I lay the tendon on the skin over the course of passage on the ankle and approximate the length accordingly. A fiber wire suture knot is inserted over the tip of the tendon, and the interference screw is inserted and tightened up to the cortical margin of the talus with the inserter device. The lateral margin of the screw must be flush with the lateral cortical margin of the shoulder of the talus. With considerable tension on the tendon, the graft, which is buried in the talar body, should not yield or be unstable (Fig. 12–1–9).

From the tip of the incision at the edge of the fibula, a guide pin is now inserted for a 4.5-mm cannulated drill bit. The guide pin is inserted through the fibula from anterior to posterior, exiting just anterior to the peroneal tendon sheath, about 1 cm proximal to the tip of the fibula. The suture at the tendon tip is pulled through a puncture over the peroneal sheath. The tendon is passed through a subcutaneous tunnel just superficial to the sural nerve and out a second small 1-cm incision, which

is made inferior to the peroneal tendons and dorsal to the sural nerve. The cannulated guide pin is then inserted, and a 4.5-mm through-and-through hole is made in the calcaneus. The tendon is now pulled down, and it is passed to the medial side of the heel through a skin puncture with a suture passer. Tension is now applied to the suture, and with the ankle placed in dorsiflexion and neutral position, the correct tension is applied on the graft for the reconstruction. Once this tension has been established, the second interference screw is inserted, which must be flush with the margin of the calcaneus. The last suture(s) is(are) now inserted into the anterior aspect of the fibula through the apex of the incision with two sutures of interrupted 0 braided Dacron. The knots must be buried to avoid any subcutaneous irritation (Fig. 12–1–10). The hamstring procedure may be combined with an open arthrotomy when intra-articular disease is simultaneously addressed (Fig. 12–1–11).

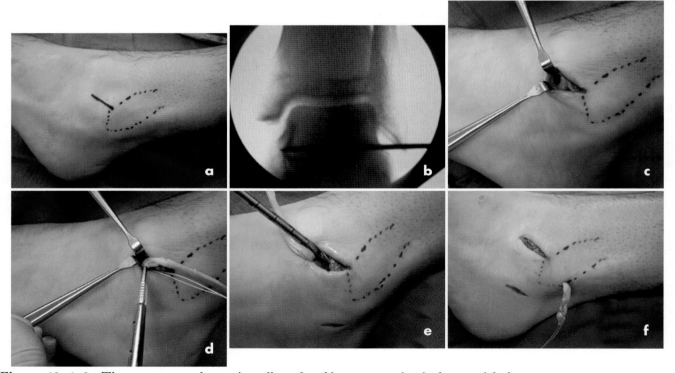

Figure 12–1–9. *The percutaneous hamstring allograft ankle reconstruction is shown with the incision marked out (a); the bone tunnel made at the junction of the neck with the body of the talus over a guide pin, which is first noted fluoroscopically (b, c); the insertion of the biointerference screw (d); the drill tunnel made in the fibula (e); and passage of the graft through a puncture behind the fibula (f). The tendon does not need to be passed out the skin behind the fibula, and the suture can be pulled through and then into the inferior incision directly.*

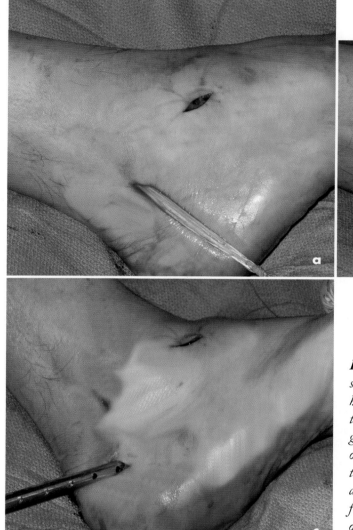

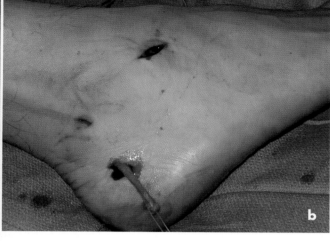

Figure 12–1–10. *In this example of a percutaneous hamstring allograft reconstruction of ankle instability, the graft has been anchored to the talus and pulled through the fibula tunnel (a). A second skin puncture is made inferiorly, and the graft is tunneled superficial to the peroneal tendons and pulled out to tension the tendon (b). A 4.5-mm drill hole is made transversely in the calcaneus, and the sutures are passed with a sucker tip technique to the medial side of the foot. With the foot held in dorsiflexion and eversion, the tendon is tensioned on the medial side of the foot while the suture is held, and the second interference screw is inserted (c).*

The foot is immobilized with a range-of-motion Walker boot, which can be applied immediately after the operation. Weight bearing is permitted at approximately 10 days after surgery, followed by range-of-motion exercise and rehabilitation, which begins at 2 weeks.

Techniques, tips, and pitfalls

1. The key to this operation is the percutaneous method. The surgeon must be familiar with the surface anatomy and the location of both the superficial peroneal and sural nerves.

2. The drill hole made in the fibula must be in the body of the fibula so as not to cause a fracture through the tip. Make sure that this is centered with a drill sleeve.

3. The location of the tendon graft as it passes from the fibula down onto the calcaneus can be either superficial to or deep to the peroneal tendons. Inserting the graft dorsal to the peroneal tendons is easier. This is not the anatomic position of the calcaneofibular ligament, which lies deep to the peroneal tendons.

4. After the reconstruction, and before closure, the stability of the ankle must be checked

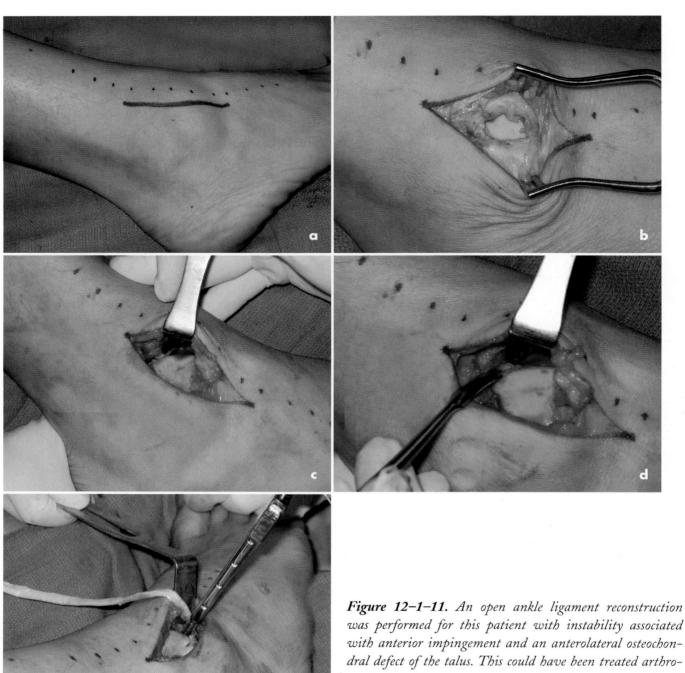

Figure 12–1–11. *An open ankle ligament reconstruction was performed for this patient with instability associated with anterior impingement and an anterolateral osteochondral defect of the talus. This could have been treated arthroscopically with a percutaneous tendon allograft as previously described and would have in fact facilitated earlier rehabilitation. The incision is marked out (a), and the copious synovitis is noted (b). The cheilectomy was performed and the lesion was probed (c, d), followed by the hamstring allograft reconstruction (e).*

fluoroscopically. When an open repair is performed, appreciation of any residual instability visually is easy.

5. If residual instability is present, with the ankle held in dorsiflexion and eversion, additional sutures are inserted at the anterior tip of the fibula to tighten the graft.

Deltoid Ligament Injury and Repair

Medial ankle pain and instability from attenuation of the deltoid ligament is an uncommon clinical entity, but one that is being increasingly identified. These injuries likely have both acute and chronic components and coexist with other foot and ankle disease, in particular flatfoot and lateral instability. Delays in diagnosis and treatment are still common. Most patients with a tear require a deltoid ligament repair that addresses the specific disease noted, such as ligament avulsion or degenerative longitudinal splits. These patients, unlike those with lateral ligament injuries, require prolonged immobilization as either primary or postoperative treatment.

Pathogenesis of Rupture

Although isolated deltoid ligament injuries are rare, we routinely treat deltoid ligament ruptures associated with ankle fractures and syndesmosis injuries, and despite radiographic and clinical evidence of deltoid ligament injury in these patients, uneventful healing is expected. Medial instability is almost unheard of after these injuries, and rarely is the deltoid ligament repaired when the injury is associated with ankle fractures. Fractures with associated deltoid ligament ruptures are easily identified, and most undergo prompt treatment with prolonged immobilization, which may be why in this setting incompetence of the deltoid ligament is rarely, if ever, a problem.

Degeneration and rupture of the deltoid ligament likely represent a spectrum of injury that results from a combination of both repetitive microtrauma and discrete trauma. Although eversion directly stresses the medial ankle and plays a role in deltoid ligament rupture, inversion injuries, which are far more common, may also be involved in the pathogenesis of deltoid ligament injury. The impingement of the deep posterior tibiotalar ligament between the talus and the medial malleolus during inversion trauma likely results in hypertrophy and degeneration. We have noted in a series of "acute" isolated deltoid ligament injuries that inversion trauma with bony impingement of the deltoid ligament occurred in most patients without evidence of articular or lateral ligament trauma. Many patients sustained the rupture as a direct result of indirect inversion trauma and had degenerative changes within the deltoid ligament. Although lateral ligament instability was not a prominent preoperative complaint in our patients, some history of inversion trauma can be assumed in most athletes. If inversion trauma has occurred, the coupling of impingement of the deltoid ligament with tensile forces from flatfoot and eversion trauma may represent a mechanism of injury.

The isolated nature of these ligament tears may be related to underlying degeneration of the deltoid ligament, which may play a role in the limited healing potential of these injuries. Ligament degeneration may explain why the deltoid ligament readily heals in patients with ankle fractures, in whom the ligament is presumably normal, and is problematic in patients with chronic deltoid ligament injuries.

Acute tension overload of the deltoid ligament from eversion injuries is the clearest mechanism of injury in these cases and likely plays some role in nearly all ruptures. The deltoid ligament also plays a role in stabilizing horizontal rotation around the ankle, and inversion trauma with resulting impingement of the deltoid ligament between the talus and the medial malleolus probably is also a cause of rupture. Although these inversion episodes may not result in overt failure, chronic impingement could result in partial tearing and degeneration, predisposing to rupture. In addition, chronic tension overload that occurs in the deltoid ligament associated with a posterior tibial tendon rupture again sets the stage for acute failure. This is probably the sequence that is associated with a stage IV rupture of the posterior tibial tendon, with degeneration, rupture, and necrosis of the ligament associated with varying degrees of flatfoot and ankle instability.

Repair of the Acute Deltoid Ligament Rupture

Repair is carried out with the patient in a supine position with a bump under the contralateral hip to facilitate medial exposure through a longitudinal incision slightly anterior to the posterior tibial tendon sheath from proximal to the medial malleolus to the level of the talonavicular joint. The tendon sheath must be opened and the posterior tibial tendon must be checked for disease. The tendon is retracted posteriorly exposing the underlying deltoid ligament, which is now explored for the orientation, location, and extent of the tear (Fig. 12–1–12).

The repair is performed according to the underlying disease and the orientation of the tear (Fig. 12–1–13). Longitudinal tears split the tendon vertically and usually involve degeneration of the central part of the tendon, which is debrided, and the repair is performed in a side-to-side fashion with nonabsorbable braided 0 suture. In cases involving avulsion of the ligament from the medial malleolus, a proximally based periosteal flap is elevated from the tip of the medial malleolus, and a trough is then made in the tip of the malleolus with a rongeur (or burr) down to bleeding bone. The sutures are then inserted either through drill holes with a K-wire in the malleolus or with a suture anchor, with a #2 nonabsorbable braided suture. These sutures are placed into the trough, and the avulsed ligament is reduced with horizontal mattress stitches. The periosteal flap is brought down over the ligament in a pants-over-vest fashion and sutured. If a midsubstance tear is present, then an end-to-end repair can be used, but the problem here is the degenerative nature of the tissue, which may need "freshening up" before repair.

Ankle Impingement Syndromes

Anterior Ankle Impingement Syndrome

Wherever possible, I treat the anterior impingement syndrome arthroscopically using a large burr (a 4-mm cylindrical burr), which is sufficient to denude the anterior osteophytes. Although open arthrotomy can be performed, additional disease is invariably associated with the anterior impingement, and this

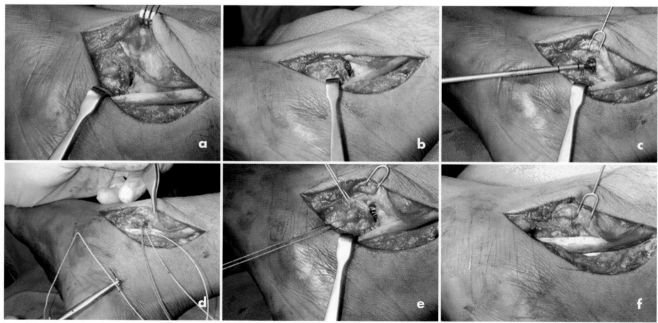

Figure 12–1–12. A 23-year-old basketball player who sustained an acute rupture of the deltoid ligament. After 4 months of conservative care, repair was performed. Note the defect in the superficial and deep deltoid ligament (a, b). The medial malleolus was debrided to bleeding bone, and the anchor was inserted (c, d). Y-shape sutures are inserted, and then they imbricate the deltoid ligament and pull it back up into the malleolus (e, f).

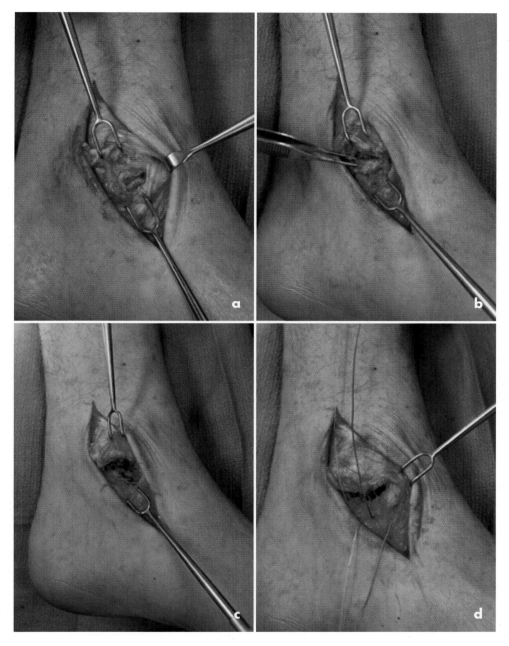

Figure 12–1–13. *Rupture of the deep deltoid ligament occurred in this 29-year-old tennis player, associated with avulsion of a bone fragment off the talus. The defect is shown (a), and the fragment is removed (b). This is a sizable defect and was repaired with sutures attached to an anchor in the talus and then imbricated up into the medial malleolus (c, d).*

syndrome is easier to address arthroscopically. When the osteophytes, however, are intracapsular, arthroscopic treatment becomes far more difficult, and an anterolateral arthrotomy is used. Bear in mind that osteophytes on the tibia are predominantly lateral, and those on the talus are predominantly medial. Even if large osteophytes are present on the talus, reaching across from the anterolateral arthrotomy for resection is not always easy. Anterior impingement with osteophyte buildup is also associated with ankle instability, and this must be evaluated. Many patients with subsequent arthritis of the ankle have recurrent instability of the ankle, which

begins with instability without osteophytes. Finally in the last stages, instability, which becomes fixed, is noted, and the tibiotalar joint is fixed in varus and is associated with marked buildup of osteophytes over the anterior joint. Correction of the impingement syndrome in these patients is much more difficult because the osteophyte resection is only part of a more complex realignment procedure of the hindfoot and ankle.

The anterior osteophytes are approached through an anterolateral arthrotomy, immediately lateral to the peroneus tertius tendon. The incision is deepened through subcutaneous tissue in the superficial peroneal nerve, which always lies immediately adjacent to the tendon, and is identified, and retracted. The extensor retinaculum is incised, and the hypertrophic capsule is incised and reflected. After a synovectomy and excision of the hypertrophied anterolateral capsule, a periosteal elevator is inserted transversely from the anterolateral distal tibia across to the more medial side. Under direct visualization, a large retractor is inserted into the joint over the distal tibia and a small fine chisel or osteotome is used to remove the osteophyte. The use of a curved quarter-inch or curved half-inch osteotome is helpful to perform this so that as the osteotome moves medially, it exits just anterior to the medial malleolus. Plantarflexing and inverting the ankle during this ostectomy are also helpful to prevent any inadvertent injury to the cartilage. At the completion of osteophyte removal, the stability of the ankle must be checked. As noted, many of these ankles are associated with chronic ankle instability, and some form of repair or reconstruction should be performed in conjunction with the osteophyte removal. If the osteophytes are intra-articular and not excessive or intracapsular, the osteophyte removal is then performed arthroscopically, followed by percutaneous ankle ligament reconstruction. If a large buildup of osteophytes is noted medially, this is usually over the talar neck and must be approached through a separate arthrotomy incision medially, just medial to the anterior tibial tendon (Fig. 12–1–14).

The problem occurs with large hypertrophic osteophytes associated with fixed varus and fixed tilting of the tibiotalar joint. In patients with these osteophytes, contracture occurs in the deep deltoid ligament, the posteromedial capsule, and at times even the posterior tibial tendon. These medial soft tissues undergo adaptive contracture, but even after resection of the osteophytes and lateral stabilization, the contracture is not always adequately released. Worse still are those patients who have, in addition to the varus tilting of the talus, an indentation that occurs in the medial tibial plafond. This is an erosion that occurs, and although these are not always painful, the talus always falls back into this eroded tibial plafond, again pushing the talus into varus, regardless of the reconstruction performed.

The only way that this erosion can be addressed is through the same procedure applied with resection of osteophytes, but instead an opening wedge osteotomy of the distal tibia in the supramalleolar region should be performed to push the medial plafond down inferiorly. Theoretically, this will increase the pressure on the medial plafond, but in biomechanical studies, it actually does not do this and the weight is distributed more evenly across the tibiotalar joint. The other option is to perform the osteophyte removal and enter a separate anteromedial incision just over the medial malleolus. A window is made in the distal tibia, and then the articular surface is tamped down with a small round tamp and

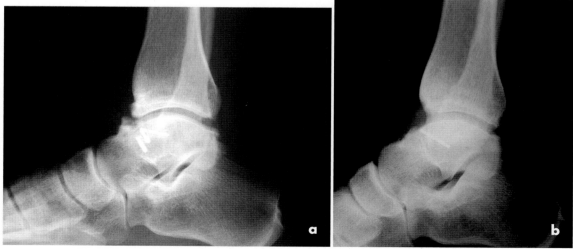

Figure 12–1–14. This patient had undergone two prior operations to correct ankle instability, with continued symptoms, but of impingement and not instability. Note the large osteophytes present on the distal tibia and on the neck of the talus (a), which were removed with an open anterolateral arthrotomy (b).

is then backfilled with bone graft, followed by replacement of the window. This procedure works well to realign the medial plafond but is also associated with early osteoarthritis, and ultimately this condition progresses, requiring more definitive treatment. One of the problems with anterior ankle cheilectomy is recurrence of the osteophyte. I have seen this in almost 75% of these patients after 5 years. More recently, I have begun using bone wax over the resected portion of the ostectomy, but it is too soon to know whether this will have any long-term beneficial effect.

Techniques, tips, pitfalls

1. Most anterior impingement syndromes can be treated arthroscopically. Large osteophytes are usually intracapsular, and full debridement of the lesion can be difficult unless an arthrotomy is made.

2. Osteophytes that are on the tibia are predominantly lateral, and those on the talus are predominantly medial; therefore arthrotomy should be planned accordingly. Assessment of the talar osteophytes without a second medial incision is difficult.

3. At the completion of debridement of the osteophytes, whether performed by arthroscopy or by arthrotomy, obtaining a lateral XR image to ensure that adequate removal has been effected is important.

4. Osteophytes seem to recur. Three to 5 years may be needed for recurrence, but I have seen this frequently enough to recognize that other treatment methods may be required, including the use of bone wax applied at the completion of the ostectomy.

5. For patients with limited ankle motion and large osteophytes, removal of the impingement may be counterproductive because the procedure will worsen the arthritis. The sudden increase in dorsiflexion simply serves to increase the range of motion, and the arthritis will deteriorate. Removal of osteophytes is a procedure performed for impingement and not for arthritis.

Posterior Ankle Impingement Syndrome

The posterior ankle pain is easily reproduced on examination with forced passive plantar flexion of the ankle. A decision has to be made whether this is arising from a hypertrophied trigonal process, from an os trigonum, or from pain from either the peroneal or flexor hallucis longus (FHL) tendons. In the case of posteromedial ankle pain, reproduction of this by forced passive dorsiflexion of the foot and then passive dorsiflexion of the hallux is usually easy. This pulls the FHL tendon deep into the retinacular tunnel and will reproduce the pain if stenosis of the fibro-osseous tunnel is present as the muscular belly of the flexor hallucis tendon is pulled distally. If the pain is present directly posteriorly with forced passive plantar flexion, this is invariably the result of an os trigonum or hypertrophy process of the talus.

Wherever possible, I use a posterolateral incision to approach the decompression. Although a posteromedial incision can be used, this should only be done when a definite diagnosis of FHL tendon disease has been made. The morbidity of the posteromedial incision is considerably greater, and even with adequate retraction of the tibial nerve, irritation and scarring of the nerve may occur, with subsequent neuritis.

The posterolateral incision is straightforward and is made over a 3-cm length posterior to the peroneal tendons. The incision is deepened through the subcutaneous tissue, and the sural nerve is immediately identified and retracted anteriorly. The peroneal retinaculum is now incised over the muscle belly posteriorly, and the peroneal tendons are retracted anteriorly (Fig. 12–1–15).

Visualization of the posterior aspect of the ankle is impossible until the retrocalcaneal fat has been excised. Retracting the fatty tissue is simply not enough; the fat and the adjacent bursal tissue need to be excised. In addition to the visualization, I find it useful to open up both the ankle and subtalar joints before performing the ostectomy. This gives me a good sense as to where the joint margin is as the ostectomy is performed. A wide periosteal elevator is used to strip the periosteum off the distal tibia and this is then left in place. A curved periosteal elevator or a Hohman retractor is inserted over the back of the tibia. Once the soft tissues are

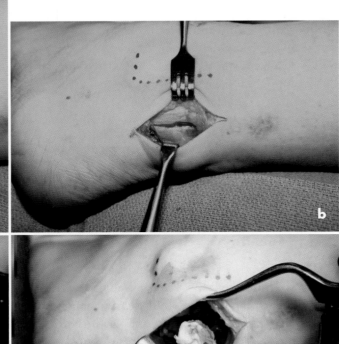

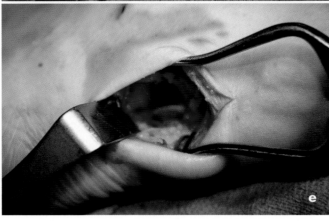

Figure 12–1–15. The approach to excision of an enlarged os trigonum. The incision is marked posterior to the peroneal tendons (a), and the peroneal sheath is incised (b). Retrocalcaneal fat is excised to expose the bone mass (c), which is cut with an osteotome and twisted off its pedicle (d). After excision of the posterior subtalar joint, the flexor hallucis longus (FHL) tendon is visible medially (e).

retracted, then the excision of the os trigonum can be performed. By now, visualizing the leading edge of the FHL tendon is important. It is muscular at this level as the muscle fibers blend in with the tendon distally. The exostectomy is performed from lateral to medial and is done with an osteotome. The use of a blunt osteotome here is actually helpful to prevent inadvertent injury to the FHL tendon, which lies immediately adjacent, on

the medial side of the posterior tubercle. Once the process has been fractured with the osteotome, it is twisted off its pedicle with a rongeur. Usually fibers, which are attached to the FHL tendon, remain medially, and these fibers need to be released sharply under direct visualization of the FHL tendon simultaneously. In this way, both the ankle and subtalar joints can be visualized, and any additional disease that may coexist in the posterior aspect of the joint can be noted (Figs. 12–1–16 and 12–1–17).

I use a similar approach as this in high-performance athletes, dancers, and gymnasts. The only difference is that a greater incidence of FHL tendon disease occurs in gymnasts and dancers and I may be more inclined to use a posteromedial incision in these patients provided I am certain that additional disease exists medially. The approach is identical, but these patients take a long time to regain full plantar flexion. During the initial phase of recovery, weight bearing is permitted as soon as comfortable in a maximally dorsiflexed position of the foot in a walker boot. This can be removed at intervals for passive range-of-motion exercises, and swimming is begun as soon as possible.

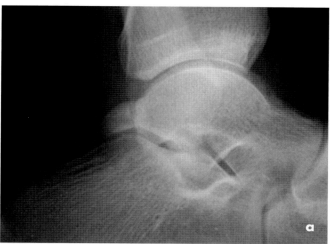

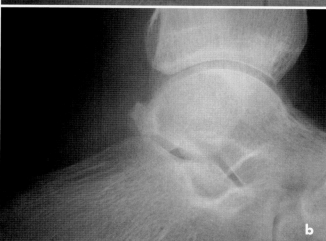

Figure 12–1–16. *The posterior bone mass of the enlarged trigonal process (a) and after its removal (b).*

Surgical Approaches to Osteochondral Lesions of the Talus

With osteochondral lesions of the talus, surgery is performed only in symptomatic cases because the lesions do not show any marked tendency for progression or typically lead to osteoarthritis. Several surgical treatment options are available that I initiate with arthroscopic debridement and with abrasion arthroplasty, subchondral drilling, or microfracture. If the lesion is too large or extensive, or if prior operations have failed, then osteochondral autograft or allograft procedures are preferable. Once a decision has been made to proceed with surgical treatment, several factors should be considered when deciding on a particular surgical approach. These include the size and depth of the lesion, the exact location of the lesion (medial versus lateral, anterior versus posterior), the history of prior surgical treatment, the stage of the disease, and the viability of the articular cartilage. Wherever possible, I treat the lesion either through arthroscopy or with an anterior or posterior arthrotomy. To this end, flexion extension lateral radiographs are useful to show the location of the lesion and its accessibility via arthrotomy as opposed to an osteotomy, which is associated with far more potential morbidity (Fig. 12–1–18).

Generally, I initiate treatment arthroscopically with abrasion, drilling, or microfracture. For lesions that are large and those that have not responded to arthroscopic treatment, an osteochondral graft should be considered. Moderate-sized defects can be filled with several small osteochondral autografts from the ipsilateral knee. Larger defects, particularly those involving the medial or lateral talar wall, may require an allograft transfer. These marginal sidewall lesions are difficult to treat with an osteochondral autograft because the graft must be inserted perpendicular to the axis of the talar dome. At times, the graft may be harvested from the corner edge of the femoral condyle, but if the lesion is on the sidewall of the talus, then autograft is not possible. For these marginal defects a medial or lateral malleolar osteotomy must be performed.

Most anterior lesions are accessible for drilling and even grafting with arthrotomy. However, if the lesion remains covered by the articular margin of the tibia, then a small window of the anterior or posterior tibia is needed for

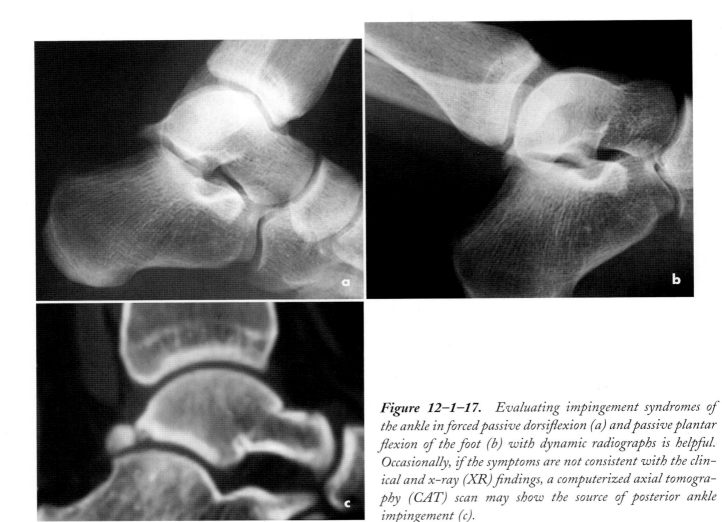

Figure 12–1–17. *Evaluating impingement syndromes of the ankle in forced passive dorsiflexion (a) and passive plantar flexion of the foot (b) with dynamic radiographs is helpful. Occasionally, if the symptoms are not consistent with the clinical and x-ray (XR) findings, a computerized axial tomography (CAT) scan may show the source of posterior ankle impingement (c).*

Figure 12–1–18. *Flexion extension lateral radiographs are shown for this patient with a large posteromedial lesion that is accessible from a posteromedial arthrotomy (a, b).*

further exposure. If extended visualization is required, this approach may be extended with an osteotomy of the anterior tibia, followed by replacement of the bone fragment and screw fixation (Fig. 12–1–19).

Approach to Lateral Talar Dome Lesions

Most lateral talar dome lesions have an anterior location, and an anterolateral incision and arthrotomy are ideal. The incision begins over the anterolateral aspect of the ankle, 2 cm proximal to the ankle joint, and is extended distally by 4 cm over the ankle joint. The intermediate dorsal cutaneous branches of the superficial peroneal nerve should be identified and protected. The extensor retinaculum is incised, the extensor digitorum longus tendon is identified and retracted medially, and the joint capsule is incised in line with the incision. Slight plantar flexion of the ankle will further facilitate exposure for access to debridement or grafting (Figs. 12–1–20 and 12–1–21).

A fibular osteotomy is rarely necessary to treat a lateral talar dome lesion and is used only for large lesions that are located posterolaterally and that cannot be accessed with arthrotomy. If a fibular osteotomy is required, then I use a 6-cm incision over the distal fibula, starting from 1 cm distal to the joint and extending proximally. The osteotomy is made with a microsagittal saw, obliquely at an angle from lateral and proximal to distal and medial, so that the distal edge is at the level of the joint line. The advantage of the oblique osteotomy is the greater surface area for healing, although a transverse osteotomy can just as easily be performed (Fig. 12–1–22). The interosseous ligaments are then incised, and the distal fibula is peeled down and retracted inferiorly to expose the lateral talar dome. The lesion will unlikely be visible or accessible once the osteotomy has been performed. For any graft procedure to be performed, the lesion must be fully visible, and any graft must be inserted perpendicular to the talar surface. For this reason, an ostectomy of the lateral wall of the distal tibia must be performed. Make this ostectomy large enough so that when the graft is reinserted this can be accomplished with screw fixation. At the completion of the intra-articular procedure, the fibular osteotomy is anatomically reduced and held with a lateral plate. The interosseous ligaments should be repaired if possible. The addition of a syndesmotic screw through the plate is necessary and

should be performed routinely. In the rare occasion when the lateral lesion has a more central location and cannot be accessed by simply inverting the ankle, an anterolateral tibial osteotomy, in addition to the fibular osteotomy, can provide excellent visualization of the lesion.

Occasionally, I use a posterolateral approach with arthrotomy when faced with a loose body, fragment, or os trigonum that cannot be removed arthroscopically. An incision is made posterolaterally, behind the peroneal sheath and anterior to the sural nerve. It is deepened through the subcutaneous tissue, the peroneal retinaculum is incised longitudinally, and the tendons are retracted anteriorly. The retrocalcaneal fat is then dissected, and this dissection provides good visualization of the ankle joint.

Approach to the Medial Talar Dome Lesions

Medial malleolar osteotomy remains a popular approach for access to medial talar dome lesions. Despite good visualization of the talus, the foot must still be forcibly everted to visualize and treat the lesion and can be improved with the use of a medially applied external distractor, with valgus manipulation of the foot, and most important with careful planning of the osteotomy. A saw is used to perform the first three quarters of the osteotomy, and the remainder should be completed with an osteotome to minimize injury to the articular cartilage. The only problem with this method is that the saw blade itself removes 1 to 2 mm of bone so that the apposition of the osteotomy may not be perfect. Nonetheless, the osteotomy should be completed with an osteotome (Fig. 12–1–23).

I use an oblique osteotomy that begins proximal to the tibial plafond and ends just distal to it. One problem with this technique is the potential for malunion because apposition of the osteotomy where the saw cut is made may not be colinear with respect to the osteotomy cut. This problem is compounded by the screw insertion, which cannot be in the traditional plane that is usually used with a fracture of the medial malleolus (Fig. 12–1–24). This may lead to malunion because of the creation of shear force at the osteotomy site. The addition of transverse screws perpendicular to the joint has been shown to biomechanically and clinically counter this

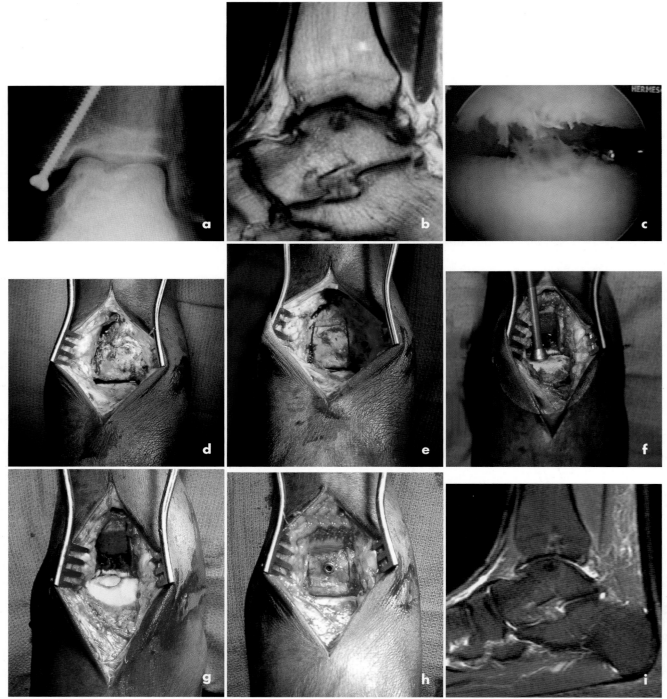

Figure 12–1–19. *The sequence of steps for a central osteotomy window of the distal tibia and an osteochondral graft for this large central lesion that had failed prior medial malleolar osteotomy and drilling of the lesion (a, b). After arthroscopic evaluation (c), a central window was marked out with cautery (d) and made with a saw and osteotome (e). The lesion was measured (f), the graft was inserted from the ipsilateral knee (g), the window was closed with a single screw (h), and the magnetic resonance imaging (MRI) picture at 1 year was noted (i).*

shearing force and help prevent translation and malunion.

The medial malleolus is exposed through subperiosteal stripping anteriorly and posteriorly approximately 1.5 cm above the joint line. The deltoid ligament is not disrupted. The tibialis posterior tendon must be protected at the posteromedial border of the tibia during the entire procedure. This tendon is more vulnerable than can be imagined. The medial malleolus is then

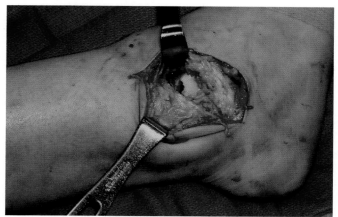

Figure 12–1–20. *The excision of this lesion was combined with an anterolateral approach to simultaneously repair an unstable ankle.*

predrilled and directed proximal and lateral, and the intra-articular space is avoided. Be careful with the starting point of the osteotomy. The starting point, which must be initiated and in the correct plane, is made after insertion of a K-wire under fluoroscopy. This ensures that the plane of the osteotomy is going to be either directly on top or lateral to the talar dome lesion. If the osteotomy is medial to the lesion, then access to graft the defect will be insufficient, even with maximum eversion stress. The cut is made along the edge of the previously inserted K-wire either dorsal or inferior to it, depending on the position of the wire. The depth of the saw cut should be monitored fluoroscopically to ensure that a small segment can be completed with an osteotome. A fine osteotome is then driven to the joint space and can be used as a lever to complete the osteotomy. The medial malleolus is reflected plantar-ward on the deltoid ligament, the medial aspect of the ankle joint is exposed, and the lesion is fully visualized with forced eversion (Fig. 12–1–25).

In the rare occasion when a medial talar dome lesion is more anterior, a standard anteromedial arthrotomy can be used, and the need for a medial malleolar osteotomy can be avoided. If the lesion is not accessible with plantar flexion of the foot to allow access to the entire margin of the lesion, the anteromedial articular surface of the tibia overlying the talar lesion is grooved with a

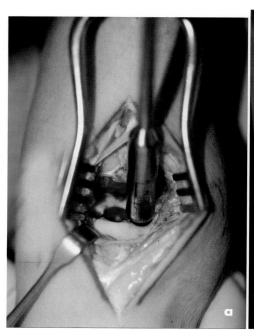
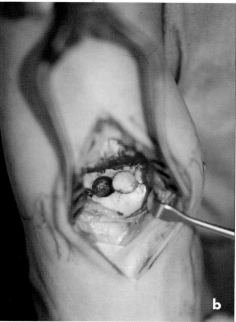

Figure 12–1–21. *Two osteochondral grafts were inserted through an arthrotomy to repair a large anterolateral defect. Note that an anterior cheilectomy has been performed to simultaneously treat an anterior impingement and resect the osteophytes.*

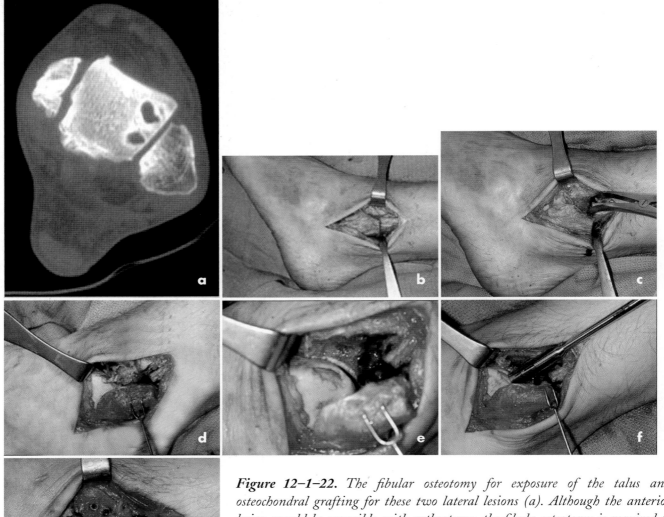

Figure 12–1–22. *The fibular osteotomy for exposure of the talus and osteochondral grafting for these two lateral lesions (a). Although the anterior lesion would be accessible with arthrotomy, the fibula osteotomy is required to approach the more posterior lesion. A transverse osteotomy is made (b), and the fibular is retracted with a laminar spreader (c) and then a skin hook (d) to access the lesion after a lateral tibial ostectomy (e). The lesion is measured perpendicular to the plane of the talus (f), and after osteochondral grafting the osteotomy is secured with a plate (g).*

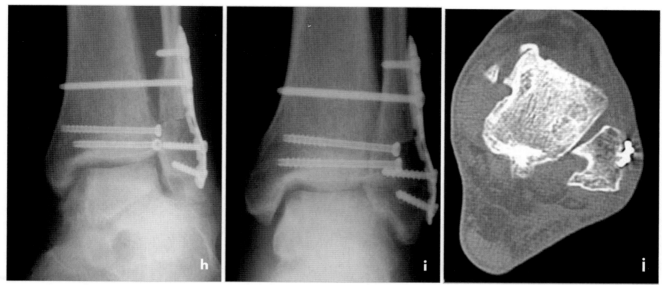

Figure 12–1–22, cont'd *The final radiographs and computerized axial tomography (CAT) scan are presented 1 year after surgery (h–j).*

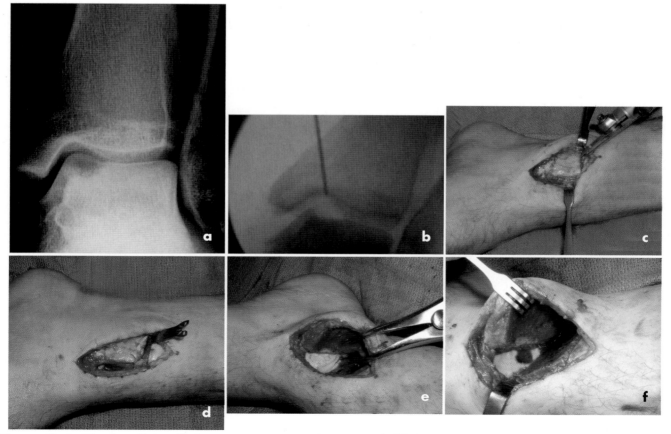

Figure 12–1–23. *A medial malleolar osteotomy was used to approach this large medial defect noted radiographically (a). The position of the osteotomy was marked fluoroscopically with a K-wire (b), the osteotomy was made with a saw (c), and the saw blade was left in the osteotomy site to verify fluoroscopically that it was in the correct plane (d). Visualization is improved with a laminar spreader (e), and the lesion is removed before grafting (f).*

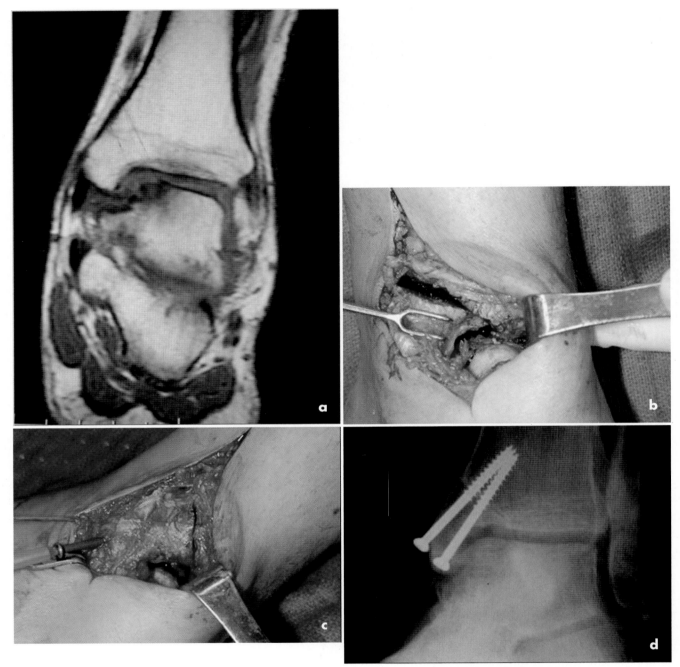

Figure 12–1–24. *This large lesion (a) could not be treated adequately with osteochondral plugs, and a bulk fresh osteochondral graft was used to replace this corner lesion. A medial malleolar osteotomy was performed (b), and after grafting, two oblique screws were used to secure the osteotomy (c). This is not the ideal plane for the screws, and despite excellent incorporation of the graft at 2 years, note the slight step off at the tibial articular surface, the result of a slight malunion of the osteotomy (d).*

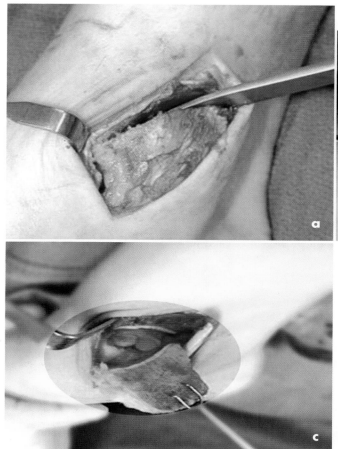

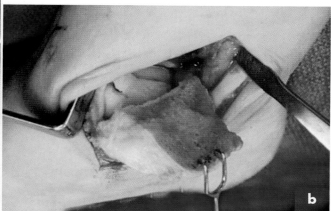

Figure 12–1–25. *A medial malleolar osteotomy was performed to access this large marginal sidewall lesion (a, b). The osteochondral grafts were inserted with maximum eversion of the foot and as perpendicular to the plane of the talus as possible (c).*

narrow gouge. The area of distal tibial articular surface that is removed is 4 to 5 mm wide anteriorly by 6 to 8 mm deep. This portion of articular surface is not replaced.

For posteromedial lesions, I prefer to perform an arthrotomy wherever possible, and this arthrotomy is indicated for any large posteromedial lesions that cannot be treated adequately with arthroscopic procedures. This is also an excellent approach in cases of prior failed operations or when lesions that involve the medial wall of the talus are addressed. When a small part of the medial wall of the talus is involved, treatment is usually limited to debridement of the lesion because a graft will not hold in this location. If the entire medial wall is involved, then use of a fresh talar allograft can be considered to replace the entire medial wall. For a posterior approach to the ankle, a standard posteromedial approach to the ankle joint is carried out (Fig. 12–1–26). The neurovascular bundle is identified and protected with minimization of the nerve retraction. The FHL

tendon is identified posterior to the neurovascular bundle and retracted posteriorly, and the tibial nerve is retracted anteriorly. The lesion is visible after capsulectomy, but the foot can be passively dorsiflexed and the posterior tibia notched with an ostectomy, with removal of a small segment of the posterior articular surface, to improve visualization of the talus and gain access for grafting (Fig. 12–1–27).

Techniques, tips, and pitfalls

1. Almost all lesions should be treated initially with arthroscopy. I have seen some patients with extremely large lesions manage indefinitely with arthroscopic debridement and microfracture.

2. I prefer arthrotomy instead of osteotomy to access the lesion. Whether this is performed for

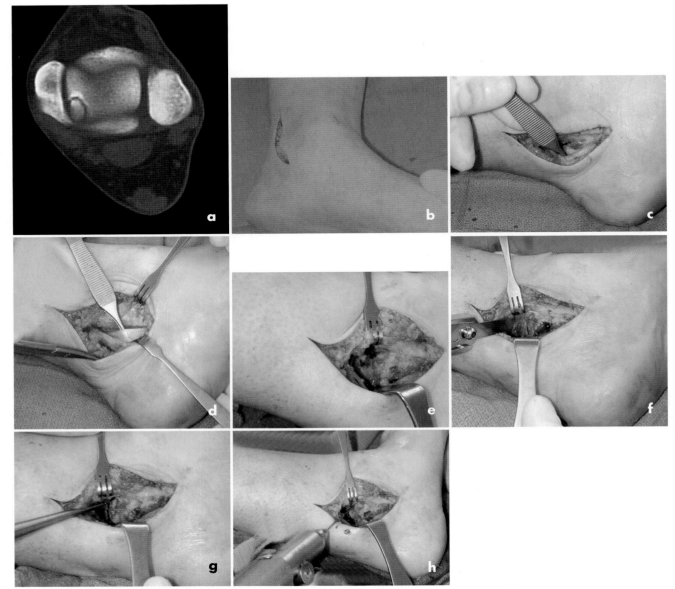

Figure 12–1–26. *This large posteromedial lesion noted on computerized axial tomography (CAT) scan (a) was approached with a posteromedial arthrotomy and drilling. The incision is noted (b), and the neurovascular bundle and the flexor hallucis longus (FHL) tendon are identified and retracted (c, d). The lesion is not easy to visualize (e) until a posterior ostectomy is performed (f), followed by curettage and drilling of the defect (g, h).*

a medial or lateral lesion, nonunion or malunion of the osteotomy and further irritation of the lesion by virtue of the plane of the osteotomy into the joint are always risks.

3. A posteromedial arthrotomy works extremely well and can be used to perform debridement or osteochondral grafting.

4. Marginal lesions are most difficult to treat with osteochondral autograft. Although the graft can be harvested from the margin of the femoral condyle, the shape and contour are never as well matched. If the lesion is large and on the margin of the talus, then a fresh osteochondral allograft may need to be used.

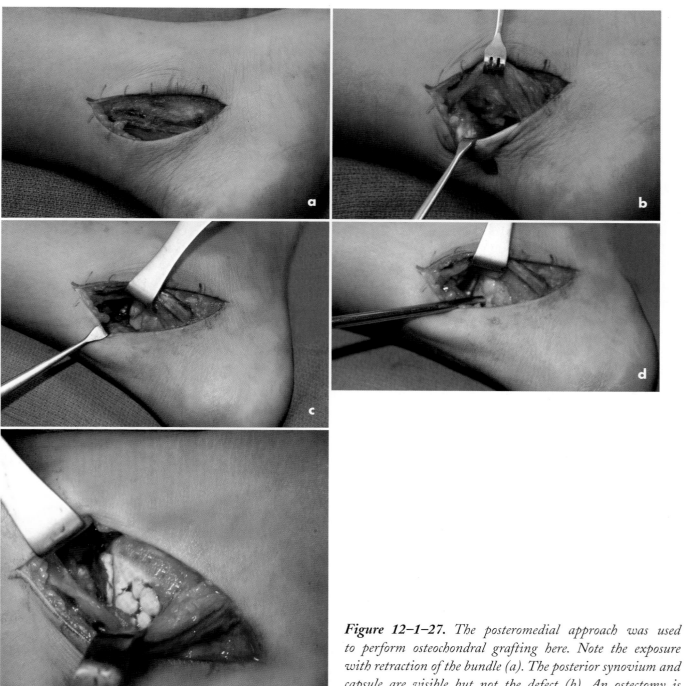

Figure 12–1–27. *The posteromedial approach was used to perform osteochondral grafting here. Note the exposure with retraction of the bundle (a). The posterior synovium and capsule are visible but not the defect (b). An ostectomy is performed to expose the defect (c), which is then probed and debrided (d), followed by insertion of four osteochondral grafts (e).*

5. Bear in mind that for all these fresh allografts, despite correct size matching, the congruence of the graft with respect to the articular surface of the tibia is never perfect. Each ankle joint has its personality, and the match of these large grafts for marginal lesions of the talus is never perfect.

Suggested Readings

Acevedo JI, Myerson MS. Modification of the Chrisman-Snook technique. Foot Ankle Int 21:154–155, 2000.

Fortin PT, Guettler J, Manoli A II. Idiopathic cavovarus and lateral ankle instability: Recognition and treatment implications relating to ankle arthritis. Foot Ankle Int 23:1031–1037, 2002.

Gautier E, Kolker D, Jakob RP. Treatment of cartilage defects of the talus by autologous osteochondral grafts. J Bone Joint Surg Br 84:237–244, 2002.

Hamilton WG, Geppert MJ. Pain in the posterior aspect of the ankle in dancers. Differential diagnosis and operative treatment. J Bone Joint Surg 78: 1491–1500, 1996.

Hamilton WG, Thompson FM. The modified Brostrom procedure for lateral ankle instability. Foot Ankle 14:1–7, 1993.

Hangody L, Kish G, Karpati Z, et al. Treatment of osteochondritis dissecans of the talus: Use of the mosaicplasty technique—a preliminary report. Foot Ankle Int 18:628–634, 1997.

Hangody L, Kish G, Modis L, et al. Mosaicplasty for the treatment of osteochondritis dissecans of the talus: two to seven year results in 36 patients. Foot Ankle Int 22:552–558, 2001.

Hintermann B. Medial ankle instability. Foot Ankle Clin 8:723–738, 2003.

Lee CH, Chao KH, Huang GS, Wu SS. Osteochondral autografts for osteochondritis dissecans of the talus. Foot Ankle Int 24:815–822, 2003.

Messer TM, Cummins CA, Ahn J, Kelikian AS. Outcome of the modified Broström procedure for chronic lateral ankle instability using suture anchors. Foot Ankle Int 21:996–1003, 2000.

Navid DO, Myerson MS. Approach alternatives for treatment of osteochondral lesions of the talus. Foot Ankle Clin 7:635–649, 2002.

Schuman L, Struijs PA, van Dijk CN. Arthroscopic treatment for osteochondral defects of the talus. Results at follow-up at 2 to 11 years. J Bone Joint Surg Br 84: 364–368, 2002.

Verhagen RA, Struijs PA, Bossuyt PM, van Dijk CN. Systematic review of treatment strategies for osteochondral defects of the talar dome. Foot Ankle Clin 8:233–242, viii–ix, 2003.

Arthrodesis of the Hallux Metatarsophalangeal Joint

Approach to Arthrodesis

Arthrodesis of the hallux metatarsophalangeal (MP) joint is indicated for correction of deformity, for arthritis of the hallux MP joint, and for unusual circumstances (e.g., in the presence of spasticity of the hallux MP joint with or without deformity). As a generalization, this is an operation that is technically easy to perform, with a predictable outcome, provided the hallux is well positioned. Any preexisting instability, hyperextension, or arthritis of the interphalangeal (IP) joint may preclude a successful outcome of MP arthrodesis. The key to this operation is in the position of the arthrodesis. The hallux must be slightly supinated into a neutral position, in slight dorsiflexion with respect to the position of the floor, and in slight valgus. Some of these parameters will need to be modified depending on patient's circumstances (e.g., the running athlete, the patient who desires to wear slightly higher heel shoes) and for any deformity of the forefoot that needs to be taken into consideration.

Alignment of Arthrodesis

The dilemma always arises as to how much dorsiflexion the hallux will tolerate in the fusion. Clearly, the greater the angle of dorsiflexion, the easier it will be to wear a high-heeled shoe, toe-off, and avoid any pressure on the IP joint. However, with a steeper MP joint angle, the tendency for rubbing on the dorsal surface of the IP joint and the nail on the underside of the shoe increases.

Furthermore over time, if the hallux MP joint is excessively dorsiflexed, a reciprocal flexion contracture will occur at the IP joint that ultimately will become fixed and may be associated with arthritis. On the contrary, too much plantar flexion of the MP joint will lead to excessive pressure under the IP joint, which is intolerably uncomfortable. Plantar flexion of the MP fusion will always ultimately lead to loosening and ultimately hyperextension of the IP joint with arthritis.

Therefore the decision as to how much dorsiflexion to incorporate into the fusion has to be made on the basis of the presence of any preexisting hyperextension and instability of the IP joint and the patient's activities, sporting interests, and shoe wear needs. Fusion of the hallux MP joint at an angle is preferable to the position of the floor rather than the metatarsal. The metatarsal declination varies considerably, and the more predictable position would be with reference to the floor. Be careful, however, with arthrodesis of the hallux MP joint in the setting of a cavus foot or a steep plantarflexed first metatarsal. This will lead to pain under the first metatarsal head and sesamoiditis. If an arthrodesis of the MP joint has to be performed in the setting of a fixed forefoot equinus or plantarflexed first ray, a dorsal wedge osteotomy of the first metatarsal may have to be performed before proceeding with the arthrodesis. The converse applies in a patient with severe elevatus of the first metatarsal. Here, position of the fusion relative to the metatarsal may be in neutral alignment, but the hallux remains elevated relative to the floor. Not much, if any, dorsiflexion can be incorporated in the hallux MP joint in patients with metatarsus primus elevatus.

The position of the hallux in the transverse plane can be difficult in the presence of a marked increase in the first to second intermetatarsal space (angle). After correction of hallux valgus with an arthrodesis of the MP joint, the decrease in the intermetatarsal angle will be almost proportionate to the magnitude of the deformity preoperatively. Therefore if the decrease of this deformity is anticipated, where is the hallux placed in the fusion intraoperatively? For example, if the hallux is placed in slight valgus, with the anticipation that a decrease in the intermetatarsal angle will occur postoperatively, the hallux is ultimately going to abut the second toe. For this reason, if I am dealing with severe deformity, I will place a temporary lag screw between the first and second metatarsal to close down the intermetatarsal space. This then reduces the deformity and allows me to predict more accurately the location for correction of the hallux with the arthrodesis. The other option is to undercorrect the hallux and leave it in a slightly more neutral position than usual, with the anticipation of the change in position of the first ray after the operation.

The alignment of the hallux in pronation and supination must be accurate. If the hallux is overpronated, pain will be present at both the medial side of the IP joint and the medial margin of the nail with an ingrown toenail occurring. Oversupination leads to pain on the medial or lateral nail fold, and an ingrown toenail can occur as well. The best way to check alignment of the hallux is to look at the way the hallux nail lines up with the adjacent toenails (Fig. 13–1–1).

Sesamoid Issues

Rarely do patients experience sesamoiditis after arthrodesis of the hallux MP joint. Sesamoid pain, if it occurs, is usually the result of a plantarflexed metatarsal and not from painful arthritis between the sesamoid and the first metatarsal head. If the latter occurs, it can be due to a hypertrophied sesamoid. It cannot always be anticipated, and a sesamoidectomy may need to be performed at a later date. However, if the patient has sesamoid pain (from pressure) preoperatively, the sesamoid can be resected in conjunction with the arthrodesis of the hallux MP joint. For these patients, I either use a direct medial approach to the MP joint and resect the sesamoid from the undersurface of the metatarsal head, simultaneously, or use the same dorsal incision to reach underneath the metatarsal head to excise the sesamoid(s).

Bone Grafting

The decision for an in situ or a bone graft interposition fusion must be made carefully. Clearly, if severe shortening of the hallux is present with transfer metatarsalgia, then an arthrodesis with a bone block graft would be ideal. Although arthrodesis is technically feasible, some shortening of the hallux always occurs, and from a functional as well as a cosmetic standpoint, this is not ideal. With a short hallux, forefoot supination occurs because of insufficient weight bearing of the hallux itself, and eventually, toe deformities will occur. One consideration is shortening osteotomies of the lesser metatarsals in conjunction with the shortening arthrodesis of the hallux MP joint. This decision is sometimes difficult because primary end-to-end arthrodesis has a considerably higher fusion rate than an interposition bone block fusion (97% versus 80%).

Approach and Joint Preparation

The incision is made medial to the extensor hallucis longus (EHL) tendon, over a length of 4 cm, with a small cuff of extensor retinaculum left for later closure. The extensor tendon is retracted laterally, and with subperiosteal dissection the entire articulation is dissected and exposed. Forcibly plantarflexing the proximal phalanx is helpful; plantar flexion facilitates dissection of the periosteum off both sides of the joint. With further plantar flexion of the hallux, the undersurface of the proximal phalanx, including the attachment of the volar plate, is easily dissected. Stripping the attachment of the sesamoids is unnecessary because they retract once the volar plate is released.

The maximum length of the hallux should be preserved when the bone cuts are planned. If a saw if used to create flat cuts, apposition of the bone surfaces is easy, but more bone is removed. Planning the ultimate position of the hallux is not as easy, and repeated shaving of either side of the joint may need to be done until the hallux is in

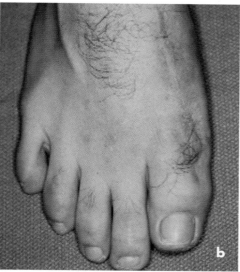
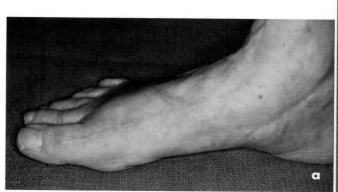

Figure 13–1–1. In both of these patients, an arthrodesis of the hallux metatarsophalangeal (MP) joint was performed with the hallux in too much pronation. The nail of the hallux does not line up with the nails of the lesser toes, and an ingrown toe nail will commonly occur (a, b).

the correct position. Alternatively, a cup and cone shape can be created to contour the joint surfaces, and I use a 5-mm burr to denude the articular surface. Commercially available reamers can be used, but these are expensive and not always available. I start with the hallux, burr into the phalanx, and preserve as much of the medial cortex of the base of the proximal phalanx for later screw fixation. Try to maintain as much of the rim of the joint as possible, but burr down to healthy bleeding cancellous bone. A reciprocal cone shape is created with the burr on the metatarsal head, and the proximal phalanx is used as a guide for the shaping of the metatarsal head. With this technique, the hallux should not cock-up because of excessive dorsal bone resection (Fig. 13–1–2).

The hallux is reduced, and the alignment of the hallux is positioned on the basis of the decision making with the patient regarding shoe wear, activities, and the shape of the forefoot. The hallux is placed in 10 degrees of dorsiflexion relative to the weight-bearing surface of the floor and supinated so that the hallux nail is now parallel with the nails of the lesser toes and slight valgus is incorporated into the position of the arthrodesis.

Before reduction and fixation of the joint, make certain that the head or phalanx has no bone defect. Even if

good bone apposition is noted, if minimal bone contact is present circumferentially, a small cancellous bone graft is required. This can be obtained from the calcaneus through a 1-cm incision on the posterior inferior heel, posterior to the sural nerve and anterior to the Achilles tendon. A small trephine can be used to harvest a cylindrical tube of cancellous bone that measures 1 cm in length, which can be contoured and placed in the defect in the MP joint. The other option is to use a mixture of allograft cancellous chips and demineralized bone matrix.

Fixation

I typically use cannulated fully threaded cancellous screws to secure the arthrodesis. I have not found that a partially threaded screw is necessary. Broad cancellous bone surfaces, which require rigidity and stability as much as compression, can be obtained manually. With the hallux in the reduced position, guide pins are introduced to cross the articular surface. The first guide pin is introduced from the plantar medial surface of the undersurface of the metatarsal neck just proximal to the metatarsal head. This is aimed distally and passed out the metatarsal head and into the lateral base of the proximal phalanx. The second guide pin is introduced from distal to proximal from the

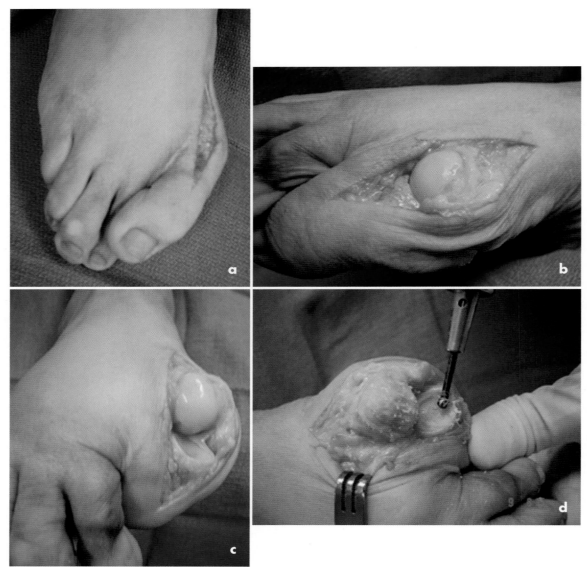

Figure 13–1–2. *This patient was treated with arthrodesis of the hallux MP joint for hallux valgus associated with spasticity. Note that the articular cartilage is healthy, and despite this, an osteotomy should not be performed. Recurrence after osteotomy for hallux valgus correction in the setting of spasticity of any kind is high. The incision used is standard (a), followed by exposure of the metatarsophalangeal (MP) joint with stripping of the periosteum off the metatarsal head and phalanx (b, c). A 4-mm burr is used to denude the articular cartilage, followed by screw fixation (d).*

medial aspect of the base of the proximal phalanx across the metatarsal head and exits slightly dorsally and laterally. If the bone on the base of the phalanx or medial head is inadequate, then the screws are introduced from the dorsal neck of the metatarsal head distally into the phalanx. Before insertion of the screws, the neck must be prepared with either a countersink or a burr to

prevent fracture. The first screw is introduced from the metatarsal head going distally. During the introduction of the first screw the hallux is compressed manually across the articular surface to provide maximum contact and compression during the screw fixation. The second screw is introduced from distal to proximal, but before insertion the medial cortex of the base of the proximal phalanx must be prepared to prevent fracture with a cannulated drill (Figs. 13–1–3 to 13–1–5).

Sometimes the standard screw fixation is not sufficient because of the plane of the metatarsal head or the proximal phalanx. This problem will occur, for example, after failed bunionectomy, when a medial eminence is not present and there is less of an anchor point for the head of the screw. If bone loss is present or the contour of the metatarsal head does not facilitate internal fixation, other means of fixation must be used instead of screws. A surgeon can use a dorsal plate, multiple threaded small K-wires, or large threaded Steinman pins. Clearly, crossing the hallux IP joint is not desired, but this is necessary with the larger threaded pins. Sometimes, however, the bone loss is so severe that the MP joint has to be anchored with the distal phalanx for support.

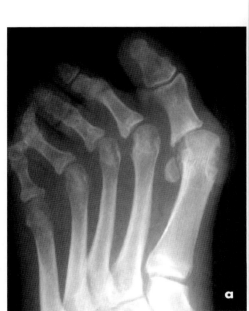
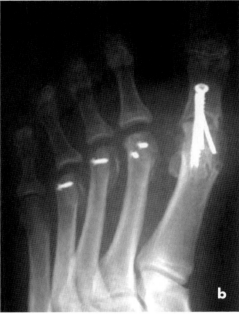

Figure 13–1–3. This patient experienced persistent pain after attempted resection arthroplasty for what appears to have been hallux valgus deformity. In addition to persistent painful arthritis of the metatarsophalangeal (MP) joint, lesser metatarsalgia was present. The fixation for the fusion was compromised because of bone loss, and in addition to a single cannulated screw, two threaded K-wires were used (b).

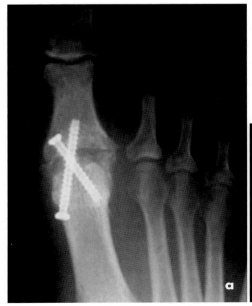

Figure 13–1–4. Note the standard position of the screws used for this arthrodesis (a, b).

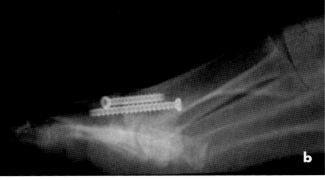

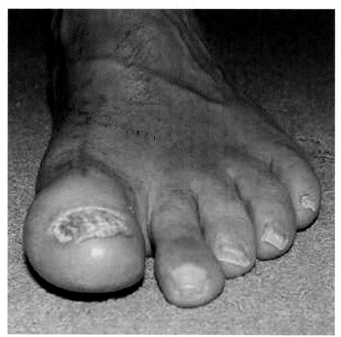

Figure 13–1–5. *The position of the hallux is not ideal. Note slight elevation of the hallux off the ground, which is expected to be present when the hallux is fused in 10 degrees of dorsiflexion relative to the floor. Neutral rotation of the hallux is present, as noted by the position of the nail, but medial translation with slight hallux varus is also present. This will cause abutment of the hallux against the shoe.*

Correction of Deformity Associated with Bone Loss

In cases with severe bone resorption or bone loss, an in situ arthrodesis is not sufficient, and structural support with an interposition graft must be considered. This is not an easy procedure to perform, and the arthrodesis rate is not as successful as that for an in situ procedure. For this reason, I will stage the surgery for selected patients, such as for those with severe bone loss and erosive synovitis associated with failed implant arthroplasty. For these patients, I will remove the implant, resect the fibrinous debris, lengthen the EHL tendon, and fill the defect with cancellous bone graft mixed with demineralized bone matrix. After 6 months, once the graft has incorporated, the second stage structural graft/fusion procedure is performed. Some patients, however, are reasonably comfortable after the first stage of the surgery, and therefore the second stage with arthrodesis is not performed. Although the hallux remains short and weak, the pain from the inflamma-

tory synovitis dissipates, and function is acceptable (Fig. 13–1–6).

Joint Exposure and Preparation for Distraction Bone Block Arthrodesis

The exposure for the arthrodesis is similar to that described previously, but the EHL tendon may need lengthening. There is no standard way to prepare the bone because irregular bone defects are frequent. In addition to flat bone cuts, the head and phalanx can be prepared exactly the same way as discussed previously with a burr, and then a reciprocal shape can be created with a slight contour and indentation in the bone graft (Figs. 13–1–7 and 13–1–8).

Considerable sclerosis of the bone margins is often present, and once the sclerosis is debrided down to bleeding bone margins, the defect can be considerable. Once the cuts at the bone ends are fashioned, a lamina spreader is inserted into the joint space with maximum distraction and the gap is measured fluoroscopically. While the laminar spreader is in place, check the perfusion to the soft tissues and the hallux because ischemia may be present. Slight adjustment to the bone cuts may need to be made with a saw or burr, and the final position of the MP joint may again need to be checked fluoroscopically. A femoral head allograft is now fashioned into shape to fill the void in the MP joint.

A saw is used to contour the graft. Once the graft has been contoured, it is fashioned repeatedly until it can easily be recessed into the prepared slot of the MP joint. This procedure is not easy and is facilitated with forcible plantar flexion of the hallux and insertion of the graft under distraction. If these do not work, then a smooth laminar spreader can be used to recreate the gap with more tension to insert the graft. No tension should be on the skin, which must close easily. The graft must be intrinsically stable at this time with minimal motion present with passive manipulation of the joint. Fixation must be stable, and a plate is invariably used. At times, however, the proximal phalanx is insufficient to apply the plate (Fig. 13–1–9), and large threaded pins are inserted across the IP joint. This type of fixation is difficult because the pins exit the metatarsal neck plantar and medial according to the dorsiflexion incorporated in the MP fusion. The pins must be

Text continued on p. 375

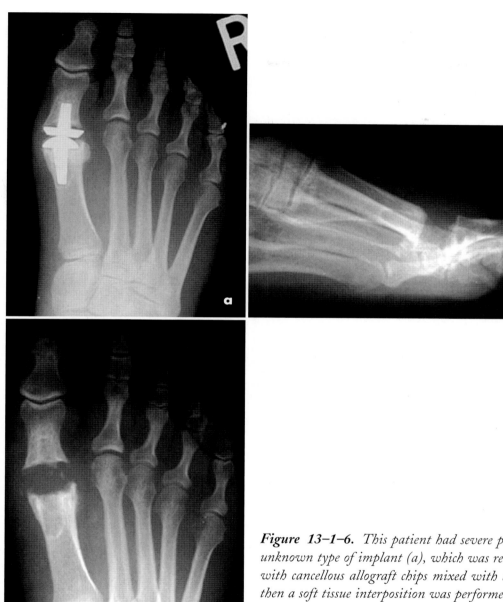

Figure 13–1–6. *This patient had severe pain associated with failure of an unknown type of implant (a), which was removed; the bone defect was filled with cancellous allograft chips mixed with demineralized bone matrix; and then a soft tissue interposition was performed with the thickened capsule and extensor hallucis brevis tendon (b, c). A subsequent structural arthrodesis was planned; however, the patient functioned reasonably without arthrodesis despite the shortening present.*

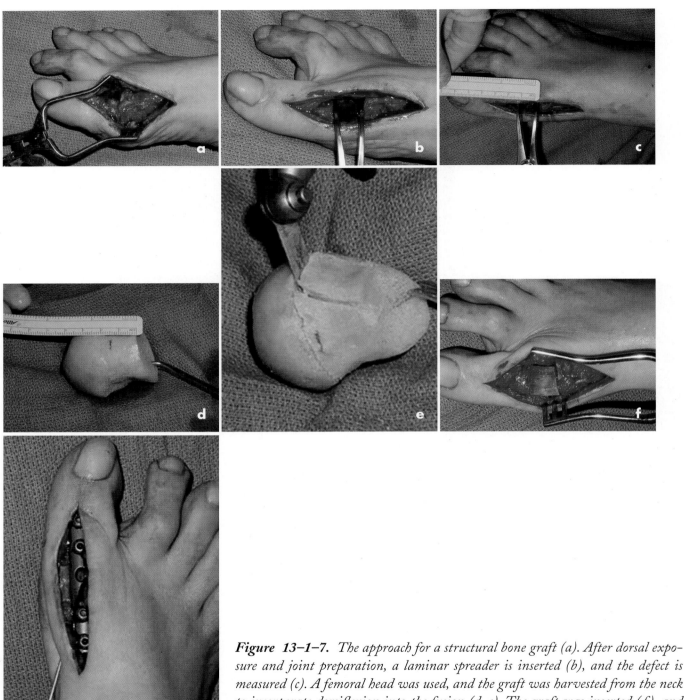

Figure 13–1–7. *The approach for a structural bone graft (a). After dorsal exposure and joint preparation, a laminar spreader is inserted (b), and the defect is measured (c). A femoral head was used, and the graft was harvested from the neck to incorporate dorsiflexion into the fusion (d, e). The graft was inserted (f), and a one-third titanium tubular plate was used in addition to an oblique cannulated 4-mm screw for fixation (g).*

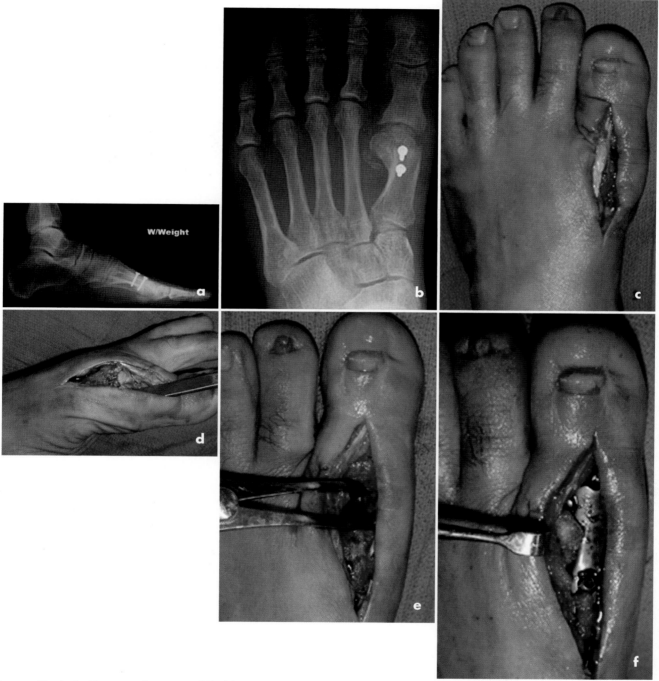

Figure 13–1–8. *Preoperative x-ray (XR) images of a patient with avascular necrosis (AVN) after what appears to have been a distal metatarsal osteotomy (a, b). Note the short first metatarsal, arthritis, and AVN. These were corrected with a bone block arthrodesis and plate fixation. Note exposure of the hallux with a dorsomedial incision. The hallux is plantarflexed with a curved periosteal elevator, and debridement is performed (c, d). A laminar spreader is inserted to measure the size of the graft. Note the slight blanching of the skin with distraction, which indicates potential skin ischemia with closure (e). The graft is cut slightly shorter from the femoral head, preventing complications of circulation, and the joint is secured with a dorsal plate (f).*

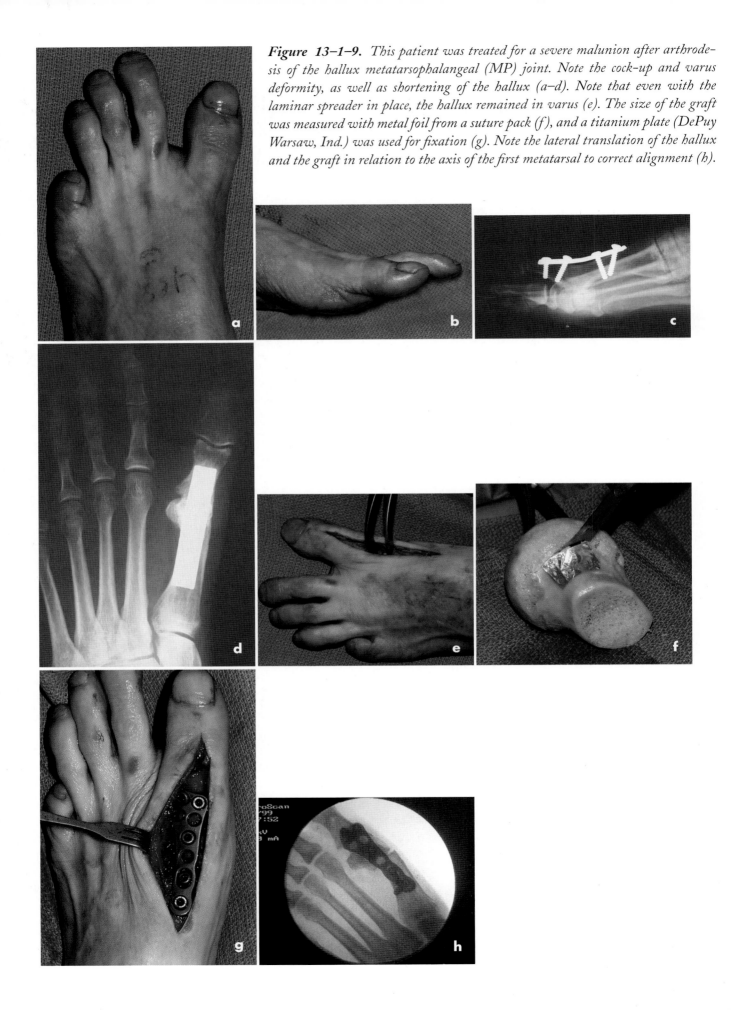

Figure 13–1–9. *This patient was treated for a severe malunion after arthrodesis of the hallux metatarsophalangeal (MP) joint. Note the cock-up and varus deformity, as well as shortening of the hallux (a–d). Note that even with the laminar spreader in place, the hallux remained in varus (e). The size of the graft was measured with metal foil from a suture pack (f), and a titanium plate (DePuy Warsaw, Ind.) was used for fixation (g). Note the lateral translation of the hallux and the graft in relation to the axis of the first metatarsal to correct alignment (h).*

inserted antegrade, and then while the hallux is compressed manually, they must be inserted retrograde across the MP joint.

Techniques, tips, and pitfalls

1. Arthrodesis of the hallux MP joint must be avoided where possible in the presence of a stiff or hyperextended IP joint. Even if the hallux MP joint is correctly positioned in slight dorsiflexion, overload of the hallux IP joint will still occur. If the hallux MP joint is fused in more dorsiflexion to accommodate for this, the tip of the hallux then becomes uncomfortable from pressure on the shoe as a result of the preexisting hyperextension of the IP joint.

2. Arthrodesis of the MP joint in the setting of a short hallux must be done carefully because the hallux will always shorten further, simply from preparation of the joint surface.

3. Nonunion after hallux MP arthrodesis is unusual. This is the result of failure of joint preparation, fixation technique, or patient compliance with mobilization postoperatively. The approach to revision can be identical with that of the primary procedure providing stable fixation is obtained and bone graft or bone graft substitutes are used to fill any defects or bone deficits.

4. If an arthrodesis of the MP joint is performed for correction of severe hallux valgus deformity associated with arthritis, the lesser toes must be corrected simultaneously. If they are not, a large, uncomfortable gap between the hallux and the second toe will occur. Generally, soft tissue releases are not sufficient and relaxation of the intrinsic tendons can only be accompanied with shortening osteotomies of the metatarsal head.

5. In the case of severe deformity of both the metatarsal and hallux associated with arthritis, positioning the hallux and the arthrodesis correctly is difficult. In these patients, intraoperatively realigning the first metatarsal with a compression screw from the first across to the second or third metatarsal is sometimes helpful. This is a temporary stabilizing screw that can be removed at some later date, after 3 months. The advantage of this screw is that it realigns the metatarsal and facilitates correct positioning of the arthrodesis. If this is not used, as the position of the first metatarsal changes after surgery, the position of the hallux may change simultaneously, and this change may lead to an abutment between the hallux and the second toe.

6. When severe hallux valgus deformity with a widened intermetatarsal space is present, an osteotomy of the first metatarsal does not need to be performed because the intermetatarsal (IM) angle will decrease after the MP fusion because of a reduction of the force of the hallux on the first metatarsal. However, when the IM deformity is severe, knowing where to position the hallux in the transverse plane is difficult because some closure of the intermetatarsal space will occur after fusion, which will then lead to abutment of the hallux on the second toe. A useful technique is to insert a lag screw between the first and second metatarsals, and this insertion will then guide the correct positioning of the MP joint (Fig. 13–1–10). The screw is left in place for 3 to 4 months and then removed.

7. If bone is avascular or the success of the arthrodesis is questionable, cancellous bone graft or demineralized bone matrix may be used to enhance the rate of fusion (Fig. 13–1–11).

8. The alignment of arthrodesis of the MP joint in the presence of hallux valgus interphalangeus is difficult, and even if positioned in slight varus, arthritis of the IP joint may ultimately occur (Fig. 13–1–12).

Arthrodesis of the Hallux Interphalangeal Joint

Arthrodesis of the hallux IP joint is indicated for correction of a claw hallux deformity, for correction of inflammatory or traumatic arthritis, or for procedures that involve the harvesting of the EHL tendon as a

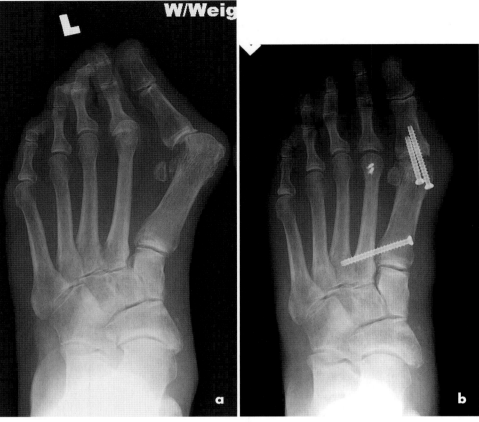

Figure 13–1–10. Severe hallux valgus associated with arthritis (a) was corrected with an arthrodesis of the metatarsophalangeal (MP) joint with a temporary lag screw between the first and second metatarsals to guide the correct position for the MP fusion (b).

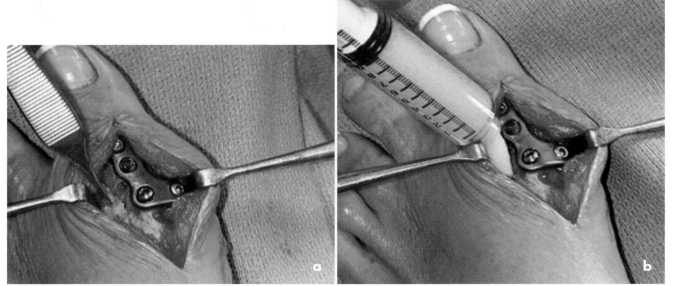

Figure 13–1–11. After realignment for this nonunion of an attempted metatarsophalangeal (MP) fusion, a defect was noted around the MP joint, which was filled with allograft cancellous bone chips, and demineralized bone matrix (DBM) (EBI, Parsipanny, NJ) was injected around the fusion mass.

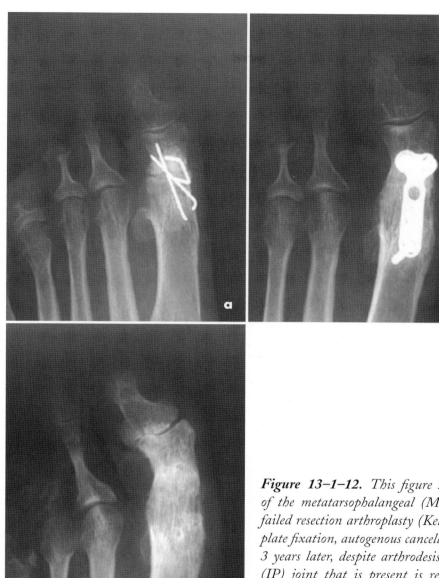

Figure 13–1–12. *This figure shows the problem of even slight malunion of the metatarsophalangeal (MP) arthrodesis, which was performed after failed resection arthroplasty (Keller arthroplasty) (a). This was revised with plate fixation, autogenous cancellous graft, and a small T-plate (b). However, 3 years later, despite arthrodesis, the severe arthritis of the interphalangeal (IP) joint that is present is related mostly to the hallux interphalangeus deformity (c). Perhaps this could have been prevented if the arthrodesis of the hallux were performed in slight overcorrection (varus) to compensate for the interphalangeus.*

tendon transfer. An incision is made dorsomedial to the EHL tendon and extends distally to end just proximal to the nail fold, and then it is cut transversely into either an L or a T shape. Maintaining some of the attachment of the EHL tendon is useful if it is not to be lengthened or used for a transfer. For some of the attachment to be maintained, the medial side of the joint is cut open, and then after subperiosteal dissection a small skin hook is used to retract the dorsal tissues and the EHL tendon. Cutting the proximal phalanx to preserve the EHL tendon attachment is easy, but cutting the distal phalanx is not as easy.

Once both the collateral ligaments are cut, the hallux is plantarflexed, the EHL tendon is retracted laterally, and the distal portion of the proximal phalanx is cut with a saw. The orientation of the cut must take into consideration the plane of the deformity. If severe rigid flexion contracture is present, then slight dorsiflexion can be incorporated into the angle of the cut. Correcting the deformity with the cut on the proximal phalanx is always the easiest because less freedom is available with the bone cut distally. Once the articular surface of the proximal phalanx is resected, the hallux is now lined up and the cut made accordingly. At this time, it is helpful to manipulate the hallux, insert a soft tissue retractor laterally to pull aside the EHL tendon, and then to completely plantarflex the hallux until the undersurface of the joint is visible. The base of the articular surface of the distal phalanx curves under the proximal phalanx, and this needs to be carefully resected. Usually, the flexor hallucis longus attachment is not disturbed. However, once the bone has been cut, visualize the attachment of the flexor hallucis longus tendon to ensure that this has not been transected (Figs. 13–1–13 and 13–1–14).

The bone is now lined up and the cut is adjusted until complete correction of the position of the distal phalanx with reference to the hallux is present. Make sure that

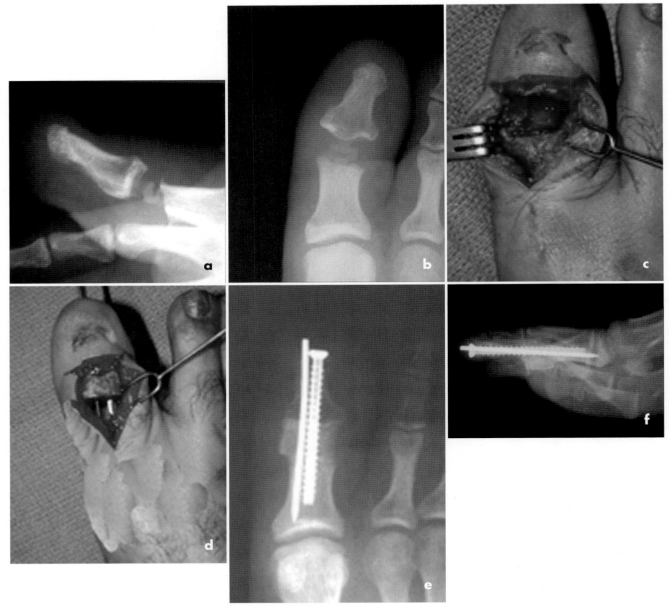

Figure 13–1–13. Arthrodesis of the hallux interphalangeal (IP) joint was performed in this patient after incorrect excision of the terminal portion of the proximal phalanx for plantar interphalangeal pain. Severe instability and hyperextension of the hallux was present with pain (a, b). Note the appearance of the IP joint with distraction (c). This was corrected with a bone block arthrodesis, and a corticocancellous graft was harvested from the ipsilateral calcaneus, cut into shape, and interposed. The guide pins were advanced out through the tip of the hallux and then back into the proximal phalanx (d). The final x-ray (XR) appearance (e, f).

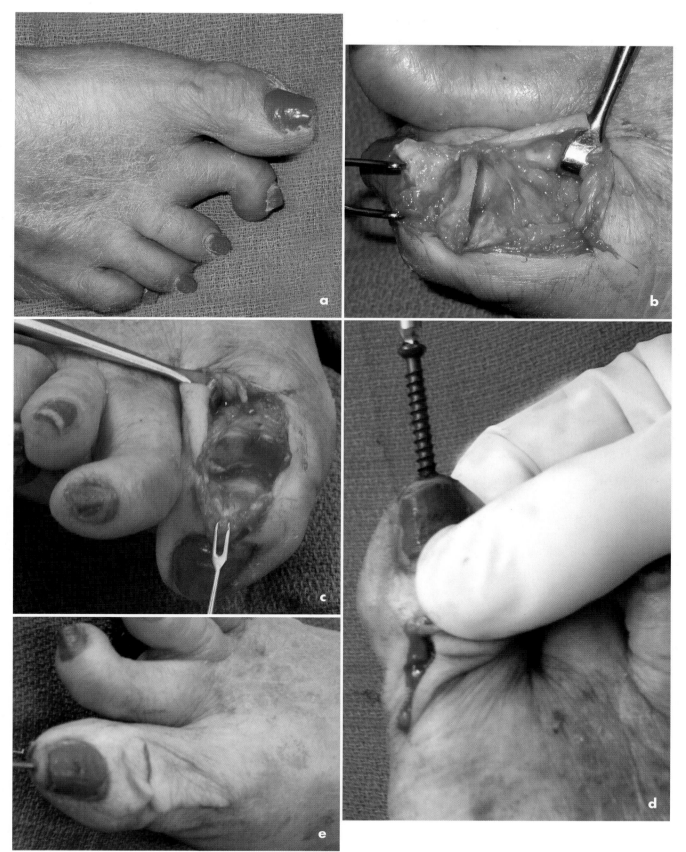

Figure 13–1–14. *The steps of arthrodesis of the hallux interphalangeal (IP) joint (a–e).*

no slight medial or lateral translation of the distal phalanx is present because either will cause a painful subcutaneous spur. If correction is performed for hallux valgus interphalangeus, then more bone will need to be removed medially, and the distal phalanx will need to be slightly translated medially to aid correction. I use a cannulated, fully threaded 4-mm cancellous screw for fixation. The guide pin is first inserted into the center of the proximal phalanx, and then a second hole is made antegrade out the distal phalanx so that it exits distally just under the nail. The guide pin is then inserted retrograde into the predrilled guide pin hole in the proximal phalanx. In this way, the hallux can be perfectly centered over the proximal phalanx. The hallux is then manually compressed as the screw is being inserted. A partially threaded screw can be used, although I have not found this to be necessary, and a fully threaded screw is sufficient, provided manual compression of the articulation is noted. If the joint slightly separates, then the screw is removed, manual compression is again applied, and the screw is reinserted.

Techniques, tips, and pitfalls

1. The incision can be made in any direction distally. The EHL tendon is always detached to some extent. One can try a straight longitudinal incision, but frequently, for exposure to be facilitated, this incision is extended distally either into the shape of a T or an L.

2. The key to the incision is to avoid the base of the nail in the germinal matrix.

3. Minimal bone should be removed from the proximal phalanx. Cutting the proximal phalanx is easier than cutting the distal phalanx, which curves under the proximal phalanx, and more bone is removed from the plantar than the dorsal distal phalanx.

4. Nonunion of this arthrodesis is unusual unless there has been a prior arthrodesis of the hallux MP joint. The added stress, with a longer lever arm on the hallux, increases the force on the joint leading to failure.

5. Fixation options are numerous, and the use of fully threaded or partially threaded screws does not appear to matter. For patients with poor bone, multiple threaded K-wires can be used and introduced along the edges of the toe, in addition to a screw.

Suggested Reading

Myerson MS, Schon LC, McGuigan FX, Oznur A. Result of arthrodesis of the hallux metatarsophalangeal joint using bone graft for restoration of length. Foot Ankle Int 21:297–306, 2000.

Arthrodesis of the Tarsometatarsal Joint

Overview

Arthrodesis of the tarsometatarsal (TMT) joint is performed for arthritis of varying extent with or without deformity, and in the setting of idiopathic osteoarthritis, of post-traumatic arthritis of the TMT joint complex, and of neuropathic deformity. Common to each of these procedures is the need to perform a realignment *and* arthrodesis. The results of arthrodesis are far better if the forefoot is correctly reduced. These results make sense because the deformity that is commonly associated with arthritis of the TMT joint is abduction of the forefoot relative to the hindfoot. With increasing abduction, the midfoot and forefoot pronate, and with this pronation, the torque increases on the medial aspect of the midfoot and on the hallux, causing hallux valgus. Note that with increasing deformity, additional procedures must be performed to obtain adequate alignment of the foot (Figs. 13–2–1 and 13–2–2). The arthrodesis should be limited to symptomatic joints. These are not always easy to determine, and a combination of the location of the patient's symptoms, the appearance on x-ray film, and findings on clinical examination will determine the joints to be fused. Then radiographic appearance of the lateral column is not helpful with the decision-making process because the lateral column is often asymptomatic in the presence of severe radiographic evidence of arthritis.

Incisions

If possible, I try to use only one incision for the arthrodesis. This, does depend on whether both the middle and medial column are included in the arthrodesis and whether deformity correction must be performed. If deformity and instability of the medial column are considerable, then I will use a separate medial incision to plantarflex the medial column (Fig. 13–2–3). I also use this incision when an extended navicular cuneiform metatarsal arthrodesis is performed that requires application of a plate from the medial side of the foot. The dorsal incision must be more lateral than is typically recognized. The base of the second metatarsal extends farther over toward the midline of the foot than is realized, and if the third metatarsal cuneiform joint is to be included in the arthrodesis, then the dorsal incision must be centered correctly over the midfoot. Once the incisions have been deepened through subcutaneous tissue, the branches of the superficial peroneal nerve must be looked for and then retracted.

A neuroma on the dorsal surface of the foot is intolerably uncomfortable and can be avoided. The tendon of the extensor hallucis brevis is used as a guide to the location of the deep neurovascular bundle. Once the tendon is identified, the bundle lies directly underneath it, and both are retracted medially. The easiest way to retract is to undermine the bundle from the subperiosteal tissue

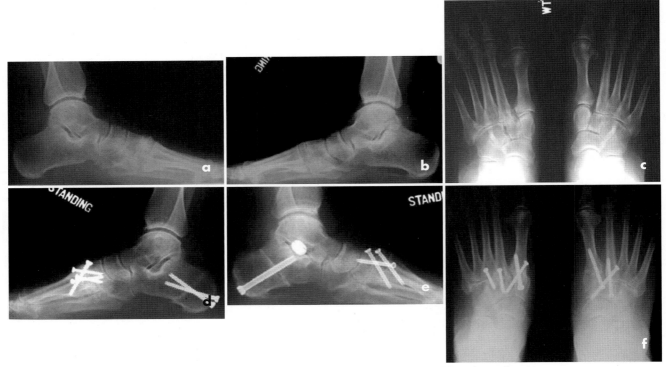

Figure 13–2–1. *This patient had arthritis of the medial and middle columns. Note how the pattern of deformity on the right foot (b) is slightly different from that of the left foot because there is more collapse of the midfoot and more hindfoot valgus. For some patients, arthrodesis of the tarsometatarsal (TMT) joints is not sufficient to correct the deformity, and correction of the secondary deformities of the hindfoot is necessary. This was accomplished with a medial translational osteotomy of the calcaneus on the left foot and additional arthroereisis of the subtalar joint on the right foot.*

over the second metatarsal and then elevate the flap with a large periosteal elevator, which includes the neurovascular bundle.

The joint is prepared with a combination of a flexible chisel, an osteotome, and occasionally a saw. I prefer to keep the anatomy of the joints completely intact and remove as little bone as possible. The problem occurs with preparation of a hard sclerotic joint, which can be associated with post-traumatic arthritis. The second metatarsal in particular can be avascular, and once this bone is debrided, the metatarsal shortens and a large gap is present in the joint. The third metatarsal usually adheres well to the second metatarsal and will follow the second metatarsal with deformity correction. If the medial and middle columns are fused, then I will try to debride the spaces between the first and second metatarsal base and between the medial and middle cuneiform and then place a bone graft in this

location to further stabilize the arthrodesis. At the completion of the joint preparation, the base of the metatarsals is then perforated with a 2-mm drill bit to facilitate some bleeding.

Fixation and Joint Stabilization

Arthrodesis must be performed with realignment. In situ arthrodesis is never ideal, and if the foot is left abducted and pronated, recurrent deformity, particularly of the forefoot, is present. Correction is therefore done first with the medial column, adducting the first metatarsal and locking this in position. For the first metatarsal to be positioned correctly, the hallux is grasped, and the base of the first metatarsal is pushed inward into the medial cuneiform, while the distal portion of the first metatarsal is pushed into adduction. At the same time, the hallux is dorsiflexed, and this dorsiflexion forces the first metatarsal into plantar flexion.

Figure 13–2–2. *Tarsometatarsal (TMT) arthritis in this patient was the primary problem, with a secondary effect on the hindfoot with abduction of the transverse tarsal joint and heel valgus. This was corrected with a TMT arthrodesis, in addition to a lengthening of the lateral column with a calcaneus osteotomy with a structural allograft.*

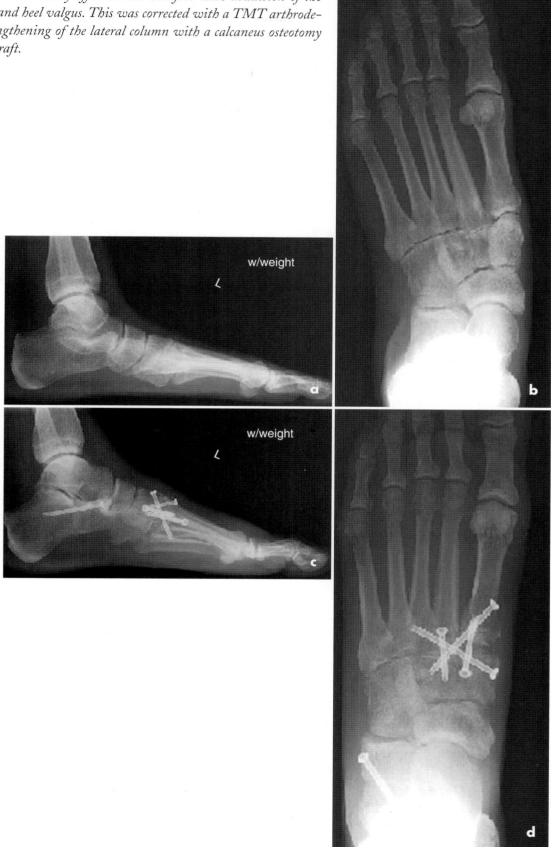

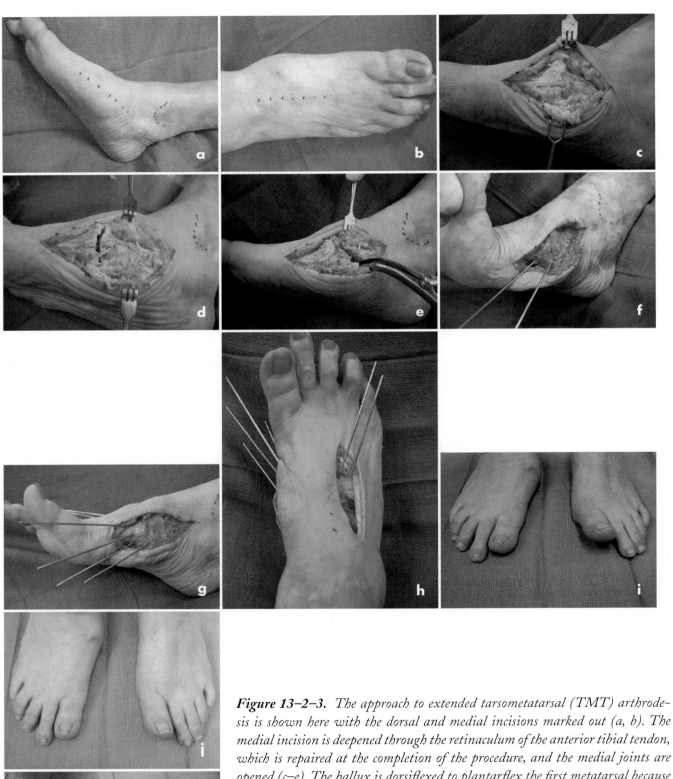

Figure 13–2–3. *The approach to extended tarsometatarsal (TMT) arthrodesis is shown here with the dorsal and medial incisions marked out (a, b). The medial incision is deepened through the retinaculum of the anterior tibial tendon, which is repaired at the completion of the procedure, and the medial joints are opened (c–e). The hallux is dorsiflexed to plantarflex the first metatarsal because the first ray is already short, and guide pins are introduced to maintain reduction (f–h). The final appearance of the foot 5 months after arthrodesis (i–k). Note the cock-up deformity of the hallux that was subsequently revised with lengthening of the extensor hallucis longus (EHL) tendon and dorsal metaphalangeal (MP) capsulotomy.*

A guide pin or K-wire is used to lock the first metatarsal in the corrected position. This can then be used as a template on which to build the rest of the foot. Once the first metatarsal is correctly positioned, then the second metatarsal can be reduced into its base and the mortise with a bone clamp, which is applied to the medial cuneiform reduction and the base of the second metatarsal. A guide pin is introduced through the medial cuneiform up and through the base of the second metatarsal to hold this in a reduced position. Alternatively, if no deformity is present, then the screw fixation for the second metatarsal cuneiform joint can be performed axially. The decision as to whether to use screws, staples, a plate, or even K-wires has to be based on the anatomy, bone loss, and the joints to be fused (Fig. 13–2–4).

Although I prefer to use screws wherever possible, sometimes they simply do not work adequately because of either the plane of the metatarsal or the paucity of bone to work with. The medial column is easier to stabilize by inserting a screw from the medial cuneiform aimed distally into the first metatarsal. Although this insertion can be made from the metatarsals directed proximally, it may split the base of the metatarsal. Therefore, after drilling, a careful countersink maneuver must be used to prevent splitting of the base of the metatarsal with insertion of the screw. Frequently a ridge is on the base of the second metatarsal as a result of hypertrophic osteophytes, which can be used to one's advantage to position the screw. However, if the entire dorsal osteophyte is left, then this will leave a dorsal ridge, which is uncomfortable. A balance has to be found between leaving a small ridge behind to facilitate screw insertion and leaving behind too large an osteophyte. Checking the plantar fixation of each metatarsal on a lateral radiograph is important. The metatarsals tend to dorsiflex with fixation because debridement of the joint is frequently performed dorsally only. These are very deep joints, and the entire base of the metatarsal cuneiform joint must be completely debrided to prevent a dorsal malunion of the arthrodesis. Insertion of a smooth lamina spreader into the joint dorsally to visualize the plantar apical surface of the joint is helpful before the arthrodesis is completed. Frequently, small bits of bone, which have not adequately been removed, remain on the plantar surface.

I do not routinely use bone graft to correct arthrodesis of the TMT joint unless a substantial defect is present.

However, insertion of small volumes of cancellous graft in the intermetatarsal and the intercuneiform space is useful if the arthrodesis is performed for more than a single metatarsal cuneiform joint. In these cases, stabilizing the medial to the middle column, including the intercuneiform space, and using bone graft are advantageous. Sometimes, after the debridement of the joint space, apposition of the joint, in particular the second metatarsal cuneiform joint, is poor. This can be addressed by inserting in a small amount of cancellous graft into the joint space with a tamp. Occasionally, large structural grafts are required to maintain alignment and provide structural support (Fig. 13–2–5).

Fixation options include screws, staples, pins, or plate. The configuration of fixation depends on the local anatomy. If the instability of the medial column is severe and the fusion is extended across to the navicular cuneiform joint, then I will consider the use of a medially applied plate. At times, I apply the plate on the tension side of the bone directly under the first metatarsal cuneiform joint, particularly in patients for whom instability and the potential for nonunion are increased (e.g., in those with neuropathy). This plantar plate has been shown to be more stable than other screw configurations for the TMT joint. Severe deformity may necessitate temporary lengthening of the lateral column with an external fixator, lengthening of the peroneal tendons, and then reduction of the medial and middle column (Fig. 13–2–6).

Management of Arthritis of the Lateral Column

The second principle is to try to maintain as much motion of the lateral column of the foot as possible. Consider the midfoot in columns: the medial column consists of the first metatarsal and medial cuneiform joint, the middle column consists of the second and third metatarsals and their corresponding cuneiforms, and the lateral column consists of the fourth and fifth metatarsals and cuboid. The second metatarsal is almost always included in the arthrodesis, which usually involves the entire middle column. This arthrodesis is performed in the setting of trauma and of idiopathic arthritis. Frequently, the middle and the medial columns need to be

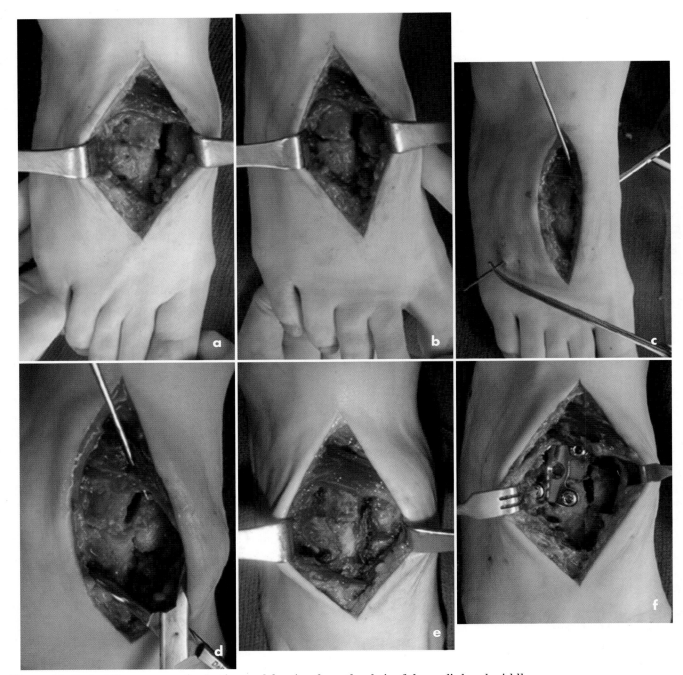

Figure 13–2–4. *The sequence of reduction and fixation for arthrodesis of the medial and middle columns is noted with one extensile incision and exposure of the subluxation and lateral deviation of the midfoot (a). The first metatarsal is pushed inward at the base, while the hallux is pulled into varus to reduce the medial column (b). The first metatarsal-medial cuneiform joint is secured with a guide pin, and a second guide pin is inserted from the medial cuneiform joint into the second metatarsal and out the skin where a clamp on the pin prevents loss of fixation when the second metatarsal is predrilled (c). The bone reduction clamp is applied to compress the medial to the middle column (d), and fixation with compression is completed (e). At this stage, instability of the middle column was noted, and a four-hole H-plate was applied to further stabilize the middle column (f).*

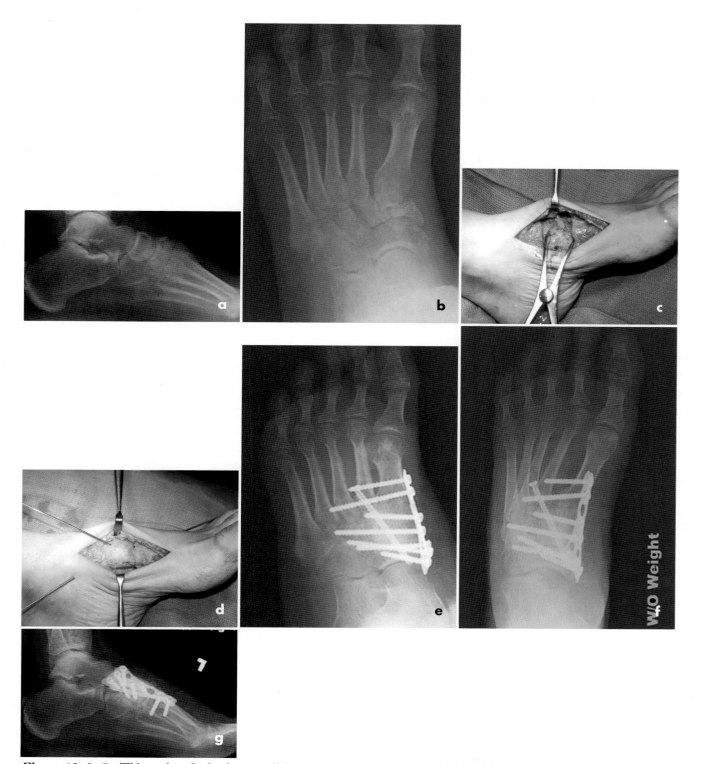

Figure 13–2–5. *This patient had a fracture dislocation of the tarsometatarsal (TMT) complex with crushing of the medial cuneiform and appeared for treatment 4 months after injury (a, b). At surgery, the cuneiform was in multiple fragments and was replaced with a structural allograft in order to maintain length of the medial column (c, d). A plate was used for stabilization (DePuy, Warsaw, Ind), and screws were inserted into the middle column for stability (e–g).*

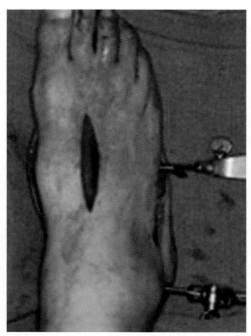

Figure 13–2–6. *The dorsal and medial incisions were completed, but before the medial and middle columns could be reduced, the lateral column had to be lengthened with a temporary external fixator with the pins in the calcaneus and fifth metatarsal.*

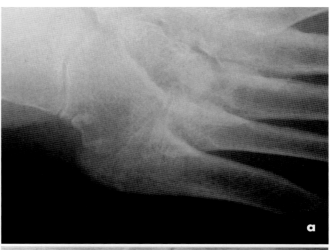

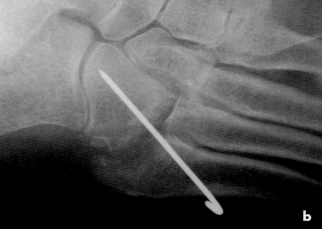

Figure 13–2–7. *Arthritis of the fifth metatarsocuboid joint only was present in this patient after trauma (a) and was treated with interposition arthroplasty with a temporary K-wire (b).*

fused at the same time. I always prefer not to fuse the lateral column, unless this is part of a neuropathic process with lateral column collapse associated with a lateral rocker bottom deformity. If arthritis of the lateral column is present and painful, arthroplasty of this joint can be considered, as opposed to arthrodesis. The foot is extremely stiff if an arthrodesis of all three columns is performed, and these arthroplasty procedures work well. Either a resection arthroplasty of the joint with interposition of soft tissues is performed, or interposition of ceramic spheres under slight distraction is performed to decrease the inflammatory arthritic process.

As previously noted, I rarely perform an arthrodesis of the metatarsal cuboid joints. In the presence of painful arthritis of all three columns, I prefer to perform an arthrodesis of the medial two columns and then an arthroplasty of some sort laterally. This can be either a soft tissue interposition arthroplasty or an insertion of ceramic spheres. The spheres are inserted under distraction so that the joint remains slightly distracted, maintaining motion. The decision as to which of these two are used depends on the availability of the ceramic spheres.

The soft tissue interposition arthroplasty is performed with a single incision located fluoroscopically between the fourth and fifth metatarsals. This location should be identified under fluoroscopy because the tendency is to make the incision too far laterally to the fifth metatarsal. Once the incision is deepened through the subcutaneous tissue, the interval between the sural nerve and the dorsal lateral cutaneous branch of the superficial peroneal nerve is used. The nerves are then retracted, and then an incision is made directly down onto the cuboid transversely, with a cut through the soft tissue envelope, including the peroneus tertius tendon (Fig. 13-2-7).

The tendon, the capsule, and periosteum are now raised as one large flap and then based distally. The flap is now raised off the base of the fourth and fifth metatarsals and used later for the interposition. The joint is now opened, distracted, and debrided. The bone can be removed off either the cuboid or the base of the metatarsals, and I prefer to resect the bone of the cuboid, keeping the soft tissue flap on the metatarsals intact. The attachment of the peroneus brevis muscle is not disturbed because this is farther proximal and more lateral than the incision and dissection. Approximately 5 mm of bone is removed from the articular surface so that full mobility, but not instability, of the metatarsal cuboid joint is noted. The flap of soft tissue is now inserted into the created joint space and then held secure with K-wires inserted transversely across the joint or with sutures.

A suture technique can be used the exact same way as soft tissue interposition arthroplasties with K-wire holes drilled through the cuboid, the sutures inserted through the cuboid, and then the soft tissue flap pulled down into the joint space. Ensuring that the soft tissue flap reaches the base of the articulation is important, and the K-wire holes must therefore exit at the underside of the cuboid. The alternative is to insert a suture anchor underneath the cuboid so that the flap can then be attached as far down on the plantar surface of the articulation as possible. Weight bearing can begin at 10 days after surgery in a walker boot with passive range-of-motion exercises starting as soon as possible.

The alternative procedure is insertion of ceramic spheres into the articulation (Figs 13–2–8 and 13–2–9). The concept of the procedure is to function as an interposition under slight distraction. An incision is made in the exact same way as the interposition arthroplasty is performed (Fig. 13–2–9a). However, no soft tissue flap is elevated. The joint is open vertically. After subperiosteal dissection, the center of each joint is located fluoroscopically, and a burr is used to remove a precise portion of the center of the joint. The burr corresponds to the size of the ceramic prosthesis. A prosthesis with a diameter of approximately 8 to 10 mm can be used (Fig. 13–2–9b, c). The key to success for this procedure is to ensure that the prosthesis has adequate coverage

dorsally, that it seats well in the prepared hole, and that it is in the center of the joint under slight distraction. Ascertaining the center of the joint is easy with a small sizer, which is part of the instrumentation for this procedure. Rehabilitation after this procedure is similar to that for the interposition arthroplasty procedure previously described.

Techniques, tips, and pitfalls

1. Realignment with the arthrodesis is essential. An in situ arthrodesis in the setting of deformity leads to continued problems, including medial midfoot pain and pronation of the forefoot with hallux valgus.

2. The reduction maneuver must begin with the first metatarsal with correction of its alignment with the talus navicular and medial cuneiform. This is a similar maneuver that is performed when a Lapidus-type bunionectomy is performed. Take a look at the example shown in the section on hallux valgus in which the hallux is dorsiflexed and the first ray is plantarflexed for guide pin and screw insertion. The only difference here would be, in addition to the dorsiflexion of the hallux, the first ray must be pushed into adduction.

3. The superficial peroneal nerve and its branches must be retracted. If a neuroma occurs, this is always painful and requires subsequent treatment.

4. If no instability is present, then the intercuneiform and intermetatarsal spaces do not require arthrodesis.

5. Bone graft is only necessary when large defects are present, and bone graft substitutes are as effective (Fig. 13–2–10).

6. Failure of TMT arthrodesis can involve the entire hindfoot and may require more extensive revision (Figs 13–2–11 to 13–2–13).

Text continued on p. 395

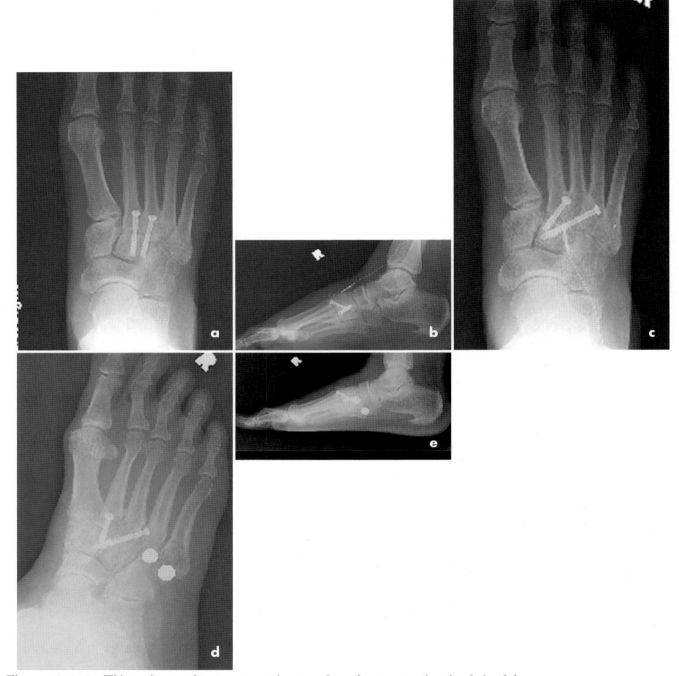

Figure 13–2–8. *This patient underwent two prior procedures for attempted arthrodesis of the tarsometatarsal (TMT) joints. The second resulted in another nonunion (a), which was revised a third time with an implantable bone stimulator (b, c). Continued pain was present in the lateral column and was treated with insertion of ceramic orthospheres into the fourth and fifth metatarsocuboid joints with ultimate success and resolution of symptoms (d, e).*

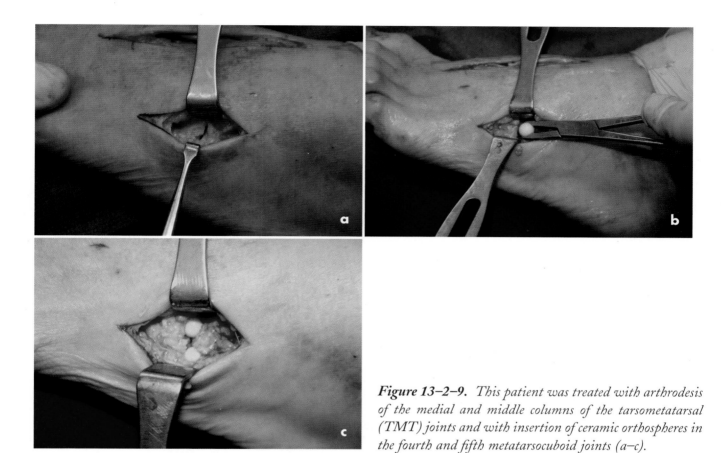

Figure 13–2–9. *This patient was treated with arthrodesis of the medial and middle columns of the tarsometatarsal (TMT) joints and with insertion of ceramic orthospheres in the fourth and fifth metatarsocuboid joints (a–c).*

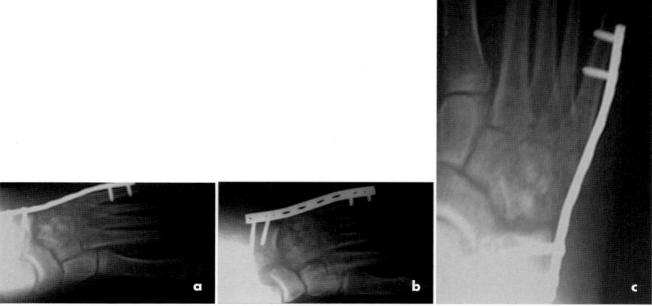

Figure 13–2–10. *This patient appeared for treatment of failure of open reduction with internal fixation (ORIF) of a midfoot dislocation with persistent subluxation of the talonavicular joint and crushing of the cuboid (a–c).*

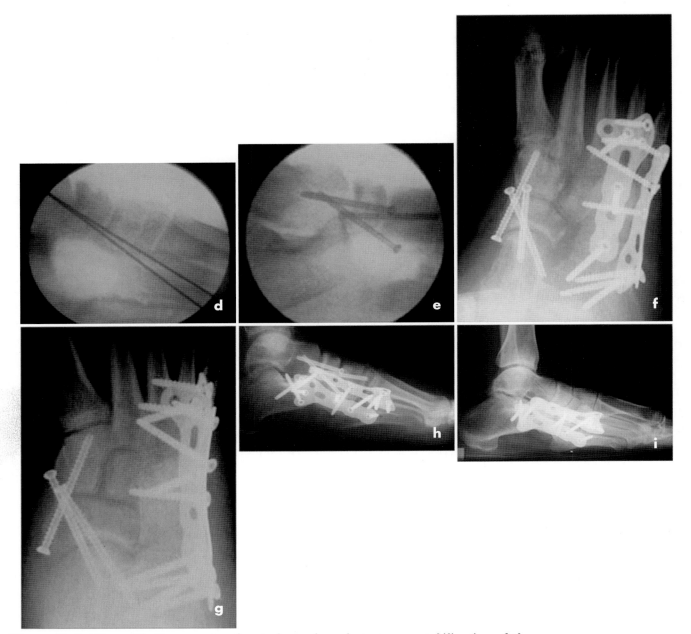

Figure 13–2–10, cont'd *For reconstruction to be performed, temporary stabilization of the medial column was performed. Note the intraoperative reduction of the talonavicular joint and the large void laterally where the comminuted bone was removed (d, e). A 4-cm structural allograft was inserted laterally to replace the cuboid, and two plates (DePuy, Warsaw, Ind) were used for the arthrodesis (f–h). The medial screws were removed at 5 months and arthrodesis was present (i).*

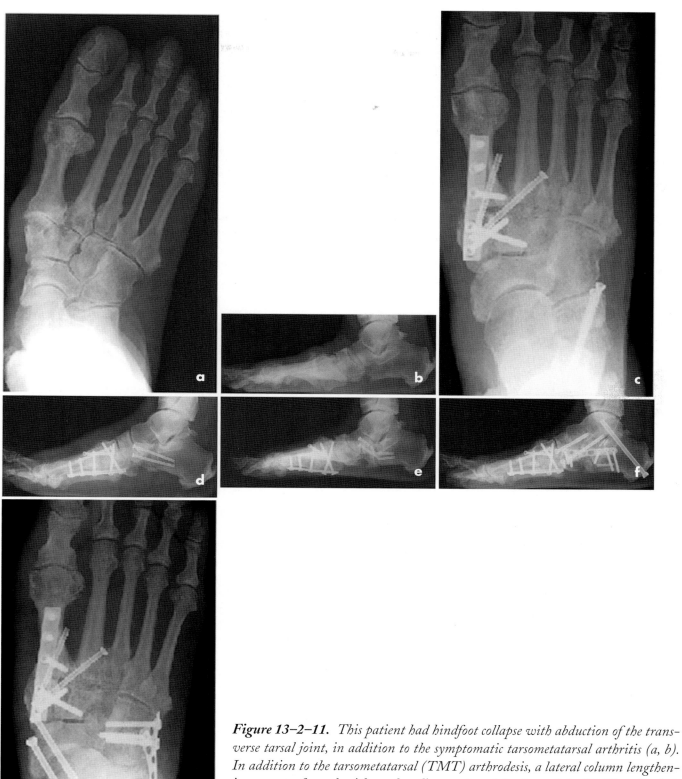

Figure 13–2–11. *This patient had hindfoot collapse with abduction of the transverse tarsal joint, in addition to the symptomatic tarsometatarsal arthritis (a, b). In addition to the tarsometatarsal (TMT) arthrodesis, a lateral column lengthening was performed with good realignment and healing of the TMT arthrodesis (c, d). Although an arthrodesis of the TMT was present, a nonunion of the lateral column occurred with worsening deformity (e), and this was corrected with structural grafting of the entire lateral column and conversion to a triple arthrodesis to improve the likelihood of arthrodesis, which occurred successfully (f, g).*

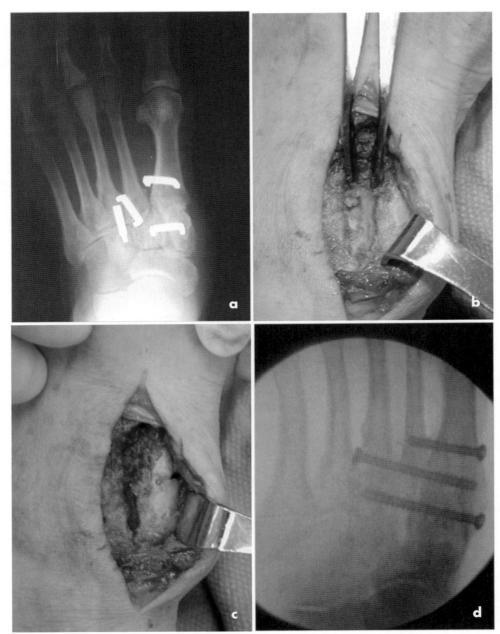

Figure 13–2–12. *Nonunion of the tarsometatarsal (TMT) joints was present in this patient for whom attempted arthrodesis was performed with staples (a). At surgery, there was complete dissociation between the medial and middle columns with bone loss at the base of the second TMT joint. The first TMT joint was fused (b, c). This was corrected with debridement and the use of demineralized bone matrix with cross screw fixation (d).*

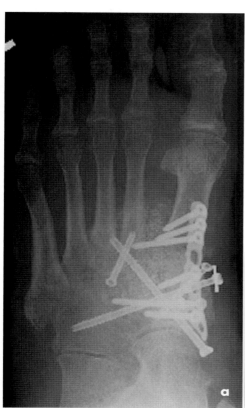

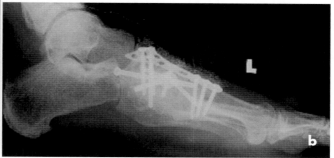

Figure 13–2–13. *This patient underwent a revision arthrodesis for failure of three prior attempts at arthrodesis for post-traumatic arthritis of the tarsometatarsal (TMT) and naviculocuneiform joints. These demonstrate the pattern of fixation and bone grafts. Note that the alignment of the foot in both projections has been maintained and that a screw was inserted across the foot from the medial cuneiform into the cuboid, although this was not part of the arthrodesis. If adequate fixation cannot be obtained, then screws may be inserted across joints where minimal, if any, motion occurs to improve stability.*

Suggested Readings

Chiodo CP, Myerson MS. Developments and advances in the diagnosis and treatment of injuries to the tarsometatarsal joint. Orthop Clin North Am 32:11–20, 2001.

Coester LM, Saltzman CL, Leupold J, Pontarelli W. Long-term results following ankle arthrodesis for post-traumatic arthritis. J Bone Joint Surg Am 83-A:219–228, 2001.

Curtis MJ, Myerson M, Szura B. Tarsometatarsal joint injuries in the athlete. Am J Sports Med 21:497–502, 1993.

Jung HJ, Myerson MS, Schon LS. The surgical algorithm for correction of idiopathic tarsometatarsal arthritis. Foot Ankle Int, 2004.

Komenda GA, Myerson MS, Biddinger KR. Results of arthrodesis of the tarsometatarsal joints after traumatic injury. J Bone Joint Surg Am 78:1665–1676, 1996.

Mann RA, Prieskorn D, Sobel M. Mid-tarsal and tarsometatarsal arthrodesis for primary degenerative osteoarthrosis or osteoarthrosis after trauma. J Bone Joint Surg Am 78:1376–1385, 1996.

Myerson MS. Tarsometatarsal arthrodesis: technique and results of treatment after injury. Foot Ankle Clin 1:73–83, 1996.

Myerson MS. The diagnosis and treatment of injury to the tarsometatarsal joint complex. J Bone Joint Surg Br 81:756–763, 1999.

Myerson MS, Fisher RT, Burgess AR, Kenzora JE. Fracture dislocations of the tarsometatarsal joints: End results correlated with pathology and treatment. Foot Ankle 6:225–242, 1986.

Sangeorzan BJ, Veith RG, Hansen ST Jr. Salvage of Lisfranc's tarsometatarsal joint by arthrodesis. Foot Ankle 10:193–200, 1990.

Subtalar Arthrodesis

Overview and Joint Preparation

The indications for subtalar arthrodesis are broad and include arthritis and deformities such as calcaneus fracture, isolated traumatic subtalar arthritis, middle facet tarsal coalition, calcaneovalgus deformity, and other isolated arthritic conditions. The approach that I take for correction of subtalar arthrodesis depends to some extent on the underlying condition. Most of these procedures are performed for post-traumatic arthritis after a calcaneus fracture, and a standard incision across the sinus tarsi is used. Complete exposure of the peroneal tendons and adequate subfibular decompression in patients with subtalar arthrodesis are essential. Impingement in the subfibular recess is common, and the bone must be removed. The easiest way to determine that an adequate decompression has been performed is to make sure that the lateral wall of the calcaneus is slightly medial to the undersurface of the overhanging talus. After completion of the procedure, I palpate the subfibular recess percutaneously and can detect whether any persistent bone is underneath the tip of the fibula.

The incision is made from the tip of the fibular extending distally down over the sinus tarsi toward the calcaneocuboid joint. On the inferior surface of the incision the peroneal tendon sheath is identified, and more distally in the incision the terminal branch of the sural nerve should be looked for. The nerve usually lies inferior to the peroneal tendons, but if the dissection extends more distally, the nerve can be at risk.

The issue often arises as to the correct incision to use after a failed open reduction with internal fixation (ORIF) of a calcaneus fracture. These extensile incisions are difficult to use for a subsequent elective arthrodesis procedure, and visualization of the entire joint can be limited because of scarring. I do not recommend using the original incision, provided 6 months has elapsed since the initial ORIF procedure, and a standard sinus tarsi approach should be used. In two situations that are faced after a calcaneus fracture treated initially with ORIF, the hardware is still in place (Fig. 13–3–1). In the first case, the hindfoot widens with collapse of the subtalar joint, and the hardware needs to be removed before the lateral wall ostectomy and arthrodesis are performed. In the other setting, arthritis is present but the overall architecture of the hindfoot has been maintained, and the hardware can be left in place. Fixation of the subtalar fusion can be more of an issue here, but the larger screws for the arthrodesis can be inserted around the plate and original screws as is done for a primary arthrodesis of the subtalar joint combined with ORIF for an acute fracture. When the hardware removal is planned, the plate and screws should be removed percutaneously with fluoroscopic imaging. Each screw can be marked with a needle, and then a 2-mm puncture incision is made directly on top of the screw through the skin and then deepened through subcutaneous tissue

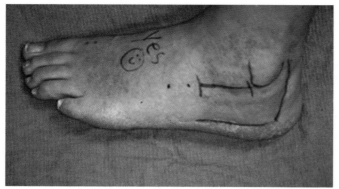

Figure 13-3-1. In this patient, the short sinus tarsi incision is used to perform the subtalar arthrodesis. The old incision, which was used for open reduction with internal fixation (ORIF) of the calcaneus, is ignored.

with a hemostat to avoid injury to the sural nerve. The plate can then be grasped with needle-nose pliers and then twisted out of the incision.

The retinaculum of the undersurface of the peroneal tendon sheath is stripped and elevated off the lateral wall of the calcaneus. Depending on the nature of the underlying disease, the peroneal tendons may be left in position or completely retracted if the lateral calcaneus has widened. After a calcaneus fracture, bone builds up under the fibula and squeezes the peroneal tendons into the fibula.

In these cases, the lateral wall of the calcaneus is completely exposed proximally toward and then posterior to the fibula, until the impingement against the lateral wall of the calcaneus is visible. A retractor is inserted into the soft tissue to pull the peroneal tendon sheath inferiorly and expose the entire lateral wall of the calcaneus (Fig. 13-3-2).

To perform the lateral wall ostectomy, I use a 2-cm curved osteotome and remove a generous amount of bone to completely expose the lateral aspect of the posterior facet of the subtalar joint and remove the lateral impingement under the tip of the fibula. Slight irregularities are often present in the lateral wall of the calcaneus after this ostectomy, and the surface should be palpated through the skin to find residual bone spikes that cause pain. The lateral margin of the posterior facet of the calcaneus should be slightly medial to the undersurface of the lateral margin of the talus. I preserve the

resected bone and cut it up with a bone cutter into 5-mm fragments for later bone graft (Fig. 13-3-3).

A retractor is then inserted into the soft tissues, and dissection is performed in the sinus tarsi. The contents of the sinus tarsi are elevated off the floor of the sinus tarsi until the anterior aspect of the posterior facet of the subtalar joint is well visualized. The insertion of a rongeur directly into the posterior facet of the subtalar joint is helpful; it should be twisted around and should loosen up the joint. The rongeur can then be pushed more medially to first open up and then debride the interosseous scar, and open up the middle facet. Once the debridement has been performed with the rongeur, a toothed laminar spreader is inserted into the sinus tarsi. With the spreader placed on stretch, the remnant of the interosseous ligament is visualized and is cut to gain access to the posterior aspect of the subtalar joint and the middle facet. I use a flexible chisel to remove and to denude the articular surface of the posterior facet, but minimal bone is removed. The posterior facet is debrided down to bleeding healthy subchondral bone. The chondral fragments are all removed with the rongeur. Final debridement is performed again with a flexible chisel on the more medial aspect of the subtalar joint with entrance into middle facet and complete denudation of the articular surface and the undersurface of the talus, as well as the dorsal surface of the middle facet (Fig. 13-3-4).

The bone graft, which had been harvested earlier from the lateral wall of the calcaneus, is used to augment the arthrodesis. The graft is now inserted into the sinus tarsi and the recesses in the subtalar joint and packed into place with a bone tamp. Be sure that no graft spills into the soft tissues, particularly under the peroneal recess laterally and then more posteriorly into the retrocalcaneal space. The cancellous bone autograft can be mixed with bone graft substitutes if a larger defect is present or when further stimulation of bone is thought to be necessary in patients at risk for nonunion.

Rarely, after an in situ subtalar arthrodesis, as previously described, a substantial defect that was not anticipated is present in the hindfoot. The technique for a distraction bone block arthrodesis of the subtalar joint is described in more detail later. If I anticipate that a defect will be present or that elevation of the height of the

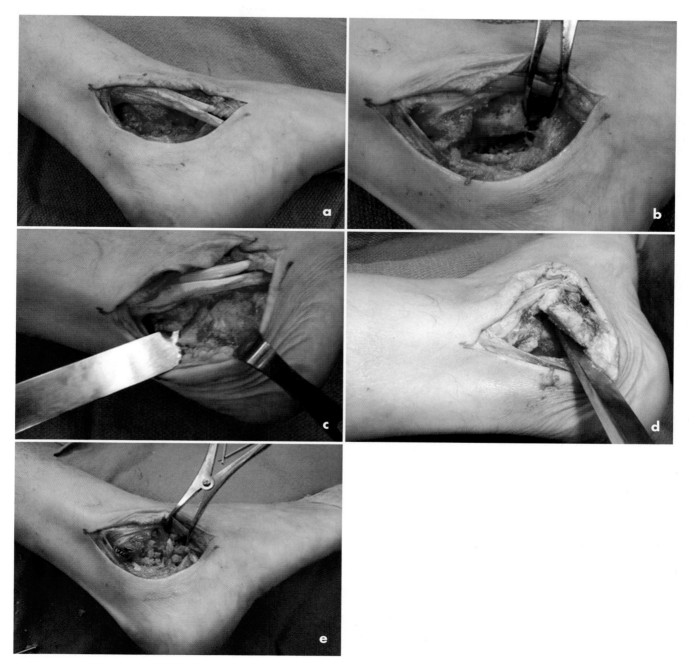

Figure 13–3–2. *In this case, the peroneal tendons are dislocated after a fracture of the calcaneus, with subfibular impingement. The incision is extended more proximally to expose the dislocated tendons (a), the joint is opened to reveal the impingement (b), and the ostectomy is performed from a posterior to anterior incision (c, d). Autograft cancellous chips are inserted and are taken from the lateral wall ostectomy (e).*

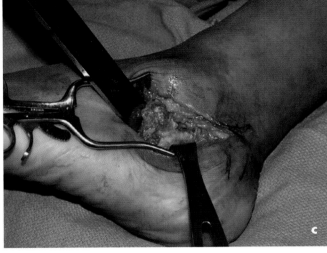

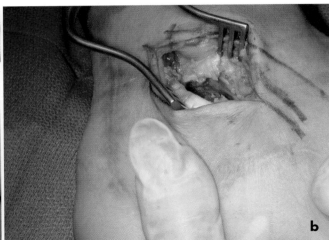

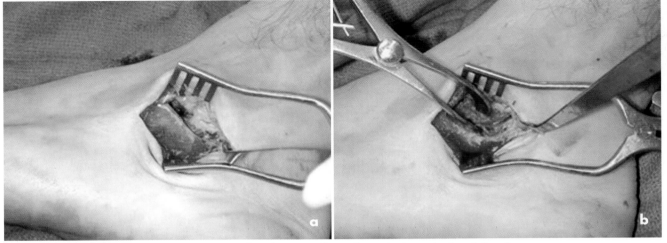

Figure 13–3–3. *Under normal circumstances the lateral wall ostectomy is performed through the short sinus tarsi incision (a, b). If the extrusion of bone extends toward the calcaneocuboid joint, the ostectomy can begin at the joint with or without an arthrodesis performed.*

Figure 13–3–4. *A lateral wall ostectomy has been performed, and the subtalar joint is not visible (a). The subtalar joint is distracted with a laminar spreader, and the joint becomes visible (b).*

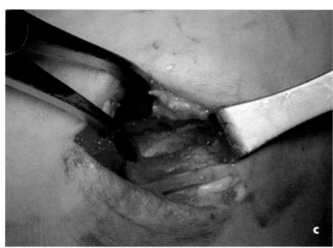
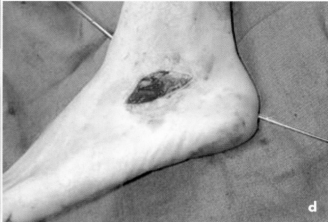

Figure 13–3–4, cont'd. With progressive joint distraction, the joint can be debrided (c), and guide pins are inserted for cannulated screw fixation (d).

hindfoot is necessary, then I will use a vertical incision. However, if I have used the standard sinus tarsi incision, then before I complete the procedure, I make sure that I can close the skin without tension. Removing some of the bulk of the bone graft may be necessary to do so. A defect will occur if avascular necrosis of the posterior facet is present, and as debridement is performed, more bone loss is present. This can be filled with either a bulk structural graft or cancellous chips. Before the graft is inserted, a laminar spreader is placed into the sinus tarsi to check the required height, and the tension on the skin is evaluated.

Fixation

I find it useful to secure the arthrodesis under fluoroscopic imaging using cannulated 6.5-mm screws. The direction of the first screw is from plantar and posterior, but the heel pad is avoided. The heel is often damaged with the impact of the hindfoot fracture, and further compromise is unwarranted with insertion of a screw too inferiorly on the heel. Approximately 5% of these screws need to be removed because of prominence or pain. Although a second screw can be inserted from the heel up into the neck of the talus, I have more recently used a second screw from a dorsal insertion directed into the neck of the calcaneus. The first guide pin is introduced in the posterior aspect of the heel off the weight-bearing surface directed up anteriorly and slightly medially toward the posterior talar body. The second guide pin is introduced dorsally immediately medial to the anterior

tibial tendon and the talar neck and is then directed inferolaterally down toward the sinus tarsi and the inferior neck of the calcaneus. Make sure that the second screw does not cause any impingement against the neck of the talus with the foot in maximum dorsiflexion (Fig. 13–3–5). The position of the screws and the alignment of the hindfoot with respect to the forefoot are checked fluoroscopically before skin closure.

Management of Subtalar Fusion Nonunion

Subtalar fusion nonunion is a frustratingly difficult problem, which unfortunately occurred in 10% of cases in a large series of patients that have been published. The incidence ranges from 9% to 33% depending on the underlying premorbid problems. Patients at high risk for this condition include those who smoke, those who have had calcaneus fractures that are associated with hard avascular bone in the region of the subtalar joint, and those in whom any areas of segmental avascular necrosis are present in the subtalar joint. If a nonunion in one of these high-risk categories is being dealt with, bone graft augmentation and supplementation with bone graft substitutes or an implantable bone stimulator will be recommended. The workup of a patient who has pain after a subtalar arthrodesis should include plain x-ray (XR) images and a computerized axial tomography (CAT) scan (Figs. 13–3–6 and 13–3–7). Sometimes the arthrodesis is solid, but an osteophyte may be present on the inferior aspect of the fibula and is projecting off the

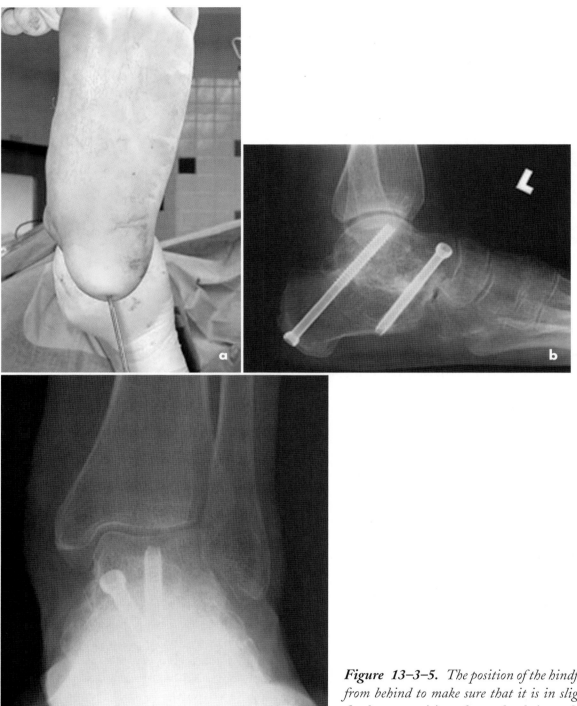

Figure 13–3–5. *The position of the hindfoot must be checked from behind to make sure that it is in slight valgus (a). The final screw position after arthrodesis on the lateral foot x-ray (XR) image (b) and on the anteroposterior (AP) ankle (c).*

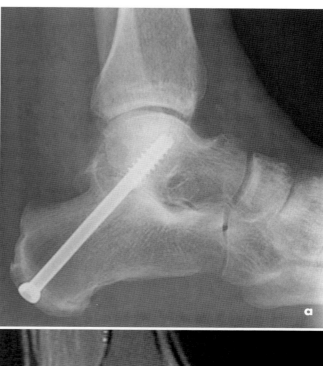

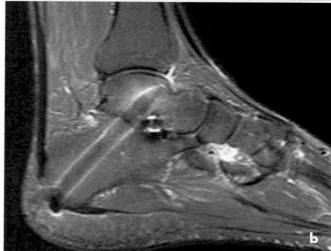

Figure 13–3–7. *Lateral x-ray (XR) image (a) and magnetic resonance imaging (MRI) picture (b) of a patient with pain after a subtalar arthrodesis. Although the computerized axial tomography (CAT) scan is usually more reliable, the lucency around the screw and in the sinus tarsi is easily visible on the MRI picture.*

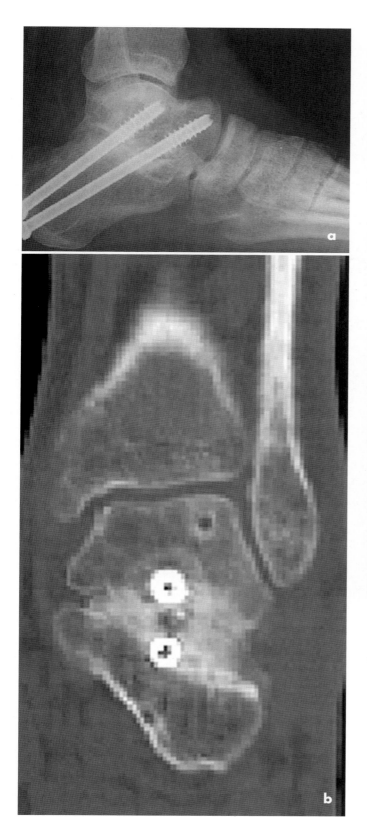

Figure 13–3–6. *Lateral x-ray (XR) image (a) and computerized axial tomography (CAT) scan (b) of a patient after a subtalar arthrodesis with pain. Note the lucency of the posterior subtalar joint on XR film but a solid fusion on the CAT scan cut through the sinus tarsi.*

arthrodesis either into the peroneal tendons or under the fibula causing subfibular impingement. The osteophyte is easily visible on a CAT scan. The arthrodesis may also be patchy, and this is also evident on a CAT scan.

The problem with correction of a nonunion is that preparation of the joint requires further debridement, and as this is performed, a large hole or defect, which needs bone graft supplementation, is frequently present (Fig. 13–3–8). This can be done with autograft or allograft, and usually cancellous allograft chips are used and are mixed with the Symphony platelet system (DePuy, Warsaw, Ind.). After this procedure, patients should be kept non–weight bearing for a prolonged period of time, up to 3 months until visible evidence of bone healing is evident radiographically. More important, these patients should have minimal swelling and no warmth in the hindfoot on palpation before initiating weight bearing.

Techniques, tips, and pitfalls

1. Sural neuritis must be avoided. The nerve is usually immediately inferior to the peroneal tendons and must be avoided during the dissection. The dorsal lateral cutaneous branch of the superficial peroneal nerve is vulnerable in the more distal portion of the incision.

2. Subfibular impingement must be avoided. This is only a problem after post-traumatic arthritis when widening of the calcaneal body is present with extrusion after calcaneus fracture. The calcaneal ostectomy with removal of the lateral wall of the calcaneus is an integral part of the subtalar arthrodesis in these cases. At the completion of the procedure and when bone graft has been packed into the sinus tarsi, make sure that no graft has slipped back between the peroneal tendon and the fibula.

3. Nonunion is a frustrating problem with this procedure. Despite all efforts to decrease this incidence, nonunion seems to occur approximately 10% of the time. Usually, nonunion occurs in higher-risk individuals, such as in those who smoke, those who have hard sclerotic subchondral bone after trauma, and those in whom slight avascular change of the posterior facet is present after calcaneus fracture. Clearly,

the use of bone graft or bone graft substitutes is useful, if not important, here. A mixture of demineralized bone matrix and cancellous bone chips is commonly used and is impacted into the sinus tarsi on completion of the joint debridement. Malunion of this arthrodesis is unusual, but if it occurs, it is due to over rotation with internal rotation of the subtalar joint during internal fixation. Malunion (by internal rotation of the subtalar joint) leads to supination of the forefoot and hindfoot varus. This can be determined visually so that when the hindfoot is held in the correct position, the heel should be in a few degrees of valgus and the forefoot plantigrade relative to the hindfoot. Be careful if the patient is lying in a lateral decubitus position because this position may make it difficult to visualize the relation among the hindfoot, forefoot, and the knee. Slight valgus positioning of the hindfoot is preferable and does not cause too much of a problem unless the arthrodesis is performed for correction of flatfoot. In these cases, the subtalar joint is intentionally internally rotated, but again, be careful that malunion with fixed forefoot has not been created.

4. The incision used for the subtalar arthrodesis is a short lateral incision from the tip of the fibula over the sinus tarsi. If any change in the position of the heel from valgus to varus is desirable with the subtalar arthrodesis, then the incision must be modified to avoid wound dehiscence postoperatively. This is particularly relevant to the bone block arthrodesis when a vertical incision is used.

5. Subtalar arthrodesis performed for correction of a middle facet coalition can be difficult if the posterior facet is completely obliterated. Although the coalition involves the middle facet, it may be difficult to visualize the posterior facet, which has to be opened gradually. The entire joint including the middle facet coalition must be opened with a laminar spreader to correct the severe valgus that can accompany this deformity. If the posterior facet is not visible, then use a small osteotome positioned fluoroscopically before attempting to open the joint.

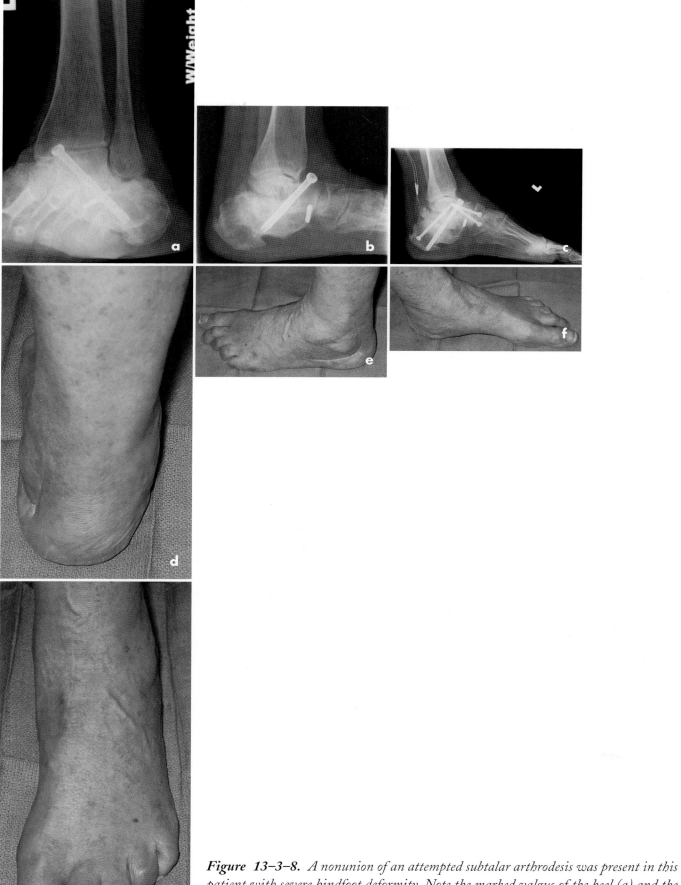

Figure 13–3–8. *A nonunion of an attempted subtalar arthrodesis was present in this patient with severe hindfoot deformity. Note the marked valgus of the heel (a) and the nonunion with subtalar collapse (b). A bone block arthrodesis was performed through a vertical posterior incision, including an implantable bone stimulator. This was not sufficient, however, to correct the remaining foot deformity, and a talonavicular arthrodesis was performed simultaneously (c–g).*

Distraction Bone Block Arthrodesis

The indications for a subtalar distraction bone block arthrodesis are fairly specific and are limited to procedures in which an arthrodesis of the subtalar joint needs to be performed but significant vertical collapse of the hindfoot is present. The traditional indication for this procedure has been after a calcaneus fracture when shortening of the heel height with painful anterior ankle impingement and weakened push-off strength are present. This subtalar distraction bone block arthrodesis can also be performed, however, for management of talar body collapse associated with either post-traumatic arthritis or avascular necrosis of the talus for which the arthrodesis is performed as a staged procedure to elevate the height of the ankle itself. This arthrodesis is particularly useful, for example, in patients with combined ankle and subtalar arthritis in which the presence of the body of the talus is insufficient to prevent subsidence when a total ankle replacement is performed. With distraction bone block arthrodesis and stabilization of the subtalar joint, both problems (i.e., the subtalar arthritis and the height of the ankle joint) are addressed, and later-stage total ankle replacement is facilitated.

Skin Incision and Dissection

The incision must be made vertically in the posterior aspect of the ankle and extend from the inferior heel up slightly posterior to the course of the sural nerve (Fig. 13–3–9). The sural nerve is identified, then the peroneal tendon sheath is identified more anteriorly, and the sheath and the nerve are retracted more anteriorly. The nerve can then be maintained in this position throughout the rest of the procedure. The nerve should be inspected, and if any severe scarring is present or the patient had symptoms of neuritis preoperatively, the nerve can be transected and buried in the fibula through a drill hole more proximally.

For visualization of the posterior subtalar joint, the subcutaneous tissues are dissected deeper on to the posterior aspect of the calcaneus. Then the back of the joint can be identified with the posterior surface of the calcaneus as a guide. The posterior aspect of the retrocalcaneal space will have to be dissected out for visualization of the calcaneus. Working now laterally with subperiosteal dissection, strip the peroneal tendon sheath and elevate the lateral wall off of the calcaneus.

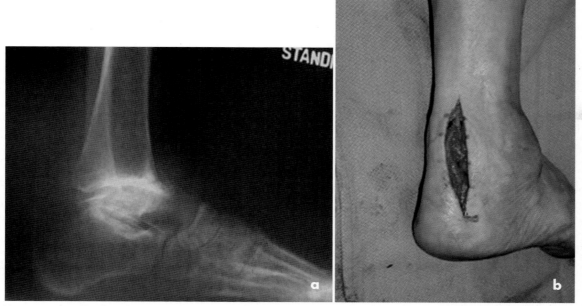

Figure 13–3–9. A subtalar bone block arthrodesis was performed in this patient for management of avascular necrosis of the talus associated with subtalar and ankle arthritis (a). The vertical incision is noted (b).

In most circumstances, subfibular impingement is present, and the lateral calcaneus ostectomy must be performed. This seems difficult, but it can be done through visualization of the hypertrophic bone laterally with bone impingement under the fibula once the peroneal tendons are elevated. The ostectomy is performed with a curved 1.5-cm osteotome, and the incision is started on the posterior margin of the tuberosity of the calcaneus inferior to the posterior facet. The entire bone mass must be removed, and about 1 cm should exist between the tip of the fibula and the calcaneus laterally.

Working posteriorly in the retrocalcaneal space, insert a curved osteotome along the posterior margin of the tuberosity of the calcaneus into the original subtalar joint. This insertion is not always easy and may have to be done fluoroscopically. If the joint is not visible, a 1-cm curved osteotome is inserted under the talar articular surface and is curved down inferior and distal. The osteotome is now gradually worked into the original joint space in order to distract the joint. Once the joint is opened, it is possible to begin the distraction with a laminar spreader, which can then be inserted deeper into the joint. I use a combination of flexible chisels and osteotomes to decorticate the entire joint. Be careful not to injure the flexor hallucis longus tendon on the posterior medial side of the joint.

The creation of a small notch or recess in the posterior tuberosity of the calcaneus with the osteotome is useful for stable insertion of the bone graft. At this time, the position of the heel should be checked because varus tilt of the calcaneus with the laminar spreader in place is common. The heel must be in slight valgus once the graft is inserted.

Bone Graft

I prefer to use structural allograft for the distraction procedure and to use a fresh frozen femoral head, cutting the graft with a saw to contour the shape of the graft for insertion into subtalar joint (Fig. 13–3–10). The graft is cut into a trapezoidal shape, is slightly higher medially than laterally, and is higher posteriorly than anteriorly. The graft size can be measured fluoroscopically, according to the space opened by the laminar spreader. Once I decide on the size of the graft, I switch the laminar spreader to one that has no teeth to extract it easily once the graft is inserted. The laminar spreader is now placed on maximum stretch to facilitate insertion of the graft, which is tamped into place securely. The graft only fills the space of the posterior facet and usually is not long enough to reach the sinus tarsi. Additional cancellous graft can be inserted into the sinus to augment the fusion. The laminar spreader is now

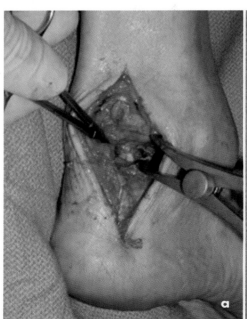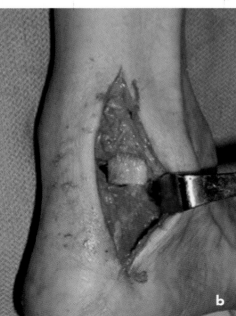

Figure 13–3–10. A laminar spreader is inserted into the incision, and the joint is distracted. Note the hemostat pointing to the flexor hallucis longus tendon on the medial aspect of the ankle(a). The graft has been tamped into place securely before fixation (b).

gradually withdrawn, and the position of the heel noted. If a varus position of the heel is persistent, the lateral calcaneus can be shaved down directly under the graft with a saw. Finally, small pieces of cancellous autograft or allograft are inserted more anteriorly into the sinus tarsi with a curved curette.

Screw Fixation

Screw fixation is easier to perform with cannulated screws. I do not think that it makes much difference whether partial or fully threaded screws are used, but the height of the graft should not be lost because of excessive compression. The same principle of position of the screws applies here as it does with the in situ fusion previously described. Rarely, the room for a large 6.5-mm screw may not be sufficient, and two or three smaller-gauge screws can be used.

Techniques, tips, and pitfalls

1. If distraction bone block arthrodesis includes any correction of deformity, be careful of the final foot position. For example, if the procedure initially involves correction of mild subtalar valgus after debridement of the posterior facet of the subtalar joint, the heel tends to fall into more valgus. For this to be corrected, the more medial aspect of the joint, including the middle facet, must be debrided.

2. If the heel tends to fall into valgus during correction, then slight internal rotation of the subtalar joint can be performed to create mild heel varus. The forefoot must not be overcorrected into supination.

3. The incision for a bone block must be vertical. If any incision in the longitudinal plane of the foot is used and an increase in the height of the hindfoot is created, a wound slough or dehiscence and likely infection will be created. With this vertical incision, however, the height of the hindfoot can be lengthened easily without risk of skin problems.

4. The incision must be posterior to the peroneal tendons and sural nerve. The nerve is retracted anteriorly, and resection of the nerve is unnecessary unless a prior neuroma from trauma or surgery is present. Retraction of the nerve anteriorly with the peroneal tendons is not difficult.

5. The back of the subtalar joint cannot be seen initially. Locate the joint fluoroscopically with a guide pin and then mark its entrance and gradually open it up with a quarter-inch osteotome until entrance inside the joint is certain. At times, this procedure is difficult, and the osteotome has to be inserted fluoroscopically, corresponding to the original joint surface. Seeing the undersurface of the talus radiographically is easier than seeing the calcaneus because the posterior facet of the calcaneus is usually severely impacted into the body of the tuberosity.

6. Once the joint has been entered, gradually prying it apart, first with the osteotome and then with the lamina spreader, is helpful. This prying cannot be done initially because bone is under the fibula and a lateral wall ostectomy needs to be performed first.

7. The biggest problem with distraction of the subtalar joint is that the lamina spreader automatically tilts the heel into varus. This is a most important problem that can be prevented. The heel varus occurs because the lamina spreader and the shape of the graft. Shaping the graft into a trapezoid that is higher medially than laterally is important, and as the graft is inserted, the heel must be manipulated into valgus before fixation.

8. Once the bone block has been inserted, dorsiflexion of the ankle is going to decrease. Even though an impingement syndrome of the anterior ankle is frequently present preoperatively, dorsiflexion motion will actually decrease intraoperatively because of the distraction and tension on the Achilles tendon. For this reason, an Achilles tendon lengthening will often need to be performed. The foot must be positioned in 10 degrees of dorsiflexion with the bone block graft in place.

Postoperative Course and Treatment

The sutures are only removed once the wound is completely healed. The wound must be watched carefully because of the stretching of the incision. The foot is immobilized in maximum dorsiflexion. If the skin's viability is in question, the foot can be positioned in slight plantar flexion to take the tension off the back of the ankle. However, this compromises later rehabilitation, and once tissue healing is present, then passive range-of-motion exercises can be started, but in dorsiflexion and plantar flexion only. Rehabilitation is only possible if a boot is being used, and if it is used, the boot must be worn at night to prevent plantar flexion and equinus contracture. Weight bearing should not begin until 8 weeks after surgery. Whether the arthrodesis is done in situ as a bone block procedure, determining whether arthrodesis is present radiographically is sometimes difficult. Frequently, monitoring of the soft tissue, swelling, pain, and in particular warmth is more helpful than the radiographic appearance, and a combination of clinical and radiographic observations is used to determine bone healing and weight-bearing

status. A limb is immobilized in either a cast or boot until evidence of full healing is evident both clinically and radiographically. Physical therapy with strengthening and rehabilitation is useful, particularly to maximize dorsiflexion and plantar flexion strength. Swelling is usually present for 6 to 12 months after the operation.

Correction of Complex Hindfoot Deformity after Calcaneus Fracture

Salvage of complex hindfoot deformity falls into a number of categories. These depend on the following: (1) the presence of widening of the hindfoot; (2) the presence of varus or valgus deformity of the calcaneus; (3) the talar declination angle; (4) the presence of hardware; (5) any secondary deformities, including abduction of the transverse tarsal joint, which may be associated with crushing of the calcaneal cuboid joint; and (6) the presence of peroneal tendon dislocation.

For all of these complex deformities, a CAT scan should be obtained (Fig. 13–3–11). Although the deformity

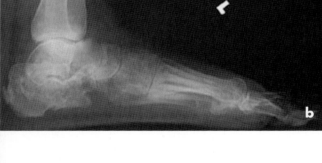

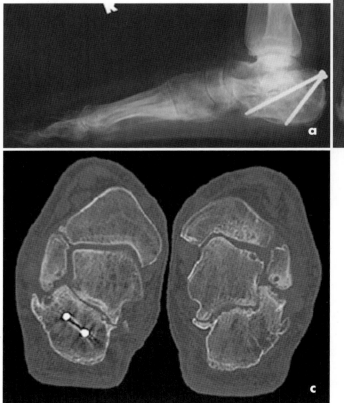

Figure 13–3–11. *Salvage of these bilateral malunited calcaneus fractures will require a subtalar arthrodesis. Note in both the lateral x-ray (XR) images (a, b) that there is marked hindfoot collapse, with overlapping of the talus and calcaneus and a severe change in the talar declination angle. Although the changes present can be anticipated, a computerized axial tomography (CAT) scan (c) is helpful in preoperative planning. Note the marked subfibular impingement and the widening and shortened height of the calcaneus.*

may be anticipated, the scan is helpful in planning the correction, particularly if an osteotomy of the calcaneus needs to be performed in conjunction with the realignment subtalar arthrodesis. These scans are performed particularly when the tuberosity of the calcaneus has slid up against the fibula and the heel remains in varus. For these patients a bone block procedure can be performed, but through the original plane of the old fracture. This procedure is more common in patients who have not been treated operatively because of a severe malunion of the calcaneal tuberosity.

If hardware is present, it must be taken into consideration because the operation may have to be staged. If the

hardware can be removed percutaneously, then a bone block procedure can still be performed. A transverse incision in the plane of the hindfoot cannot be made when lengthening of the height of the hindfoot is performed, and for this reason, if a plate is present, it may need to be removed through the posterior incision in conjunction with percutaneous stab incisions directly over the screws. This would be my preferred approach rather than staging the operation. The combination of an osteotomy of the calcaneus and a subtalar arthrodesis can be performed either through a vertical incision posteriorly, as for a subtalar bone block arthrodesis, or through a more standard incision following the peroneal tendons (Figs. 13–3–12 and 13–3–13).

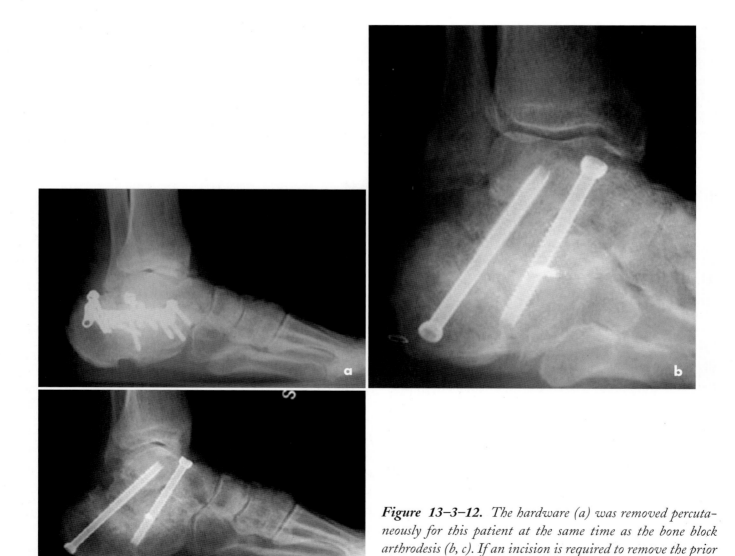

Figure 13–3–12. The hardware (a) was removed percutaneously for this patient at the same time as the bone block arthrodesis (b, c). If an incision is required to remove the prior hardware, then the operation should be staged to avoid wound dehiscence.

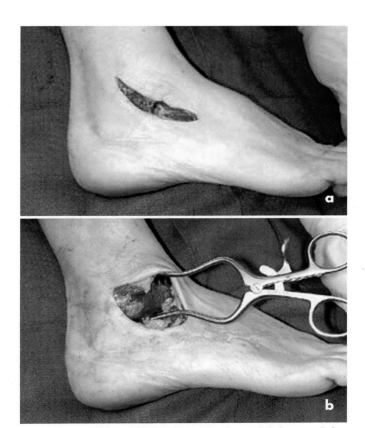

Figure 13–3–13. After open reduction with internal fixation (ORIF) of a calcaneus fracture, arthritis was present, and a sinus tarsi incision was used to perform the subtalar arthrodesis. Note the original incision and the excellent exposure of the subtalar joint with this approach (a, b).

The latter incision is much easier to use because visualization of the plane of the osteotomy from the site of the calcaneus is complete. If a bone block procedure is performed in addition to the osteotomy, as illustrated in the following case, the osteotomy can still be performed with a large osteotome inserted in the plane of the fracture. Regardless of the type of incision used, the osteotome must be inserted fluoroscopically. After removal of the overhanging bone, which is lying underneath the fibula, a guide pin is inserted in the plane of the deformity. This is usually from dorsolateral to plantar and medial at approximately an angle of 30 degrees. The guide pin is inserted and then the position checked with an axial view of the hindfoot fluoroscopically.

Minor adjustments are made to the guide pin until the pin is exactly in the plane of the original fracture and then the osteotomy performed. I use a large broad

osteotome to initiate the osteotomy, and the guide pin is then removed. The progress of the osteotomy should be checked fluoroscopically also with an axial image of the calcaneus. Cracking the osteotomy open on the inferior medial aspect of the calcaneus at the completion of the osteotomy is easier than perforating through with the osteotome; this perforation risks injury to the medial soft tissues. Once the osteotomy is complete, the tuberosity now needs to be levered down inferiorly back into its corrected position. Usually the tuberosity has to be distracted distally and then pulled into valgus. The tuberosity is freed up with an osteotome, and then I insert a lamina spreader into the osteotomy site to open it up completely. The osteotome is then levered laterally into the osteotomy site, and then the tuberosity is forced down inferiorly. With this method the tuberosity tends to be pushed into more varus, so guide pins are usually necessary to control the position of the calcaneus as it is being pulled into valgus while it resumes a more normal height. Multiple guide pins are inserted into the tuberosity to maintain this position. At times, the use of adjunctive bone graft is not necessary because of the plane of the osteotomy, which is in a sense sliding the calcaneus distally and into valgus simultaneously. This procedure is always performed, however, in conjunction with the subtalar arthrodesis, which can be done either as an in situ procedure or as a bone block procedure, depending on the extent of the subtalar collapse. If a bone graft procedure is being performed, the trick is to insert the graft and not lose the reduction of the calcaneal osteotomy. For this reason, I use multiple guide pins in the tuberosity extending up into various parts of the calcaneus and the more anterior portion of the talar neck and head, and then I insert a lamina spreader into the subtalar joint while the guide pins are maintaining the reduction. The graft is inserted in much the same way as that described for the subtalar distraction bone block arthrodesis, and then some of the guide pins can be realigned to cross through the osteotomy site and the subtalar joint simultaneously (Fig. 13–3–14).

Sometimes the deformity is severe, and in addition to a standard bone block of the subtalar joint, lengthening of the lateral column needs to be performed simultaneously with a second bone block to correct crushing of the calcaneocuboid joint. In Fig. 13–3–15, a double bone block was performed. The biggest problem with these procedures is planning the incision. This is the one time where

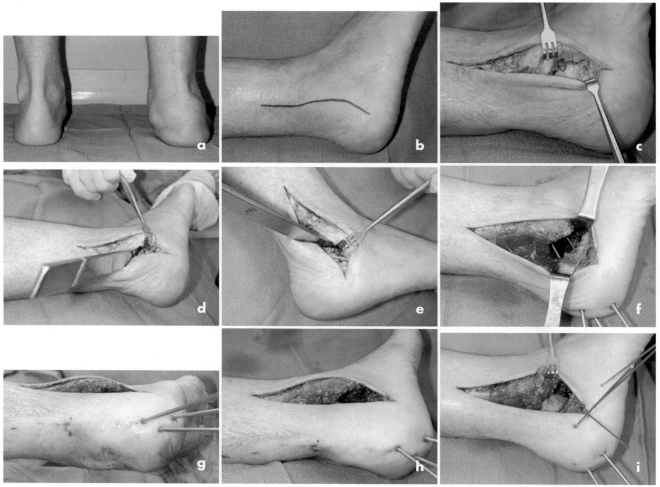

Figure 13–3–14. *This patient had severe hindfoot malunion after a nonsurgically treated calcaneus fracture. Note the widening and valgus of the heel (a). For correction of the hindfoot collapse, a bone block arthrodesis was planned, but a calcaneus osteotomy through the original fracture plane was performed to correct the valgus collapse of the heel (b, c). An osteotome was inserted under fluoroscopy into the calcaneus in the plane of the original fracture line (d, e), and the calcaneal tuberosity was levered inferiorly and medially with the osteotome and a laminar spreader and then held in place with multiple guide pins and K-wires (f–h). Once the position and reduction were verified, a structural bone graft was inserted into the subtalar joint (i).*

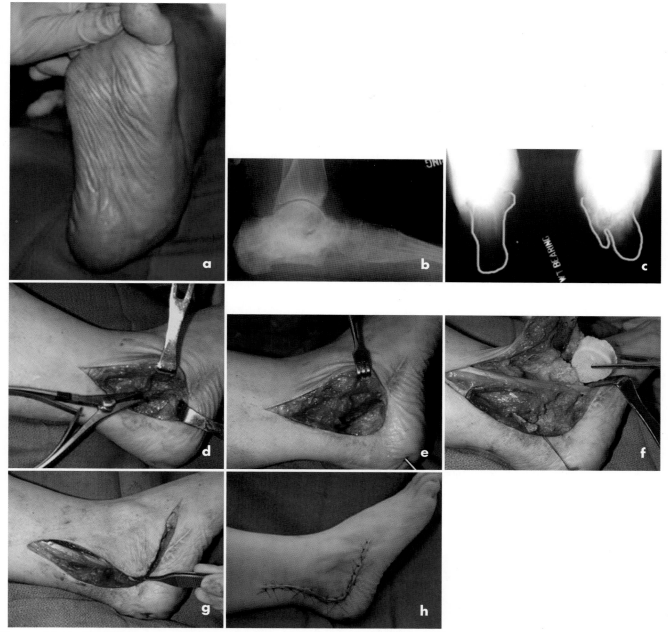

Figure 13–3–15. *With severe hindfoot valgus associated with abduction of the transverse tarsal joint, a double osteotomy/arthrodesis was performed for this patient. Note the hindfoot valgus (a) and the collapse on x-ray (XR) film and computerized axial tomography (CAT) scan (b, c). Although a strictly vertical incision would have been preferable, a curved incision was used to approach the calcaneus, the dislocated peroneal tendons, and the hindfoot valgus. A calcaneus osteotomy in the plane of the original fracture was performed, and the subtalar joint was distracted (d), followed by reduction with slight medial translation of the tuberosity (e). Once this was secured, a second structural graft was inserted into the calcaneocuboid joint. Note the dislocation of the peroneal tendon. The suture under the fibula is attached to half of the peroneus brevis tendon, which was used to perform a modified Chrisman-Snook procedure to correct the dislocated peroneal tendons (f). As anticipated, using an incision like this with distraction is associated with tension; however, this incision closed uneventfully (g, h).*

an extensile incision can be used, but the elasticity and the tension of the skin must be tested during the operation to avoid excessive tension with skin closure.

Techniques, tips, and pitfalls

1. Sometimes the calcaneal tuberosity is markedly displaced proximally and lies at the level of the talus (Fig. 13–3–16). Correction of this type of deformity requires an open lengthening of the Achilles tendon, and the tuberosity has to be levered down inferiorly before the bone block graft can be inserted.

2. A bone block graft does not always need to be performed in the setting of a decrease in the talar declination angle. If no anterior ankle pain is present and the pain is limited to the subtalar joint, then an in situ arthrodesis can be considered. This is particularly the case when a nonunion is present, in addition to the collapse of the height. In these patients, correction of the nonunion takes precedence over restoring height of the hindfoot (Fig. 13–3–17).

3. I prefer to use a short sinus tarsi incision rather than the original incision used for ORIF of the fracture. Elevation of the flap, which is thick-ened and scarred, is difficult. Exposure of the joint with the original incision is also difficult.

4. Removal of hardware is not necessary before arthrodesis. If a lateral wall ostectomy must be performed, then the hardware can be removed percutaneously. This applies in particular to a bone block distraction, in which the incision cannot be made along the length of the calcaneus to remove hardware.

5. Obtaining arthrodesis in this group of patients is not predictable. Bone sclerosis; segments of avascular bone; and other factors, including the skin, mitigate against a successful fusion. These patients should stop smoking before undergoing arthrodesis.

6. Arthrodesis should be performed as soon as possible if the patient has symptoms. Many of these individuals are construction workers, and the longer they do not return to work with post-traumatic arthritis, the less likely it is that they will ever return to an active lifestyle. I have not found that these patients improve substantially after 9 months following calcaneus fracture.

7. If a symptomatic tarsal tunnel syndrome is present, then the subtalar fusion should be performed first and the tarsal tunnel release staged to facilitate rehabilitation after the nerve operation.

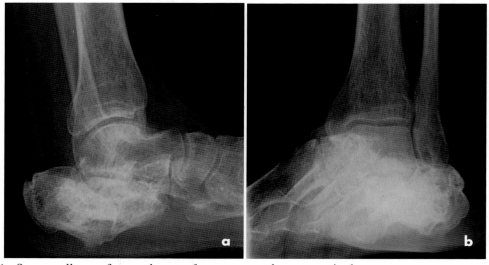

Figure 13–3–16. *Severe collapse after a calcaneus fracture treated nonoperatively was present in this patient with marked anterior ankle pain, limited push-off strength, and subtalar arthritis. Note the marked valgus deformity of the hindfoot with subfibular impingement (a, b).*

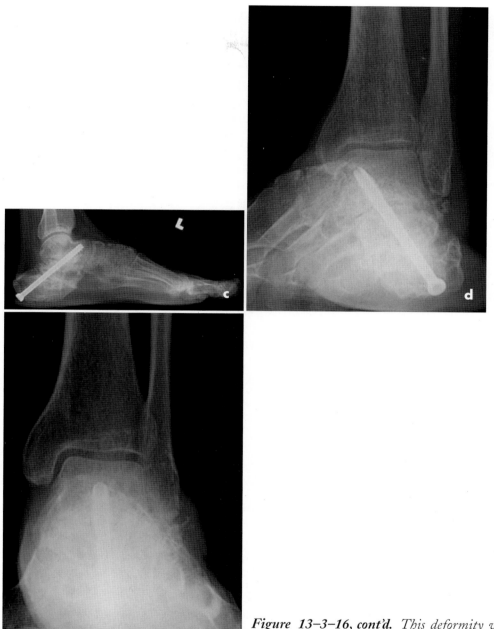

Figure 13–3–16, cont'd. *This deformity was corrected with a subtalar distraction bone block arthrodesis with structural allograft, with good realignment of the hindfoot and ankle (c–e).*

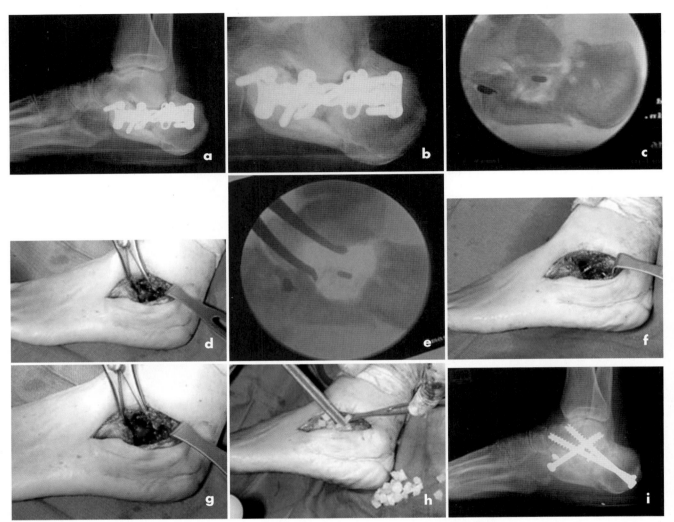

Figure 13–3–17. *This patient had a severe malunion and nonunion of a calcaneus fracture after attempted open reduction with internal fixation (ORIF). Note the position of the tuberosity, the incorrect position of the plate, and the failure of the plate to hold the fracture aligned. Despite the marked change in the talar declination, no anterior ankle pain was present, and a bone block graft was not performed (a, b). The nonunion was corrected through a short sinus tarsi incision, followed by realignment with joint distraction and use of cancellous allograft chips to fill the defect (c–h). During insertion of the laminar spreader, the skin should be checked to be sure it can be closed without any tension.*

Suggested Readings

Buch BD, Myerson MS, Miller SD. Primary subtalar arthrodesis for the treatment of comminuted calcaneal fractures. Foot Ankle Int 17:61–70, 1996.

Easley ME, Trnka HJ, Schon LC, Myerson MS. Isolated subtalar arthrodesis. J Bone Joint Surg Am 82:613–624, 2000.

Myerson MS. Fractures and dislocations of the calcaneus. In Helal B, Rowley DI, Cracchiolo A, III,

Myerson MS (eds): The Foot and Ankle. London, Martin Dunitz, 1996.

Myerson MS. Primary subtalar arthrodesis for the treatment of comminuted fractures of the calcaneus. Orthop Clin North Am 26:215–227, 1995.

Myerson M, Multhopp-Stephens H. Fractures of the calcaneus. In Myerson M (ed): Current Therapy in Foot and Ankle Surgery. St Louis, Mosby-Year Book, 1993, pp 249–257.

Myerson M, Quill GE, Jr. Late complications of fractures of the calcaneus. J Bone Joint Surg 75A:331–341, 1993.

Stamatis E, Myerson MS. Percutaneous removal of hardware following open reduction and internal fixation of calcaneus fractures. Orthopedics 25:1025–1028, 2002.

Trnka HJ, Easley ME, Lam PW, et al. Subtalar distraction bone block arthrodesis. J Bone Joint Surg Br 83:849–854, 2001.

Trnka HJ, Myerson MS, Easley ME. Preliminary results of isolated subtalar arthrodesis: Factors leading to failure. Foot Ankle Int 20:678–678, 1999.

Triple Arthrodesis

Overview and Approach

The triple arthrodesis is a reliable procedure for correction of hindfoot deformity and arthritis. In a series of 183 triple arthrodesis procedures, I reported on 152 patients who were examined with rigid screw fixation and a mean follow-up of 5.7 years after the arthrodesis. Three nonunions occurred, and the prevalence of ankle arthritis, the cause of which is discussed later, was fairly high. A triple arthrodesis is performed if a simpler hindfoot arthrodesis will not be sufficient. Indications for triple arthrodesis include a severe flexible flatfoot deformity, a rigid flatfoot deformity, post-traumatic arthritis, severe tarsal coalition associated with arthritis or uncorrectable deformity of the subtalar and transverse tarsal joint, congenital and neuromuscular deformity, and inflammatory arthritis. I try not to overuse the triple arthrodesis in the setting of the flexible flatfoot because osteotomy combined with tendon transfer is usually sufficient for correction of deformity and maintains joint motion. Generally, post-traumatic arthritis follows a talus or calcaneus fracture, but for most of these patients with this arthritis, a subtalar arthrodesis is the procedure of choice, not a triple arthrodesis. A triple arthrodesis is usually the preferred procedure after a talar neck fracture with malunion and involvement of both the talonavicular (TN) and subtalar joint. In the presence of a middle facet tarsal coalition, a subtalar arthrodesis is sufficient, and a triple arthrodesis is preferred only in the setting of arthritis or deformity that is typically associated with a naviculocuneiform coalition. For patients with inflammatory arthritis, be careful in selecting an isolated TN fusion, even when this is the only involved hindfoot joint. Isolated TN arthrodesis has a higher incidence of nonunion, and once this occurs, correction is far more difficult because of bone loss and erosion, even with a triple arthrodesis. For this reason, I rarely perform an isolated TN arthrodesis for correction of rheumatoid arthritis.

The Lateral Incision

The incision is made from the tip of the fibular extending distally down over the sinus tarsi toward the calcaneocuboid (CC) joint (Fig. 13–4–1). On the inferior surface of the incision the peroneal tendon sheath is identified, and the terminal branch of the sural nerve must be looked for more distally in the incision. Both the peroneal tendons and sural nerve are retracted inferiorly, and the incision can be deepened down on the periosteum directly over the calcaneus. The incision is extended distally toward the CC joint and then further toward the base of the fourth metatarsal. In the terminal aspect of the incision, care must be taken to ensure that no branches of either the sural or lateral cutaneous branch of the superficial peroneal nerve are present. The retinaculum of the undersurface of the peroneal tendon sheath is stripped and elevated off the lateral wall of the calcaneus. I prefer to save the contents of the sinus tarsi because in the event of a wound dehiscence, sufficient

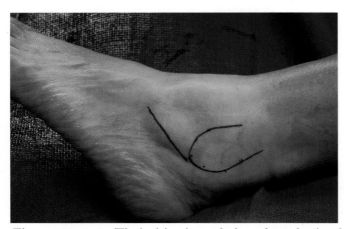

Figure 13–4–1. *The incision is marked out from the tip of the fibula across the sinus tarsi.*

tissue is always covering the peroneal tendons. The soft tissues are elevated sharply off the floor of the sinus tarsi until the anterior aspect of the posterior facet of the sub-talar joint is visualized.

Calcaneocuboid Joint Preparation

The incision is deepened directly onto the periosteum along the CC joint, and a large periosteal elevator is used to strip the lateral aspect of the calcaneus and then the cuboid. The peroneal retinaculum is retracted inferiorly, and a knife blade is inserted directly into the CC joint and then manipulated dorsally to cut the cervical ligament. The knife blade is swept vertically through the CC joint, and then it is rotated dorsally across the bifurcate ligament and directly into the posterior facet with one maneuver. The cuboid bone should now be freely mobile, and the articular surface of the entire joint is denuded with a 2-cm flexible chisel, as well as with a rongeur and curette. Removal of more than 2 mm of bone and cartilage on either side of the joint is unnecessary. Remember that regardless of the type of deformity, a lateral bone wedge is not removed, and the position of the hindfoot is corrected with translation and rotation, not with resection of bone wedges. A smooth laminar spreader is inserted into the CC articulation to ensure that all the cartilage has been removed. Care must be taken to ensure that a minimal amount of bone is resected to minimize any shortening of the lateral column.

Subtalar Joint Preparation

A toothed laminar spreader is inserted into the sinus tarsi, and when it is placed on stretch, the interosseous ligament is easily visualized and cut to gain access to the posterior aspect of the subtalar joint and the middle facet. A 1-cm flexible chisel is used to denude the articular surface of the posterior facet. As with the CC joint, minimal bone is removed. The posterior facet must be debrided down to bleeding healthy subchondral bone (Fig. 13–4–2). Be careful in the posteromedial corner of the joint, where the flexor hallucis longus tendon is at risk for injury from the chisel. Finally, the more medial aspect of the subtalar joint and the middle facet must be completely denuded, including the undersurface of the talus and the dorsal surface of the middle facet. Before the medial incision is made, the space between the navicular and the cuboid is debrided with a rongeur. This debridement adds another segment and bone surface to the fusion mass and makes the triple arthrodesis a "quadruple arthrodesis" (Fig. 13–4–3).

Talonavicular Joint Preparation

The TN joint is clearly the most difficult of the three joints to visualize and to debride adequately. For either a varus or valgus deformity, the TN joint is only partly visible, but it must be distracted to visualize the entire joint (Fig. 13–4–4). Do not be tempted to approach the TN joint from the lateral incision. Visualizing only one third of the joint laterally, perhaps more, is possible if the hindfoot is fixed in varus. However, the TN joint is the one joint that will end up in nonunion if the joint debridement is not performed carefully. The only time I use a single incision for a hindfoot fusion is to revise a malunion of a triple arthrodesis. This procedure is discussed later. The medial incision is made immediately adjacent (medial) to the anterior tibial tendon, extending from the ankle toward the medial cuneiform bone. The extensor retinaculum is incised, and the anterior tibial tendon is retracted laterally, exposing the deep subcutaneous tissue. Partially cutting into the extensor retinaculum and the medial edge of the anterior tibial tendon more distally may be necessary at times because the tendon blends into the fibers of the retinaculum.

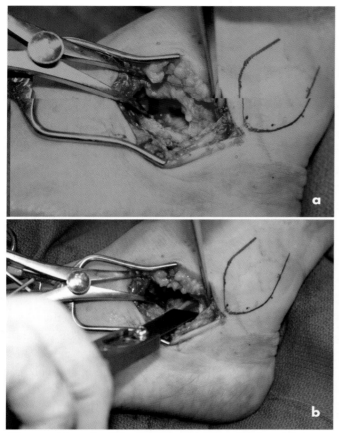

Figure 13–4–2. *The subtalar joint is visible with insertion of a laminar spreader, which pushes the joint anteriorly (a), and debridement is performed with a flexible chisel (b). Note the protection of the peroneal tendons with a curved retractor behind the subtalar joint.*

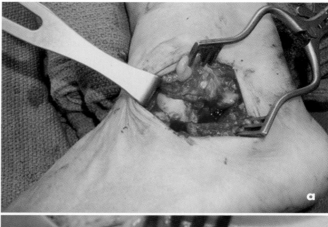

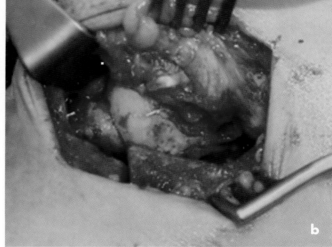

Figure 13–4–3. *The local anatomy of the junction between the talus, navicular, cuboid, and calcaneus is presented (a, b). It is the junction of these four bones and is referred to as the fourth joint, hence a quadruple arthrodesis.*

After the dissection a retractor is inserted to retract the anterior tibial tendon and the medial soft tissues. The periosteum along the navicular bone is stripped, and then the TN joint is fully exposed with a curved periosteal elevator. Inserting an elevator directly into the joint to fully expose the head of the talus and then to strip further the soft tissue dorsally and laterally is useful. When a severe valgus deformity is corrected, pushing the midfoot into varus and then loosening the tension of the medial TN joint are helpful. I then cut around the medial joint from the outside in, through the remnant of the posterior tibial tendon and spring ligament into the TN joint. This makes opening and distraction of the joint far easier. A smooth laminar spreader or rongeur is inserted into the joint and then interchanged with a toothed laminar spreader to facili-

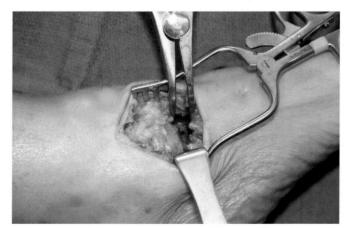

Figure 13–4–4. *Exposure of the talonavicular joint (TN) is facilitated with a laminar spreader followed by joint debridement with a flexible chisel.*

tate distraction of the joint. The entire joint is denuded of cartilage with a 1-cm flexible chisel. Be careful of the navicular because this bone can be hard and can fragment if not debrided gently. If the bone is sclerotic, then a 4-mm burr may be better than a chisel to debride the navicular bone because the contour of the bone must be maintained. The same contour must be maintained with debridement of the talar head while a small flexible chisel is used. Be careful if osteopenia is present because the lamina spreader may crush into the talus. At the completion of the joint debridement, it should appose well, maintaining the overall joint contour. If excessive bone is resected, the medial column of the foot will be shortened, followed by a varus malunion.

Reduction of Deformity and Screw Fixation

The reduction maneuver of the hindfoot relative to the forefoot is critical. I think that for most deformities, the hinge point is the TN joint and therefore this is the joint that I reduce and fix first. The foot is rotated around the axis of the TN joint, and as the forefoot is adducted, the first metatarsal is plantarflexed to correct the forefoot relative to the hindfoot (Fig. 13–4–5). This maneuver is only unsuccessful when the subtalar joint is rigid and the calcaneus is laterally translated, in which case I fix the subtalar joint first. If the latter is done, then the TN joint may not line up perfectly, although clinically the forefoot may seem to be corrected.

I use 6.5-mm cannulated screws for the subtalar joint and 5-mm screws for the CC and TN joints. I generally begin with the TN joint fixation. Two guide pins are inserted into the TN joint: the first is inserted from the inferior medial tuberosity, and the second is inserted slightly more dorsally, immediately adjacent to the anterior tibial tendon. The head of the second more dorsal screw will be close to the naviculocuneiform joint. On the undersurface of the calcaneus, but off the weight-bearing surface of the heel, a guide pin for a 6.5-mm screw is inserted directly into the body of the talus.

The position of the guide pins is checked fluoroscopically, and the screws are inserted. Make sure that the heads of the screws are all well buried flush with the margin of the bone and are not protruding into the naviculocuneiform joint or the heel pad. The CC joint is fixed last, and the approach is from posterior to anterior.

For the insertion of the guide pin to be facilitated into the CC joint, the lateral aspect of the calcaneus is notched with a chisel 1 cm proximal to the articular surface (Fig. 13–4–6). This step is important in the fusion, and the lateral foot must be elevated across the CC joint. Although the TN and subtalar joints are already fixed, some lateral mobility will still be present, and if the cuboid bone drops down, weight bearing will be painful as a result of a malunion. Be sure therefore to elevate the inferior aspect of the cuboid and create a plantigrade lateral weight-bearing surface. The guide pin for a 5-mm screw is inserted across the notched surface into the CC joint, followed by a 35-mm screw. Two 5-mm screws were used for the TN joint and measured approximately 50 mm in length (Fig. 13–4–7).

Before completion, checking the stability of the ankle joint is helpful. Although not common, ankle instability, either to varus or valgus stress, leads to accelerated arthritis and should be stabilized intraoperatively. In Figure 13–4–8, gross instability was noted after screw fixation and was repaired with a modified Chrisman-Snook procedure.

Techniques, tips, and pitfalls

1. Two incisions should be used; they permit access to all of the bones of the hindfoot.
2. The concept of a triple arthrodesis is expanded to a quadruple arthrodesis to include the recess between the navicular and the cuboid.
3. Minimal bone should be resected, and under no circumstances should large wedges of bone be removed because removal will only add to shortening of the foot and possibly malunion.
4. Correction of deformity is obtained by translation and rotation and not by resection of wedges of bone.
5. Rigid internal fixation is preferable, and I have found that cannulated screws are more accurate to maintain reduction than staples or pins.
6. I have not found it necessary to use bone graft because of the good bleeding cancellous bone surfaces, which are always well apposed. Bone

Text continued on p. 427

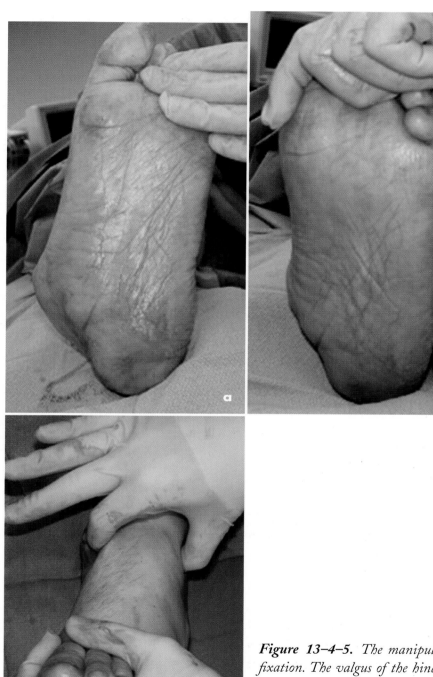

Figure 13–4–5. *The manipulation of the hindfoot is demonstrated before fixation. The valgus of the hindfoot is noted (a), and with manipulation of the hindfoot around the axis of the talonavicular (TN) joint, the heel assumes a neutral position (b). The forefoot is adducted and pronated around the TN joint while the index finger palpates the TN joint for reduction (c).*

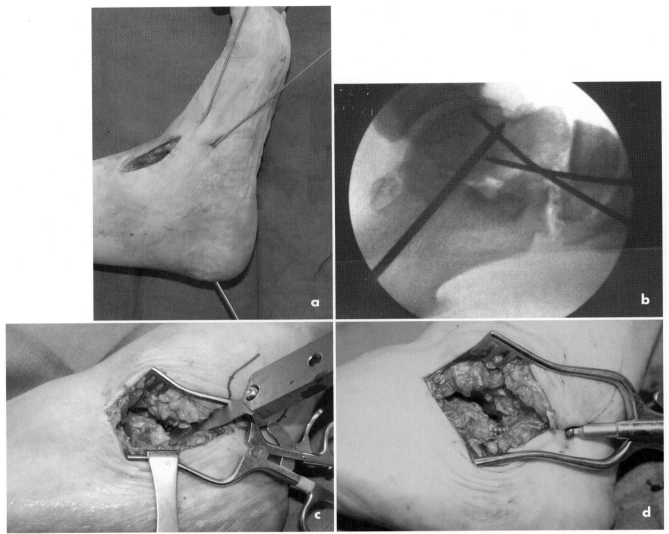

Figure 13–4–6. *The guide pins across the subtalar and talonavicular (TN) joints are noted (a, b). For a screw to be inserted across the calcaneocuboid (CC) joint without fracture, a notch is cut in the lateral calcaneus 1 cm proximal to the joint (c). The screw is inserted percutaneously into the notch that is created (d).*

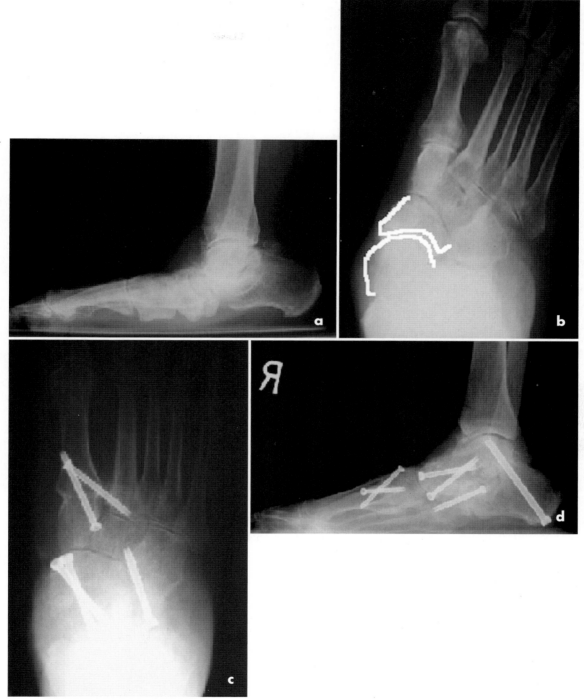

Figure 13–4–7. *Note the first tarsometatarsal instability on the preoperative lateral x-ray (XR) image (a). There is a gap on the plantar surface of the first tarsometatarsal (TMT) joint. Severe subluxation of the talonavicular (TN) joint with marked uncovering of the head of the talus is noted (b). This was corrected with a triple arthrodesis and an arthrodesis of the first TMT joint. This leaves an open naviculocuneiform joint, which will likely undergo increased stresses. Another option may be to perform an opening wedge osteotomy of the medial cuneiform. This procedure will correct the dorsiflexed first ray, but not the first TMT arthritis.*

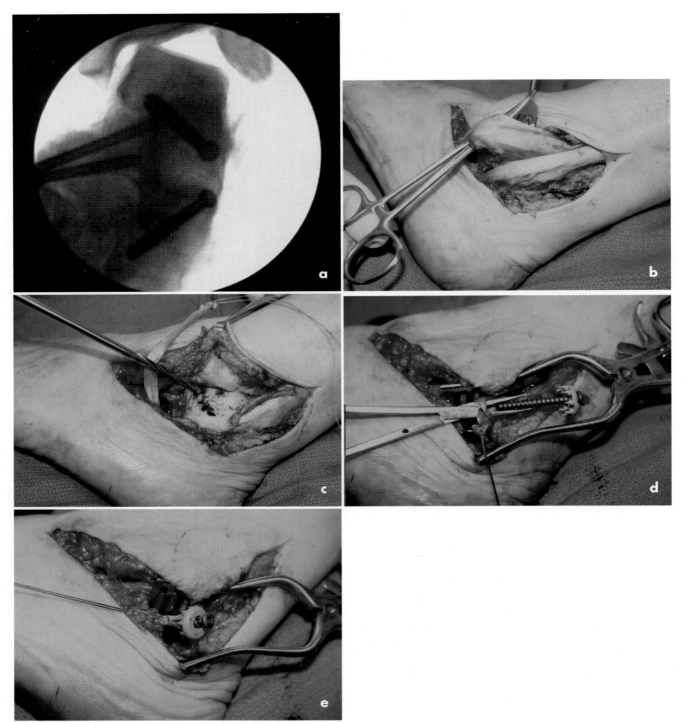

Figure 13–4–8. *After the screw fixation, gross instability on inversion stress was noted (a). The incision for the triple arthrodesis was extended proximally, and the peroneus brevis tendon was identified (b). The tendon was split, and a 4.5-mm drill hole was made in the fibula (c). The tendon was pulled through posteriorly, and a screw was pulled through the tendon over a spiked ligament washer (d) and then fixed into the calcaneus under tension (e).*

graft may be used in cases of severe deformity with a nonunion of a prior attempted triple arthrodesis where a void exists after the debridement and realignment. If one is concerned about a defect, then cancellous allograft chips may be used and impacted into the sinus tarsi. If I use allograft chips, I will mix the graft with the Symphony platelet system (DePuy, Warsaw, Ind.) for patients who are at higher risk for nonunion.

7. The reduction maneuver prior to insertion of the cannulated guide pins is important, and the hinge of the TN joint is the key to correct alignment. If a severe fixed valgus deformity of the subtalar joint is present, then I fix this joint first, followed by the TN joint, which then has to be more forcibly adducted and plantarflexed.

8. Severe abduction of the forefoot with marked subluxation of the TN joint may require a structural bone graft with lengthening of the CC joint for correction (Fig. 13–4–9).

9. Although isolated CC or TN arthrodesis may be sufficient to correct deformity or arthritis of that joint, correction of a hindfoot deformity is rarely sufficient, and a triple arthrodesis is preferred (Fig. 13–4–10).

10. After the screw fixation, check the ankle dorsiflexion and perform a gastrocnemius muscle recession or lengthening of the Achilles tendon as required (Fig. 13–4–11).

The Medial Approach to Triple Arthrodesis

For correction of severe fixed valgus deformity, particularly in the setting of rheumatoid arthritis, I use a single medial incision to perform the triple arthrodesis. Any incision on the lateral foot in the setting of severe rigid hindfoot valgus is at jeopardy for dehiscence. The approach to triple arthrodesis with a medial incision is performed through an extensile incision that begins at the naviculocuneiform joint and then extends proximally behind the medial malleolus. The incision must be dorsal to the neurovascular bundle at all times. Imagine using a portion of this incision for excision of a middle facet

tarsal coalition and then extending it proximally and distally. The plane of the dissection runs between the flexor hallucis longus and the flexor digitorum longus tendons.

Pulling the flexor hallucis longus tendon inferiorly protects the neurovascular bundle during the dissection. Starting at the TN joint is the easiest way to identify the joints. Because of the severe abduction that is present across the TN joint, the head of the talus is always easily visible. The dissection is then deepened down onto the head of the talus, and then the middle facet can be identified with the working under the head of the talus. Once the middle facet is visualized between the talar head and the anterior aspect of the calcaneus, it should be opened with a curved osteotome. With the curved osteotome in place, the opening of the anterior aspect of the subtalar joint is then facilitated with insertion of a lamina spreader. The posterior facet is now denuded of the articular cartilage with a flexible chisel, followed by exposure of the TN joint. Stripping of the entire dorsomedial aspect of the joint is necessary.

By this time, the lamina spreader can be inserted into the TN joint followed by debridement as needed. Removal of a wedge from the head of the talus is sometimes necessary to adduct the foot around the transverse tarsal joint. An osteotome is used to cut all the way across into the CC joint, which can be verified fluoroscopically. A guide pin can be inserted across from the head of the talus into the CC joint to verify the position of the joint before cutting it with the osteotome. Realigning the subtalar joint is fairly easy also with the removal of slightly more bone on the medial side with the joint debridement. I correct the deformity by first bringing the heel into neutral and then fixing this with a cannulated guide pin. The midfoot is then passively pronated, adducted, and then plantarflexed across the transverse tarsal joint, and the TN joint is then fixed. Extending the fixation across into the naviculocuneiform joint is also sometimes necessary because not much navicular bone is present to facilitate fixation itself (Fig. 13–4–12).

Triple Arthrodesis and Medial Ankle Instability

The approach to triple arthrodesis with an unstable medial ankle has to be performed cautiously. This is usually in the setting of a flatfoot deformity associated

Text continued on p. 432

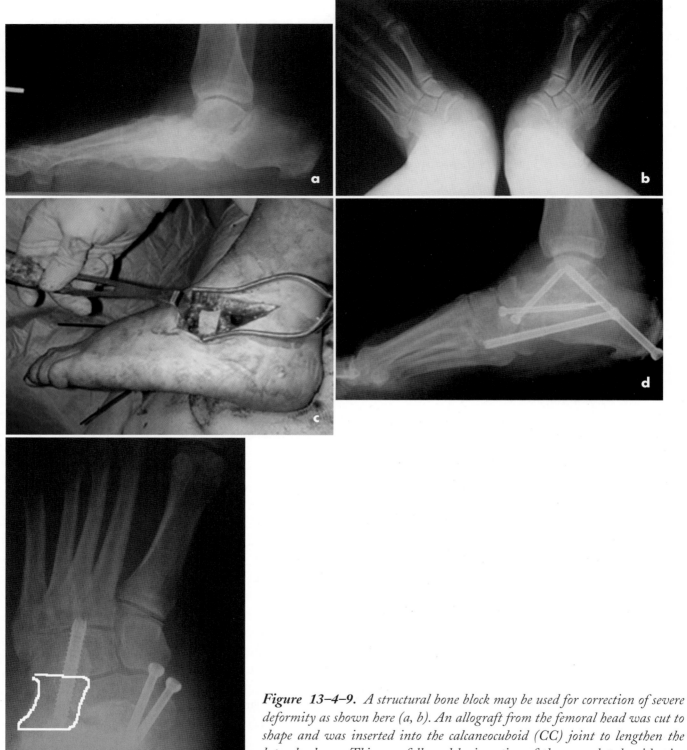

Figure 13–4–9. *A structural bone block may be used for correction of severe deformity as shown here (a, b). An allograft from the femoral head was cut to shape and was inserted into the calcaneocuboid (CC) joint to lengthen the lateral column. This was followed by insertion of the cannulated guide pins (c). The postoperative appearance is noted (d, e), with the bone block graft outlined on the anteroposterior (AP) view.*

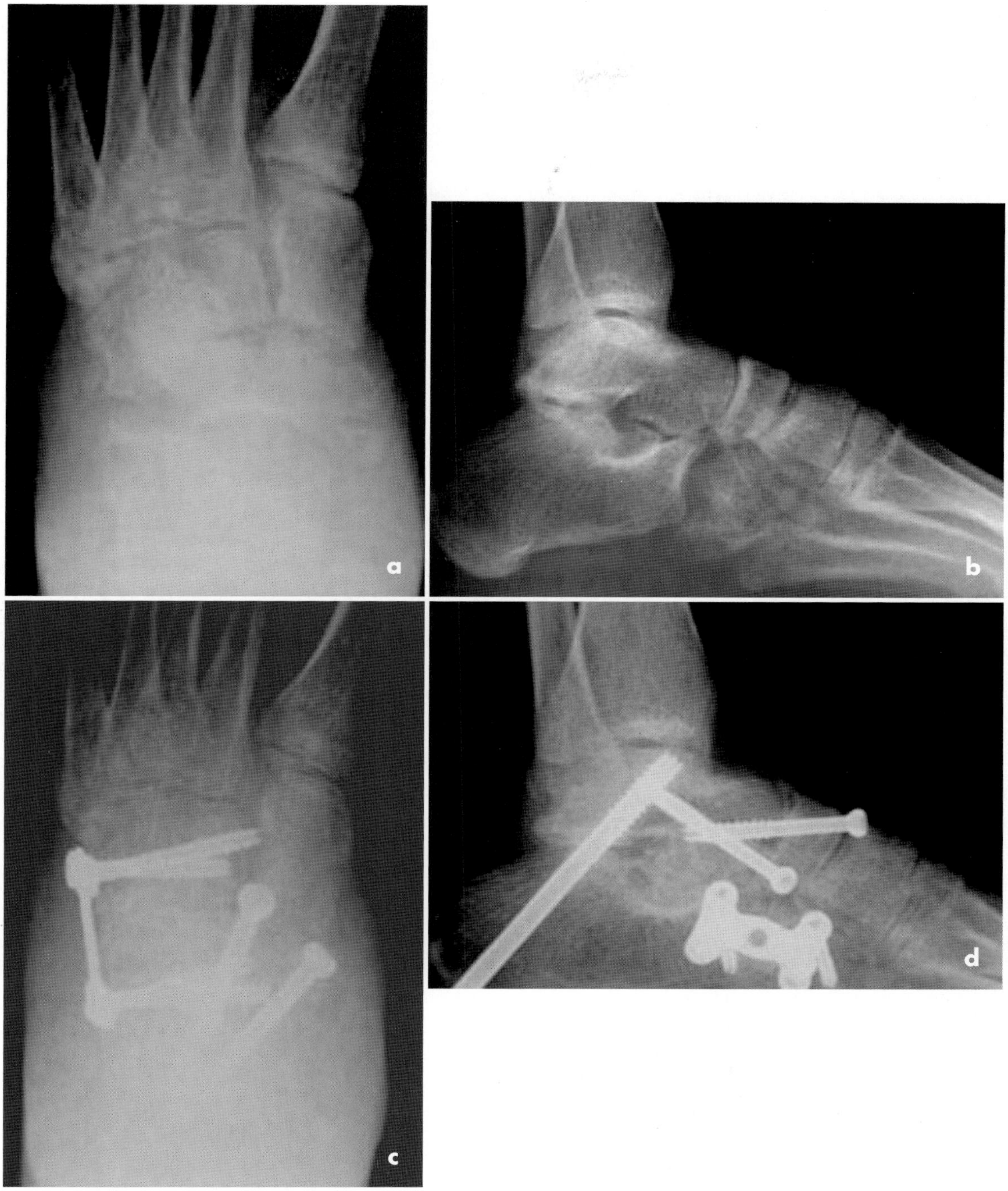

Figure 13–4–10. *The preoperative (a, b) x-ray (XR) images show severe hindfoot deformity after a crush injury of the cuboid bone, associated with bone loss and a cavovarus position of the hindfoot. Although the disease was located laterally in the calcaneocuboid (CC) joint, correction of the deformity without a triple arthrodesis was not considered possible. For correction of the deformity, a structural bone block graft was inserted into the CC joint to lengthen the lateral column as part of the arthrodesis (c, d).*

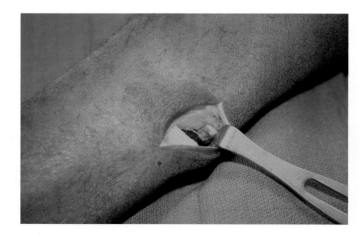

Figure 13–4–11. *A gastrocnemius muscle recession was performed in this patient after the triple arthrodesis. An incision is made laterally, and the sural nerve is identified and retracted. The fascia is cut transversely with a knife, and the muscle belly is noted below.*

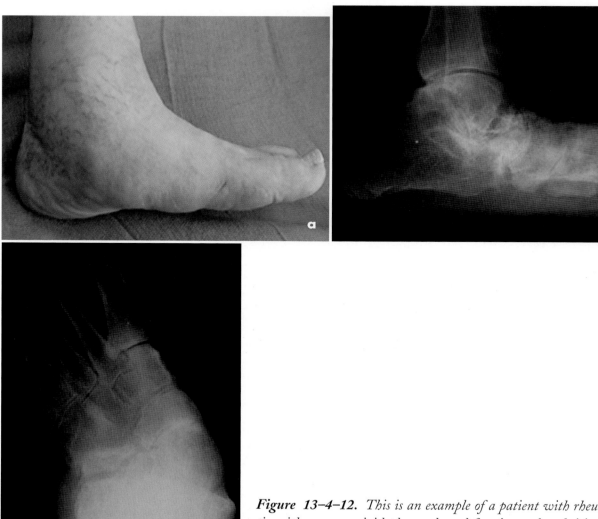

Figure 13–4–12. *This is an example of a patient with rheumatoid arthritis with a severe rigid planovalgus deformity and arthritis of the hindfoot (a–c).*

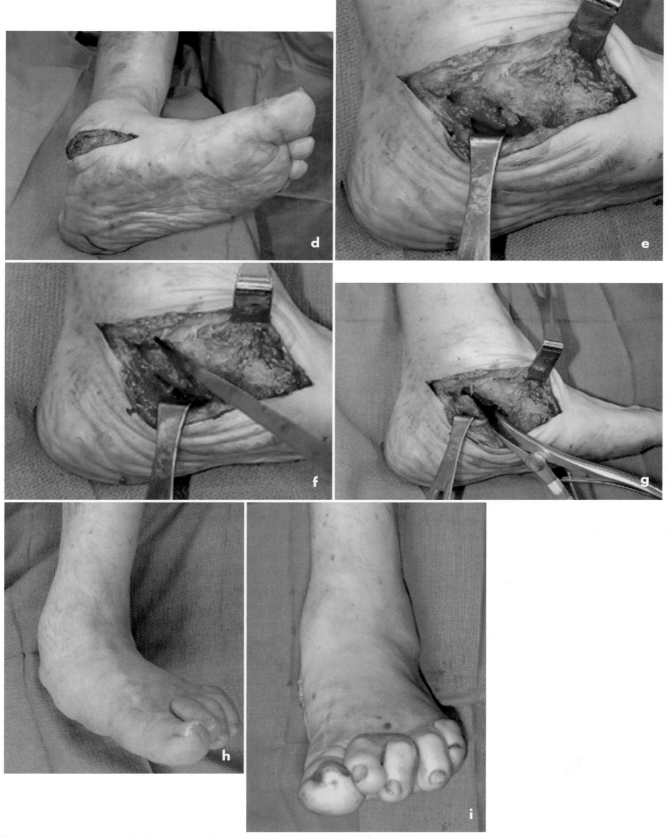

Figure 13–4–12, cont'd. *Note that this is an extensile approach (d) and that the neurovascular bundle is retracted inferiorly with the flexor hallucis longus tendon (e). This is followed by the opening of the subtalar joint with the osteotome (f) and insertion of a laminar spreader to visualize the entire subtalar joint (g). The preoperative and immediate postoperative clinical appearance is noted (h, i).*

with a rupture of the deltoid ligament. A number of alternatives for correction of this deformity are available, including a triple arthrodesis with reconstruction of the deltoid ligament, a triple arthrodesis followed by an ankle replacement, and a pantalar arthrodesis. With each of these procedures, medialization of the calcaneus is important to balance the weight-bearing forces under the ankle more effectively. With a medial shift of the calcaneus, the occurrence of an increased load on the medial ankle takes stress off the deltoid ligament reconstruction. For a more extensive discussion of the correction of the deltoid rupture, see the chapter on correction of flatfoot deformity (Ch. 7–2). A simple repair of the deltoid ligament has not seemed to be adequate, and some sort of reconstruction must be performed. More importantly, a triple arthrodesis cannot be performed without some sort of reconstruction of the deltoid ligament. The technique that is described in the chapter on flatfoot deformity includes a hamstring allograft reconstruction of the deltoid ligament (Fig. 13–4–13).

Laterally, the incision needs to be modified for the triple arthrodesis when a calcaneal osteotomy is performed simultaneously. I prefer to use two separate incisions. The first is for the calcaneal osteotomy, and the second is a slightly shorter incision in the sinus tarsi but is slightly more dorsal than one would normally make. The calcaneal osteotomy is performed first, and the calcaneus is shifted medially by 10 mm. The guide pin for fixation of the calcaneal osteotomy is then inserted through the tuberosity and into the body of the calcaneus. The same guide pin, however, will be used to insert across the subtalar joint once the subtalar joint has been debrided so that one screw is used that will incorporate both the calcaneal osteotomy and a fixation for the subtalar arthrodesis (Fig. 13–4–14).

Because of the medialization of the calcaneus from the osteotomy, the screw needs to be inserted slightly more laterally on the undersurface of the posterior heel so that the screw enters the body of the talus correctly. I have not encountered skin-healing problems with these two incisions laterally. If for any reason the use of these two incisions causes concern, then certainly one more extensile incision can be used directed posteriorly underneath the peroneal tendons. My only concern with this approach is the stretch on the skin as the calcaneus is shifted medially. When I use two incisions, the poste-rior incision for the calcaneal osteotomy is slightly more posterior and vertical so that little stress is placed on this incision with medialization of the calcaneus (Fig. 13–4–15).

Revision Triple Arthrodesis

The foot must be inspected immediately before the start of the revision triple arthrodesis and must be carefully examined in the weight-bearing position to determine the exact location of the apex of the deformity. The position of the calcaneus (neutral, varus, or valgus) and the location of pressure anywhere along the lateral plantar surface of the foot must be examined. The location of the apex (or apices) of the deformity must be determined. Once this is done, the revision can be planned. As a generalization, for correction of a varus deformity, the incisions are made laterally, and for revision of a valgus deformity, the primary incision is medial.

An example of a revision is a varus malunion of a previous triple arthrodesis. The use of any of the original incisions is unnecessary and often not advantageous because placement of the incision is critical to gain maximum access for correction. These incisions must be extensile and will often cross the original incision. Remember that the incision is on the side of the apex of the deformity so that with resection of a wedge of bone from that side, the chance of skin-healing problems is less likely. The incision is deepened, creating large thick skin flaps, with elevation of the entire dorsal, lateral, and plantar tissues off the hindfoot.

Malunion seems to occur as a result of inappropriate positioning of the foot intraoperatively with fixation. This does not occur in the postoperative period as a result of inappropriate casting. Varus or valgus malunion seems to occur with increased frequency when the TN joint is not lined up correctly. Further problems can occur when wedges of bone are resected from either the medial or lateral transverse tarsal joint (Fig. 13–4–16).

Correction of malunion is actually far easier than correction of a nonunion after a triple arthrodesis. After a nonunion, avascular bone loss is frequent, and with the loosening of fixation, the ability to secure the arthrodesis the second time around is far less. These problems

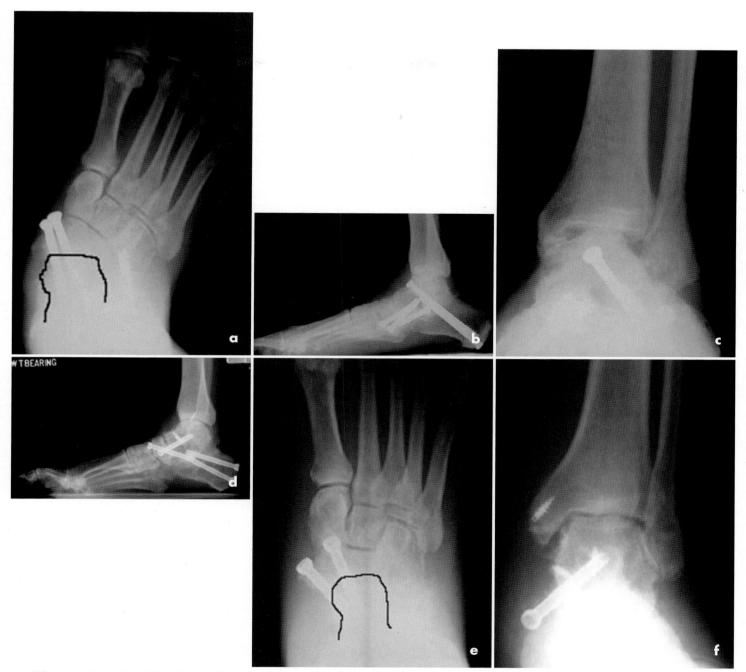

Figure 13–4–13. *After this triple arthrodesis, severe abduction of the foot persisted (a) despite reasonable alignment on the lateral radiograph (b). The major problem, however, was the marked valgus deformity of the tibiotalar joint with associated arthritis (c). This was corrected with a transverse tarsal medial wedge rotational osteotomy with a medial incision and with reconstruction of the deltoid ligament with a hamstring allograft attached to the talus, medial malleolus, and calcaneus with bone suture anchors (d, e, f).*

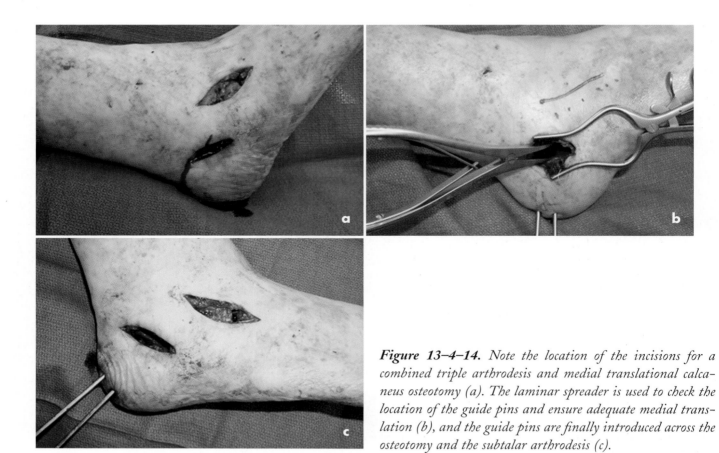

Figure 13–4–14. *Note the location of the incisions for a combined triple arthrodesis and medial translational calcaneus osteotomy (a). The laminar spreader is used to check the location of the guide pins and ensure adequate medial translation (b), and the guide pins are finally introduced across the osteotomy and the subtalar arthrodesis (c).*

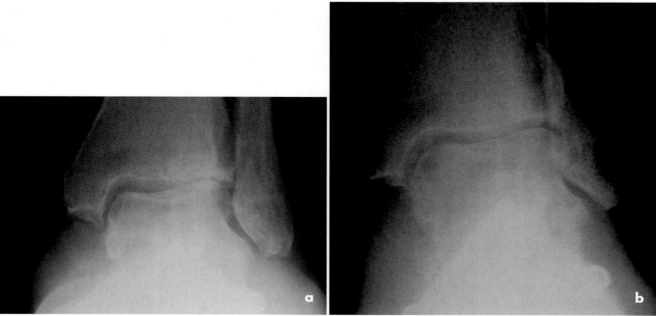

Figure 13–4–15. *Note the valgus tilting of the tibiotalar joint on the preoperative anteroposterior (AP) ankle view (a). This was associated with a severe flatfoot deformity and rupture of the deltoid ligament. The triple arthrodesis was combined with a medial translational osteotomy of the calcaneus and a deltoid ligament reconstruction. Note the postoperative AP ankle with good correction of the tibiotalar alignment (b).*

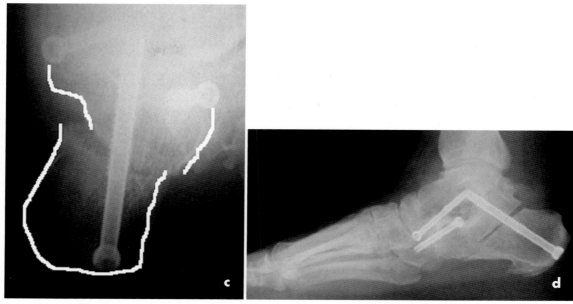

Figure 13–4–15, cont'd. *And the medial translation of the calcaneus on the axial and lateral views (c, d).*

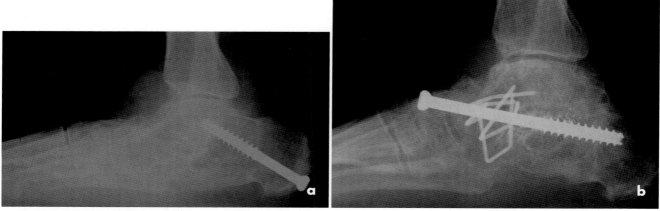

Figure 13–4–16. *Valgus malunion after this unsuccessful triple arthrodesis was corrected with a medial translational osteotomy of the calcaneus, and a transverse tarsal osteotomy with a medial closing wedge from a medial incision (a, b).*

do not occur, however, with a varus or valgus malunion when arthrodesis is present. However, the problem with correction of malunion is the inevitable slight shortening of the foot that occurs.

The size of the wedge of bone that is resected depends entirely on the location of the apex of the deformity. For example, if the apex of the deformity is at the base of the fifth metatarsal and the calcaneus is in slight valgus, then no wedge needs to be resected. For this deformity, an osteotomy can be made directly across the transverse

tarsal joint, and the entire midfoot can be rotated around the osteotomy without resection of the wedge. If, however, the apex of the deformity is at the level of the cuboid bone or the CC joint, then a wedge of bone usually needs to be resected. Therefore a varus malunion and an equinovarus malunion do differ. With an equinovarus deformity, the wedge that is resected will be slightly more dorsal than lateral. For correction of varus malunion, a second deformity may exist in the calcaneus itself in addition to the primary deformity, which is in the transverse tarsal joint. If a double deformity is present and the calcaneus is indeed in varus, then a calcaneal osteotomy must be performed, in addition to a transverse tarsal osteotomy.

For correction of a varus malunion, a biplanar osteotomy is performed at the apex of the deformity. A lateral incision is used and can be extended all the way posteriorly to include the calcaneus, if a calcaneal osteotomy is necessary. Because the plane of correction is from varus to valgus, an incision on the lateral aspect of the foot is not at jeopardy, and the single skin incision can be made extending from the base of the fourth metatarsal all the way to the back of the calcaneus. A decision has to be made before the incision is started as to the necessity for a calcaneal osteotomy. Therefore the foot has to be carefully inspected preoperatively to note whether the calcaneus is in varus; the more significant deformity at the transverse tarsal joint must also be inspected.

For exposure, the incision is deepened through the subcutaneous tissue, and an extensile thick flap is created across the entire transverse tarsal joint. The peroneal tendons and sural nerve are reflected inferiorly, and a large malleable retractor is inserted underneath the calcaneus at the level of the CC joint extending all the way underneath the arch of the foot. The soft tissues need to be stripped off both the dorsal and plantar surface of the transverse tarsal joint. The soft tissues are then protected with the malleable retractor both on the dorsal and plantar surfaces so that full visualization and access to the lateral aspect of the foot are available for the wedge osteotomy.

A guide pin is now inserted across the transverse tarsal joint under fluoroscopy. Locating the position of the osteotomy with this guide pin is important. Although the lateral foot and the apex of the deformity are easy to see, the medial extent of the wedge is not that predictable. I use two guide pins if I am performing a wedge resection or one pin if a rotational osteotomy across the transverse tarsal joint is performed. Make sure that the guide pins meet at the appropriate point on the medial side of the foot. A triangular, not a trapezoidal, wedge that will shorten the foot even further, should be resected. The osteotomy is then initiated on either the inside or outside of the guide pin depending on its location. Remember that the thickness of the saw blade itself will remove an extra 2 mm of bone with each cut. Do

not be tempted to use an osteotome for removal of this wedge; it is not nearly as precise. The osteotome cannot be controlled medially, and it can perforate into the soft tissues. Once the osteotomy is completed, the forefoot is rotated, as well as translated, to gain the correction. Note that as the transverse tarsal joint is rotated from varus to valgus, plantar flexion of the first metatarsal will occur. At times, this can be severe, and if it is, a dorsal wedge osteotomy of the first metatarsal or medial cuneiform must also be performed. The focus of the correction must be, however, on the lateral side of the foot for correction of the hindfoot and then any secondary deformities corrected subsequently. Once the hindfoot has been corrected, guide pins are then inserted to maintain the position of the foot, which should be inspected fluoroscopically before screws are inserted. Generally, the plane of the osteotomy is such that screws will be inserted from distal to proximal across the osteotomy. For example, as the foot is rotated into pronation and translated slightly laterally, an elevated dorsolateral segment will be present, and it can be used for insertion of the guide pins and screws. Frequently, however, these need to be inserted across additional joints, and therefore the screws will ultimately need to be removed at a later date. The other option for fixation is to use staples. However, because of the offset, which is usually created as a result of this osteotomy, unless one uses an offset staple, these are not ideal to use (Fig. 13–4–17).

Once the incision has been deepened down further through subcutaneous tissue, the entire dorsal and lateral periosteal surface is elevated off the calcaneus and cuboid. The peroneal tendons are reflected and retracted inferiorly, and then with subperiosteal dissection the entire dorsal surface of the original CC joint and then the TN joint are exposed. The talus and navicular should be easily visible from the lateral aspect of the foot. Large soft tissue retractors are inserted on the underside of the CC joint and dorsally over the original TN joint to protect the soft tissue structures.

A guide pin(s) is inserted transversely across the original transverse tarsal fusion mass to determine the location of the bone cut. Before the bone cut is initiated, a longitudinal mark along the length of the calcaneus and cuboid bone is made with electrocautery. After the osteotomy, when the shift of the hindfoot position is started, the exact amount of translation and rotation can

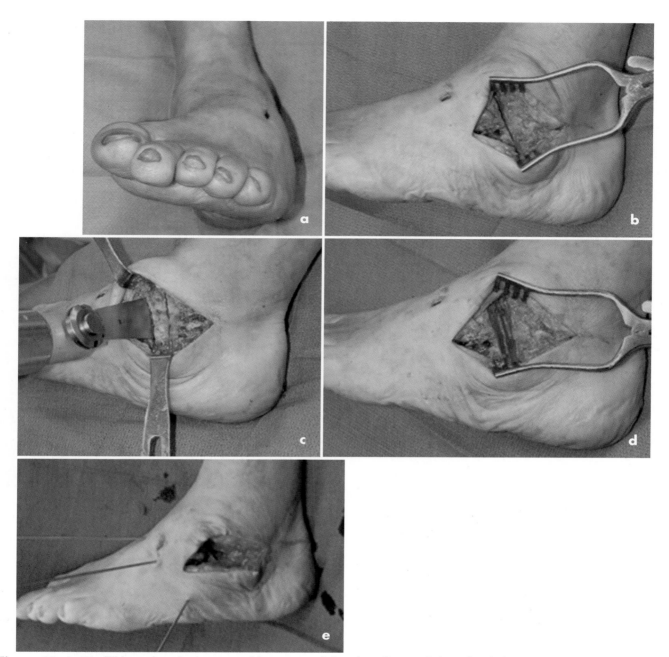

Figure 13–4–17. *This patient had severe adductovarus deformity after a triple arthrodesis, with plantar lateral foot pain (a). The heel was not in varus, and a calcaneus osteotomy was unnecessary. The apex of the deformity was dorsolateral directly over the calcaneocuboid (CC) joint, with more adduction, and for this reason the wedge was removed with the apex directly lateral (b–d). The hindfoot is reduced, and the guide pins inserted (e).* Continued

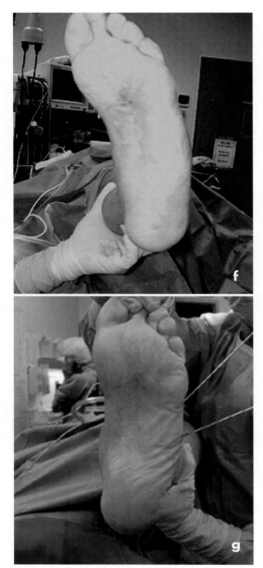

Figure 13–4–17, cont'd. *The preoperative and intraoperative appearance of the foot from the plantar surface shows the correction (f, g).*

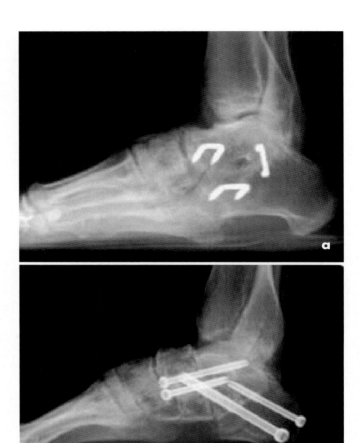

Figure 13–4–18. *Note how this equinovarus malunion of a triple arthrodesis has been corrected. The heel was in varus, with supination of the midfoot, and excessive pressure under the fifth metatarsal base (a). This was corrected with two osteotomies: one, with the calcaneus into valgus, and the other, a transverse tarsal osteotomy. Note the elevation of the midfoot with restoration of a plantigrade forefoot. The transverse tarsal osteotomy could have been made a few more millimeters distally; however, this did not influence healing or motion in this case.*

be visualized. A saw blade, not an osteotome, is used to cut across the original transverse tarsal joint. The first cut is made parallel with the position of the guide pin, approximately three quarters of the way across the foot. The guide pin is now removed, and the second bone cut performed. The size of the wedge cut is of course variable, but it is usually approximately 8 to 10 mm in height at the apex dorsolaterally. The foot should rotate nicely out of the deformed position, and in addition to the rotation, some dorsal translation of the lateral aspect of the foot can be created to totally unload the cuboid and fifth metatarsal pressure (Fig. 13–4–18).

Techniques, tips, and pitfalls

1. With fixation, I generally begin with the TN joint, which I think is the "key" to the reduction of any hindfoot deformity. The foot, particularly the planovalgus foot, pivots around the TN joint. Once this is locked in position, the rest of the joints fall into place. This is, however,

a generalization. I do not believe it is wrong to begin with the subtalar joint. Indeed, sometimes the primary fixation of the TN joint does not adequately reduce the heel valgus. In this instance, I will start with the subtalar joint fixation first. If this is done, however, the midfoot needs to be forcibly pronated around the head of the talus. If this maneuver is used for correction of severe hindfoot valgus, while the position of the foot may be correct, the anteroposterior (AP) radiograph shows slight overcorrection of the TN joint with the navicular protruding slightly medial to the head of the talus. This is not abnormal and results from primary correction of the subtalar joint followed by forcible pronation, adduction, and plantar flexion of the midfoot around the head of the talus.

2. Under normal circumstances, because I start correction with fixation of the TN joint, I can feel with my thumb and index finger around the joint as the foot is swiveled from valgus into the neutral position. This is an important maneuver, and although some "feel" to this step is present, this technique must be mastered to prevent undercorrection and overcorrection of the arthrodesis.

3. When naviculocuneiform arthritis or first tarsal metatarsal arthritis is present and a triple arthrodesis is performed, the decision has to be made whether to include these joints in the arthrodesis. This makes the foot extremely stiff and will inevitably lead to overload of the remaining "open" medial joint. In addition to arthritis, instability of one of these joints will presumably necessitate arthrodesis because no subluxation of the joint appears on the lateral x-ray (XR) image with a gap on the plantar surface. For these patients, I try to perform an opening wedge osteotomy of the medial cuneiform to realign either the naviculo-cuneiform or cuneiform metatarsal joint *without* performing an arthrodesis. Joint instability is invariably corrected, and although arthritis may be present and mild, it seems to

be preferable to an arthrodesis. I will wait and see what happens with this joint and perform an arthrodesis at a later date, if necessary.

4. Although bone graft is not necessary for filling in the void in the sinus tarsi, I will on occasion use a structural bone graft for correction of severe deformity. Sometimes, because of abduction across the transverse tarsal joint with crushing of either the cuboid or the calcaneus, a structural graft in the CC joint for purposes of lengthening is useful.

5. A triple arthrodesis is rarely necessary after calcaneal fracture because a subtalar arthrodesis is usually sufficient. However, when severe collapse of the hindfoot with abduction across the transverse tarsal joint has occurred, then a triple arthrodesis is preferable. Under these circumstances, however, correcting the position of the calcaneus is necessary, and usually an osteotomy of the calcaneus in addition to the arthrodesis is necessary. If an osteotomy is performed, be careful of the incision because any elongation of the height or length of the foot must be in the plane of the incision itself.

6. Planning the triple arthrodesis in the presence of pantalar arthritis can be tricky. The triple arthrodesis is usually done as a staged procedure to be followed by either a total ankle replacement or possibly an arthrodesis, depending on the outcome of the triple. Perfect position at the hindfoot is essential if this is being planned as a staged triple arthrodesis before a total ankle replacement.

7. Motion is lost after a triple arthrodesis. This is not only in inversion and eversion, but also in dorsiflexion and plantar flexion. This occurs whether or not the triple arthrodesis is performed for correction of a flatfoot or a cavus foot deformity. Needless to say, significant stresses are placed on the ankle joint after a triple arthrodesis whether or not it is performed correctly. Generally, a valgus stress is placed on the ankle in the setting of a preexisting flatfoot deformity, where laxity or elongation of the

deltoid ligament may have been present preoperatively.

8. With severe valgus deformity, the Achilles tendon moves laterally with the calcaneus, and the gastrocnemius-soleus muscle shortens. Once the heel has been returned to a neutral position, this contracture will be unmasked. Wherever possible, I try *not* to lengthen the Achilles tendon because of inevitable weakening of the muscle. If the deformity can be corrected, I am more inclined to do so without lengthening.

9. Some deformities cannot be corrected with a triple arthrodesis without additional osteotomy or arthrodesis. Figure 13–4–19 shows one such deformity, with marked rigidity in this adolescent foot associated with a middle facet coalition and fixed elevation of the first metatarsal. Compensatory contracture of the hallux in plantar flexion with contracture of the short flexor of the hallux is present. In addition to the triple arthrodesis, a lengthening of the anterior tibial tendon and plantar flexion osteotomy of the first metatarsal was performed.

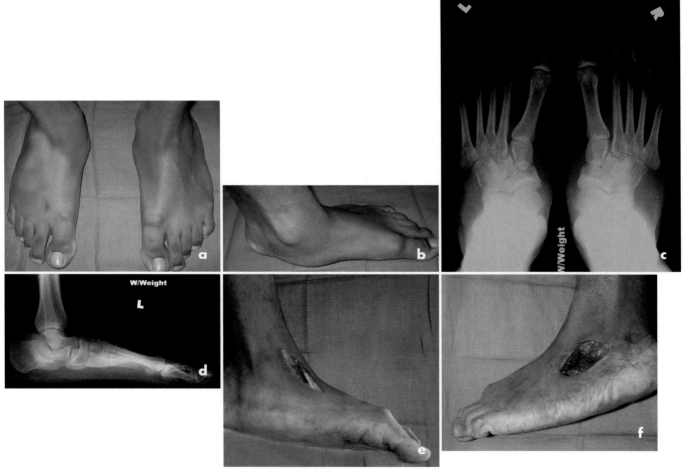

Figure 13–4–19. *This triple arthrodesis was performed in a 19-year-old patient for severe rigid flatfoot associated with a middle facet coalition (a–d). Note the marked elevation of the first metatarsal and the fixed flexion of the hallux (b, d). After the standard medial and lateral incisions (e, f).*

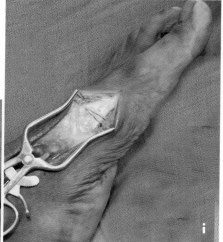

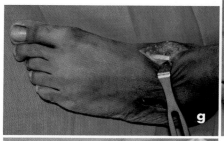

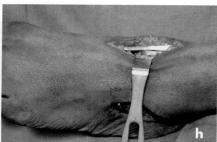

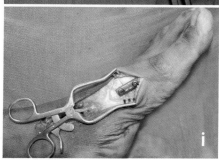

Figure 13–4–19, cont'd. *The anterior tibial tendon was exposed (g) and length-ened with a Z-step cut incision in the tendon (h). Once the fixation of all three joints was complete, the elevation of the first metatarsal was corrected with a plantar flexion osteotomy with removal of a small wedge of bone from the base of the first metatarsal (i) and fixation with a two-hole one-third tubular plate (j).*

Suggested Reading

de Heus JA, Marti RK, Besselaar PP, Albers GH. The influence of subtalar and triple arthrodesis on the tibio-talar joint. A long-term follow-up study. J Bone Joint Surg Br 79:644–647, 1997.

Fortin PT, Walling AK. Triple arthrodesis. Clin Orthop Relat Res Aug (365):91–99, 1999.

Haddad SL, Myerson MS, Pell RF 4th, Schon LC. Clinical and radiographic outcome of revision surgery for failed triple arthrodesis. Foot Ankle Int 18:489–499, 1997.

Jeng C, Vora A, Myerson MS. The medial approach to triple arthrodesis for correction of severe hindfoot deformity. Foot Ankle Int, 2004.

Pell RF 4th, Myerson MS, Schon LC. Clinical outcome after primary triple arthrodesis. J Bone Joint Surg Am 82:47–57, 2000.

Raikin SM. Failure of triple arthrodesis. Foot Ankle Clin 7:121–133, 2002.

Saltzman CL, Fehrle MJ, Cooper RR, et al. Triple arthrodesis: Twenty-five and forty-four-year average follow-up of the same patients. J Bone Joint Surg Am 81:1391–1402, 1999.

Sullivan RJ, Aronow MS. Different faces of the triple arthrodesis. Foot Ankle Clin 7:95–106, 2002.

Ankle Arthrodesis

When an ankle arthrodesis is performed, a technique should be used that is predictable, has a high rate of fusion, and can be applied to most patients. This technique should consist of internal fixation, which is stable both clinically and biomechanically. I have demonstrated that the mini-arthrotomy approach with three crossed screws for fixation has been reliable and versatile and has an arthrodesis rate of 96%. I originally described this approach for use in ankles without much deformity and without bone defects or the presence of avascular segments of the talus and distal tibia. This approach is certainly advantageous, and ankles without deformity are easier to correct with the mini-arthrotomy approach. However, arthrodesis can be performed with the mini-arthrotomy, even in the presence of significant deformity. Little periosteal stripping is present with this approach, and this approach is associated with rapid bone healing and an increased likelihood of arthrodesis as a result of maintaining the periarticular blood supply.

The range of motion following arthrodesis depends on the preexisting deformity and, in particular, the motion of the remaining joints. The true sagittal motion of the tibiotalar joint accounts for about 70% of the sagittal plane motion. The sagittal motion after arthrodesis is predominantly in plantar flexion through the transverse tarsal joints (Fig. 13–5–1).

Incision and Joint Exposure

Two incisions are used for the approach to the ankle. The first incision is made medially, medial to the medial malleolus in between the notch of the malleolus and the anterior tibial tendon, over a 2.5-cm length. On the lateral side of the ankle, the interspace between the peroneus tertius tendon and the fibula is identified, lateral to the lateral cutaneous branch of the superficial peroneal nerve. The nerve should be identified and retracted medially with the peroneus tertius tendon. On the medial side of the ankle the incision is deepened through subcutaneous tissue through the capsule that is incised down to the periosteum, and a retractor is inserted. Stripping the anterior distal periosteum off the tibia is helpful; then, the articular debris, osteophytes, and loose bodies should be removed. Both gutters should be debrided extensively, with a focus on the lateral gutter between the talus and the fibular. Either a rongeur or a smooth nontoothed laminar spreader is inserted in the medial incision, followed by insertion of a toothed laminar spreader laterally (Fig. 13–5–2).

The joint is debrided with a flexible chisel, not a saw or a burr, which burns the bone. With the laminar spreader alternating between the medial and the lateral side of the joint, the articular surface of the talus and tibia is completely denuded. Use a lot of irrigation to ensure

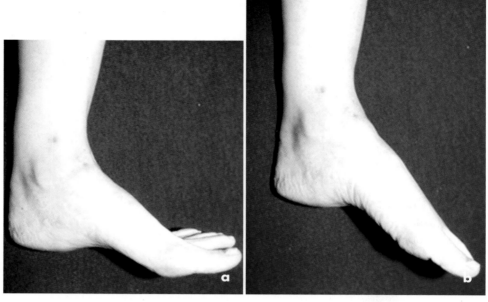

Figure 13–5–1. This is the range of motion of the ankle in dorsiflexion (a) and plantar flexion (b) following the mini-arthrotomy fusion. The motion is in the transverse tarsal joint.

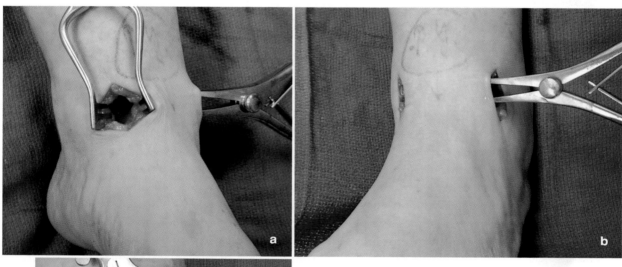

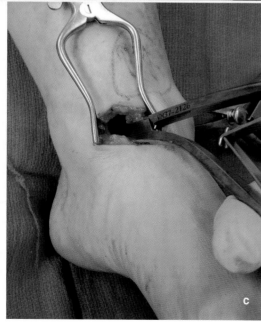

Figure 13–5–2. A rongeur is inserted medially and twisted vertically to open the joint so that a laminar spreader can be inserted laterally (a, b). Once this is done, a retractor is inserted medially to facilitate debridement (c).

that good articular apposition is obtained and that a good bleeding cancellous bone is present. With the laminar spreaders now removed, the position of the joint is checked fluoroscopically, and the guide pins are inserted (Fig. 13–5–3).

Screw Fixation

Crossing the plane of the screws is important. No screw construct should be present where all of the screws are perpendicular to the axis of the joint. Parallel screw fixation should be avoided because this is ineffective in controlling torsion and rotational forces. The fixation is performed with three screws over cannulated guide pins. The first guide pin is introduced from the posterior leg adjacent to the Achilles tendon between the tendon and the sural nerve (Fig. 13–5–4). The second guide pin and screw is inserted from the medial malleolus and extends obliquely down toward the anterior aspect of the sinus tarsi (Fig. 13–5–5).

The third pin is introduced from the anterolateral tibia immediately adjacent to the fibula, but this insertion depends on whether a slight bone shoulder is present.

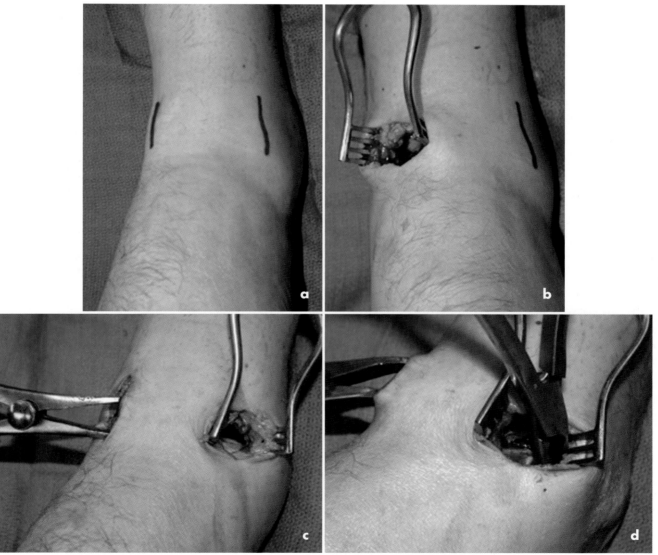

Figure 13–5–3. *The mini-arthrotomy approach to ankle arthrodesis is demonstrated with the incisions (a), the exposure of the joint with a retractor (b) and the alternation of the retractor with a laminar spreader between the medial and lateral incisions (c). Attention is paid to the medial and lateral gutters by debridement with a rongeur (d).*

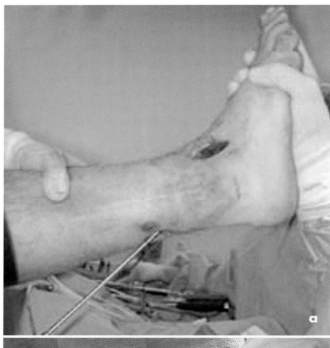

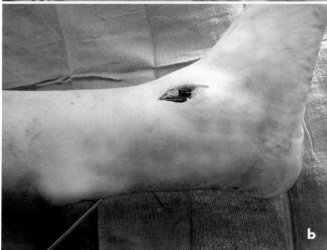

Figure 13–5–4. *The first guide pin (and screw) is shown in these two patients (a, b) and is inserted from the distal tibia into the medial neck of the talus.*

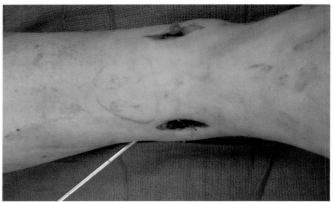

Figure 13–5–5. *The second guide pin is inserted from the medial malleolus toward the sinus tarsi, with the posterior facet avoided.*

enter the subtalar joint, and I rarely use a screw longer than 40 mm here. The third screw is introduced either from the anterolateral distal tibia or through the fibula (Fig. 13–5–6).

Always check for motion in the ankle after each screw insertion. This procedure provides a "feel" for the quality of fixation and the contribution of each screw to the arthrodesis construct. Aiming for the first metatarsal with the first posterior screw is important. The position of the guide pin should be checked fluoroscopically on the lateral view but, more importantly, on an anteroposterior (AP) view of the foot to make sure that the guide pin is in the center of the talus. The pin is often inserted too far laterally so that it may appear to be in the correct position on a lateral image but may be completely out the neck of the talus. When using the mini-arthrotomy approach, leave existing hardware in place unless it blocks the location of the arthrodesis screw. Note that sometimes fixation is more important than compression in ankles with osteopenia, and fully threaded screws can be used as needed, in this case, across the medial malleolus (Fig. 13–5–7).

Correction of Deformity

If bone defects are present, they will be noticeable with the foot held in a neutral position. A bone graft should be used. Provided the defect is not substantial, it can be filled with cancellous chips, and I routinely use allograft bone.

Once the guide pins are introduced, their position is checked fluoroscopically, and minor adjustments can be made to their position until it is perfect. The "best" screw here is the posterior axial screw, and this is introduced first, from the posterior aspect of the tibia into the anteromedial neck of the talus with a 6.5-mm partially threaded screw that usually measures 65 mm. The second screw is introduced from the medial aspect of the medial malleolus and extends down inferolaterally into the lateral body of the talus. The second screw must not

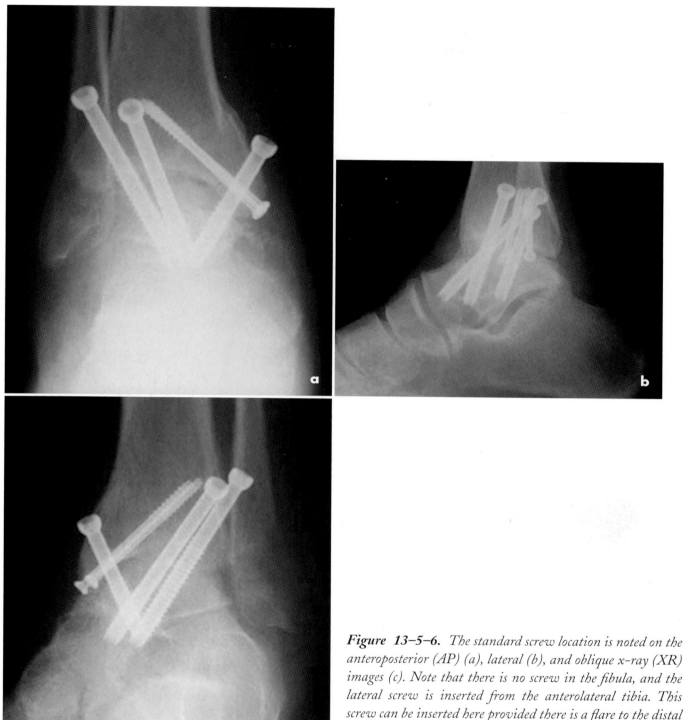

Figure 13–5–6. *The standard screw location is noted on the anteroposterior (AP) (a), lateral (b), and oblique x-ray (XR) images (c). Note that there is no screw in the fibula, and the lateral screw is inserted from the anterolateral tibia. This screw can be inserted here provided there is a flare to the distal lateral tibia. If it is not present, the third screw is inserted through the distal fibula.*

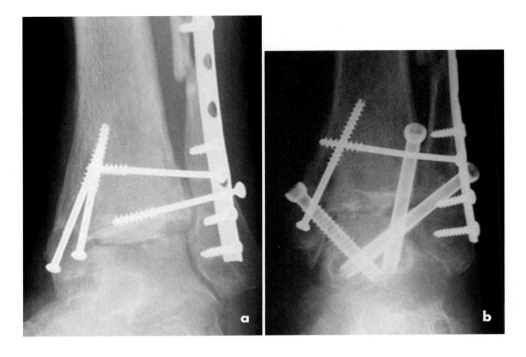

Figure 13–5–7. Existing hardware was left in place to perform this arthrodesis (a, b). Note the use of a fully threaded screw across the medial malleolus to improve purchase (b).

The joint is contoured and further debrided down to healthy bleeding cancellous bone, and then the allograft chips are inserted with a tamp. Once the foot is dorsiflexed, the graft is then compressed. If the vascularity of the joint surface is in question, then demineralized bone matrix can be added, in addition to the graft. I use a combination of the Symphony platelet system (DePuy, Warsaw Ind.), demineralized bone matrix, and even an implantable bone stimulator (EBI, Parsippany, NJ) in patients at high risk for conditions such as neuropathy or avascular necrosis.

The position of the ankle is fused relative to the forefoot, not the lateral position of the talus. Equinus deformity should be corrected with the bone contour within the ankle. However, if this deformity persists despite the joint debridement and bone resection, an Achilles tendon lengthening is performed percutaneously. Maintaining slight equinus and forcing the foot into dorsiflexion with the tightness of the posterior ankle (soft tissues) to create a tension band effect with the internal fixation are useful. The use of these methods presumes that some fixation is used in the anterior ankle to minimize any anterior toggle. Unless a cavus or calcaneus hindfoot deformity is present, the foot should never be left in equinus. The position of the ankle is determined according to the position of the forefoot, and although this may correlate with the declination angle of the talus, this is not necessarily the case with forefoot equinus. Do not over-dorsiflex the ankle to position the forefoot in neutral position. Such movement will put the hindfoot in calcaneus, which causes a painful heel strike. For these patients, positioning the ankle correctly and then adding a dorsiflexion osteotomy of the calcaneus is preferable.

If a large defect is in the ankle, then a tricortical structural allograft is preferable to a cancellous graft. I use a structural allograft, using a fresh frozen femoral head, which is contoured with a saw to fit into the joint space. The same technique is used after arthrodesis for failed total ankle replacement (Fig. 13–5–8).

Occasionally when a bone defect is present, apposition of the surfaces of the ankle is good, and a structural graft is not necessary. Fusion of the ankle joint only and preservation of the subtalar and transverse tarsal joints, wherever possible, are preferable. The graft is cut, shaped, and inserted into the ankle, and then the posterior and medial screws are inserted. Because these screws are not usually enough to compress the joint, an anterior plate is used for fixation. The plate is applied to the tibia first; then, the foot is forcibly dorsiflexed and the graft compressed. While the foot is held in this position, small screws are inserted through the plate into the talus (Fig. 13–5–9).

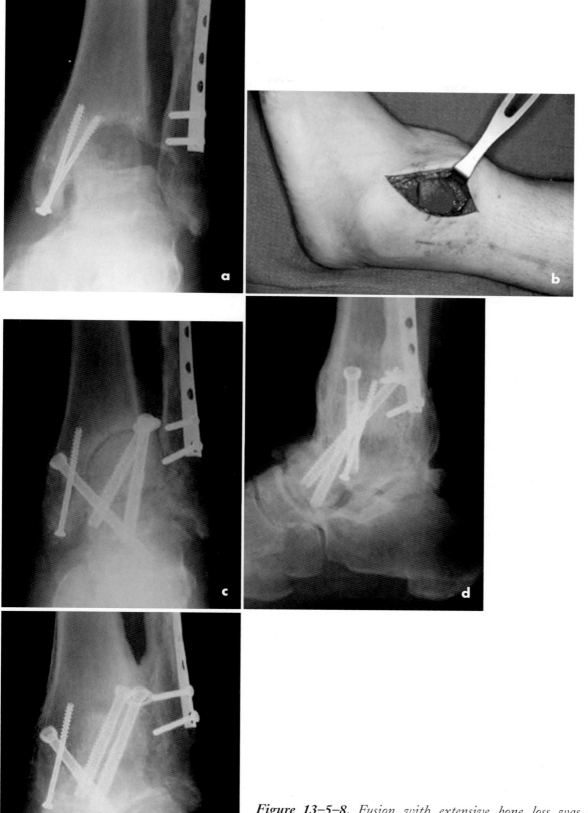

Figure 13–5–8. Fusion with extensive bone loss was performed with a modification of the mini-arthrotomy approach (a, b) by extending the lateral incision for insertion of a tricortical allograft from a femoral head. The early x-ray (XR) appearance is noted (c) with final healing occurring at 16 weeks (d, e).

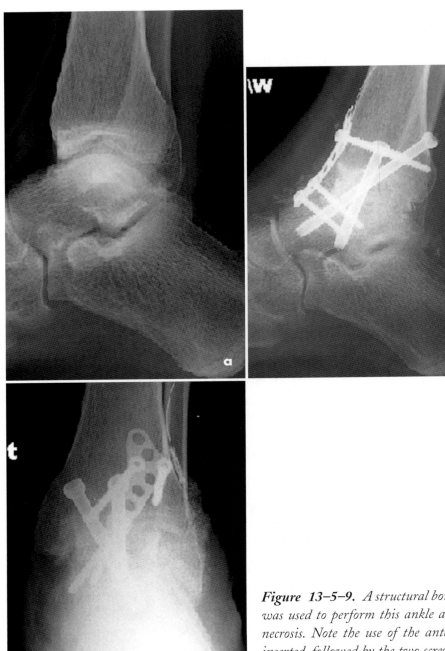

Figure 13–5–9. *A structural bone graft (fresh frozen femoral head allograft) was used to perform this ankle arthrodesis in the setting of severe avascular necrosis. Note the use of the anterior plate. The cannulated screws are first inserted, followed by the two screws through the plate into the tibia. Then the foot is forcibly dorsiflexed, compressing the ankle, and the two screws are inserted into the talus.*

Correction of Nonunion

Nonunion associated with bone loss and deformity requires a more extensile lateral incision, although the medial incision may be the same as that used for the mini-arthrotomy approach. In one patient with nonunion, a laminar spreader was inserted into the joint to push the medial dome of the talus into the notch (Fig.

13–5–10, *d*). It was then compressed first with lag screws introduced with a power, not manually, while the position was held with the laminar spreader laterally. Two plates were used anterolaterally, although one plate would be sufficient (Fig. 13–5–10, *e, f*).

When planning correction of equinus malunion of the ankle, consider that if a wedge is removed from the

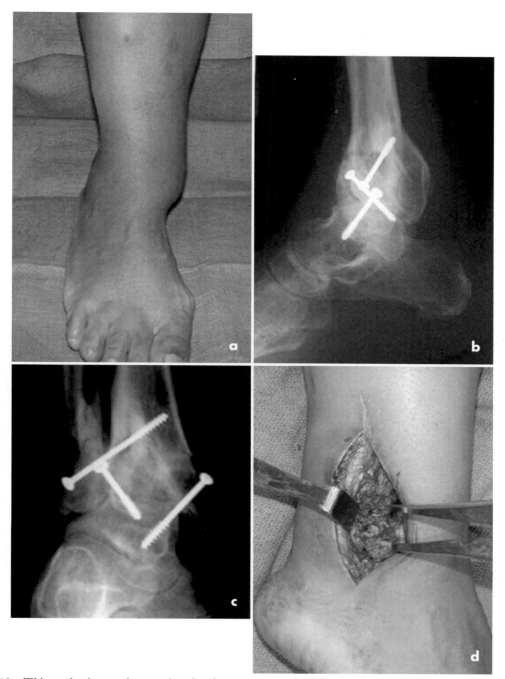

Figure 13–5–10. *This malunion and nonunion (a–c) were corrected with a laminar spreader used to realign the joint (d).*

Continued

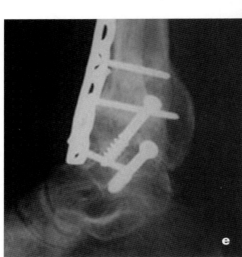

Figure 13–5–10, cont'd.
Followed by the use of cancellous screws inserted with power and two plates to maintain alignment (e, f).

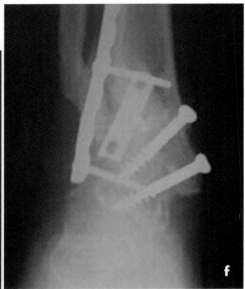

Figure 13–5–11. Resection of an anterior-based wedge is not appropriate to correct this equinus malunion.

anterior distal tibia and the foot brought up into dorsiflexion, the foot will fall forward relative to the tibia, and push-off is compromised (Figs. 13–5–11 and 13–5–12). Before fixation and after removal of this wedge, the foot must be translated posteriorly under the tibia. The alternative technique is to make a flat cut (without a wedge), push the foot posteriorly, and then impact the foot into the tibia to prevent loss of length of the limb. The foot must be translated back posteriorly under the tibia and left in a neutral position. This principle applies to revision of an equinus malunion, as well as the primary arthrodesis procedure. In correction of equinus malunion of an ankle fusion, the surgeon may be tempted to remove an anterior-based wedge from the distal tibia, dorsiflex the foot, and complete the arthrodesis. The foot may now be in neutral position, but a secondary translational deformity will occur and cause difficulty with gait.

Correction of Failed Ankle Arthrodesis

An important question that should be asked here is whether the ankle should be converted to a tibiotalar calcaneal arthrodesis. This is not just a matter of a nonunion or malunion, but bone loss, bone sclerosis, and possibly subtalar arthritis may be associated. If the motion in the subtalar joint is good, I will avoid a tibiotalar calcaneal arthrodesis. With appropriate fixation, revising the ankle, even in the presence of bone loss, is always possible. Prepare to add bone graft, to add bone graft supplements, to add implantable bone stimulation,

and to use varied types of rigid fixation. Frequently, compression across the joint is no longer possible because screw failure may have led to large voids in the tibiotalar joint space and larger fully threaded screws will need to be used (Fig. 13–5–13).

Wherever possible, I preserve the fibula. If a fibulectomy has been previously performed, then a lateral approach to the nonunion or malunion may be used. However, if the fibula is present, then revision is focused anteriorly. Incorporating the fibula into the arthrodesis process is

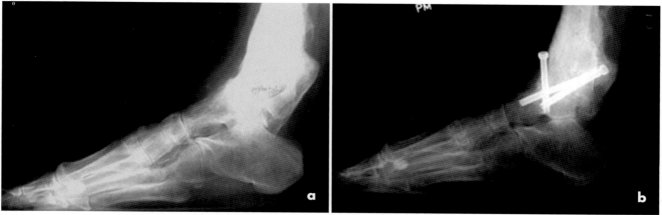

Figure 13–5–12. *This severe equinus deformity was not well corrected. Although the foot has been bought up into a slightly better position, the forefoot is still in equinus relative to the tibia (a, b). In addition, the talus should have been translated more posteriorly under the tibia to prevent vaulting over the foot.*

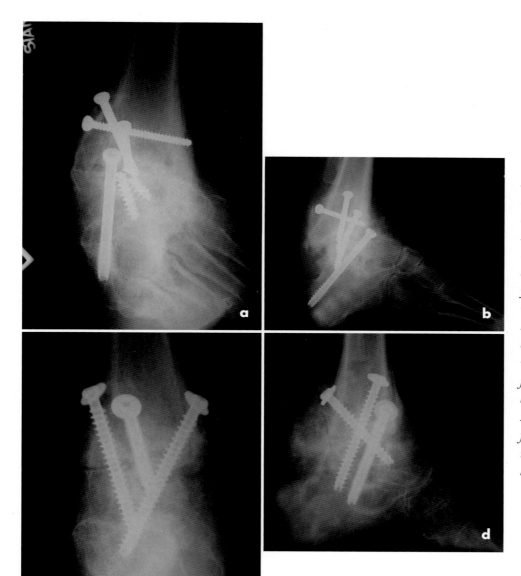

Figure 13–5–13. *A revision of this poorly positioned ankle arthrodesis was performed with screw fixation. The patient had undergone a prior subtalar arthrodesis successfully, and 24 years later an ankle arthrodesis was attempted. This left the hindfoot in severe varus and equinus (a, b). This deformity was corrected with a partial fibulectomy, and a transfibular approach to the ankle with screw fixation. Note the use of fully threaded screws to maximize purchase in this poor bone (c, d).*

useful, particularly in the presence of bone loss in the region of the lateral tibial plafond. In this case, adding graft to the entire syndesmosis and in the fibular gutter, and then adding a fibular plate with lag syndesmosis screws increases the stability of the construct and hence arthrodesis (Figs. 13–5–14 and 13–5–15). If patients undergo an arthrodesis for bone loss anteriorly, the foot tends to dorsiflex during the fixation maneuver, and the heel is positioned in calcaneus. This movement can be extremely painful and is a difficult position for the foot for ambulation with an inefficient gait.

Techniques, tips, and pitfalls

1. Removal of preexisting hardware before this arthrodesis is unnecessary. This hardware adds to the dissection and periosteal stripping, and screws can be inserted around this fixation. This procedure is much easier when cannulated screws are used because the guide pins will facilitate the correct passage of the screw.

2. Three-point fixation of an ankle arthrodesis is essential. The screws must come in at oblique angles to each other. Parallel screws cannot possibly control the rotation and torque on the ankle, and this method has been well demonstrated biomechanically. Crossed screw fixation is biomechanically superior.

3. As with other arthrodesis procedures, patients should avoid COX-2 nonsteroidal anti-inflammatory medication postoperatively. These have been demonstrated to inhibit bone formation and can lead to the presence of a delayed union or nonunion.

4. The mini-arthrotomy approach can be applied to revision procedures for correction of nonunion of an ankle arthrodesis or even for those in whom a slight avascular necrosis of the talus is present. One relies on the anterior

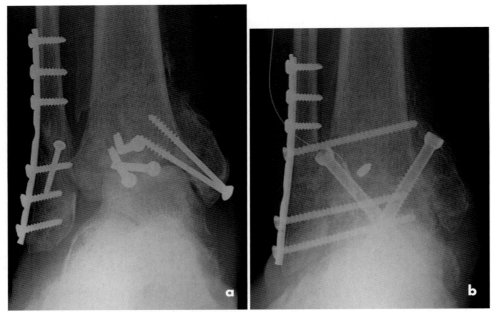

Figure 13–5–14. This arthrodesis was performed for the sequelae of a severe distal tibia fracture. Note the implosion of the talus into the distal tibia, the nonunion of the medial malleolus, and the fibula syndesmosis diastasis (a). The approach to arthrodesis was to maximize the contact of the tibia to the talus and involved a syndesmosis arthrodesis, inclusion of the medial malleolus in the arthrodesis, and an implantable bone stimulator. Note the markedly improved alignment, healing of the malleolar nonunion, and arthrodesis. The only problem with this fusion is the level of the malleolar tips and the potential for impingement on the shoe.

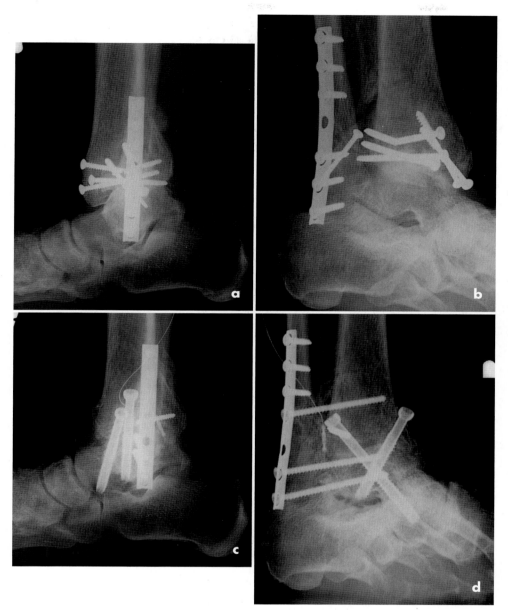

Figure 13–5–15. *This fracture fixation was inadequate and resulted in arthritis with impaction of the talus into the distal tibia. Hindfoot valgus and pes planus were coincidental (a, b). The arthrodesis was performed with cannulated screw fixation and was supplemented with arthrodesis of the syndesmosis (c, d). An alternative treatment here could have been a tibiotalocalcaneal arthrodesis to simultaneously address the hindfoot valgus, which was asymptomatic, however.*

vascularized portion of the tibia and the neck of the talus for arthrodesis. Vascularity of the talus is often patchy, and fusion of the talus may be sufficient enough to warrant joint debridement, as is normally performed. This will need to be augmented with bone graft or bone graft substitutes.

5. I find it useful to completely denude and debride the malleolar gutters and fill this with bone graft. This procedure applies particularly to the fibula and the lateral aspect of the talus

in cases of diastasis in which the fibula separates from the tibia as a result of old syndesmosis injuries.

6. If ankle deformity is present preoperatively, the mini-arthrotomy approach can still be used with the addition of bone graft to neutralize the position of the talus under the tibia; for example, when erosion of the distal lateral tibia is present with valgus deformity, as a result of collapse of the plafond. Preserving the notch of the medial malleolus under these

circumstances and using the medial corner of the ankle as a template for the position of the talus under the tibia are ideal. Once these have been done after the debridement, then the distal lateral portion of the tibia can be grafted by tamping the graft into place. This is followed by secure fixation.

7. Correction of cavus foot deformity with the mini-arthrotomy fusion is not difficult. Be careful of the position of the heel because the forefoot tends to be brought out of equinus and the hindfoot is put in too much calcaneus. The deltoid ligament may need to be released for correction of severe varus deformity (Fig. 13–5–16).

8. Correction of a valgus deformity begins by realigning the ankle after debridement and inserting a guide pin medially from the medial

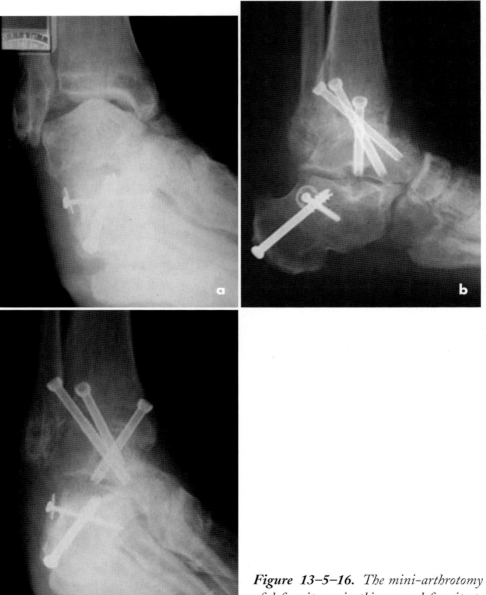

Figure 13–5–16. The mini-arthrotomy approach can be used for correction of deformity, as in this cavus deformity previously treated unsuccessfully with calcaneus osteotomy and ankle ligament reconstruction (a–c).

malleolus into the talus. This procedure maintains the position of the medial ankle in the mortise, and this can then be followed by secure grafting and completion of the internal fixation as previously described.

9. This is one type of fusion in which attention to detail after surgery is important. I do not permit weight bearing until the fusion is evident on x-ray (XR) film. This can at times be difficult because the articular apposition may be excellent early on when fusion cannot have taken place. I therefore use the presence of swelling, induration, and warmth of the ankle to determine the present of arthrodesis. I do not use a walking boot here, but instead keep the foot in a cast until I am certain that arthrodesis is present. The walking boots permit too much torque on the ankle, and I prefer to use a cast with an elevated rubber heel under the axis of the leg.

10. If infection is present and arthrodesis is still planned, then external fixation should be used as either a single or staged procedure to correct the infection and obtain arthrodesis. A multiplanar ring fixator may be used to debride and excise the infection; then tibial lengthening and docking into the ankle is planned to obtain arthrodesis. If the infection is extensive, then the arthrodesis may ultimately include the subtalar joint as well (Fig. 13–5–17).

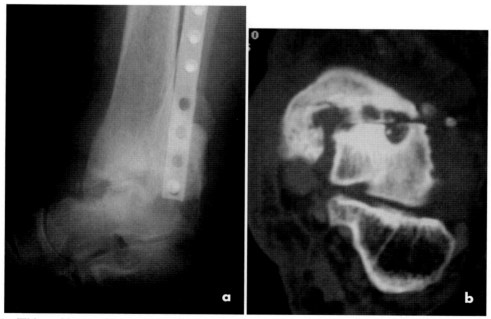

Figure 13–5–17. *This ankle was infected after open reduction and internal fixation, and by the time the patient was referred for treatment, severe erosive lytic changes were present (a, b).*

Continued

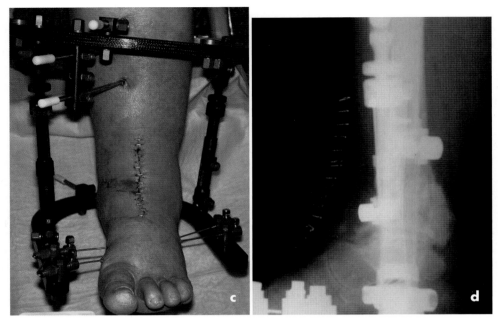

Figure 13–5–17, cont'd. *A single-stage arthrodesis was planned with joint debridement and external fixation (c), but although the infection was eradicated, nonunion occurred and was ultimately treated with intramedullary fixation (d).*

Suggested Readings

Cooper PS. Complications of ankle and tibiotalocal-caneal arthrodesis. Clin Orthop Oct(391):33–44, 2001.

Glick JM, Morgan CD, Myerson MS, et al. Ankle arthrodesis using an arthroscopic method: Long-term follow-up of 34 cases. Arthroscopy 12:428–434, 1996.

Levine SE, Myerson MS, Lucas P, Schon LC. Salvage of pseudoarthrosis after tibiotalar arthrodesis. Foot Ankle Int 18:580–585, 1997.

Miller SD, Myerson MS. Tibiotalar arthrodesis. Foot Ankle Clin 1:151–161, 1996.

Muir DC, Amendola A, Saltzman CL. Long-term outcome of ankle arthrodesis. Foot Ankle Clin 7: 703–708, 2002.

Myerson MS, Quill G. Ankle arthrodesis. A comparison of an arthroscopic and an open method of treatment. Clin Orthop Jul(268):84–95, 1991.

Neufeld SK, Uribe J, Myerson MS. Use of structural allograft to compensate for bone loss in arthrodesis of the foot and ankle. Foot Ankle Clin 7:1–17, 2002.

Paremain GD, Miller SD, Myerson MS. Ankle arthrodesis: Results after the miniarthrotomy technique. Foot Ankle Int 17:247–252, 1996.

Paremain GP, Myerson MS. Vascularity of the ankle joint after arthrodesis: A cadaveric study. Foot 5:127–131, 1995.

Raikin SM. Arthrodesis of the ankle: Arthroscopic, mini-open, and open techniques. Foot Ankle Clin 8:347–359, 2003.

Van Bergeyk A, Stotler W, Beals T, Manoli A 2nd. A functional outcome after modified Blair tibiotalar arthrodesis for talar osteonecrosis. Foot Ankle Int 24:765–770, 2003.

Tibiocalcaneal and Tibiotalocalcaneal Arthrodesis

As a rule, I always prefer to perform a tibiotalocalcaneal (TTC) arthrodesis instead of a pantalar arthrodesis. The addition of the transverse tarsal joint to the arthrodesis adds far more rigidity to the foot, which has been noted both biomechanically and clinically in previous publications. Even when performing a TTC arthrodesis, I prefer to leave the navicular bone free of the anterior aspect of the remnant of the talus. The same concept applies to the tibiocalcaneal (TC) arthrodesis after a cheilectomy of the anterior tibia when the anterior aspect of the tibia may abut the navicular bone. In some patients with neuropathy and after correction of a Charcot deformity, including the navicular bone in this arthrodesis is tempting, but I do not consider it advisable. The more motion one has, particularly in the setting of a neuropathy, the better the function of the foot. A pantalar arthrodesis is then only performed when severe pantalar arthritis is corrected or when the deformity is of such magnitude that the correction cannot be obtained through the TTC complex alone. The approach to pantalar arthrodesis is almost identical with that of combined incisions used for an ankle and a triple arthrodesis. In fact, I start out with the ankle joint using the mini-arthrotomy approach with two anterior incisions and then extend these distally once the ankle is completely debrided. The medial incision is in line with the approach of the talonavicular joint. Laterally, however, if the incision for the ankle arthrodesis is extended distally, then one incision is slightly anterior or dorsal to the calcaneocuboid joint. The incision should not be too far lateral over the fibula, although performing the subtalar and calcaneocuboid fusion is easier when this incision is indeed more lateral.

A fibulectomy should not be performed. The same concept applies to pantalar arthrodesis as it does to the ankle arthrodesis, and preservation of the fibula is preferable. The same applies to the medial malleolus, although at times, correction of the ankle cannot be accomplished without either an osteotomy or a resection of the medial malleolus.

As for fixation, the approach is similar to that outlined for the following screw technique for TTC arthrodesis. The only difference here is that the fixation of the talonavicular joint can be extended proximally into the tibia with screws started at the inferior pole of the navicular bone, which cross both the talonavicular and tibiotalar joints into the back of the tibia.

Fixation Alternatives for the Tibiocalcaneal and Tibiotalocalcaneal Arthrodesis

The fixation options for a TC arthrodesis include screws, a blade plate, or an intramedullary (IM) rod. To some extent, the choice of fixation may depend on personal preference, but at times a more stable fixation with either a blade plate or IM fixation is preferable because of significant bone loss and deformity. When any erosive changes or avascular necrosis of the ankle is present, then I find that screws are not usually strong enough. This is particularly the case with neuropathic deformity. A blade plate has been biomechanically demonstrated to be superior to an IM rod in torsion and bending strengths, and frequently I use a blade plate for fixation (Fig. 13–6–1).

Historically, use of the blade plate was more important, when the IM rod did not have the capacity for posterior to anterior screw fixation. Under those circumstances, even though the rod could be used, little stability existed between the calcaneus and the tibia because of the paucity of fixation in the calcaneus. With the advances that have been made in IM fixation, posterior to anterior screws, which engage the rod and the posterior calcaneal tuberosity, are now possible. However, if a rod is being used, a sufficient amount of bone in the calcaneus must be present distally and be distal to the rod itself for stable fixation. If a minimum

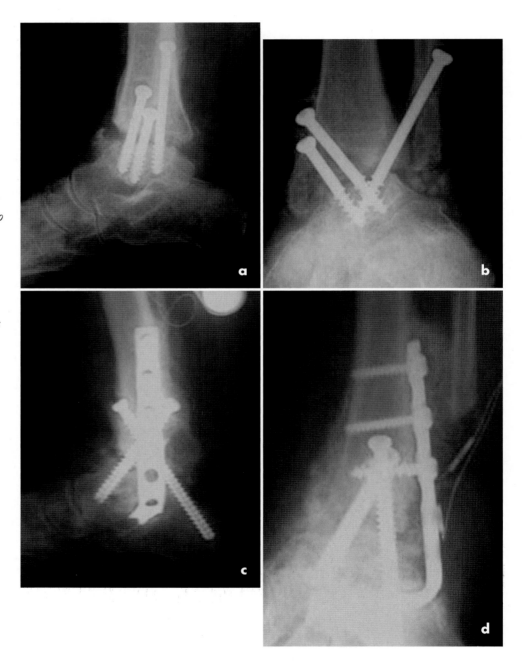

Figure 13–6–1. *A blade plate was selected for this patient who had a failed ankle fusion, an avascular talus, and lateral erosion of the talus (a, b). Although an isolated revision ankle arthrodesis could have been attempted, the patient was obese; the screws penetrated into the subtalar joint; and with the deformity present, it was thought that a tibiotalocalcaneal (TTC) arthrodesis would be more reliable and it was performed with a blade plate (c, d).*

amount of bone in the calcaneus is present, the screws can be inserted across the calcaneocuboid joint into the cuboid bone. Postoperative weight-bearing status may also be a consideration, and if I am concerned about the ability of a patient to remain non–weight bearing, then I may prefer to use an IM rod. Although the locking screws may break, a nonunion is not as worrisome in the setting of neuropathic deformity, provided the foot remains axially aligned under the tibia. I do use screws alone for a TTC fusion, and I rarely use them when the talus is missing and the overall alignment of the limb is satisfactory without much defect between the distal tibia and calcaneus. Generally, I use the IM rod for a TTC arthrodesis and a blade plate for a TC arthrodesis.

Transfibular Approach

A lateral transfibular approach to the ankle and hindfoot can be used. Although this will devascularize the lateral ankle, an alternative is often unavailable for correction of severe deformity when a fibulectomy is necessary. The incision is made vertically, directly over the fibula, extending down distally over the sinus tarsi toward the inferior aspect of the calcaneus. The sural nerve must be identified and then retracted inferiorly with the peroneal tendons. A fibulectomy is performed with an acetabular reamer, which is used to completely denude and decorticate the fibula. The reamings that are obtained for later bone graft are preserved (Fig. 13–6–2).

If a blade plate is used for fixation, the distal 8 cm of the fibula must be removed, and following use of the reamer, the more proximal 4 cm of the fibula is cut with a saw. I prefer to use a chisel and not a saw to denude the ankle and subtalar joints. If severe deformity is present, however, then the distal tibia may have to be cut at the plafond with a saw. Often the foot cannot be centered under the ankle because the medial malleolus blocks the shift of the talus. If this seems to be a problem, then the malleolus is removed with an oblique osteotomy through a separate medial incision. The dissection in the sinus tarsi and subtalar joint is performed as that described for a subtalar arthrodesis.

When a talectomy and TC arthrodesis are performed, the necrotic remnants of the talus are completely excised. A sizable defect remains, and either it can be filled with bone graft or the talus can be apposed directly onto the calcaneus. Usually, despite the contouring of the posterior aspect of the calcaneus and the undersurface of the distal tibia, joint apposition cannot be easily obtained. The dilemma is that for apposition of the calcaneus against the tibia, the hindfoot tilts up into dorsiflexion, leaving a calcaneus position. Filling the defect adequately with cancellous graft is possible, but I prefer a tricortical structural allograft. A fresh frozen femoral head is used, defrosted in saline for 20 minutes, and then cut with a saw into the appropriate trapezoidal shape to fill the defect. The graft is difficult to fit in place. One alternative is to fix the hindfoot with guide

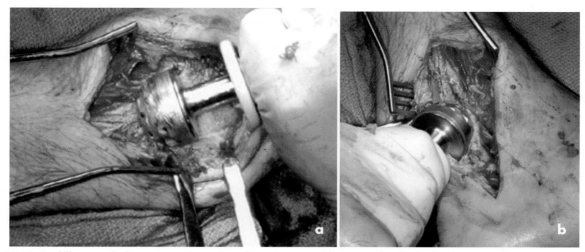

Figure 13–6–2. *The acetabular reamer is used to decorticate and harvest the fibula for bone graft (a, b).*

pins and then to force the foot into plantar flexion while the pins are in place. With the foot plantarflexed, the TC gap opens and the graft is inserted and tamped into place securely. The foot is now maximally dorsiflexed, and the bone graft is compressed between the calcaneus and the tibia, followed by definitive fixation. If the gap is not significant, then I use allograft cancellous bone chips and compress the graft in with a tamp, as previously stated.

Fixation: Blade Plate

I first align and stabilize the hindfoot using percutaneous guide pins. The first guide pin is introduced from the plantar aspect of the heel into the anterior distal tibia, and the second pin is introduced from the posterior inferior tibia into the anterior midfoot. The alignment of the blade plate is now secured by placing it laterally against the calcaneus and the tibia. Guide pins are introduced through the cannulated holes or through the screw holes while the plate is in a reversed position, flush with the bone. The plate must be flush with the lateral aspect of the calcaneus and the distal tibia, which may have to be shaved or abraded with a saw to have the blade plate appose correctly. The plate may have to be rotated or angulated to have maximum purchase in the calcaneus. If the blade enters the calcaneus perpendicular to its axis, then the blade must be under the subchondral plate of the posterior facet. Alternatively, the blade can be angled into the calcaneus from a posterior to anterior insertion so that it enters the sustentaculum tali. The plate is removed and then reversed onto the guide pins and then tamped with a large mallet into place securely (Fig. 13–6–3). Be sure that the blade enters the calcaneus in a smooth plane. A small instrument placed under the plate is helpful while banging on the blade with the tamp to prevent angulation. Fingers can be used to support the plate, but be careful. Once the plate is 1 cm from the bone, use a tamp over the distal screw hole. Apposition of the plate against the calcaneus and the tibia should be good. In addition to the screws through the plate, I may use supplemental cannulated screw fixation from the inferior aspect of the calcaneus into the distal tibia or the distal tibia posteriorly into the navicular bone anteromedially (Fig. 13–6–4).

At times, a decision has to be made as to the technical aspects of a TC arthrodesis to restore height of the hind-

foot with a structural graft. For example, a TC arthrodesis can be performed with no structural graft if apposition of the calcaneus against the posterior tibia is good. A large defect, which varies in size from a trapezoid to a large triangle depending on bone erosion, is always present between the undersurface of the tibia and the dorsal surface of the posterior facet. At times, if the apposition between the tibia and calcaneus is very good and the defect not too large, then it can be filled with cancellous graft only. The alternative is to use a large structural graft, which is contoured to the exact size of the defect. This is highlighted in Figure 13–6–5.

Fixation: Intramedullary Rod

The key to IM fixation is correct alignment of the foot under the tibia. According to an anatomic model of the foot, the calcaneus is slightly lateral to the longitudinal axis of the tibia. Therefore inserting the rod through the center of the calcaneus and being in the center of the tibia at the same time are not physically possible. If this alignment is going to be accomplished, then the medial malleolus needs to undergo osteotomy, and the talus (if present) needs to be moved medially. In this manner, a more vertical access to the tibia is possible. This may, however, not be entirely necessary depending on the length of the screws through the calcaneus. Even if the rod is slightly medial, it is invariably located close to the sustentaculum so that at least one screw will be in good bone medially. However, if only the lateral x-ray (XR) images are viewed, the screws may appear to be in the calcaneus when, in fact, they are protruding medially into the soft tissue and can cause tendonitis and neuritis. Therefore each situation has to be monitored according to the anatomy and the deformity. Monitoring is also important when placing screws from a posterior to anterior insertion because the premise for a screw of this nature is that it must enter the calcaneal tuberosity and not exit the soft tissues medially. Therefore an effort should be made to make sure that the rod is indeed in as much of the calcaneus as possible, whether the screws are put in from a lateral or from a posterior to anterior insertion through the calcaneus.

The key to IM fixation is correct alignment of the foot under the tibia. The same principles apply to the incision and exposure as for the blade plate fixation. Once adequate debridement and alignment has been obtained,

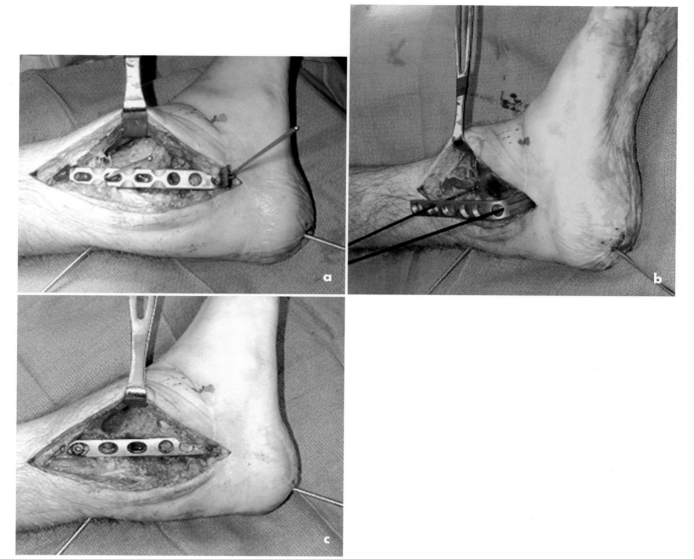

Figure 13–6–3. *A blade plate was used for a tibiocalcaneal (TC) arthrodesis. Note the temporary guide pin fixation obtained to maintain limb alignment and the cannulated blade applied with the flat plate surface to the side of the ankle (a). Guide pins are inserted through the distal cannula and one of the screw holes (b), and the plate is then reversed and positioned over the preinserted guide pins, then tamped firmly into place (c).*

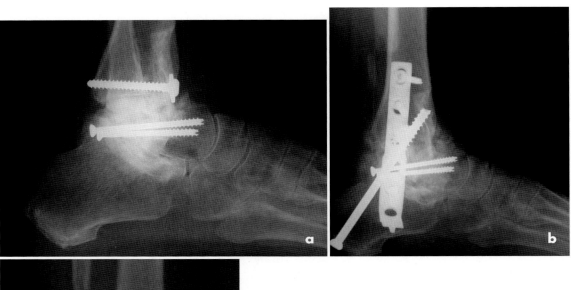

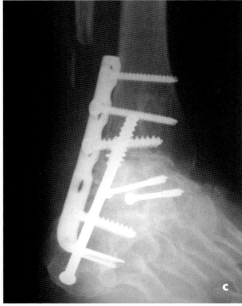

Figure 13–6–4. *Avascular necrosis of the talus with collapse of the body only was present in this patient (a), and a blade plate was used for arthrodesis (b, c). Note the use of an additional screw from the calcaneus into the distal tibia, which is at times necessary to control rotation of the ankle.*

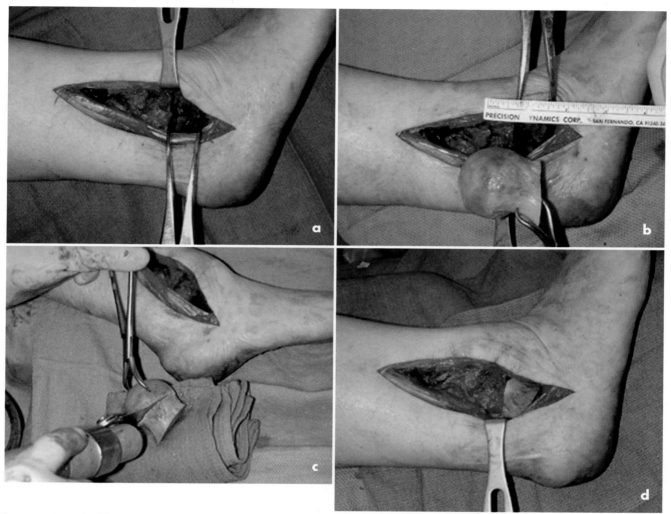

Figure 13–6–5. *The steps in planning a tibiocalcaneal (TC) arthrodesis with interposition structural graft for this patient with avascular collapse of the talus. Note the laminar spreader in place that measures the size of the defect (a). The femoral head allograft was measured (b) and cut with a large saw (c) and inserted under compression (d). These procedures were followed by stabilization with an intramedullary (IM) rod (VersaNail, DePuy Ace, Warsaw, Ind.).*

the IM guide pin is selected. A 2-cm incision is made on the plantar aspect of the hindfoot immediately anterior and slightly medial to the heel pad. The guide pin is inserted through the inferomedial calcaneus through the talus (if present) and into the tibia and checked fluoroscopically. Before proceeding with the reaming, I use a large cannulated drill bit, passed over the IM guide pin, followed by the reamers up to 1 mm greater than the diameter of the rod selected. Generally, I use a rod that is 11 mm in diameter by 20 cm in length. The rod is now inserted and gradually tamped into place with the external alignment guide, and the inferior portion of the

guide is used to gently tamp the rod into position. The position of the rod must be checked fluoroscopically each step of the way to ensure adequate positioning on the plantar surface of the heel. If any motion is noted at the rod interface with rotational stress on the foot, a cannulated screw can be inserted from the distal medial tibia into the inferior tuberosity of the calcaneus. Surprisingly, the rod does not interfere with insertion of this screw (Figs. 13–6–6 and 13–6–7).

Wherever possible, I use 6.5-mm cannulated screws for fixation of any hindfoot or ankle arthrodesis, and a TTC

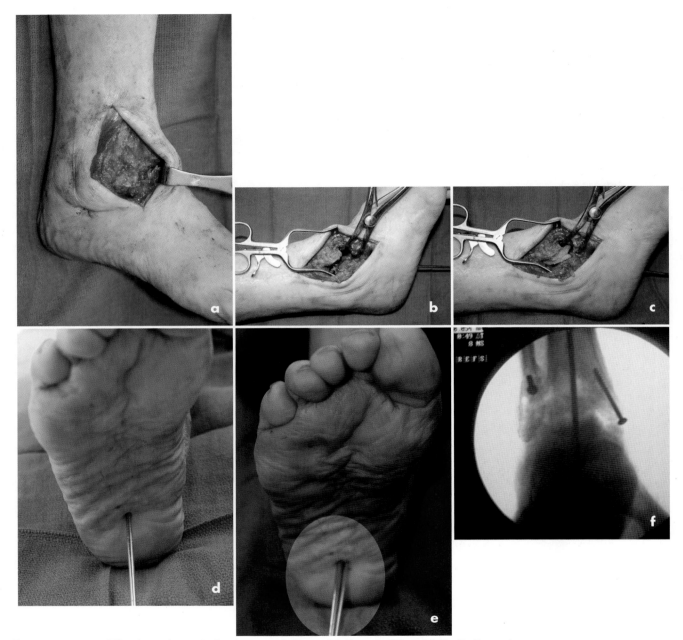

Figure 13–6–6. *The insertion of the intramedullary (IM) rod (VersaNail, DePuy Ace, Warsaw, Ind.). A transfibular approach is used (a), the joint is exposed, and the surfaces are prepared for arthrodesis. Once good cancellous bone is exposed, any defect is filled with bone graft, in this case with cancellous allograft chips mixed with demineralized bone matrix (b, c). The guide pin is inserted slightly medial to the undersurface of the calcaneus (d) and checked fluoroscopically. If the position of the guide pin is not ideal, a second pin can be inserted adjacent to it, instead of reinserting the first guide pin with a new position, which may again be incorrect (e). The position is again checked fluoroscopically (f).*

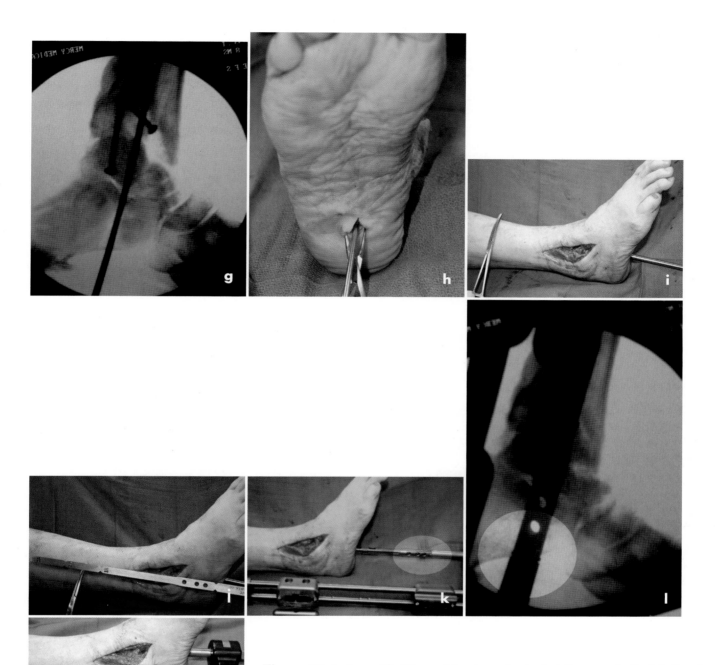

Figure 13–6–6, cont'd. *The position is again checked fluoroscopically (g). On the lateral view, note that there is good contact between the tibia and talus, and although the foot could have been translated further anteriorly, this puts too much forward pressure on the fusion and is mechanically incorrect. A longitudinal incision is made, the tissue is spread to push aside the lateral plantar nerve (h), and the reaming is begun. Once reaming is complete, the length of the rod can be determined according to a clamp applied to the limb (i) with a ruler (j). Ideally, the longer the rod, the better the stability. The inserter device is locked (k), and the position of the rod is checked at the inferior surface of the calcaneus to ensure that it is in far enough and not protruding (l). In this patient, the fixation screws in the calcaneus are inserted lateral to medial, although with the locking system of this device, the alignment guide can be rotated posteriorly for posteroanterior insertion of the screws (m).*

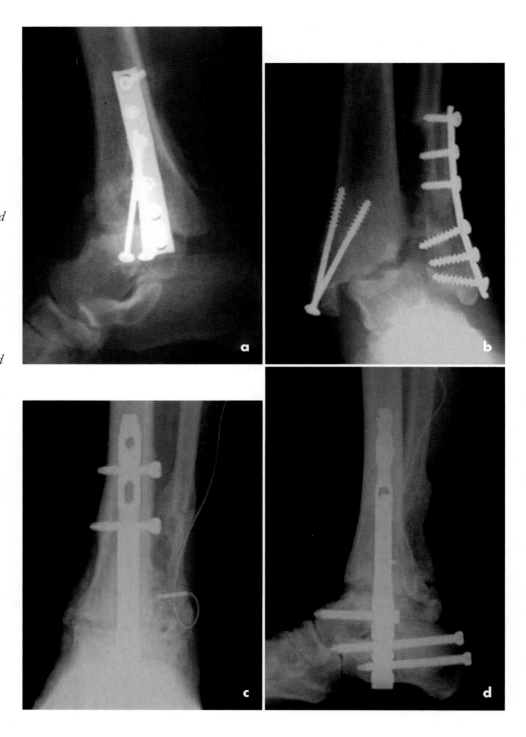

Figure 13–6–7. An intramedullary (IM) rod was used to correct the deformity and perform a tibiotalocalcaneal (TTC) arthrodesis in this patient with post-traumatic deformity. As in the example in Figure 13–6–1, a decision had to be made regarding the procedure. In this instance, the patient was morbidly obese, and it was thought that the enhanced stability with a TTC arthrodesis would be preferred (a, b). Note the removal of the medial malleolus, which was necessary to translate the talus medially under the tibia and to correctly position the rod centrally (c). An implantable bone stimulator was used to enhance the arthrodesis (c, d).

arthrodesis is no exception. The ideal patient for this type of fixation has arthritis, has reasonable bone quality, has minimal deformity, and is able to comply with postoperative care and restricted bearing of weight (Fig. 13–6–8). However, as seen Figure 13–6–9, cannulated screws were used to correct severe ankle arthritis in a patient who had previously undergone a triple arthrodesis.

Techniques, tips, and pitfalls

1. A fracture of the distal tibia has been seen above a blade plate, a rod, or screws. A stress riser is at the tip of the hardware, and the chance of a fracture can be minimized with

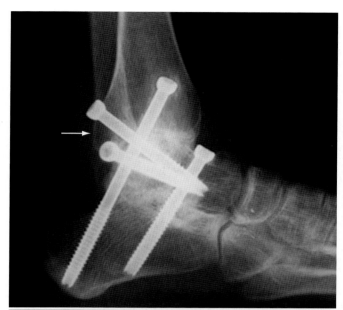

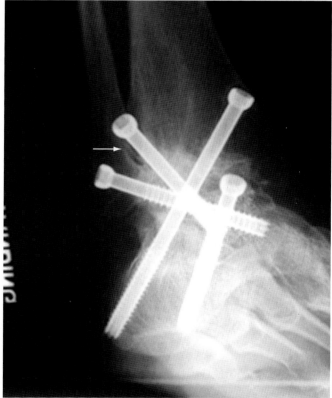

Figure 13–6–8. Cannulated screws were used to perform this tibiotalocalcaneal (TTC) arthrodesis (a, b). The bone quality was good, alignment was not compromised, and no avascular necrosis was present. The posterior and lateral screws in the ankle (white arrow) are in the same location as for an isolated ankle arthrodesis.

a longer rod. I rarely use a 15-cm rod for this reason.

2. The lateral plantar nerve may be injured with the IM fixation. The potential for injury has been demonstrated anatomically. Nonetheless, even though the rod is in proximity to the nerve, I have rarely seen the nerve injured. IM fixation can, however, cause neuritis, particularly if the rod is left slightly prominent. If the screws are fractured and the rod migrates distally in the calcaneus, then irritation against the lateral plantar nerve certainly can be a problem.

3. Compression of an IM rod may be helpful. Compression devices are available with most of the commercially used rods. If devices are available, they probably should be used where a gap is present before insertion of the tibial screws. The problem with the all compression systems is that they tend to cause migration of the rod distally out below the calcaneus, and this has to be estimated before the compression is started. Alternatively, if compression is used with the Ace IM system VersaNail (VersaNail, DePuy, Warsaw, Ind.), then the guide holes for the tibial screws may be slightly offset as a result of this compression.

4. Internal and external rotation of the foot and of the leg can become a problem with the IM rod system. This is purely a visual problem.

5. If tension is present on the skin margins during closure, the skin flap has to be modified. Tension may occur because of compression across the ankle and a "concertina" effect of the skin. In addition to modification of the skin closure, the peroneal tendons can be transected and both tendons removed to facilitate wound closure.

Pantalar Arthrodesis

For the most part, the procedure for pantalar arthrodesis is an extension of the principles of an ankle and a triple arthrodesis. The same can be said for a TTC arthrodesis in which a correction of the transverse tarsal

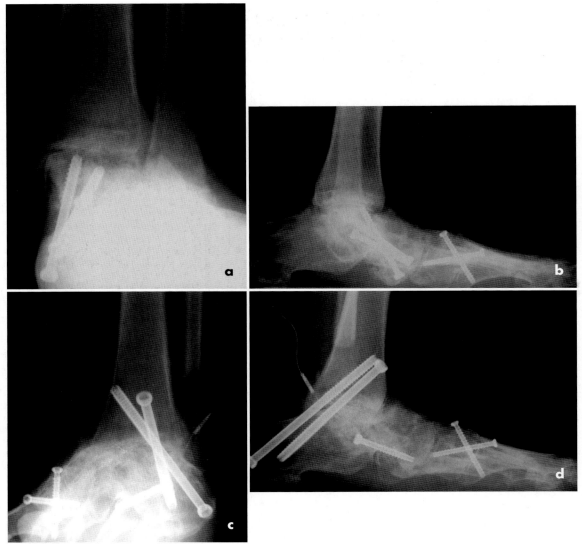

Figure 13–6–9. *This patient with rheumatoid arthritis underwent a tibiocalcaneal (TC) arthrodesis with cannulated 6.5-mm screws. Note the avascular necrosis of the talus, valgus deformity, and arthritis (a, b). Although the foot remains slightly collapsed, marked improvement in the alignment was present with the correction (c, d).*

joint is added. Ideally, I prefer to use the same incisions for an ankle arthrodesis and then extend them down over the talonavicular joint medially and the subtalar and calcaneocuboid joints laterally. These incisions can, of course, be modified according to the presence of deformity, but, by and large, this is the approach that I would use. Occasionally, when the deformity is significant, a fibulectomy is performed with an extended lateral incision. Rarely, when the hindfoot has severe varus deformity, the head of the talus is pointing laterally and barely articulating with the navicular bone. In these instances, a single lateral incision can be used to perform the arthrodesis. The head of the talus is visible in the sinus tarsi, and most of the talonavicular joint preparation and debridement can be performed from the lateral incision. At times, the posterior tibial tendon needs to be cut from its attachment to the navicula for correction, and this cutting can be done percutaneously. For practical purposes, however, the approach to the pantalar arthrodesis should include two incisions for maximal exposure and joint preparation (Figs. 13–6–10, 13–6–11, and 13–6–12).

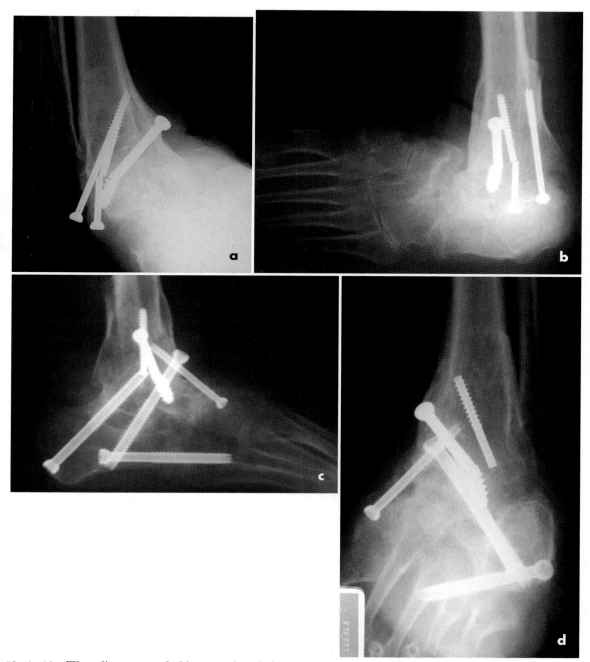

Figure 13–6–10. *The alignment of this pantalar fusion was important. The arthrodesis needed to correct the predominant supination deformity in the transverse tarsal joint but also to revise the prior attempted ankle arthrodesis to bring the ankle and hindfoot out of varus (a, b). Severe deformity of this nature can only be corrected reliably with screws, and this procedure was performed through an extensile lateral approach to the hindfoot and an accessory medial incision over the talonavicular joint (c, d).*

Continued

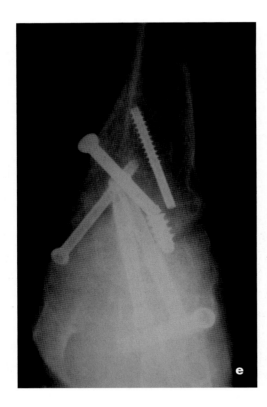

Figure 13–6–10, cont'd. Severe deformity of this nature can only be corrected reliably with screws, and this procedure was performed through an extensile lateral approach to the hindfoot and an accessory medial incision over the talonavicular joint (e).

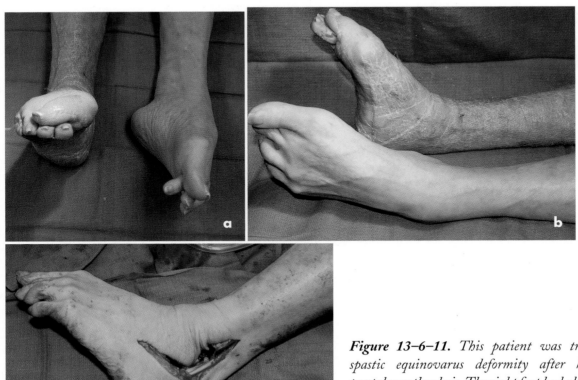

Figure 13–6–11. This patient was treated for bilateral spastic equinovarus deformity after head injury with pantalar arthrodesis. The right foot had already been corrected. Note the equinovarus present on the left foot (a, b), which was corrected with screws through a single extensile lateral incision (c).

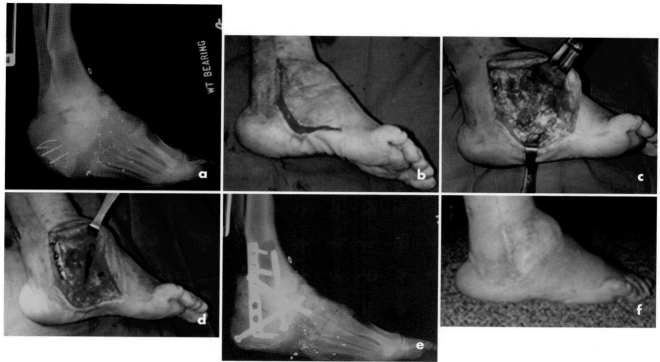

Figure 13–6–12. *A pantalar arthrodesis was performed in this patient after a shotgun injury to the hindfoot. He had undergone multiple operations and had a cavus foot, marked pain under the lateral foot, and calcaneus (a). Because of the paucity of good lateral skin, a staged procedure was performed. The first procedure was a tibiotalocalcaneal (TTC) arthrodesis performed with a blade plate, and this was followed by the second stage, when a transverse tarsal rotational wedge was removed to correct the varus hindfoot (b–d). The final appearance of the foot and x-ray (XR) image is noted (e, f).*

Talectomy

The various arthrodesis procedures of the hindfoot that have been described are performed as an alternative to amputation or the use of some sort of a brace if at all feasible. Talectomy must be considered as an alternative to arthrodesis in the adult patient. The motion present makes it an appealing procedure when used in conjunction with a brace. In adults, talectomy has been used for salvage involving nonunion of ankle fusions, failed total ankle arthroplasty, inflammatory arthropathy, neuroarthropathy, failed talar prostheses, failed pantalar fusions, adult neglected clubfoot, post-traumatic avascular necrosis talus, and deformities due to sciatic nerve palsy and compartment syndrome. His-

torically, total talectomy has been largely used to treat children with congenital diseases such as arthrogryposis or myelomeningocele, and today it is used most often in adults to treat talar trauma. Although its indications continue to evolve, severe deformity correction can be achieved with its use. The severe and often recalcitrant nature of the problems that warrant consideration of talectomy place the procedure in the category of a salvage operation. The effort of the surgeon must be to obtain a painless, plantigrade, "braceable" foot and ankle. With this in mind, good results can be obtained when patient expectations and surgical goals are realistic for the use of talectomy in the adult patient (Figs. 13–6–13 and 13–6–14).

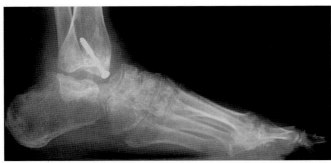

Figure 13–6–13. This talectomy followed severe trauma in an adult patient. Although the patient functioned reasonably with minimal pain, she required an ankle foot orthosis (AFO) for daily activities.

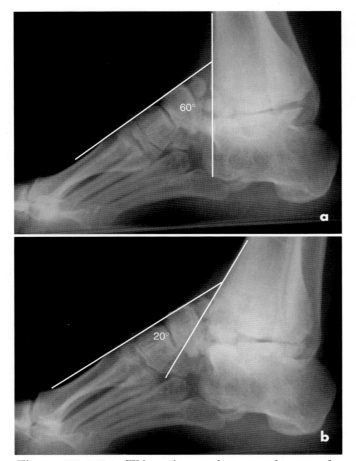

Figure 13–6–14. This patient underwent talectomy after trauma as an adolescent and functioned extremely well without a special shoe or brace. Approximately 40 degrees of sagittal motion, which is sufficient for function, remained in the hindfoot (a, b).

Suggested Readings

Levine SE, Myerson MS, Lucas P, Schon LC. Salvage of pseudoarthrosis after tibiotalar arthrodesis. Foot Ankle Int 18:580–585, 1997.

Myerson MS, Alvarez RG, Lam PW. Tibiocalcaneal arthrodesis for the management of severe ankle and hindfoot deformities. Foot Ankle Int 21:643–650, 2000.

Papa J, Myerson M, Girard P. Salvage, with arthrodesis, in intractable diabetic neuropathic arthropathy of the foot and ankle. J Bone Joint Surg Am 75: 1056–1066, 1993.

Papa JA, Myerson MS. Pantalar and tibiotalocalcaneal arthrodesis for post-traumatic osteoarthrosis of the ankle and hindfoot. J Bone Joint Surg Am 74: 1042–1049, 1992.

The Rheumatoid Foot and Ankle

Forefoot Reconstruction

The standard approach for correction of rheumatoid forefoot deformity has involved resection of the metatarsal heads with realignment of the lesser toe deformities and arthrodesis of the hallux metatarsophalangeal (MP) joint. Over the years, in my hands, this has been the most reliable procedure for correction of deformity particularly associated with erosive changes of the MP joint with destruction of bone, in particular the metatarsal head.

Modifications of the procedure may include resection of the lesser metatarsal heads with resection arthroplasty of the hallux MP joint (as an alternative to arthrodesis). This is certainly an option, although this resection does not appear to be as stable a procedure as the arthrodesis. However, the resection arthroplasty can be considered in the presence of arthritis of both the MP and the interphalangeal (IP) joints of the hallux. If the arthritis is associated with deformity of both joints, then one alternative is to perform an arthrodesis of the IP joint in conjunction with a resection arthroplasty of the MP joint. I am, however, opposed to performing a resection arthroplasty of the hallux in the patient with rheumatoid arthritis and hallux valgus because soft tissue laxity associated with erosive changes and ligamentous instability will lead to a recurrence of deformity.

Other options for correction of the deformity at the MP joint of the lesser toes include synovectomy and shortening osteotomies of the metatarsal head or shaft. Synovectomy is certainly an option to consider in the presence of severe synovitis associated with minimal joint deformity and the absence of metatarsalgia. However, once subluxation or dislocation of the MP joints occurs, then synovectomy is not of any benefit. The concept of joint preservation of the MP joint is a good one in patients with inflammatory joint disease. The synovitis surprisingly decreases with mechanical offloading of the MP joint as a result of the shortening osteotomy. Although this is a reasonable procedure to be performed in a patient with rheumatoid arthritis, it is not easily accomplished because of the paucity of good bone around the metatarsal head, the erosive changes typically associated with joint subluxation and dislocation, and the difficulty of performing this operation and maintaining a salvageable joint. Nonetheless, in patients who have involvement of one or two joints without severe erosions present, shortening osteotomy is an option. This is more the case where one or two of the lesser MP joints are involved, and one is reluctant to resect all of the metatarsal heads.

Many intermediate stages of deformity of the rheumatoid forefoot exist in which arthrodesis of the MP joint may not be considered necessary. For example, a healthy joint is still present but is associated with hallux valgus.

A standard operation for correction of hallux valgus (e.g., bunionectomy and metatarsal osteotomy) may not be as successful as, for example, a tarsometatarsal arthrodesis (the modified Lapidus procedure). If hallux valgus is not present initially and metatarsal head resections are performed, then the hallux deformity will always increase as a result of shortening of the lesser toes and the absence of a lateral buttress to the hallux. Preservation of the hallux MP joint is even more relevant if joint preservation osteotomy procedures of the lesser metatarsal heads are performed.

Incisions and Dissection

The choice of incisions used for the metatarsal head resections or the metatarsal head osteotomies is determined by the magnitude of deformity. In general, I prefer two longitudinal incisions made in the second and fourth web spaces. However, the incisions have to be balanced against the possibility of wound dehiscence and problems with skin healing after the dorsal longitudinal skin incisions. The option of a dorsal transverse incision is available, but this cannot be performed if dislocation of the MP joints is present with shortening and contracture of the soft tissues. Although this is an easier incision to perform, the surgeon must be certain that sufficient bone has been resected to facilitate soft tissue closure. The other option is for a plantar-based elliptical incision. Although I have used this incision on occasion, the dilemma is the management of the contracted dorsal soft tissues, including the extensor tendons and capsule. I see no advantage of a plantar-based incision other than the proximity of the metatarsal heads. The soft tissue hypertrophy, callus, or bursae are always resorbed once the metatarsal heads have been resected, and the excision of an ellipse of tissue on the plantar surface does not seem warranted.

I generally use two dorsal longitudinal incisions that are made in the second and the fourth web spaces but maintain as wide a skin bridge between them as possible. The metatarsals are resected first, followed by the MP fusion. In this way, inadvertent manipulation of the hallux MP joint is avoided. Both incisions should be as long as possible and extend from the cleft of the web space proximally for a length of 4 cm. Care must be taken not to overretract the tissue to prevent bruising and ecchymosis of the tissue during the dissection. When one side of

the skin is retracted, the other is relaxed. I find it easier to start with the more lateral fourth web space incision because the fifth metatarsal is always the easiest to remove. In each case, the extensor tendons of the toes are transected 2 cm proximal to the metatarsal neck and are clamped and pulled distally. This clamping of the tendons facilitates the exposure of the MP joint through retraction of the tendon all the way up to the dislocated joint (Fig. 14–1–1).

The dissection is deepened, and a capsulectomy is performed until the MP joint is identified. This is not always easy to see if the joint is dislocated, but the joint must be reduced before the osteotomy of the neck is performed. I use a curved periosteal elevator inserted over the dorsal surface of the MP joint, and then with plantar-directed pressure the remnant of the metatarsal head is delivered into the dorsal surface of the wound. The proximal phalanx is depressed underneath the metatarsal head for further exposure. Soft bone, where the metatarsal head is crushed, is the problem encountered. The soft bone does not create a problem with the resection of the head, but remnants of the metatarsal head must be sought after it is removed. This problem also applies to the base of the proximal phalanx, which can be fractured, with fragments left behind. I do not resect the base of the proximal phalanx, even with severe dislocation. This resection unnecessarily shortens the toe and adds to dorsal instability.

The metatarsal neck is cut at the level of the flare between the metaphysis and the diaphysis of the metatarsal with a saw. Do not use an osteotome, which will fracture the metatarsal in an irregular manner, leaving irregular bone spikes present. The cut is directed in a slightly plantar direction obliquely to avoid any plantar spike that creates metatarsalgia. I use a clamp or towel clip to hold, rotate, and then pull out the head, but cutting the collateral ligaments, and remnant of the plantar plate.

A choice can be made as to what to do with the extensor tendons. These can be left cut or repaired. However, these choices are not my preference because I do not want any dorsiflexion contracture to occur postoperatively. To prevent this contracture, I perform a plantar tenodesis of the extensor tendons. Each extensor tendon is grasped with a hemostat and then passed underneath the metatarsal neck. A wire is then directed antegrade

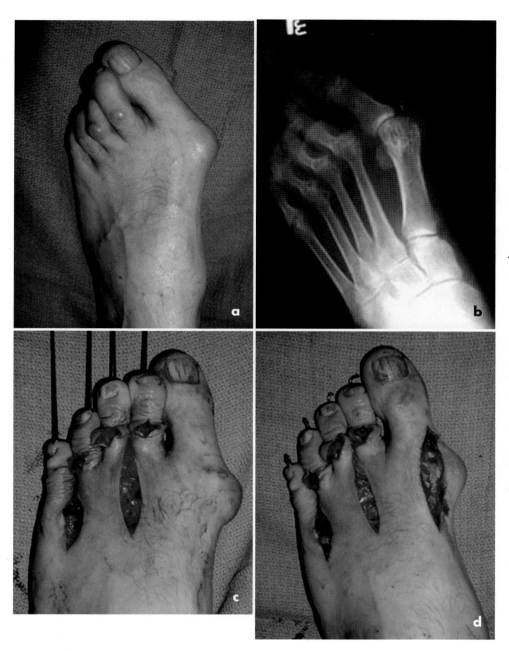

Figure 14–1–1. This patient has typical forefoot disease and was approached with standard forefoot incisions (a, b). Note that there is slight bruising of the forefoot skin as a result of retraction (c, d). The medial eminence of the first metatarsal head is not resected. Rarely, a large bursa or rheumatoid nodule must be resected simultaneously. However, be careful with medial skin retraction. If a large nodule or sesamoid must be excised, an additional medial incision is preferable.

and then retrograde across the MP joint and through the tendons into the metatarsal itself. This wire holds the extensor tendons under the metatarsal neck, and the tenodesis effect prevents dorsal extension contracture. The K-wires are never stable enough in osteopenic bone. However, this stability can be ensured with insertion of the K-wire as proximal as possible into the cuneiforms or cuboid bone. Wound closure is performed with nylon sutures only because the subcutaneous tissue is rarely thick enough to hold a suture. No tension should exist on the skin incisions at all (Fig. 14–1–2).

The correction of the claw toe deformities has often been described as unnecessary. However, if the toes are left deformed at the proximal IP joint, MP joint deformity tends to recur later as well. These contractures should be addressed either with manual manipulation of the joint or resection arthroplasty. Manual manipulation of the joint will work, provided this is not a rigid contracture. However, I have seen many recurrences of the manual manipulation, even when followed with the use of a K-wire for the appropriate time.

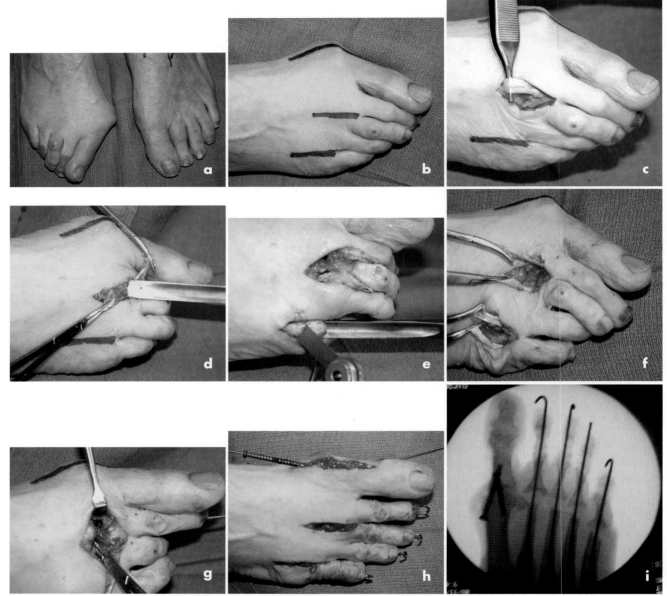

Figure 14–1–2. *The forefoot reconstruction with arthrodesis of the hallux metatarsopha-langeal (MP) joint and resection of the lesser metatarsal heads in a patient who had undergone a prior successful similar procedure (a). The incisions are marked out as widely spaced as possible (b), and the extensor tendons to the second toe are cut transversely (c). A curved shmogler is inserted under the metatarsal head to expose the neck (d). Note the slightly oblique plane of resection of the fifth metatarsal (e), and after resection of all of the metatarsal heads, the extensor tendons are clamped (f). The extensor tendon is then passed under the metatarsal neck, and a K-wire is passed through the extensor tendon into the metatarsal shaft (g). The arthrodesis of the MP joint is performed with cannulated fully threaded 4-mm screws (h), and the final intra-operative fluoroscopic appearance is noted (i).*

I prefer to leave the K-wires in for 6 weeks to gain as much stability at the posterior interphalangeal (PIP) and MP joint as possible. Subsequently, these K-wires will loosen and need to be removed prematurely. The K-wires are inserted as far back posteriorly into the cuneiforms as possible to prevent early loosening.

Techniques, tips, and pitfalls

1. Management of the toe deformity can be frustrating. Try to preserve as much length of the toe as possible. If severe deformity or contracture is present, the patient is far better off with an isolated toe amputation.

2. The toes rarely function with any grip strength after head resection, and if recurrent contracture develops, it is more difficult to correct subsequently than if a primary toe amputation is performed.

3. If infection or ulceration under the metatarsal head is present, a more urgent operation is performed. I use a similar approach to resect the metatarsal head(s) from the dorsal incisions but pass an antibiotic-soaked sponge through the incision from dorsal to plantar (almost like flossing teeth) and then leave the plantar ulcer open but close the dorsal incision (Fig. 14–1–3).

4. For deformity of the hallux and the MP joint but minimal arthritis, a joint preservation procedure may be ideal. A modified Lapidus procedure is a good procedure that gives lasting relief and maintains alignment. This can be performed with either resection of the metatarsal heads or shortening osteotomies (Fig. 14–1–4).

5. Resection of the lesser metatarsal heads is a good procedure but should not be performed indiscriminately. Shortening osteotomies of the metatarsal relieve the pressure on the joint and decrease the pain from erosive disease (Fig. 14–1–5).

6. For profound disease, resection of all the metatarsal heads can be performed through a

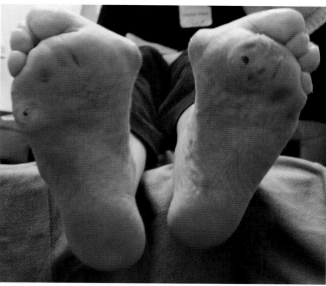

Figure 14–1–3. *Plantar ulceration as a result of erosion of the metatarsal head is addressed urgently with resection to prevent osteomyelitis.*

transverse dorsal (Fig. 14–1–6) or plantar (Fig. 14–1–7) incision.

7. For severe deformity with marked hallux valgus with dislocation of the MP joint, the soft tissue contracture is so severe laterally that even with an adequate lateral adductor and capsular release, the tension on the lateral soft tissue is still excessive so that tearing of the skin can occur. If the hallux is not reducing easily without tension laterally, then further bone should be resected.

8. Fixation of the MP joint can be difficult because of osteopenia. If the screws do not appear able to hold, then use a plate or large threaded pins. Most of these patients have some IP joint disease as well, and crossing the IP joint with the Steinmann pins is not as problematic as in patients with a normal joint.

9. Positioning the MP joint with pins is difficult. For positioning of the MP joint with the use of pins, the declination angle of the first metatarsal has to be considered because the pins usually exit the metatarsal neck and do not engage the entire shaft of the metatarsal. If the hallux is plantar flexed to have better fix-

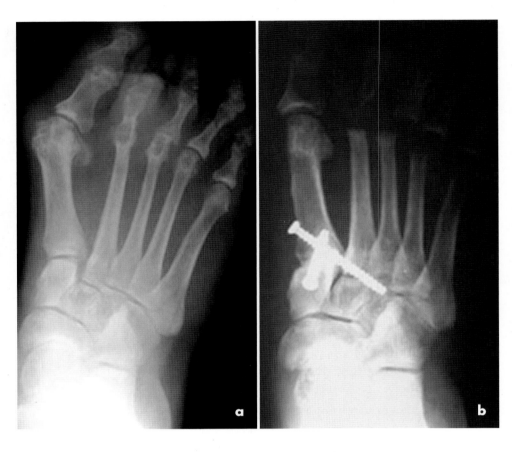

Figure 14–1–4. This patient had erosive disease of the lesser metatarsophalangeal (MP) joints but no involvement of the hallux MP joint (a). Arthritis of the hallux interphalangeal (IP) joint was present, and avoiding arthrodesis of the MP joint if the IP joint is already deformed is preferable. Although shortening osteotomies of the lesser metatarsals could have been performed, resection of the heads in conjunction with a Lapidus procedure was performed (b).

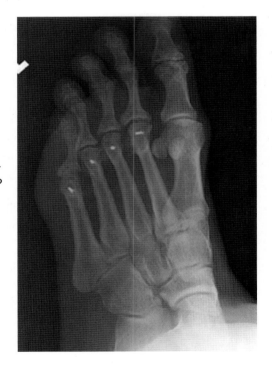

Figure 14–1–5. This patient was an ideal candidate for lesser metatarsophalangeal (MP) joint preservation, particularly because the hallux MP joint is relatively normal, although the interphalangeal (IP) joint is affected.

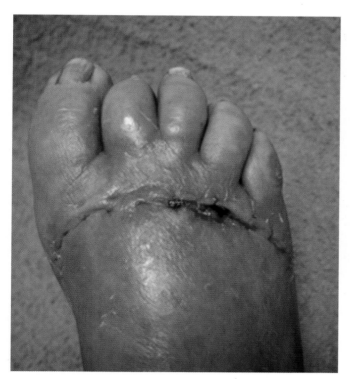

Figure 14–1–6. This is the immediate postoperative appearance after a transverse incision was used in this elderly patient with severe forefoot deformity and a resection of all of the metatarsal heads including the first was performed. This procedure is an option for patients who are more debilitated and for whom a more lengthy recovery after arthrodesis may not be warranted. This incision should be used carefully in association with severe dislocations, due to concern for wound healing problems.

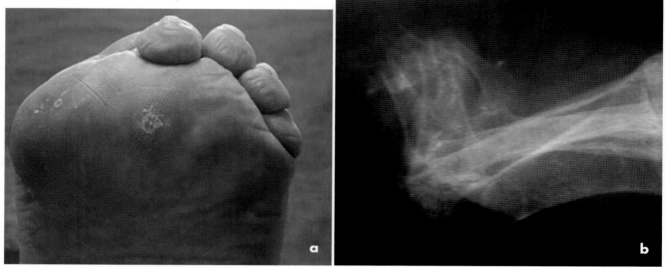

Figure 14–1–7. In an elderly patient with severe deformity and potential ischemia, approaching the head resection from the plantar surface may be preferable (a–c).

Continued

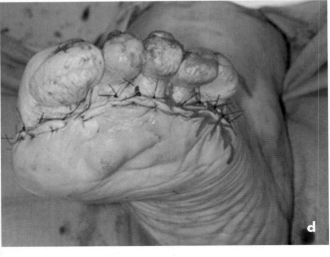

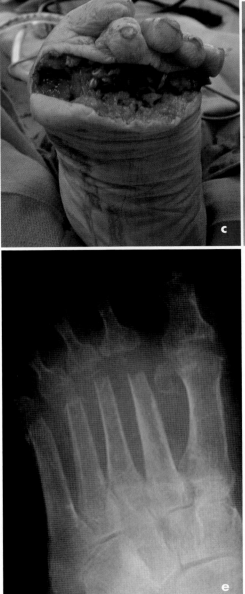

Figure 14–1–7, cont'd. *Although this is not conducive to a "cosmetic" reconstruction, in this patient, all of the metatarsal heads, including the first, were removed from the plantar incision, followed by resection of an ellipse of tissue (c, d). Note the improved alignment of the hallux and toes following resection (e).*

ation with the threaded pins, then this will lead to a plantar flexion malunion with the hallux being too straight and will eventually lead to IP joint disease.

10. Alignment of the hallux MP arthrodesis is important. If any valgus is present, an increased incidence of subsequent IP joint arthritis is present (Figs. 14–1–8 and 14–1–9).

Correction of Rheumatoid Hindfoot and Ankle Deformity

Arthrodesis is the predominant operation used for correction of rheumatoid hindfoot and ankle deformity. The complication rate in this group of patients with this deformity is, however, significantly increased as a result of wound healing problems from immune suppression, dysvascularity and skin fragility, and bone instability as a result of osteopenia. These potential complicating fea-

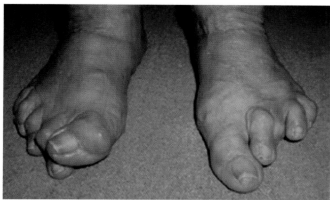

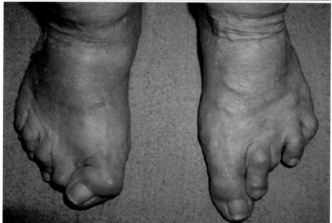

Figure 14–1–8. *Recurrent deformity here is difficult to treat. Hallux interphalangeal (IP) arthritis is present after arthrodesis and metatarsal head resection. Arthrodesis of the IP joint is difficult to attain in this situation. Toe deformities persist in both feet after prior reconstruction. Deformities can be minimized by arthroplasty of the proximal interphalangeal (PIP) joints combined with the tenodesis of the extensor tendons as above.*

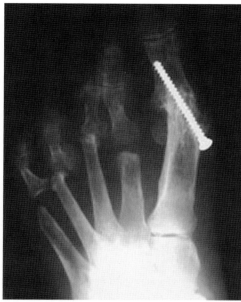

Figure 14–1–9. *Valgus of the MP fusion. This will lead to increased incidence of valgus deformity of the hallux and interphalangeal (IP) arthritis. Note also the irregular resection of the level of the metatarsal heads, which leads to recurrent pain and deformity.*

tures have to be taken into consideration, and efforts to prevent wound complications, infection, and ultimate failure including amputation must be undertaken at all times. Wherever possible therefore, I try to use one operation that has a higher rate of success. This is important, for example, in patients with talonavicular arthritis because I rarely use an isolated arthrodesis of this joint for correction of arthritis, even in the absence of deformity. Even if the arthritis is limited to the talonavicular joint, performing an isolated joint arthrodesis is not advantageous because the remaining minimal motion in the subtalar and calcaneal cuboid joints does not compensate for the potential failure of nonunion.

The approach to correction is no different from that described in the section on triple arthrodesis. Generally, two incisions are used. However, in certain situations a single incision is used medially to avoid lateral incision in a setting of severe deformity. Some patients have profound deformity with talonavicular dislocation, anterior subluxation of the talus, and associated rigid valgus deformity of the hindfoot. In these patients a lateral incision is more likely to lead to wound dehiscence because of the traction on the lateral foot as it is corrected into neutral position. A single incision is therefore used to approach the entire hindfoot arthrodesis, as described in the section on triple arthrodesis.

Although total ankle replacement has been performed successfully for patients with rheumatoid arthritis, I approach this procedure with caution because of an increased incidence of subsidence, fracture, and malalignment in patients with osteopenia. For patients who have good limb alignment and have maintained the overall axis of the foot relative to the tibia, a total ankle replacement is a reasonable procedure. Total ankle replacement should not, however, be performed if a planovalgus deformity is present. This procedure can be staged; a triple arthrodesis can be performed first and then 6 months later, the total ankle replacement. This staging of surgery in the patient with rheumatoid disease must be performed carefully because the potential for wound complications is a constant concern. Although I personally do not discontinue immunosuppressive med-ication at the time of hindfoot surgery, some rheuma-tologists prefer to do so. For these patients who undergo frequent and staged operations, the repeated cessation of medication leads to a flare-up of the arthritis, decreases mobility, and increases generalized debility. These staged operations need to be carefully considered (Figs. 14–1–10 and 14–1–11).

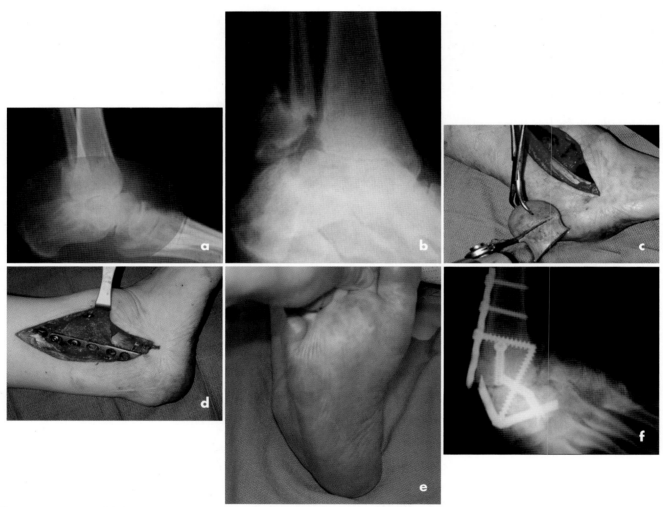

Figure 14–1–10. *This patient with rheumatoid arthritis underwent treatment of severe hindfoot collapse with fracture of the fibula and painful arthritis of the ankle and subtalar joints (a, b). Although a tibiocalcaneal arthrodesis was attempted, adequate contact between the distal tibia and calcaneus could not be obtained, and a bone block arthrodesis with femoral allograft was used to perform a tibiotalocalcaneal arthrodesis (c, d). The patient returned 1 year later with broken hardware (e–g).* Continued

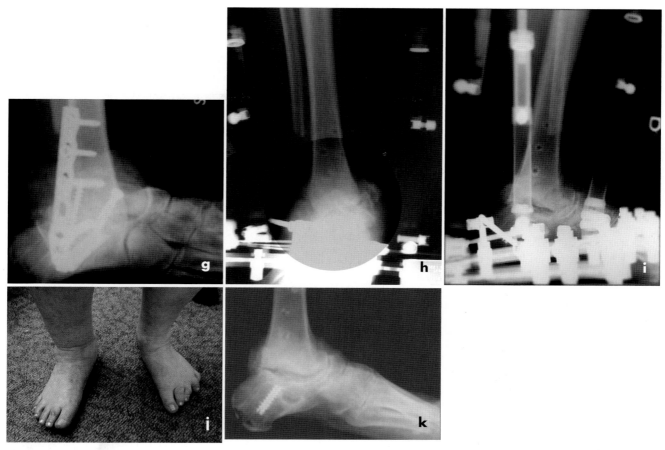

Figure 14–1–10, cont'd. *The patient returned 1 year later with broken hardware (f) and an open draining sinus laterally, which was confirmed as osteomyelitis on debridement and biopsy. An external fixator was applied, hardware was removed, and the fixator was left in place for 4 months (h, i). The final outcome 2 years later was satisfactory with good alignment and stability. The hindfoot was not painful, and a brace was worn for outdoor ambulation (j, k).*

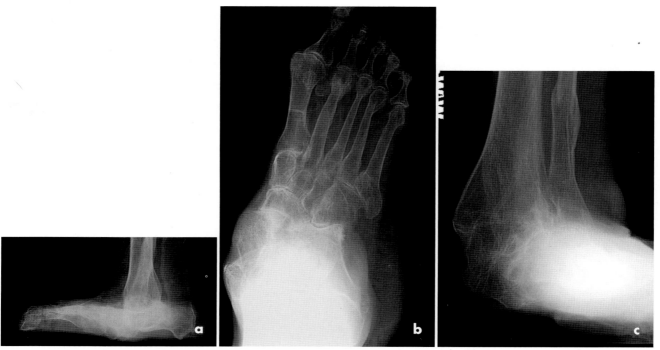

Figure 14–1–11. *A pan-talar arthrodesis was performed with screw fixation for correction of this severe hindfoot and ankle deformity (a–c) associated with a prior stress fracture of the fibula.*

Continued

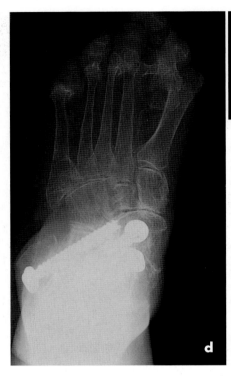

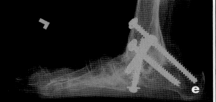

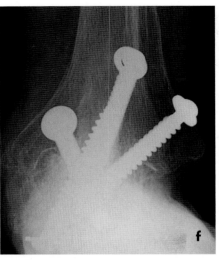

Figure 14–1–11, Cont'd. *Note the use of fully threaded screws to gain maximum purchase (d–f).*

Suggested Readings

Coughlin MJ. Rheumatoid forefoot reconstruction. A long-term follow-up study. J Bone Joint Surg Am 82: 322–341, 2000.

Cracchiolo A 3rd. Rheumatoid arthritis. Hindfoot disease. Clin Orthop 340: 58–68, 1997.

Nassar J, Cracchiolo A III. Complications in surgery of the foot and ankle in patients with rheumatoid arthritis. Clin Orthop Oct(391): 140–152, 2001.

Toolan BC, Hansen ST Jr. Surgery of the rheumatoid foot and ankle. Curr Opin Rheumatol 10: 116–119, 1998.

Stockley I, Betts RP, Rowley I, et al. The importance of the valgus hindfoot in forefoot surgery in rheumatoid arthritis. J Bone Joint Surg Br 72: 705–708, 1990.

Thordarson DB, Aval S, Krieger L. Failure of hallux MP reservation surgery for rheumatoid arthritis. Foot Ankle Int 23: 486–490, 2002.

Weinfeld SB, Schon LC, Myerson MS. Controversies and perils: Fusions of the foot and ankle in patients with rheumatoid arthritis. Tech Orthop 11: 224–235, 1996.

Index

Page numbers with "f" denote figures; those with "t" denote tables